Handbook of
INFERTILITY AND ULTRASOUND
for Practicing Gynecologists

Handbook of
INFERTILITY AND ULTRASOUND
for Practicing Gynecologists

Second Edition

Chaitanya Nagori MD DGO
Director
Dr Nagori's Institute for Infertility and IVF
Ahmedabad, Gujarat, India

Sonal Panchal MD
Ultrasound Consultant
Dr Nagori's Institute for Infertility and IVF
Ahmedabad, Gujarat, India

JAYPEE

JAYPEE BROTHERS MEDICAL PUBLISHERS
The Health Sciences Publisher
New Delhi | London

Jaypee Brothers Medical Publishers (P) Ltd

Headquarters
EMCA House
23/23-B, Ansari Road, Daryaganj
New Delhi 110 002, India
Landline: +91-11-23272143, +91-11-23272703
+91-11-23282021, +91-11-23245672
E-mail: jaypee@jaypeebrothers.com

Corporate Office
4838/24, Ansari Road, Daryaganj
New Delhi 110 002, India
Phone: +91-11-43574357
Fax: +91-11-43574314
E-mail: jaypee@jaypeebrothers.com

Overseas Office
J.P. Medical Ltd
83 Victoria Street, London
SW1H 0HW (UK)
Phone: +44 20 3170 8910
E-mail: info@jpmedpub.com

EU GPSR Authorised Representative
Logos Europe, 9 rue Nicolas Poussin
17000, La Rochelle, France
Phone: +33 (0) 6 67 93 73 78
E-mail: contact@logoseurope.eu

Website: www.jaypeebrothers.com
Website: www.jaypeedigital.com

Inquiries for bulk sales may be solicited at: jaypee@jaypeebrothers.com

Handbook of Infertility and Ultrasound for Practicing Gynecologists

First Edition: 2015

Second Edition: 2021

Reprint: 2026

ISBN 978-93-90020-76-8

Printed at: Samrat Offset Pvt. Ltd.

Dedicated to

My Patients
and
My Students

Preface to the Second Edition

The obstetrician and gynecologist have to deal with infertility patients and also has to use ultrasound for one's own patients. But unfortunately the knowledge of infertility and ultrasound is insufficient as these are the two aspects of gynecologists' practice to which they are not much exposed during their studies. The information available in big books of infertility and ultrasound is so wide that it is not possible for a practicing obstetrician and gynecologist to spare that time. We decided so, to write a book, that is handy, to the point, includes practical tips; and makes the gynecologist confident when dealing with a patient with infertility or doing an ultrasound scan, *Handbook of Infertility and Ultrasound for Practicing Gynecologists* as the first stepping stone to successful infertility and ultrasound practice.

First edition of this book has proved its worth as a quick guide for an Obstetrician and Gynecologist for their infertility patients and ultrasound scans. We here present the second edition of this book. We have tried to include all the new updates in every topic of this book, and still maintain it basic purpose to present to the point and practical information with tips and tricks to help in day-to-day practice.

Chaitanya Nagori
Sonal Panchal

Preface to the First Edition

We have been into infertility and ultrasound practice since more than two decades now and have seen more than 13,000 to 14,000 cases so far. Both learning and teaching has remained our passion for all our lives. It is not feasible for a busy gynecologist to go through lots of books with elaborate descriptions to treat their infertility patients.

We thought, today when we have a lot of experiences to share with you all that can be of help, we should take an opportunity to put it into words. We have tried to make the book short, precise and to the point, so that it can be used as a quick reference for all our friends, colleagues and students. We have tried to include the common topics which may be of help to a practicing gynecologist for infertility treatment and ultrasound. Though we have tried to make it as practical as possible, we have also tried to put the explanations, wherever required so that it becomes easy to digest and apply.

We hope this will be of great help to you all.

Chaitanya Nagori
Sonal Panchal

Contents

Section 1: INFERTILITY

1. **Counseling of an Infertile Couple** 3

   Chaitanya Nagori
   - When to Start the Treatment? *4*
   - Counseling for Semen Analysis *4*
   - Counseling for Cervical Factor *5*
   - What Information do we get from a Normal Postcoital Test? *6*
   - Counseling for Uterine Factor *7*
   - Counseling for Tubal Factor *7*
   - Counseling for Ovarian Causes *8*
   - Unexplained Infertility *8*
   - Counseling for Intrauterine Insemination *8*
   - Counseling for In Vitro Fertilization *9*

2. **Hormonal Assessment of an Infertile Couple** 11

   Chaitanya Nagori

   Investigations for the Infertile Women *11*

3. **Clomiphene Citrate** 26

   Chaitanya Nagori
   - Mechanism of Action *26*
   - Indications of Clomiphene Citrate *26*
   - Unexplained Infertility *27*
   - Contraindications *27*
   - Treatment Regimes *27*
   - Monitoring *28*
   - Results *29*
   - Side Effects *29*
   - Treatment Alternatives *31*

4. **Letrozole** 38

   Chaitanya Nagori
   - Mechanism of Induction of Ovulation *38*
   - Indications *39*
   - Characteristics of Letrozole *39*
   - Advantages *39*
   - Doses *40*
   - Side Effects (Drawbacks) *41*
   - Future Uses *41*
   - Author's View *42*
   - Letrozole + Gonadotropins *42*
   - Letrozole + Clomiphene Citrate *42*

5. Gonadotropins..45

Chaitanya Nagori

- Physiology *45*
- Follicle-stimulating Hormone Preparations Available *46*
- Principles of Gonadotropin Therapy *46*
- Physiology of Ovulation *46*
- Different Regimes of Gonadotropin Therapy *46*
- Recombinant Follicle-stimulating Hormone *49*
- Protocols for Assisted Reproductive Technology *53*
- Predictors of Ovarian Response *55*
- Luteinizing Hormone Supplementation: For Whom, When, and Why? *56*
- Recombinant Luteinizing Hormone *57*

6. Intrauterine Insemination 62

Chaitanya Nagori, Sonal Panchal

- Indications of Intrauterine Insemination *62*
- Steps of Intrauterine Insemination *63*
- Our Experiences *70*

7. Sperm Preparation..73

Chaitanya Nagori

- Collection of Semen Sample *73*
- Sperm Preparation Methods *75*

8. Luteal Phase Defect 84

Chaitanya Nagori, Sonal Panchal

- Luteal Phase Physiology *84*
- Pathophysiology of Luteal Phase Defect *85*
- Rescue of Corpus Luteum in Infertile Patient *86*
- Diagnosis of Luteal Phase Defect *87*
- Controversies in Diagnosis *88*
- Luteal Phase Support *89*
- Progesterone Resistance *100*
- Onset of Luteal Support *100*
- Duration of Luteal Support *101*

9. Ovulation Induction in PCOS 106

Chaitanya Nagori

- Principles of Treatment *106*
- Treatment Modalities in Polycystic Ovary Syndrome *106*

10. Medical Management of Male Infertility 120

Chaitanya Nagori

- Preventive Measures *120*
- Criteria for Medical Management in Male Infertility *121*
- Treatment Options *122*

- Antioxidants *128*
- Dosage of Drugs *131*
- Dosage of Antioxidants *132*

11. Recurrent Pregnancy Loss 137

Chaitanya Nagori

- Causes of Recurrent Pregnancy Loss *137*
- Investigations for Recurrent Pregnancy Loss *161*

12. Practical Tips for Infertility Management 166

Chaitanya Nagori

- Drugs *166*
- Investigations *167*
- Procedures *168*
- In Vitro Fertilization and Intracytoplasmic Sperm Injection *169*
- Ultrasonography *169*
- Prescription *169*
- For Beginners *170*

Section 2: ULTRASOUND

13. Optimizing the Image and Basic Transvaginal Sonography..173

Sonal Panchal

- Equipment Settings *173*
- Optimizing the Image *173*
- Doppler Settings *177*
- Method *184*
- Basic Probe Movements *186*
- Orientation, Observation, and Interpretation of Transvaginal Scan *187*

14. Ultrasound in Uterine Diseases 198

Sonal Panchal

- Müllerian Duct Abnormalities *198*
- Acquired Uterine Abnormalities *208*
- Endometrial Pathologies *215*
- Endometrial Malignancy *221*
- Uterine Scar *225*
- Cervical Lesions *225*

15. Ultrasound in Gynecology: Adnexal Diseases 230

Sonal Panchal

- Ovarian Lesions *231*
- Tubal Lesions *242*
- Miscellaneous Lesions *247*
- Tips to Reach to Correct Diagnosis *249*

16. Cycle Assessment for Infertility Treatment by Ultrasound 251

Sonal Panchal

- Baseline Scan *251*
- Baseline Scan of Ovaries *252*
- Ultrasound and Doppler Features for Polycystic Ovaries *253*
- Uterus *261*
- Preovulatory Scan *261*
- Features of a Mature Follicle *262*
- Application of 3D US for Follicular Assessment *264*
- Features of a Mature Endometrium *264*
- Endometrial Grading *265*
- Secretory Scan *270*
- Luteinized Unruptured Follicle *271*
- Luteal Phase Defect *272*

17. Normal and Abnormal First-trimester Pregnancy 277

Sonal Panchal

Confirmation of Pregnancy *279*

18. Normal Fetal Anatomy in Second Trimester 297

Sonal Panchal

- Head *298*
- Trunk *310*

19. Fetal Screening for Chromosomal Anomalies 321

Sonal Panchal

- Ultrasound as a Screening Modality *323*
- Neural Tube Anomalies *324*
- Facial Anomalies *327*
- Ocular Abnormalities *328*
- Cardiac Abnormalities *329*
- Abdominal Abnormalities *330*
- Skeletal Abnormalities *333*
- Miscellaneous Abnormalities *334*
- Chromosomal Markers *334*
- Noninvasive Prenatal Tests *354*

20. Systematic Examination of Fetal Central Nervous System: How Much Should an Obstetrician Know? 362

Sonal Panchal

- Time of Examination *362*
- Equipment and Approach (According to ISUOG Guidelines) *363*
- Method of Transvaginal Scan *363*
- Imaging Specifications *363*
- Qualitative Examination of the Head *366*

- Study of the Cerebral Vasculature *373*
- Qualitative Evaluation of Fetal Spine *374*
- Quantitative Assessment of Head *375*
- Fetal Spine Examination in High-risk Patients Demands Study of all the Three Planes *384*

21. Fetal Echocardiography for Obstetrician 391

Sonal Panchal

- Equipment Settings *392*
- Evaluation of the Heart *397*
- Study of Internal Cardiac Anatomy *402*
- Classification of Cardiac Diseases *415*

22. Role of Ultrasound in Diagnosis and Management of Fetal Growth Restriction 435

Sonal Panchal

- Definition *435*
- Classifications *440*
- Risk Factors for Intrauterine Growth Restriction *441*
- Ultrasound Diagnosis of Intrauterine Growth Restriction *441*
- Prediction of PIH and FGR *444*
- Silent Period of Increased Resistance *450*
- Obstetric Management Depending on Doppler Findings *459*

23. Ultrasonography in Male Infertility 465

Sonal Panchal

- Scrotal Ultrasound *465*
- Varicocele *466*
- Common Testicular Abnormalities *469*
- Transrectal Ultrasound *473*

24. 3D and 4D Ultrasound in Obstetrics and Gynecology 482

Sonal Panchal

- Volume Ultrasound in Obstetrics *486*
- Nuchal Scan *488*
- Ovarian Lesions *507*
- Preovulatory Scan *509*

Index 515

Section 1

Infertility

- **Counseling of an Infertile Couple**
  Chaitanya Nagori
- **Hormonal Assessment of an Infertile Couple**
  Chaitanya Nagori
- **Clomiphene Citrate**
  Chaitanya Nagori
- **Letrozole**
  Chaitanya Nagori
- **Gonadotropins**
  Chaitanya Nagori
- **Intrauterine Insemination**
  Chaitanya Nagori, Sonal Panchal
- **Sperm Preparation**
  Chaitanya Nagori
- **Luteal Phase Defect**
  Chaitanya Nagori, Sonal Panchal
- **Ovulation Induction in PCOS**
  Chaitanya Nagori
- **Medical Management of Male Infertility**
  Chaitanya Nagori
- **Recurrent Pregnancy Loss**
  Chaitanya Nagori
- **Practical Tips for Infertility Management**
  Chaitanya Nagori

CHAPTER 1

Counseling of an Infertile Couple

Chaitanya Nagori

INTRODUCTION

Counseling is the backbone of infertility management. The correct explanation about reproduction and dialog with the patients helps them conceive. Insler has mentioned in his book that "many patients conceive when they are sitting outside the consulting room". This means that there should be literature placed in the waiting room, handouts given to patients, and there should be elaborative explanatory displays placed in the waiting room, that patients can read and would help them clear a lot of their misconceptions about reproduction, which they might be reluctant to clear in person.

In the busy outpatient department (OPD), it is very difficult for a practicing gynecologist to spend time with the patients for counseling. I shall put forward a few suggestions from my side:

- There should be informative and illustrative posters placed in the waiting room explaining the physiology of conception.
- Attractive and interesting literature regarding reproductive physiology, causes of infertility, and outline of management should be placed in the waiting room, which should be easily accessible to them.
- We have prepared a small booklet regarding the same and is given to every patient once I have done a detailed consultation about their problems with them. This booklet helps the patient to go through the things that are discussed, once again and take a correct decision about the management of their problem.

Such explanation or literature allows the patient to know what would be the management strategy for their problem and how are we going to follow it and therefore they appreciate the treatment that is given. This transparency also builds patient's confidence in you.

Moreover, it also would be a great means of propagating the correct knowledge about infertility through patients as they would discuss whatever they have read and understood by reading the book, with their friends.

One very important suggestion that I would like to give to very busy practitioners is, please allot a specific and separate time slot for patients with fertility problems, so that you can patiently listen to them and discuss the solutions or treatment strategy with them. Remember that the initial counseling and the time spent with them plays a very vital role in management of the patient.

Now I shall try to elaborate as to how I discuss about various aspects of causes of infertility, and management of infertility with the patient.

As infertility is a social stigma in our culture, not only the couple (I mean the husband also) but concerned relatives should also be involved in counseling, so that they would allow and co-operate with the couple to take the correct treatment. The refusal of treatment in majority of cases is by in laws or parents. Therefore, it is very vital that all the people concerned and all those who are going to play a role in decision making as to whether to continue the treatment or not should know about infertility and the correct treatment option for that particular couple.

WHEN TO START THE TREATMENT?

About 85% of the couples conceive within 1 year of unprotected intercourse and 95% in 2 years. Therefore, if a patient comes for treatment, earlier than a year and a half of continuous unprotected intercourse (active married life), which is very common in rural areas of India and in lower socioeconomic class of people, explaining the above said fact will increase their faith in you and your treatment and will also prevent unnecessary investigations, anxiety and frustrations for the patient.

No invasive investigations like laparoscopy should be done within these 2 years and nature should be given enough time to work for the couple to achieve pregnancy.

Among noninvasive investigations, semen analysis and midcycle/preovulatory scan are the two investigations that may be done. These will more or less prove the normalcy of the couple and then counseling only can help them conceive.

We have observed that couples do conceive very often after the treatment is stopped. This is because the stress and anxiety of treatment is removed and the patient is relaxed. Moreover, when we are treating these couples, we become very enthusiastic doing some invasive investigation/procedure in every cycle one after the other like Rubin's test (RT), hysterosalpingography (HSG), dilatation and curettage (D&C), laparoscopy, etc., and do not allow an opportunity for conception. Therefore, when this patient is exhausted and abandons treatment, she conceives spontaneously.

Therefore, remember that counseling is more important than overenthusiastic invasive investigations.

COUNSELING FOR SEMEN ANALYSIS

In 40–50% of couples presenting with fertility problems, male factor is responsible either partially or completely. In our social setup even today, males do not accept this fact and therefore they do not agree for examination or investigations. This problem is more prevalent in people who are less educated. Proper counseling is a must with the male partner before subjecting the female partner for treatment of infertility.

The couple must be explained that according to the recent World Health Organization (WHO) criteria 2012,[1] 15 million sperms/mL, 30% motility, and 4% sperms with normal morphology are considered normal physiological semen criteria. In spite of this even today, we read several laboratories quoting 60 million count as normal in their reports. Because of this wrong information and ignorance of laboratory officials and clinicians, several patients unnecessarily have to take medicines for long periods to increase their sperm count. Remember, when sperm count is 15 million/mL or more, no treatment is required. Up to 86% abnormal sperms is normal and physiological and even patient with 4–14% normal sperms can conceive either naturally or by intrauterine insemination (IUI). Only when <4% of sperms are normal, in vitro fertilization/intracytoplasmic sperm injection (IVF/ICSI) may be required.

When the sperm count is <15 million/mL, semen analysis must be done at least three times—2 weeks apart and 2 months apart to confirm the diagnosis. These patients should directly not be subjected to IVF or ICSI. Instead we must try medical treatment for these males to improve the sperm count, so that they can conceive naturally or with IUI. The whole moto of medical management of a subfertile male is not to increase the sperm count five to ten times or to achieve excellent semen parameters. It is to increase the count by a few million so that ICSI can be converted to IVF, IVF to IUI, and perhaps IUI into natural conception. Medical management has been discussed in the chapter on male infertility of this book.

COUNSELING FOR CERVICAL FACTOR

The cervical factor of infertility is rare at present as surgeries on cervix are not often done. Frequent D&Cs may damage endocervical glands and epithelium. Cauterization of cervix should be discouraged.

I believe that even today, postcoital test (PCT) is very useful in infertility management. When more than seven sperms are seen per high-power field of microscope, 10–12 hours after intercourse, it is considered an excellent PCT according to WHO standards.[2]

Majority of assisted reproductive technology (ART) textbooks opine that PCT has no significance. I have found it very useful for counseling of the husband. He gets assured that he is normal when PCT is normal, so does not feel guilty and becomes more cooperative for the treatment. It may not have much role for ART, but it has place for regular infertility treatment.

These are the patients for whom even timed intercourse can be an option. Many a times when the couple changes the gynecologist, semen analysis is asked for. If patient already has a few semen analysis reports, I will depend on PCT. The satisfaction of the couple is of the highest level and the confidence increases when the couple sees the moving spermatozoa in cervical secretions under the microscope after 10–12 hours of intercourse before doing the test it must be confirmed that it is preovulatory period for the female, considering the cycle length and also that the intercourse was done the previous night.

WHAT INFORMATION DO WE GET FROM A NORMAL POSTCOITAL TEST?

- Preovulatory cervical mucus is normal
- Sperm count is normal.

Moreover when the patient (the couple) is shown these moving sperms under microscope even after 12 hours of intercourse, it gives them confidence that both the partners are normal and that helps them conceive.

Patient is explained that these sperms may remain alive for 48–72 hours in cervix in most patients and in few they have also been seen till 7 days. There is a misconception in majority of the couples that intercourse must be done when ovulation occurs. Showing PCT to patients removes this misconception. Cervix acts as a reservoir for sperms, so after the intercourse even if ovulation occurs in 2–3 days, conception can occur. We can explain the patient that if for conception the intercourse was needed exactly when ovulation occurs, hardly any raped girl would conceive. Couple should therefore be advised intercourse at least once in 2–3 days during 10–20 days of 28–30 days cycle. The couple should be clearly told that abstinence of more than 3 days is not advisable during this period, in natural cycle as well as in stimulated cycles for IUI.

Majority of the couples believe that if IUI is done, it is better to have abstinence before that to get good sperm count. But this is not true. An abstinence of more than 3–4 days does not increase the count; instead the percentage of dead sperms in this semen increases. Therefore, intercourse should not be planned; it should be absolutely voluntary and can be done irrespective of the day of IUI.

Abstinence is one of the causes for failed IUI. Let me explain, why and how!! In majority of gynecology clinics, where there is no IVF setup, the semen preparation laboratory is not adequately equipped, and so the semen preparation is suboptimal and so chances of conception are less. Moreover, patient observes abstinence before IUI, so the chance of natural conception also is denied. As a result patient does not conceive when she is on treatment but conceives spontaneously when she abandons treatment.

Remember therefore intercourse at regular intervals in the fertile period is absolutely essential.

Majority of couples with long-term infertility have lost the charm of their marital relations. Their sexual relations are only planned and compulsory, only targeted for childbearing. They must be explained that child is only a by-product. Main thing is the love and affection, intercourse is just an expression of this feeling and results in conception. Counseling can help them regain the charm of their marriage. All myths regarding intercourse must be discussed and sorted out, e.g., posture, position, timing, washing, etc.

COUNSELING FOR UTERINE FACTOR

This is to be discussed with the patient after a three-dimensional (3D) ultrasound as 3D ultrasound is now a gold standard for congenital uterine malformations and endometrial pathologies. Patient also can see and understand these 3D pictures and the optimum management then can be easily explained. Fibroids less than 4–5 cm in size and not touching the endometrium do not require removal. Patient can also be convinced and explained this by explaining them how the embryo comes from the tube to the uterus and implants in the endometrium.

Majority of the patients have a wrong concept that D&C helps conception. This is a myth and should be clarified. D&C should not be done in modern infertility practice. The only role today of D&C is to exclude endometrial tuberculosis (TB) by either histopathology or TB polymerase chain reaction (PCR) of the endometrial sample along with culture. D&C must not be done to diagnose luteal phase defect or to check whether the endometrium is in proliferative phase or secretory phase. It has a higher chance of damaging the endometrium and resulting into infertility.

COUNSELING FOR TUBAL FACTOR

Patient must be explained that fertilization occurs in fallopian tube and after 4–5 days, embryo comes to settle in the uterus. This explanation is also useful to counsel if the patient gets an ectopic pregnancy. Tubal evaluation is very important in infertility practice. RT for tubal evaluation should be discarded. Laparoscopy is the gold standard for evaluation of the tubes.

Patient should be explained that at the time of ovulation, fimbrial end of the tube covers the ovary, a negative pressure of –1 mm Hg (mercury) develops due to movements of the cilia, this sucks the ovum from the follicle, into the tubal lumen. So ovum does not separate and release from the follicle to roll into the tubal lumen, but tube is vital and instrumental. Therefore, it is important that tubo-ovarian relation should be healthy, a patent tube is not sufficient. HSG gives us only incomplete information, about the patency of the tube. This can be replaced by sonosalpingography (SSG).

Now microsurgery is almost replaced by ART for pathological tubes. Results of microsurgery are very good in tubotubal anastomosis in patients with tubal ligation (TL), especially laparoscopic tubal ligation. Therefore, in young patients where TL is done microsurgery should be offered as an alternative to ART as it is a onetime procedure and patient gets a breathing time for up to 2 years and also has a chance to conceive more than once if the couple wishes so.

COUNSELING FOR OVARIAN CAUSES

Patient should be counseled that ova is released from the ovary only once in a month and it survives for 6–8 hours. Sperms that are stored in the cervix can reach the ova and conception can occur. Ovulation can be confirmed by serum progesterone levels assessed on Day 21–22. Daily sonography is not required just to confirm whether the ovulation has occurred or not if no active treatment or intervention is planned. Basal body temperature record and cervical mucus does not help much in management.

UNEXPLAINED INFERTILITY

About 5–10% of patients are infertile in spite of everything being normal. They have normal semen analysis, normal endoscopy, normal luteal phase, and normal endocrinological reports. These are the ideal patients for IUI. Six cycles of superovulation with IUI must be tried for these couples before subjecting the them for ART. The IUI is the choice of treatment for idiopathic infertility rather than IVF.

COUNSELING FOR INTRAUTERINE INSEMINATION

Intrauterine insemination is very effective method for fertility treatment. But the couple must be explained that it is not IUI procedure alone that gives pregnancy, selection of the patient, correct stimulation protocol, precise ultrasound monitoring, and optimum luteal support are all equally important to get pregnancy. So six cycles of properly and dedicatedly done IUI must be tried in patients of <35 years of age and at least three to four cycles in patients up to 40 years of age. It gives excellent pregnancy rate provided all the steps mentioned earlier are done correctly.

There should not be any abstinence of more than 48 hours before IUI, otherwise it decreases pregnancy rate. Gynecologists should have good setup for IUI to get excellent results. In-house laboratory should be established in gynecologist's setup.

COUNSELING FOR IN VITRO FERTILIZATION

There are lots of misconceptions prevailing for IVF treatment regarding three aspects:

1. Indications
2. Results
3. Cost

Indications

It must be clearly understood that IVF is the first choice in only those patients who have bilateral tubal block, severe endometriosis or severe male factor infertility. IVF may be done in patients with unexplained infertility only when six well-tried superovulation with IUI cycles have failed to give pregnancy. Dysovulatory infertility like polycystic ovaries (PCO) is not an indication of IVF.

Results

Patients believe that IVF is like a fast food and a sure shot solution to infertility. They have been misled about the same. They must be explained that the results of IVF in the best centers of the world are:

- 30% in first cycle
- 40–45% in second cycle
- 50–55% in three cycles
- 60–65% in four cycles
- 65–70% in five cycles
- 70–73% in six cycles.

Therefore, in patients who do not have absolute indications for IVF should be given a chance of IUI instead of taking them for IVF because about six superovulation with IUI cycles cost the same as one IVF cycle, with more chances of success.

Cost

IVF is a very expensive procedure. Its cost includes charges for gonadotropins and medicines, which comprises the largest amount, nearing ₹ 60,000–80,000 depending on the requirement of the patient. The second highest cost is of disposables and media. This is also about ₹ 10,000–15,000. Over and above this the cost also includes consulting fees of the IVF consultant, embryologist, anesthetist, etc. Therefore, it must be understood when we try to cut off the cost, one has to compromise on drug quality and disposables. This would definitely compromise with the results also.

With fixed packages, it is likely to do compromise with the quality of treatment therefore.

Carry Home Message

- Counseling plays very important role in infertility management.
- About 15 million count with 30% motility with 4% normal sperms are new WHO 2012 criteria.
- Seven motile sperms/high-power field (HPF) are excellent PCT.
- Dilatation and curettage is done only to rule out tuberculosis.
- Laparoscopy is gold standard for tubal evaluation.
- Serum progesterone on Day 21 indicates ovulation.
- Six cycles of IUI should be tried in unexplained infertility before ART.
- When taking patients for ART, results and cost must be discussed with the patient.

REFERENCES

1. Morshedi M. New 2010 WHO standards (5th edition) for the evaluation of human semen. (2010 WHO Guidelines for Semen Analysis).
2. Moghissi KS. Postcoital test: physiologic basis, technique and interpretation. Fertil Steril. 1976;27(2):117-129.

CHAPTER 2

Hormonal Assessment of an Infertile Couple

Chaitanya Nagori

INTRODUCTION

It is extremely important to ask for precise investigations. Otherwise it may cause more confusion and patient has to spend unnecessarily for investigations. This chapter will tell us exactly which investigation should be requested for and when. It is unfortunate, that investigations are given more preference than clinical acumen. Clinical acumen is vanishing because of easily available investigations. If I remember days on undergraduate studies, there was a popular book of Clinical Surgery, that had mentioned the sequence as: Provisional diagnosis → Investigations → Final diagnosis. But the sequence followed today is Investigations → Provisional diagnosis → Final diagnosis. This should be strongly discouraged. Provisional diagnosis must be written when an investigation is asked for. Clinician should never diagnose a condition based on investigations alone.

We have seen patients taking tablet bromocriptine for months or years at a stretch for a borderline high prolactin levels. Patient should be treated not the reports. Remember that the clinician should be the ultimate person to make the diagnosis and decide the treatment. I would humbly request and strongly recommend pathologists not to comment on further investigations, diagnosis or management. Profiles and packages offered by laboratories are of no use. Clinician must evaluate the requirement of each investigation individually. Moreover as far as infertility is concerned, any hormonal assessment has clinical value, only if done at a particular time of the cycle and therefore packages and profiles are absolutely meaningless for infertility management. Moreover, it is also essential to understand the physiology of the hypothalamopituitary ovarian axis **(Fig. 1)**. Here we have emphasized the need for investigations for routine infertility practice and investigations especially required for in vitro fertilization (IVF) are separately discussed.

INVESTIGATIONS FOR THE INFERTILE WOMEN

Serum Follicle-stimulating Hormone

- Day 2–3 follicle-stimulating hormone (FSH) is done along with luteinizing hormone (LH) for diagnosis of polycystic ovarian syndrome (PCOS).

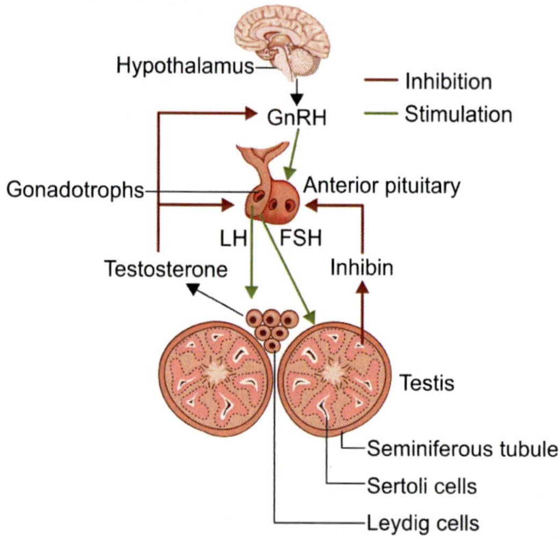

Fig. 1: Hypothalamo-pituitary testicular axis (FSH: follicle-stimulating hormone; GnRH: gonadotropin-releasing hormone; LH: luteinizing hormone)

This should not be done as it does not change the line of treatment. PCOS can be diagnosed by history, clinical examination, and ultrasound (US). US diagnosis of polycystic ovaries (PCO) has been discussed in the Chapter 16 of this book. We have never used FSH/LH ratio for diagnosis of PCOS. Because abnormal value of this ratio only indicates anovulation, which is otherwise also evident by history.

- Day 2–3 FSH is done before IVF. Higher FSH indicates lower chances of pregnancy.[1,2] Serum FSH levels up to 10–12 IU/L is considered normal. We do not get Day 2–3 serum FSH done as age + antral follicle count (AFC) gives better idea for assessing the ovarian reserve. However, systematic reviews from most studies have failed to define a single threshold or cut off value of serum FSH to describe poor ovarian function.[3]
- Occasionally for diagnosis of menopause, when progesterone withdrawal bleeding is absent, serum FSH can be used to confirm the diagnosis.
- Earlier serum FSH was assessed in several cycles to decide which cycle can be used for fertility treatment but raised serum FSH in anyone cycle can be an indicator of extremely low or no possibility of ongoing pregnancy.[4] Treatment should not be started in selected cycles also when serum FSH is normal.
- Basal FSH provides predictive value for pregnancy which can be judged by baseline scan. High FSH suggests poor ovarian reserve and that can be diagnosed by baseline scan. High FSH is a direct pituitary compensation for the older and less responsive ovary, where reduced oocyte numbers and reduced ovarian hormone production are present and lead to

attenuated negative feedback on hypothalamic/pituitary secretion of FSH. High basal FSH levels should be used for counseling women as regards their outcome rather than exclude them from IVF cycles. FSH above 15 IU/L in young women still show fair pregnancy rates, indicating that quality can compensate for quantity of oocytes.[5] Cycling women with high FSH should be offered treatment without further delay.[6] We, therefore, routinely do not recommend serum FSH assessment but rely more on baseline scan.

Serum Luteinizing Hormone

- Day 2–3 LH along with serum FSH is done to diagnose PCOS. But high LH indicates only anovulation which can be judged by history. So routine LH is not done.
- *Day 8–9 LH in clomiphene citrate (CC) cycles:* CC stimulates hypothalamus to secrete FSH and LH both. High LH is detrimental to ova and gives poor pregnancy rate with CC in spite of good ovulation rates. So, when LH is more than 10–12 IU/L, CC should not be given for the second cycle and patients should be switched over to gonadotropins.

Serum Estradiol Level

- *Follicular maturity*: Serum estradiol (E2) helps to decide the maturity and quality of the follicle. Especially when the follicle looks mature but the endometrium appears thin, it is E2 level that can decide whether it is the follicular immaturity or local endometrial cause for the same. Normal E2 level for a mature follicle is 150 pgm/mL/follicle. Serum level of E2 less than this indicates a bad quality or immature follicle. Normal serum E2 level with thin endometrium indicates a local cause. Though in today's practice if color Doppler is used for assessment of follicular and endometrial quality, E2 level is not required to assess physiological maturity of the follicle.
- *For poor responder*: For IVF cycles E2 is done on Day 2. If E2 is > 80 pgm/mL, it indicates poor IVF outcome as it indicates early follicular recruitment due to high FSH and poor ovarian reserve.[7,8] This is not required for intrauterine insemination (IUI) cycles and in majority of assisted reproductive technology (ART) cycles.
- *To assess ovarian suppression*: In IVF cycles with long agonist protocol, gonadotropin-releasing hormone agonist (GnRHa) is started from Day 21 of previous cycle. This downregulates pituitary and FSH, LH levels are therefore very low. In turn it also brings E2 to baseline levels. To assess downregulation therefore, E2 is done on Day 2 of the cycle and stimulation may be started if E2 <30 pgm/mL, or some may also allow <50 pgm/mL. In patients who are on downregulation with oral

contraceptive pills, E2 levels are checked after 12 days of oral contraceptive pills to start stimulation.

- *For suspected risk of hyperstimulation*: After superovulation in IUI cycles or when gonadotropins are used for ovulation induction, ovaries may develop multiple follicles. Ovarian hyperstimulation syndrome (OHSS) is feared in such patients. E2 level can be measured for these patients. In non-IVF cycles, E2 >1,600 pgm/mL and in IVF cycles E2 levels > 4,000 pgm/mL on the day of ovulation trigger can cause OHSS. But risk of OHSS can also be judged by three-dimensional (3D) US and has been discussed at length in the US section of the book. We, therefore, do not get E2 levels done to assess the risk of OHSS.

  We always prefer a chronic low dose protocol for superovulation with IUI in PCOS patients. In spite of that if we get four to five follicles in each ovary, we would use GnRHa for ovulation trigger to avoid OHSS. E2 level assessment is not required to decide the ovulation trigger if proper US assessment with Doppler is done.

  In IVF/intracytoplasmic sperm injection (ICSI) cycles, OHSS is common for PCOS patients. In these patients therefore antagonist protocol is preferred to long agonist protocol and agonist is used for ovulation trigger in these patients. This protocol is almost 100% OHSS proof. If we get multiple follicles unexpectedly in an agonist downregulated cycle, ovarian volume on US can give a clue to the risk of OHSS. This is if total ovarian volume (of both ovaries) is more than approximately 180 cc.[9] In these cases, hCG is withheld. Therefore to avoid OHSS:
  - Use chronic low dose protocol in PCOS patients
  - Use antagonist protocol instead of long agonist protocol for down-regulation and agonist as ovulation trigger
  - In doubtful cases, ovarian volume is calculated by 3D US and when ovarian volume is huge, hCG is withheld.

We use US to assess the risk of OHSS, but E2 can be used by a gynecologist, if facility of 3D US is not available.

Serum Progesterone

Most of progesterone is secreted by corpus luteum in second half of the cycle. Otherwise it is an intermediate hormone for other steroid hormones.

Normal values:

- *Follicular phase*: 1 ng/mL
- *LH surge*: 1–2 ng/mL
- *Ovulation*: 3 ng/mL

Midluteal serum progesterone, i.e., a week before menses is approximately 10 ng/mL. A level of >3 ng/mL indicates ovulation. Therefore if only ovulation is to be documented and no intervention is planned, repeated US scans are not required. In the same way endometrial biopsy is not required to confirm secretory changes in endometrium and serum progesterone estimation suffices for the same.

Ultrasound with color Doppler is a better modality to assess the secretory phase of the cycle. It can define all luteal phase problems—luteal phase defect (LPD)/luteinized unruptured follicle. This has been discussed in detail in Chapter 16 of this book. So, it is the inevitable conclusion that random serum progesterone has little value beyond documenting ovulation.

Serum Prolactin

Prolactin is the hormone secreted by anterior pituitary and is regulated by prolactin inhibitory factor, which is secreted from hypothalamus.

- Normal level of prolactin is 10–25 ng/mL.
- In microadenoma it is between 100 and 200 ng/mL
- In macroadenoma it is >200 ng/mL
- Immunoassay for prolactin does not reflect the bioassay always
- Many times patients have no symptoms in spite of high prolactin level because of presence of macromolecules which are big prolactin molecules that account for 10–12% of normal patient otherwise but showing hyper-prolactinemia on laboratory investigation.

Galactorrhea with Normal Prolactin Levels

Patients may come with complaint of galactorrhea and may present with normal serum prolactin levels. This may be mucoid discharge and not actual galactorrhea. Any discharge therefore from the breast should be checked under microscope. If it contains fat globules, only then it is galactorrhea.

When ovulation induction is done, in many patients E2 leads to rise in prolactin levels in first half of the menstrual cycle. These patients are known as spikers. This is transient hyperprolactinemia. The clinical presentation is poor endometrium in spite of good follicles. This condition is difficult to diagnose, but bromocriptine can be given in a dose of 1.25 mg/BD in these patients in first half of the cycle. It is a therapeutic test. If endometrium improves, it is continued in the subsequent cycle, otherwise it is stopped. If patient is a spiker, she needs treatment; otherwise this condition also deteriorates oocyte quality and causes LPD as certain amount of prolactin is essential for development of good follicle and also for corpus luteal function.

Marginally high prolactin levels are also found in PCOS patients due to high E2 and high dehydroepiandrosterone sulfate (DHEAS). In these cases bromocriptine or cabergoline is not the treatment, only PCOS is to be treated.

Table 1: Sources of testosterone.	
Hormone	***Source***
Testosterone	• 50% peripheral conversion • 25% ovary • 25% adrenal
Androstenedione	• 50% ovary • 50% adrenal
Dehydroepiandrosterone (DHEA)	• 90% adrenal • 10% ovary
Dehydroandrosterone (DHA)	• 100% adrenal

17-OH-Progesterone

This investigation is done in all patients with hirsutism. It is increased due to 21-hydroxykase deficiency. Because of 21-hydroxylase deficiency in patients of heterogeneous carrier, late onset of congenital adrenal hyperplasia is observed. 17-OH-progesterone (17-OH-P) is a weak androgen and manifests as hirsutism, acne, clitoral enlargement, and menstrual irregularity at puberty.

Normal level of 17-OH-P is <200 ng/dL. Whenever the level is between 200 and 800 ng/dL, it requires adrenocorticotropic hormone (ACTH) testing. Level of >800 ng/dL is diagnostic of 21-hydroxylase deficiency.[10] These patients are treated with dexamethasone 0.5 mg daily at bedtime.

Serum Testosterone

Normal value of serum testosterone is 20–80 ng/dL. Its normal production is 0.2–0.3 mg/day. Out of this 80% binds to sex hormone binding globulin (SHBG) and 19% to albumin. Only 1% is free testosterone **(Table 1)**. Testosterone may rise in PCOS and tumors. Tumor is suspected if there is sudden onset of symptoms due to increased testosterone. PCOS patients show gradual rise in testosterone levels.[11] Routine estimation of serum testosterone is not required as it does not change the line of treatment.

Serum Dehydroepiandrosterone Sulfate

Dehydroepiandrosterone sulfate is exclusively secreted from adrenal glands. The normal value is 350 ngm/dL. It increases with hyperprolactinemia. Therefore in patients with PCOS, prolactin and DHEAS are slightly on higher side which do not require any specific treatment except the treatment of PCOS. This rise is secondary to E2 because of anovulation.

Whenever DHEAS is very high, it is due to adrenal tumor. So US is a better guide to diagnose adrenal tumor. Serum testosterone and US suffices to rule out adrenal tumors.

If there is moderate rise in PCOS and it does not require any treatment. If 17-OH-P is normal there is no need to search for adrenal enzyme defect. DHEAS > 700 µgm/dL is accepted as a marker for adrenal dysfunction. This is rarely found and does not change the management. Therefore, routine testing of DHEAS is not required.

Inhibin A and B

Inhibin B is predominantly secreted by antral follicles. Low, Day 3 inhibin B level of <45 pgm/mL has poor response to superovulation and patient is less likely to conceive. Same thing can be judged by raised serum FSH, raised serum anti-Müllerian hormone (AMH) or low AFC and so routine use of inhibin B estimation is not justified.

Inhibin A is secreted from preovulatory follicles. Both inhibin A and B are secreted from granulosa cells and regulate FSH by negative feedback mechanism. Routine estimation of inhibin A does not add any information that may change the management of the patient.

Serum Anti-Müllerian Hormone

It is a member of transforming growth factor (TGF). It is produced from granulosa cells. The expression of AMH is localized in granulosa cells of primary preantral and small antral follicles and has important role in human folliculogenesis. AMH expression in follicle decreases when antral follicle size is >8 mm in size. In follicles undergoing atresia and in corpus lutea also the AMH expression is completely lost.[12]

Anti-Müllerian hormone levels in women are low until the age of 8 years, rise rapidly until puberty and decline steadily from the age of 25 years until menopause, when AMH production ceases **(Table 2)**.

It is now well established that serum AMH concentrations reflect the number of preantral and small antral follicles in the ovary, this would account for raised AMH levels found in both polycystic ovarian morphology (PCOM) and PCOS.[13]

Table 2: Anti-Müllerian hormone: Values and implications.

Ovarian fertility potential	*pmol/L*	*ng/mL*
Optimal fertility	28.6–48.5	4.0–6.8
Satisfactory fertility	15.7–28.6	2.2–4.0
Low fertility	2.2–15.7	0.3–2.2
Very low/undetectable	0.0–2.2	0.0–0.3
High level	>48.5	>6.8

Physiology

Anti-Müllerian hormone has an inhibiting role in the ovary, contributing to follicular arrest.[14] It lowers the sensitivity of follicles to FSH, that is required for normal folliculogenesis. In vitro studies have shown that the action of FSH in promoting follicular growth is counteracted by AMH.[15] It has a steady level throughout the cycle except for a slight dip just after LH peak.[16] Though some investigators have recorded cyclical fluctuations in AMH with rapid decrease in early luteal phase.[17]

Anti-Müllerian Hormone and Polycystic Ovary

The reported property of AMH to counteract the actions of FSH implies that the high production of AMH by polycystic ovary (PCO) may have an important role in the pathophysiology of the syndrome.[14] In anovulatory PCOS, the failure of follicle development is due to an intrinsic inhibition of FSH action and this inhibition is due to the high concentration of AMH.[18] Increased ovarian stromal blood flow in PCOS may be because of over expression of vascular endothelial growth factor (VEGF), which modulates the permeability of theca cells and increase insulin-like growth factor 1 (IGF-1).[19,20] This in turn enhances gonadotropin-stimulated steroid production in granulosa cells and theca cells resulting in increased ovarian androgen production and subsequently increased AMH production.[21] AMH levels are two to three times higher in PCOS than in healthy controls.[22] This has been attributed not only to increased number of antral follicles, but also to higher production of AMH per follicle in patients with PCOS as compared to size-matched counterparts from normal ovary.[23]

In addition a positive correlation between AMH and serum concentration of both LH and testosterone in PCOS has been reported.[24]

Each individual follicle in a PCO in women with PCOS produces significantly more AMH than its sized-matched counterpart from a normal ovary.[23] Moreover, it has also been shown that metformin administration in PCOS patients is associated with reduction in AMH concentration in follicle and serum, suggesting that the measurement of AMH can be used to evaluate the treatment efficacy with insulin sensitizers.[25]

It can predict ovarian response. It can predict menopause by low levels. If AMH is very high in PCOS, then it predicts OHSS.

Anti-Müllerian Hormone and In Vitro Fertilization

In IVF patients, serum AMH value can predict the response of ovary and so it is useful for counseling the patient. When calculated optimal AMH cutoff of <1.26 ng/mL was used to predict responses to controlled ovarian stimulation (COS), it was found to have a 97% sensitivity for predicting poor responses

Table 3: AMH group.

AMH group (pmol/L)	*GnRH analog*	
<1.0	375 Antagonist	(Modified natural cycle)
1.0 to <5	375 Agonist	300 Antagonist
5.0 to <15	225 Agonist	225 Agonist
≥15.0	150 Agonist	150 Antagonist

(<4 oocytes retrieved) and 98% accuracy in predicting a normal COS response.[26] Nelson et al. suggested AMH-based strategy for deciding the COS protocol **(Table 3)**.[27]

But we have found AFC equally effective and more precise for prediction of ovarian response. We routinely do not assess AMH levels either in IVF or non-IVF cycles. With extremely low serum AMH levels, moderate, but reasonable pregnancy and live birth rates are still observed in our practice. Extremely low AMH level does not seem to represent an appropriate marker for withholding fertility treatment. Younger women are likely to have better pregnancy rates than their older counterparts with equally low AMH.[28]

Constant AMH and inhibin B levels suggest that neither AMH nor inhibin B is an accurate marker of ovarian response after low dose gonadotropins ovulation induction in patients with PCOS.[29] Mashiach et al. have also shown a relationship between follicular fluid AMH concentrations and the quality of embryos in patients with PCOS.[30]

Routine use of AMH does not help in managing non-ART patients. We require one to two follicles for superovulation with IUI and AMH will not help us in changing the line of treatment. Poor responding ovary or low reserve ovary can be very well judged by US.

Serum AMH estimation is indicated in:[31]

- Predicting both over and under response in controlled ovarian hyperstimulation (COH)
- Determining the most appropriate treatment regimen
- Pretreatment counseling for couples to make an appropriate and informed choice
- Predicting long-term fertility
- Predicting the age of menopause
- Predicting ovarian aging prior to or following chemotherapy/surgery
- Screening for polycystic ovaries.

The inhibitory effect of AMH on folliculogenesis may in future be used for hormonal contraception.

Clinical applications of AMH apart from fertility assessment are as follows:

- To confirm presence of testicular tissue in children with low testosterone levels

- Differential diagnosis of intersex disorders
- In patients with bilateral nonpalpable gonads
- Females with granulosa cell tumors.

Insulin Resistance

Now it has been proved that in patients of PCOS there is high androgen because of increased insulin level and its sensitivity. It indicates the severity of PCOS. Clinically waist circumference of 35 inches or 90 cm is predictive of abnormal endocrinology and metabolic function.

There are various methods to diagnose insulin resistance. But 2 hours glucose and insulin response is the most reliable one.

2 hours glucose tolerance test (after 75 g of glucose):
- *Normal*: <140 mg/dL
- *Impaired*: 140–190 mg/dL
- *Noninsulin-dependent diabetes mellitus (DM)*: ≥200 mg/dL

2 hours insulin response (after 75 g of glucose):
- *Insulin resistance very likely*: 100–150 μU/mL
- *Insulin resistance*: 151–300 μU/mL
- *Severe insulin resistance*: >300 μU/mL

In clinical practice, patients with high insulin resistance are the ones who require ovarian drilling. They have tonically high LH levels and therefore drilling helps. Alternatively they may also be benefitted by GnRH antagonist.

Antagonist decreases LH levels, prevents premature luteinization and improves oocyte quality.

Patients with insulin resistance who do not want immediate pregnancy are the patients for Metformin therapy. 3D US is a novel way to diagnose insulin resistance, based on assessment of stromal volume.[32] But for all those who do not have volume US, 2 hours glucose and 2 hours insulin test is the best alternative. So for chronic anovulation only three investigations are required:

1. Serum prolactin
2. Serum thyroid-stimulation hormone (TSH)
3. Insulin resistance

Thyroid Function Tests

- Normal level is 0.5–2.5 mIU/mL
- If TSH is high, measure free T4
- Any woman after the age of 35 years should be assessed for thyroid function
- Presence of antithyroid antibodies indicates future hypothyroidism

- During pregnancy or in recurrent pregnancy loss, it is done every 2 months
- Requirement of thyroxine decreases with age
- For hyperthyroidism T4 is measured and if it is normal, T3 is measured.

Laboratory Investigations for Male Infertility

In patients of male infertility, there are three important hormonal investigations: serum TSH, serum LH, and serum testosterone used for diagnosis and treatment plan. There are various permutation combinations of these hormones.

- *High FSH, high LH, and low/normal testosterone*: This indicates primary testicular failure, due to spermatogenic and Leydig cell damage. Treatment option for these patients will be only donor insemination or adoption. These patients cannot even provide sufficient number of sperms for ICSI. Though microdissection testicular sperm extraction (micro-TESE) may help.
- *High FSH, normal LH, and normal testosterone*: This combination indicates primary spermatogenic failure. As LH is normal, there is no Leydig cell damage. This is due to inhibin deficiency. Treatment option to these patients is again donor insemination or adoption. Micro-TESE may be tried.

  In both these groups, FSH is high. Therefore, instead of assessing these three hormones, one can assess only serum FSH and if that is high evaluation of other two hormones is not required. But if serum FSH is normal, LH and testosterone levels need to be assessed.

  In patients with high FSH, with normal LH and testosterone, the possible diagnosis is varicocele. In grade 3 varicocele, because of testicular damage, FSH is borderline high. In these patients varicocele ligation + gonadotropins + antioxidants can improve spermatogenesis in many cases.
- *Normal FSH, high LH, and high testosterone*: Normally LH and testosterone are regulated by negative feedback mechanism. But in this case, LH and testosterone both are high, as testosterone is not perceived by receptors. This is known as partial androgen resistance. High androgen will be converted into E2 and so E2/testosterone ratio will be high. This high E2 will cause gynecomastia, that is a diagnostic criterion. It also causes oligoasthenoteratozoospermia, which does not respond to drugs. ART is advised in these patients or adoption if the patient is not affording, after proper counseling.
- *Normal FSH, normal LH, and normal testosterone*: This is a very common finding in our patients. It may be due to organic cause like obstruction

in ductal system, retrograde ejaculation, varicocele or germ cell failure. The treatment is according to the cause.

- *Obstruction*: Surgery or ICSI after percutaneous epididymal sperm aspiration/testicular sperm aspiration (PESA/TESA)
- *Retrograde ejaculation*: α-adrenergic blocking drugs + IUI or ART
- *Varicocele*: Surgery + gonadotropins + antioxidants
- *Germ cell failure*:
  - *Spermatogonia arrest:* Donor insemination
  - *Spermatid arrest:* FSH + ICSI

But most commonly patients having azoospermia with normal FSH, LH, and testosterone do not have any pathological cause. These patients have qualitative failure causing azoospermia or severe oligozoospermia.

As discussed in the chapter on medical management of male infertility, these patients can be treated with FSH or human menopausal gonadotropin (hMG) 75–150 international units (IU) thrice a week and hCG 5000 IU twice a week. It has given excellent results in many cases. In these cases endogenous bioactivity is poor in spite of normal immunological levels [radioimmunoassay (RIA) test]. This is why exogenous FSH, LH, and hCG are useful.

- *Low FSH, low LH, and low testosterone*: These are the patients having hypogonadotropic hypogonadism. These patients can be treated by hCG 5,000 IU every fifth day for 5–7 weeks till testosterone becomes normal as it is required for initiation of spermatogenesis. After testosterone becomes normal, FSH 75 IU is added thrice a week for maturation of sperms. This is given for 3–6 months. But results are excellent and it initiates spermatogenesis.

There may be panhypopituitarism which require replacement of thyroid, corticotrophin, and growth hormone (GH).

There may be Kallmann syndrome which is congenital. Prolactinoma is normally macro type which requires surgery.

Hyperprolactinemia

Most diagnostic symptom of hyperprolactinemia is loss of libido. There is no galactorrhea or gynecomastia. Cause of low testosterone is macroadenoma leading to hyperprolactinemia, and this macroadenoma must be removed surgically. If there is no macroadenoma, oligospermia is because of androgen resistance. Therapy of choice for these patients is long-term bromocriptine or cabergoline.

Thyroid Dysfunction

Autoimmune thyroiditis is the most common condition. Hypothyroidism can cause oligospermia and hyperprolactinemia because of high TSH.

Hyperthyroidism also causes oligospermia. Therefore, thyroid function assessment is required in patients of oligospermia.

Adrenal Dysfunction

Infertility may be the only manifestation of adrenal dysfunction. It leads to feminization and softening of testis. Raised DHEAS also leads to increased prolactin levels. These are also associated with signs and symptoms of adrenal insufficiency. Risk is high in patients with family history of congenital adrenal hyperplasia.

Endocrine Workup

- Serum FSH
- Serum LH
- Serum testosterone
- Serum prolactin
- Serum TSH and T4
- Serum DHEAS
- Serum E2
- Serum 17-OH-P
- Serum cortisol
- Sex hormone-binding globulin

Carry Home Message

- Investigation is requested for confirmation of provisional diagnosis.
- FSH >15 IU/L indicates poor quality and quantity of ova.
- In CC cycle, Day 8–10 FSH should be <10 IU/L.
- E2 >1600 pgm/mL in IUI cycle may lead to OHSS.
- S. Progesterone >3 ng/mL documents ovulation.
- S. Prolactin >100 IU indicates adenoma.
- Prolactin is high in PCOS patients.
- 17-OHP is recommended in all patients with hirsuitism.
- Low AMH indicates poor ovarian reserve.
- High FSH in male indicates testicular failure.
- Hypogonadotrophic hypogonadism has good fertility prognosis after treatment in both the partners.
- When FSH, LH and testosterone are normal in men, it is mostly qualitative failure.

REFERENCES

1. Muasher SJ, Oehniger S, Simonetti S, Matta J, Ellis LM, Liu HC, et al. The value of basal and/or stimulated serum gonadotropin levels in prediction of stimulation response and in vitro fertilization outcome. Fetil Steril. 1988;50:298-307.

2. Scott RT, Toner JP, Muasher SJ, Oehninger S, Robinson S, Rosenwaks Z. Follicle-stimulating hormone levels on cycle day 3 are predictive of in vitro fertilization outcome. Fertil Steril. 1989;51:651.
3. Bancsi LF, Broekman FJ, Mol BW, Habbema JD, te Valde ER. Performance of basal follicle stimulating hormone in prediction of poor response and failure to become pregnant after in vitro fertilization: a meta-analysis. Fertil Steril. 2003;79:1091-100.
4. Pearlstone AC, Fournet N, Gambone JC, Pang SC, Buyalos RP. Ovulation induction in women age 40 and older: the importance of basal follicle stimulating hormone level and chronological age. Fertil Steril. 1992;58:674-9.
5. van Rooji IAJ, de Jong E, Broekmans FJM, Looman CWN, Habbema JDF, te Velde E. High follicle stimulating hormone levels should not necessarily lead to the exclusion of subfertile patients from treatment. Fertil Steril. 2004;81:1478-85.
6. Abdalla H, Thum MY. Repeated testing of basal FSH levels has no predictive value for outcome in women with elevated basal FSH. Hum Reprod. 2006;21(1):171-4.
7. Smotrich DB, Widra EA, Gindoff PR, Levy MJ, Hall JL, Stillman RJ. Prognostic value of day 3 estradiol on in vitro fertilization outcome. Fertil Steril. 1995;64:1136-40.
8. Licciardi FL, Lui HC, Rosenwaks Z. Day 3 estradiol serum concentrations as prognosticators of ovarian stimulation response and pregnancy outcome in patients undergoing in vitro fertilization. Fertil Steril. 1995;64:991-4.
9. Oyesanya OA, Parsons JH, Collins WP, et al. Total ovarian volume before human chorionic gonadotrophin administration for ovulation induction may predict the hyperstimulation. Hum Reprod. 1995;10:3211-2.
10. Kuttenn F, Couillin P, Girard F, Billaud L, Vincens M, Boucekkine C, et al. Late onset adrenal hyperplasia in hirsutism. New Engl J Med. 1985;313:224-31.
11. Easterling Jr WE, Talbert LM, Potter HD. Serum testosterone levels in the polycystic ovary syndrome. Am J Obstet Gynecol. 1974;120:385.
12. Elvin JA, Clark AT, Wang P, Wolfman NM, Matzuk MM. Paracrine actions of growth differentiation factor-9 in the mammalian ovary. Mol Endocrinol. 1999;13(6): 1035-48.
13. Fanchin R, Maria SL, Righini C, Guibourdenche J, Frydman R, Taieb J. Serum AMH is more strongly related to ovarian follicle status that serum inhibin B, oestradiol, FSH and LH on the day 3. Hum Reprod. 2003;18:323-7.
14. Pellat L, Rice S, Mason HD. Anti-Müllerian hormone and polycystic ovarian syndrome: a mountain too high? Reproduction. 2010;139:825-33.
15. Durlinger AL, Gruijters MJ, Kramer P, Karels B, Kumar TR, Matzik MM. Anti-Müllerian hormone attenuates the effect of FSH on follicle development in the mouse ovary. Endocrinology. 2001;142:4891-9.
16. La Marca A, Stabile G, Artenisio AC, Volpe A. Serum anti-Müllerian hormone through out the human menstrual cycle. Hum Reprod. 2006;21(12):3103-7.
17. Streuli J, Fraisse T, Chapron C, Bijaoui G, Bischof P, de Ziegler D. Clinical uses of anti-Müllerian hormone assays: pitfalls and promises. Fertil Steril. 2009;91(1): 226-30.
18. Pellat L, Rice S, Dilaver N, Heshri A, Galea R, Brincat M, et al. Anti-Müllerian hormone reduces follicle sensitivity to follicle-stimulating hormone in human granulosa cells. Fertile Steril. 2011;96:1246-51.
19. El Behery MM, Diab AE, Mowafy H, Ebrahiem MA, Shehata AE. Effect of laparoscopic ovarian drilling on vascular endothelial growth factor and ovarian stromal blood flow using three dimensional power Doppler. Intern J Gynecol Obstet. 2011; 112:119-21.
20. Abd El, Aal DE, Mohamed SA, Amine AF, Meki AR. Vascular endothelial growth factor and insulin-like growth factor 1 in polycystic ovary syndrome and their relation to ovarian blood flow. Eur J Obstet Gynecol reprod Biol. 2005;118:219-24.

21. Willis D, Mason H. Gilling-Smith C, Franks S. Modulation by insulin of follicle stimulating hormone and luteinizing hormone actions in human granulosa cells of normal and polycystic ovaries. J Clin Endocrinol Metab. 1996;81:302-9.
22. Pigny P, Merlen E, Robert Y, Cortet-Rudelli C, Decanter C, Jonard S, et al. Elevated serum level of anti-Müllerian hormone in patients with polycystic ovary syndrome: relationship to the ovarian follicle excess and to the follicular arrest. J Clin Endocrinol Metab. 2003;88:5957-62.
23. Pellat L, Hanna L, Brincat M, Galea R, Brain H, Whitehead S, et al. Granulosa cell production of anti-Müllerian hormone is increased in polycystic ovaries. J Clin Endocrinol Metab. 2007;92:240-5.
24. Carlsen SH, Vanky E, Fleming R. Anti-Müllerian hormone concentrations in androgen suppressed women with polycystic ovary syndrome. Hum Reprod. 2009; 24:1732-8.
25. Piltonen T, Morin Papunen L, Koivunen R, Perheentupa A, Ruokonen A, Tapanainen JS. Serum anti-Müllerian hormone levels remain high until late reproductive age and decrease during metformin therapy in women with polycystic ovary syndrome. Hum Reprod. 2005;20(7):1820-6.
26. Gnoth C, Schuring AN, Friol K, Tigges J, Mallmann P, Godehardt E. Relevance of anti-Müllerian hormone measurement in a routine IVF program. Hum Reprod. 2008;23:1359-65.
27. Nelson SM, Yates RW, Lyall H, Jamieson M, Traynor I, Gaudoin M, et al. Anti-Müllerian hormone-based approach to controlled ovarian stimulation for assisted conception. Hum Reprod. 2009;24:867-75.
28. Weghofer A, Dietrich W, Barad DH, Gleicher N. Live birth chances in women with extremely low serum anti-Müllerian hormone levels. Hum Reprod. 2011;26(70):1905-9.
29. Fong SL, Schippe I, de Jong FH, Themmen APN, Visser JA, Laven JSP. Serum anti-Müllerian hormone and inhibin B concentrations are not useful predictors of ovarian response during ovulation induction treatment with rFSH in women with polycystic ovary syndrome. Fertil Steril. 2011;96(2):459-63.
30. Mashiach R, Amit A, Hasson J, Amzalzg S, Almog B, Ben-Yosef D, et al. Follicular fluid levels of anti-Müllerian hormone as a predictor of oocyte maturation, fertilization rate, and embryonic development in patients with polycystic ovarian syndrome. Fertil Steril. 2010;93(7):2299-302.
31. Loh JS, Maheshwari A. Anti-Müllerian hormone—is it a crystal ball for predicting ovarian ageing? Human Reprod. 2011;26(11):2925-32.
32. Panchal S, Nagori CB. Correlation of ovarian and stromal volumes to fasting and postprandial insulin levels in polycystic ovarian syndrome patients. Int J Infertil Fetal Med. 2014;5(1):12-4.

CHAPTER 3

Clomiphene Citrate

Chaitanya Nagori

INTRODUCTION

Clomiphene citrate (CC) is a mixture of two isomers, enclomiphene (trans) 62% and zuclomiphene (cis) 38%. Enclomiphene is more potent, more estrogenic, and responsible for ovulation inducing actions. Enclomiphene has a shorter duration of action and disappears within few days while zuclomiphene is detected over a month because of its slow clearance rate. It accumulates cycle after cycle. Enclomiphene is antiestrogenic centrally and estrogenic peripherally and zuclomiphene is the other way round (estrogenic centrally and antiestrogenic peripherally). CC is in clinical use since 1967 for dysovulatory infertility. The efficacy of the drug varies in clinical practice if the proportion of enclomiphene and zuclomiphene are not maintained.

MECHANISM OF ACTION

It acts purely as antagonist or antiestrogenic agent. It binds with estrogen receptors at hypothalamus signaling lack of estrogen to hypothalamus. This in turn releases gonadotropin-releasing hormone (GnRH) which causes pituitary to secret more follicle-stimulating hormone (FSH) and luteinizing hormone (LH). This stimulates the ovarian follicular development. As the duration of action is longer, it allows FSH and LH secretion for a longer period and so causes multifollicular development. Clomiphene has direct effect on ovary to stimulate follicular estradiol (E2) synthesis. It increases the GnRH pulse frequency in ovulatory patients[1] and pulse amplitude in anovulatory patients like polycystic ovary syndrome (PCOS).[2] Clomiphene does not display progestational, corticotropic, androgenic or antiandrogenic properties.

INDICATIONS OF CLOMIPHENE CITRATE

WHO Group II Patients

It is extremely effective in anovulatory patients in whom hypothalamo-pituitary ovarian axis is normal. Normal thyroid function tests and prolactin should be confirmed before starting the treatment. It is not effective in hypogonadotropic hypogonadism, i.e., WHO group I as there is no negative feedback mechanism of estrogen.

Luteal Phase Defect

Short luteal phase is associated with low levels of FSH in follicular phase causing luteal phase defect (LPD). CC will increase FSH and LH in follicular phase, develop the good follicle and correct the abnormality in luteal phase. So CC is the drug of choice for LPD due to short luteal phase.[3]

UNEXPLAINED INFERTILITY

The rationale of using CC in unexplained infertility is that it corrects subtle hormonal defects due to deficiency of FSH and LH. It increases the number of follicles available for fertilization and corrects LPD. Cochrane database supports the use of CC in unexplained subfertility. Former belief of cervical dysmucorrhea and decreasing endometrial receptivity in unexplained infertility is not accepted and instead of contraindication, it is now considered the indication for CC in modern era for unexplained infertility. CC with intrauterine insemination (IUI) is beneficial as compared to expectant management.[4] Though there are some studies in which CC has not been found to increase pregnancy rates in ovulatory patients.[5]

CONTRAINDICATIONS

- Large ovarian cyst >5 cm in diameter. The cycle can be started when size of the cyst is <5 cm on Day 5 of the cycle
- Liver disease
- Hypogonadotropic hypogonadism—as the hypothalamic-pituitary-ovarian axis is highly dysfunctional
- Hypergonadotropic hypogonadism
- Before starting CC:
  - Thyroid function tests should be normal
  - Serum prolactin should be normal
  - Male partner should be evaluated
  - Progesterone withdrawal bleeding should be present in otherwise amenorrhoic patients
  - Adrenal function should be normal.

TREATMENT REGIMES

CC is given as 50 mg dose daily between Day 2 and Day 5 (both inclusive) for 5 days after spontaneous or induced bleeding. Ovulation, conception, and pregnancy rates are same independent of the day when CC is started.

Table 1: Dose of clomiphene citrate and ovulation rate.

Dose	Ovulation rate
50 mg	52%
100 mg	22%
150 mg	12%
200 mg	7%

But Day 5 is the most accepted day for starting the treatment. On Day 5 of the cycle there is a physiological decrease in serum FSH concentration, which provides the means for selection of the dominant follicle.

Most women (up to 74%)[6] respond to clomiphene with maximum 100 mg daily dose. Higher doses have very poor pregnancy rate. Professor Bruno Lunenfeild and Professor Roy Homburg have recommended only one dose to start with and maximum, 100 mg daily. The advantage of using this dose is that it can diagnose clomiphene resistant cases earlier and will cut down superfluous cycles of treatment till ovulation occurs. Dose more than 100 mg is not approved by US Food and Drug Administration (FDA) and adds only a little to pregnancy rates. Higher doses do not increase the ovulation rate or follicular recruitment.[7] **Table 1** shows the ovulation rates with different doses of CC. Even though clomiphene is not deposited in adipose tissue, the dose required for obese patient is higher. This is due to high androgen level which inhibits ovulation in obese patients.

Royal College of Obstetricians and Gynaecologists (RCOG) guidelines with American College of Obstetricians and Gynecologists (ACOG) recommendation is that CC can be used maximum for 12 months in lifetime and maximum for 6 months continuously. Therefore, monitoring for evidence of ovulation is a must when patient is on CC.[8,9]

MONITORING

- Serum progesterone in midluteal phase if is >3 ng/mL, it is an evidence of ovulation. It is done to confirm ovulation with CC.
- LH detection kit can help to know the LH surge. Normally, LH surge occurs after 7 days of the last dose of CC.
- Serial sonography just for documenting ovulation is not justified. It does not help to change the line of treatment. It is very inconvenient for the patient as compared to serum progesterone levels assessment done a week before expected date of menstruation.
- If LH on Day 8–9 is >10 IU/mL success rate is very low because of poor quality ova and embryo.

- Endometrial biopsy (EB) should not be done to know the proliferative or secretory phase as it is an invasive test.

Monitoring during CC treatment is must because it can be used only for 3-6 months. Majority of conceptions occur within first 3 months.

RESULTS

- CC will induce ovulation in approximately 75-80% of cases.
- Up to 70-75% of cumulative pregnancy rate can be achieved in 6-9 months.[6]
- In many series only up to 40% pregnancy rates have been achieved because of antiestrogenic effect on cervical mucus, endometrium, ova and embryo causing thick cervical mucus, thin endometrium and antioestrogenic effect itself that causes high LH and is detrimental to ova and embryo also.[10]
- About 75% of conceptions occur in the first 3 months. So in clinical practice, many consultants use it only for 3 months. After 6 months of therapy, only few pregnancies are recorded in literature.
- So, if the patient has not conceived within 3-6 months with CC, re-evaluation of the patient and switching over to further management is required.

  High ovulation rate and low pregnancy rate[11] with CC is because of:
  - Its antiestrogenic effect on cervix
  - Its antiestrogenic effect on endometrium
  - High LH, that deteriorates the ovum quality
  - Decreased uterine blood flow and decreased PP14, that are required for implantation
  - Direct effect on oocytes

SIDE EFFECTS

- Serious side effects are extremely rare.
- Transient hot flushes, mood swings, breast tenderness, nausea, and pelvic pain may occur.
- Visual disturbances may occur which are reversible after cessation of treatment.

  Alternative treatment is tried if patient complains of visual disturbances.

Antiestrogenic Effects of Clomiphene Citrate

Antiestrogenic effect on cervix, endometrium,[12] ovary, ovum, and embryo have been described but there is no objective evidence that these effects occur or have clinical consequences. Enclomiphene is a more potent antiestrogenic isomer and has a half-life of few days.[13] Though endometrial thickness is within normal range in majority of cases. This is because clomiphene is a selective estrogen receptor modulator and has a negative effect only on few patients. Very rarely endometrium suppression is observed which is less than 6 mm in spite of a good mature follicle. In this case, CC is not given, instead patient is to be shifted over to other therapy because usually endometrial suppression is repeated in subsequent cycles. This is because zuclomiphene component of CC, has a very long half-life and its accumulation from cycle to cycle leads to depletion of estrogen receptors, so much so that it may also cause hot flushes, postmenopausal syndrome like symptoms, visual scotomata and also cervical dysmucorrhea.[14] CC can be stored in body fat and accumulate in the body around crucial times of implantation, organogenesis, and embryogenesis.[15] Cervical dysmucorrhea can be overcome by IUI. In these patients having antiestrogenic effect, even though ovulation rate is 80%, conception rate is only 40%. Exogenous estrogen supplementation has no effect. Exogenous estrogen should not be used to correct cervical dysmucorrhea or increase endometrial thickness as receptors are already occupied by CC and exogenous estrogen will also not be perceived. Tamoxifen and letrozole can be used instead of CC to overcome these side effects. No significant difference in ovulation rates was found with raloxifene and CC.[16]

Risks of Clomiphene Citrate

- Multiple pregnancy (5–8%)—but most are twins or triplets—higher order pregnancies are rare (0.08–1.1%).[17]
- *Miscarriage*: It does not increase spontaneous miscarriage rate.[18]
- *Congenital anomalies*: There is no substantial evidence that CC causes any particular birth defects or increases the incidence of birth defects.[19] Neural tube defects and hypospadias are the ones most often found in babies of CC treated mothers. Other defects that were found to be associated with CC were Dandy-Walker malformation, muscular ventricular septal defect (VSD), cloacal exstrophy, anencephaly, all septal heart defects combined, coarctation of aorta, esophageal atresia, craniosynostosis and omphalocele. Another study though shows that CC is not associated with increased incidence of craniosynostosis.[20]
- *Ovarian hyperstimulation syndrome (OHSS)*: Mild OHSS may occur in a few cases of PCOS, which requires only conservative management. Severe OHSS is rare and I have not seen any in my practice of 30 years.
- *Breast and ovarian cancer*: Previous studies suggested that if CC is used for more than 12 months, it can increase the incidence of ovarian malignancy. But subsequent studies have proved that fertility drugs are not associated with any invasive cancers. CC does not increase the risk of breast cancer.

Women on clomiphene therapy must be counseled that no causal relationship has been established between ovulation inducing drugs and breast or ovarian cancer. However, prolonged treatment with CC is futile and should be avoided because it has little success.

TREATMENT ALTERNATIVES

Extended Clomiphene Treatment

- CC is given for 7–10 days.
- 150 mg of CC is given for 8 days.
- 50 mg/day is given for 5 days and increment of 50 mg/day is done every 5 days to reach 250 mg/day.

No factors have been identified that can predict which patient will respond to extended regime. Such extended regimes have extremely poor pregnancy rates and are not much helpful in clinical practice.

Clomiphene Citrate + Glucocorticoids

This combination is very useful in chronic anovulatory patients. It is also given to those patients who have high dehydroepiandrosterone sulfate (DHEAS). It can be given to all the patients who show increase in adrenal androgen production. It has given good results even with normal DHEAS and unselected population having clomiphene resistance due to increased androgen. Two large trials evaluated CC-resistant anovulatory patients with normal DHEAS levels. Those treated with dexamethasone on cycle days 3–12 and CC, showed 75–88% ovulation rates and 40% conception rates as compared to 15–20% and 5% respectively, without dexamethasone.[21] Those patients who are resistant to 100–150 mg of CC, start ovulating when glucocorticoids are added. Glucocorticoids are given in the form of dexamethasone 0.5 mg daily or prednisolone 5 mg daily continuously for 30 days at bed time. It can be given continuously for 3–6 months. No serious side effects are seen, though water logging and weight gain have been documented. The dose can be reduced to 0.25 mg/day or can be stopped in secretory phase of the cycle. As the drug is very cheap and effective and does not have any major disadvantage it should be tried in chronic anovulatory patients. Glucocorticoids improve response of follicles to stimulation and the health of developing oocytes.[22]

Clomiphene Citrate + Estrogen

Estrogen was tried to improve cervical mucus and endometrial thickness. But these effects are not due to the dosage and duration of treatment of CC.

It is idiosyncratic response in subgroup of CC which may reduce conception rate. So combination with estrogen is not of any help and should not be used in clinical practice. Empirical treatment with estrogen has no role.

Clomiphene Citrate + Bromocriptine

Bromocriptine is given to the patients of hyperprolactinemia. But there are two definite indications even with normal prolactin level.

1. *Galactorrhea with normal prolactin level*: In these cases, galactorrhea must be confirmed by presence of fat globules under the microscope in the secretions expressed from the breast. It must be differentiated from simple mucoid discharge that does not have fat globules.
2. There are patients who are known as spikers. In these patients, prolactin is increased in the first half of the cycle when CC is used for ovulation induction. These patients are given bromocriptine in first-half of the cycle. It is not to be continued in second half of the cycle as normal level of prolactin is required for maintenance of corpus luteum. Clinically these patients show poor endometrium even though there is no local cause and follicle is very good and meets all parameters on B-mode and color Doppler for optimum maturity. Bromocriptine can be tried in these patients and if endometrium improves, it can be continued for 3–6 months.

Clomiphene Citrate + Human Chorionic Gonadotropin

Routine use of human chorionic gonadotropin (hCG) for rupture of the follicle is not justified. If the follicle is mature it will reflect as serum E2 level of 150 pgm/mL or more. This will initiate the LH surge which in turn will cause rupture of the follicle and exogenous hCG is not required. But if the follicle is not mature and if hCG is given as a trigger for ovulation, it will lead to premature luteinization or atresia. Therefore, hCG must not be given just for follicular rupture.

Human chorionic gonadotropin must be combined with clomiphene when IUI is to be done. hCG in these cases is done to time IUI as follicle ruptures at 34–36 hours after hCG injection. A meta-analysis of seven studies comparing triggering ovulation with hCG (1,461 patients) with urinary LH testing to identify endogenous LH surge (1,162 patients) for timing IUI for women with unexplained infertility treated with CC, reported lower odds of pregnancy when hCG trigger was used as compared to endogenous LH surge.[19] hCG can also be given in patients proved to have absent, inadequate or delayed LH surge. This is a common occurrence in endometriosis. hCG, therefore must be used for timed intercourse, to time IUI and in cases of delayed LH surge.

Clomiphene Citrate + Gonadotropin

Gonadotropins are often combined with clomiphene with the idea that it would decrease the requirement of gonadotropins. Clomiphene citrate by its direct effect on ovary, increases the sensitivity of ovary to gonadotropins. This combination has risk of ovarian hyperstimulation and multiple pregnancies. Increased LH secretion induced by CC, may also reduce the likelihood of conception.[20]

I am personally never convinced by this combination and would never use it. It does not increase the pregnancy rate. The argument is that CC increases FSH and LH both. The poor pregnancy rate with CC is because of high LH which will remain inspite of adding gonadotropins. The effect of high LH will decrease the implantation and pregnancy rate. So even though we get a follicle after adding gonadotropins, in many of these patients, the follicular quality is not good and pregnancy rates are only comparable to CC alone and much less than gonadotropins alone. Instead letrozole is a better drug to be combined with gonadotropins. This will be discussed in chapter 4. Low dose FSH protocol is recommended by Professor Roy Homburg as a first line of treatment for ovulation induction instead of CC. The study has shown to double the pregnancy rates, with reduced treatment pregnancy interval and more singleton pregnancies.[25]

Gonadotropin-releasing Hormone Agonist

Gonadotropin-releasing hormone agonists are not used routinely in IUI cycles and are reserved only for in vitro fertilization (IVF) cycles. Agonists are used for downregulation and this in IUI cycles only increases the requirement of gonadotropins, without increasing the pregnancy rate.

Clomiphene Citrate + Antagonist

This makes a good combination in thin lean PCOS patients where LH is tonically raised. It improves the quality of ovum and also the conception rates. For patients on clomiphene therapy, serum LH levels are checked on Day 8–9 of the cycle. If it is >10 IU/mL, it is an indicator of poor pregnancy rates. These are the ideal patients to start antagonist. Regular use of antagonist with CC is not justified because it sharply decreases LH and quality of follicle is changed and it causes regression of follicle as well as luteal phase defects.

Clomiphene Citrate + Metformin

Several workers have shown that metformin is inferior to CC for ovulation induction and metformin alone should not be used for ovulation induction.[26]

But in CC resistant cases of PCOS when metformin is combined with CC, it increases ovulation four to nine times than clomiphene alone. Metformin is a very useful drug when patient does not want to conceive immediately. If metformin is taken for 6 months, it will normalize hormonal milieu. It will decrease LH and androgen. So if CC is given when patient wants to conceive, ovulation will occur and will decrease the incidence of multiple pregnancies also. Pretreatment with metformin for patients to be treated with CC has shown to improve ovulation rates[27] and conception rates[28] in several studies. Though another study has clearly shown that metformin pretreatment does not improve the pregnancy rates or extended metformin therapy does not reduce the required dose of CC.[29,30] A meta-analysis of 17 randomized controlled trials (RCTs) in PCOS women has shown both increased ovulation and pregnancy when metformin was added to CC. This effect was found to be statistically significant in obese women with PCOS, whereas it failed to reach significance in nonobese women with this condition. It is therefore logical to routinely use metformin with CC in obese women with PCOS and glucocorticoid as the first adjunct of choice for nonobese PCOS women failing to respond to CC.[31]

Clomiphene Citrate + Drilling

It is done in CC resistant PCOS cases. Drilling is also done before switching over to gonadotropins.

Clomiphene + Low Dose Aspirin

Aspirin may be used to increase the blood flow by vasodilatation which may counter the effect of stress in reducing pelvic blood flow.[32] Though in a meta-analysis this benefit has not been established.[33]

Prior Treatments

- *Clomiphene after prior treatment with oral contraceptive (OC) pills*: The mechanism of action of OC pills is to decrease LH. High LH will cause high androgen, which in turn will cause anovulation. So OC pills when given for 2–3 months will decrease the LH and in turn androgen improves the sensitivity to clomiphene with the same dose. Therefore, in PCOS patients prior treatment with OC pills was given routinely in CC resistant cases and did show good results.
- *Micronized progesterone*: If it is given for 5 days, it modulates LH pulsatility, reducing LH concentration and induces more favorable environment for CC.

Carry Home Message

- Clomiphene citrate should be used for 3–6 months, 100 mg/day starting from Day 5.
- Clomiphene citrate + estrogen has no role.
- Clomiphene citrate + dexamethasone is useful in chronic anovulatory patient and when DHEAS is high.
- Clomiphene citrate + bromocriptine is used in patients with normal prolactin levels with galactorrhea and spikers when prolactin is high in first half of the cycle.
- Routine use of hCG is not justified.
- Clomiphene citrate + GnRH agonist for downregulation has no role in IUI cycles.
- Clomiphene citrate + antagonist must be used in thin lean PCOS patients.
- Clomiphene citrate + gonadotropins do not improve pregnancy rates.
- Clomiphene citrate + metformin can be used in CC resistant PCOS patients.
- Metformin, OC pills, and progesterone are useful prior to CC.
- Clomiphene citrate without IUI does not increase the fecundity rates in patients with unexplained infertility but does definitely increase the fecundity rates with IUI.[34]
- Ovarian drilling is offered to CC resistant PCOS.

REFERENCES

1. Kerin JF, Liu JH, Phillipou G, Yen SS. Evidence for a hypothalamic site of action of clomiphene citrate in women. J Clin Endocrinol Metab. 1985;61:265-8.
2. Kettel LM, Roseff SJ, Berga SL, Mortala JF, Yen SS. Hypothalamic-pituitary-ovarian response to clomiphene citrate in women with polycystic ovary syndrome. Fertil Steril. 1993;59:532-8.
3. The practice committee of American Society for Reproductive Medicine. The clinical relevance of luteal phase deficiency. Fertil Steril. 2012;98:112-7.
4. Deaton JL, Gibson M, Blackmer KM, Nakajima ST, Badger GJ, Brumsted JR. A randomised controlled trial of clomiphene citrate and intrauterine insemination in couples with explained infertility or surgically corrected endometriosis. Fertil Steril. 1990;54:1083-8.
5. Guzick DS, Carson SA, Coutifaris C, Oversheet JW, Factor-Litvak P, Steinkampf MP, et al. Efficacy of superovulation and intrauterine insemination in the treatment of infertility. N Engl J Med. 1999;340(3):177-83.
6. Thessaloniki ESHRE/ASRM-sponsored PCOS consensus workshop group. Consensus on infertility treatment related to polycystic ovary syndrome. Fertil Steril. 2008;89:505-22.
7. Dickey RP, Taylor SN, Curole DN, RYe PH, Lu PY, Pyrzak R. Relationship of clomiphene dose and patient weight to successful treatment. Hum Reprod. 1997;12:449-53.
8. Gysler M, March CM, Mishell DR Jr, Bailey EJ. A decade's experience with an individualized clomiphene treatment regimen including its effect on the post-coital test. Fertil Steril. 1982;37:161.
9. Gorlitsky GA, Kase NG, Speroff L. Ovulation and pregnancy rates with clomiphene citrate. Obstet Gynecol. 1978;51:265.
10. Homburg R. Clomiphene citrate-end of an era? Hum Reprod. 2005;20:2043-51.

11. Out HJ, Coelingh Bennink HJ. Clomiphene citrate or gonadotrophins for induction of ovulation? Hum Reprod. 1998;13:2358-61.
12. Gonen Y, Casper RF. Sonographic demonstration of an adverse effect of clomiphene citrate on endometrial growth. Hum Reprod. 1990;5:670-4.
13. Young SL, Opsahl MS, Fritz A. Serum concentration of enclomiphene and zuclomiphene across consecutive cycles of clomiphene citrate therapy in an ovulatory infertile women. Fetil Steril. 1999;71:639-44.
14. Ghobadi C, Mirhosseini N, Shiran MR, Moghadamnia A, Lennard MS, Ledger WL, et al. Single dose pharmacokinetic study of clomiphene citrate isomers in an ovular patients with polycystic ovary disease. J Clin Pharacol. 2009;49:147-54.
15. Mikkelson TJ, Kroboth PD, Cameron WJ, et al. Single-dose pharmacokinetics of clomiphene citrate in normal volunteers. Fertil Steril. 1986;46:392-6.
16. de Paula Guedes Neto E, Savaris RF, von Eye Corleta H, de Moraes GS, do Amaral Cristovam R, Lessey BA. Prospective, randomized comparison between raloxifene and clomiphene citrate for ovulation induction in polycystic ovary syndrome. Fertil Steril. 2011;96(3):769-73.
17. Reefhuis J, Honein MA, Schieve LA, Rasmussen SA, National birth defects prevention study. Use of clomiphene citrate and birth defects. National birth defects prevention study, 1997-2005. Hum Reprod. 2011;26:451-7.
18. Badawy A, Shokeir T, Allam AF, Abdelhady H. Pregnancy outcome after ovulation induction with aromatase inhibitors or clomiphene citrate in unexplained infertility. Acta Obstet Gynecol Scand. 2009;88:187-91.
19. Correy JF, Marsden De, Schokman FC. The outcome of pregnancy resulting from clomiphene-induced ovulation. Aust N Z J Obstet Gynaecol. 1982;22:18-21.
20. Reefhuis J, Honein MA, Show GM, Romitti PA. Fertility treatments and craniosynostosis: California, Georgia and Iowa. 1993-1997. Pediatrics. 2003;111:1163-6.
21. Elnashar A, Abdelageed E, Fayed M, Sharaf M. Clomiphene citrate and dexamethasone in treatment of clomiphene citrate resistant polycystic ovary syndrome: a prospective placebo-controlled study. Hum Reprod. 2006;21:1805-8.
22. Thurston LM, Norgate DP, Jonas KC, Gregory L, Wood PJ, Cooke BA, et al. Ovarian modulators of type 1 11 beta-hydroxysteroid dehydrogenase (11 beta HSD) activity and intra-follicular cortisol: cortisone ratios correlate with the clinical outcome of IVF. Hum Reprod. 2003;18:1603-12.
23. George K, Nair R, Tharyan P. Ovulation triggers in anovulatory women undergoing ovulation induction. Cochrane Database Syst Rev. 2008;3:CD006900.
24. Sagle MA, Hamilton-Fairley D, Kiddy DS. A comparative, randomized study of low dose human menopausal gonadotrophin and follicle-stimulating hormone in women with polycystic ovarian syndrome. Fertil Steril. 1990;53:792-7.
25. Homburg R, Hendriks ML, Konig TE, Anderson RA, Balen AH, Brincat M, et al. Clomiphene citrate of low dose FSH for the first-line treatment of infertile women with anovulation associated with polycystic ovary syndrome: a prospective randomized multinational study. Hum Reprod. 2012;27(2):468-73.
26. De Leo V, la Marca A, Ditto A, Morgante G, Cianci A. Effects of metformin on gonadotropin-induced ovulation in women with polycystic ovary syndrome. Fertil Steril. 1999;72:282-3.
27. Kocak M, Caliskan E, Simsir C, Haberal A. Metformin therapy improves ovulation rates, cervical scores and pregnancy rates in clomiphene citrate resistant women with polycystic ovary syndrome. Fertil Steril. 2002;77:101-6.
28. Khorram O, Helliwell JP, Katz S, Bonpane CM, Jaramillo L. Two weeks of metformin improves clomiphene citrate induced ovulation and metabolic profiles in women with polycystic ovary syndrome. Fertil Steril. 2006;85:1448-51.

29. Silbert TI, Kruger TF, Lombard C. Evaluating the equivalence of clomiphene citrate with and without metformin in ovulation induction in PCOS patients. J Assist Reprod Genet. 2009;26:165-71.
30. Cataldo NA, Barnhart HX, Legro RS, Myers ER, Schlaff WD, Carr BR, et al. Extended-release metformin does not reduce the clomiphene citrate dose required to induce ovulation in polycystic ovary syndrome. J Clin Endocrinol Metab. 2008;93:3124-7.
31. Creanga AA, Bradley HM, McCormick C, Witkop CT, et al. Use of metformin in polycystic ovary syndrome: a meta-analysis. Obstet Gynecol. 2008;111:959-68.
32. Ebbesen SMS, Zachariae R, Mehlsen MY, Thomsen D, Højgaard A, Ottosen L, et al. Stressful life events are associated with poor in vitro fertilization (IVF) outcome: a prospective study. Hum Reprod. 2009;24:2173-82.
33. Khairy M, Banerjee K, El-Toukhy T, et al. Aspirin in women undergoing in vitro fertilization treatment: a systematic review and meta-analysis. Fertil Steril. 2007;88:822-31.
34. Practice committee of American Society of Reproductive Medicine. Use of clomiphene citrate in infertile women: a committee opinion. Fertil Steril. 2013;100(2):341-8.

CHAPTER 4

Letrozole

Chaitanya Nagori

INTRODUCTION

Letrozole is an aromatase inhibitor used for ovulation induction. It is the third generation of aromatase inhibitor. First and second generations of aromatase inhibitors are not used in clinical practice. The main advantage of letrozole is that it is a reversible enzyme inhibitor. It was for the first time used in 2001 for ovulation induction.

MECHANISM OF INDUCTION OF OVULATION

- *Central mechanism*: Estrogen withdrawal centrally causes increase in activins produced from pituitary and several other tissues.[1] This stimulates synthesis of follicle-stimulating hormone (FSH) by a direct action on gonadotropes.[2]
- *Peripheral mechanism*: Androgens have stimulatory role in early follicular growth[3] mediated directly through testosterone augmentation of follicular FSH receptor expression[4,5] and directly through androgen stimulation by insulin-like growth factor 1 (IGF-1), which may synergize with FSH to promote folliculogenesis.[6,7]

Aromatase, a cytochrome P450 dependent enzyme acts as ultimate step in synthesis of estrogen, catalyzing the conversion of androgen to estrogen. This conversion occurs at peripheral sites such as muscle, fat, and liver. Letrozole inhibits aromatase enzyme by completely binding to the heme of cytochrome P450 subunits of enzyme, so that androgen is not converted to estrogen.

The end result is low estrogen causing negative feedback at hypothalamus and pituitary releasing FSH and luteinizing hormone (LH) releasing factors resulting in high FSH and LH causing folliculogenesis.

As androgen is not converted into estrogen, there is slightly higher level of androgen which also helps folliculogenesis. Letrozole has no effect on estrogen receptors and acts on hypothalamus. So, it has no deleterious effect on LH surge, cervical mucus and endometrium.

As FSH and LH stimulate folliculogenesis, estrogen will rise and will cause negative feedback on FSH release so FSH will decrease. This decrease in FSH is responsible for monofollicular development as other follicles will not grow. This is not the case with clomiphene citrate (CC), which binds to estrogen receptors and FSH will go on rising in spite of high estrogen, leading to multifollicular development. Another important advantage is that along with FSH, LH will not increase and so quality of ova is not disturbed and does not affect implantation. This is another advantage over CC which causes persistent high LH along with FSH.

INDICATIONS

- *Clomiphene citrate resistant cases*: When 100–150 mg of CC fails to induce ovulation, letrozole should be tried.
- *Polycystic ovary syndrome (PCOS)*: In these patients baseline estradiol (E2) is elevated which blocks hypothalamus causing anovulation. Letrozole will reduce estrogen and stimulate hypothalamus to release luteinizing hormone-releasing hormone (LHRH) to secrete more FSH and induces folliculogenesis.
- It is useful in cases where CC induces cervical dysmenorrhea and poor endometrium. Letrozole is devoid of antiestrogenic effect as it does not bind to estrogen receptors.
- When LH is elevated on Day 8 or Day 9 after CC, letrozole should be tried.
- It is useful in poor responders along with gonadotropins.

CHARACTERISTICS OF LETROZOLE

- It causes total suppression of estrogen (up to 97–99%) with doses up to 5 mg/day. Maximum suppression occurs between Day 5 and 7.
- After Day 7 estrogen level will rise due to folliculogenesis because of increasing FSH after negative feedback of estrogen due to letrozole.
- This rise of estrogen will continue for 5–7 days. This E2 peak will cause LH surge for ovulation. So LH surge occurs after 12 days unlike CC when it occurs early.
- High estrogen rise after 7 days will decrease FSH, which is responsible for monofollicular development.
- It has no antiestrogenic effect on cervical mucus or endometrium.
- Temporary rise of androgen improves the sensitivity of follicle to gonadotropin. Patient, therefore, requires lower dose of gonadotropins when it is combined with letrozole.

ADVANTAGES

- It is almost free from side effects and is well tolerated.
- Monofollicular development.
- No antiestrogenic effect leading to higher pregnancy rates.
- Low multiple pregnancy rate due to monofollicular development.
- Low abortion rate because of no effect on endometrium.

- Higher androgen stimulates follicle and so lower doses of gonadotropins are required.

  There is a transient accumulation of androgens in the ovary when letrozole is given for ovulation induction. This creates an androgenic microenvironment in the maturing follicle that enhances the follicular sensitivity to FSH for a short duration (half-life of letrozole is approximately 45 hours). This action is of help in poor responders in whom ovarian aging has already reduced ovarian androgens.
- It is useful in patients with high body mass index (BMI).[8]
- It improves the level of marker of endometrial receptivity better than CC.[9]
- The incidence of cardiac anomalies in the letrozole group was slightly lower than the 1 in 400 rate quoted in general population,[10] whereas the cardiac anomaly rate in fetuses of mothers with CC stimulation was about seven times higher.
- Letrozole also leads to reduction in secretion of estrogen from granulosa cells leading to less circulating estrogens, therefore less chances of thrombosis in hyperestrogenic states during controlled ovarian hyperstimulation (COH) and also an additional safely for women with hormone-dependent cancers undergoing fertility therapy.[11]
- Aromatase inhibition may potentially improve endometrial receptivity, especially in patients with endometriosis.[11]
- Concomitant use of aromatase inhibitors with gonadotropins reduces the doses of gonadotropins required[12] and improve the response of gonadotropins in poor responders.[13] It also reduces the supraphysiological levels of estrogen seen with development of multiple ovarian follicles and improves treatment outcome. Low estrogen levels decrease ubiquitination to allow upregulation of estrogen receptors and increasing sensitivity to subsequent estrogen rise.[14] This in turn leads to improved endometrial blood flow and faster proliferation of the endometrium, which might have a positive impact on implantation.[15]
- Endometrium of PCOS females is dysfunctional.[16] Estrogen receptors in the endometrium, which should normally reduce in the midsecretory phase[17] are not reduced, with altered status of other receptors also. This functional derangement leads to progesterone resistance. This is why antiestrogenic agents for ovulation induction may be beneficial in PCOS patients. Moreover, these agents would also improve endometrial receptivity by suppressing the action of ERα and also has a positive impact on endometrial expression of $\alpha v\beta 3$.[18]

DOSES

- Recommended dose is 2.5 mg from Day 3 to 7.
- Some workers suggest 5 mg dose. The disadvantage of 5 mg dose routinely is not justified as 2.5 mg can suppress 97–99% of estrogen.

5 mg may suppress more estrogen causing more FSH to be secreted. So it may not cause monofollicular development. As it is a chemotherapeutic agent, it may be toxic to ovum and embryo.

- *20 mg on Day 3*: It has advantage having short half-life and reduces embryotoxic effect. But symptoms of hypoestrinism may develop.
- It is superior to anastrozole 1 mg from Day 3 to 7 or anastrozole 5 mg single dose.

New Regimes

- *Extended letrozole therapy*: 2.5 mg letrozole is given from Day 1 for 10 days in CC resistant PCOS patients. It may produce more follicles and may give better pregnancy rates.[19]
- *Letrozole step-up protocol*: One, two, three, and four tablets of 2.5 mg of letrozole is given respectively on Day 2, 3, 4, and 5. This gives multifollicular development and higher pregnancy rate. The mechanism of action in this regime is longer duration of FSH exposure, prevention of estrogen secretion from granulosa cells, so estrogen does not rise and FSH does not get suppressed.[20] But in both these cases the actual advantages of letrozole, unnecessary exposure of ovum to LH and monofollicular development are lost. As both lead to longer duration of FSH and LH secretion and also lead to multifollicular development. Therefore, larger and more robust studies are required to accept these protocols in routine practice.

SIDE EFFECTS (DRAWBACKS)

- It increases intrafollicular androgen which may arrest the growth of follicle. But optimum level of androgen is not yet decided.
- As it is chemotherapeutic agent for carcinoma breast, it may be teratogenic to ovum and embryo. But it is not proved.

FUTURE USES

- Letrozole helps to improve implantation in in vitro fertilization (IVF). Some women have high levels of aromatase P450 in endometrium and are related to poor IVF results. It can be useful to them.
- Decreased supraphysiological estrogen and decreased aromatase will improve implantation.
- It stimulates follicles for in vitro maturation (IVM) in PCOS.
- Letrozole may reduce the chronic pelvic pain of endometriosis.[21]
- Letrozole may be used to reduce the risk of ovarian hyperstimulation syndrome (OHSS) and thrombosis due to hyperestrinism—when given on Day 4–7 and 10 after human chorionic gonadotropin (hCG) trigger

in an IVF patient, it reduces estrogen levels and thus reduce the risk of OHSS.[22]

- Letrozole challenge test may be used for predicting the ovarian response to gonadotropin stimulation. This test is done by evaluating FSH on Day 3 and Day 7 of a letrozole cycle. Ratio of Day 7 and Day 3 FSH is >1.5 which predicts poor response to gonadotropins.[23] Aromatase inhibitors are also used to treat male subfertility.
- Anastrozole 1 mg/day or letrozole 2.5 mg/day is the recommended dose for patients with high aromatase activity and increased testosterone to estrogen ratio in nonobstructive azoospermic patients. Therefore, in patients with low testosterone levels, use of aromatase inhibitors is justified.[24]

AUTHOR'S VIEW

Should letrozole replace CC: I strongly believe that letrozole should be used as the first line of drug. The argument is that it has comparable pregnancy rate with CC and it does not increase congenital malformations. The main advantage is, it has no antiestrogenic effect on cervical mucus and endometrium and so it will cut down superfluous cycles of treatment. No antiestrogenic effect is the single most important benefit with letrozole that prevents the use of CC.

LETROZOLE + GONADOTROPINS

We have found letrozole + recombinant FSH (rFSH), a very useful combination for giving equivalent pregnancy rates like gonadotropins with advantage that lower number of ampoules are required. Apart from this, it gives lower rate of multiple births. It sensitizes ovary by rise in androgen level, is an added advantage that reduces number of gonadotropin ampoules. We have used this combination routinely in superovulation with intrauterine insemination (IUI).

So, letrozole is superior to CC in PCOS and poor responders.

Other aromatase inhibitors especially anastrozole was also tried for ovulation induction. It appears from clinical studies that anastrozole is less effective than letrozole for ovulation induction.[25,26]

LETROZOLE + CLOMIPHENE CITRATE

As letrozole and CC have different mechanism of action, combination of both may improve the ovulation rate than letrozole alone. Mejia et al. gave letrozole 2.5 mg and CC 50 mg from Day 3–7 in PCOS patients. Patients who received both the drugs had higher ovulation rate. But there was no difference in pregnancy rate, multiple pregnancy rate or abortion rate.

Patients who ovulated showed no difference in endometrial thickness, size of the follicle or serum progesterone levels. But absolute difference of 34% in ovulation was noted.[27]

Hajisafi et al. used 100 mg of CC and 5 mg of letrozole in resistant cases of CC and letrozole.[28] This observation requires further studies. LH which is already high in PCOS will be increased further when both the drugs are used. This LH will not come down because of receptors occupied by CC even after high estrogen after follicular development. This may reach the "ceiling level of LH". This is the only reason that like CC, ovulation rate is high with this combination but pregnancy rate is not increased and perhaps it may decrease instead, than when giving only letrozole. Instead letrozole + FSH is a better combination.

Carry Home Message

- Letrozole causes monofollicular development.
- It has no antiestrogenic effect.
- It is a drug of choice in PCOS and poor responders.
- Letrozole + gonadotropins is an excellent combination.
- Letrozole may replace CC as first line of treatment in future.

REFERENCES

1. Roberts V, Meunier H, Vaughan J, J Rivier, C Rivier, W Vale, et al. Production and regulation of inhibin subunits in pituitary gonadotropes. Endocrinology. 1989;124:552-4.
2. Weil SJ, Vendola K, Zhou J, Adesanya OO, Wang J, Okafor J, et al. Androgen receptor gene expression in the primate ovary: cellular localization, regulation and functional correlations. J Clin Endocrinol Metab. 1989;837:2479-85.
3. Mason AJ, Berkemeier LM, Schmelzer CH, Schwall RH. Activin B: precursor sequences, genomic structure and in vitro activities. Mol Endocrinol. 1989;3:1352-8.
4. Weil S, Vendola K, Zhou J, Bondy CA. Androgen and follicle-stimulating hormone interactions in primate ovarian follicle development. J Clin Endocrinol Metab. 1999;84:2951-6.
5. Vendola KA, Zhou J, Adesanya OO, Weil SJ, Bondy CA. Androgens stimulate early stages of follicular growth in the primate ovary. J Clin Invest. 1998;101:2622-9.
6. Vendola K, Zhou J, Wang J, Famuyiwa OA, Bievre M, Bondy CA, et al. Androgens promote oocyte insulin-like growth factor I expression and initiation of follicle development in the primate ovary. Biol Reprod. 1999;61:353-7.
7. Giudice LC. Insulin like growth factors and ovarian follicular development. Endocr Rev. 1992;13:641-69.
8. McKnight KK, Nodler JL, Cooper JA, Chapman VR, Cliver SP, Bates GW Jr. Body mass index-associated differences in response to ovulation induction with letrozole. Fertil Steril. 2011;96(5):1206-8.
9. Wallace KL, Johnson V, Sopelak V, Hines R. Clomiphene citrate versus letrozole: molecular analysis of the endometrium in women with polycystic ovary syndrome. Fertil Steril. 2011;96(4):1051-6.

10. Hoffman JI. Incidence of congenital heart disease: I. Postnatal incidence. Pediatr Cardiol. 1995;16:103-13.
11. Garcia-Valesco JA. The use of aromatase inhibitors in in vitro fertilization. Fertil Steril. 2012;98(6):1356-8.
12. Mitwally MF, Casper RF. Aromatase inhibition reduces the dose of gonadotropin required for controlled ovarian hyperstimulation. J Soc Gynecol Investig. 2004;11:406-15.
13. Mitwally MF, Casper RF. Aromatase inhibition improves ovarian response to follicle stimulating hormone in poor responders. Fertile Steril. 2002;77:776-80.
14. Mitwally MF, Witchel SF, Casper RF. Troglitazone: A possible modulator of ovarian steroidogenesis. J Soc Gynecol Investig. 2002;9:163-7.
15. Nirmala PB, Thampan RV. Ubiquitination of the rat uterine oestrogen receptor: dependence on oestradiol. Biochem Biophys Res Commun. 1995;213:24-31.
16. Giudicel C. Endometrium in PCOS: implantation and predisposition to endocrine CA. Best Pract Res Clin Endocrinol Metab. 2006;20:235-44.
17. Lessey BA, Killam AP, Metzger DA, Haney AF, Greene GL, McCarty KS Jr. Immunohistochemical analysis of human uterine estrogen and progesterone receptors through the menstrual cycle. J Clin Endocrinol Metab. 1988;67:334-40.
18. Lessey BA, Palomino WA, Apparao KBC, Young SL, Lininger RA. Estrogen receptor-alpha (ER-alpha) and defects in uterine receptivity in women. Repro Biol Endocrinol. 2006;4(Suppl 1):S9.
19. Badawy A, Mosbah A, Tharwat A, Eid M. Extended letrozole therapy for induction of ovulation in CC resistant PCOS patients: a novel protocol. Fertil Steril. 2009;92:236-9.
20. Mitwally MF, Said T, Galal A. Letrozole step-up protocol: a successful superovulation protocol. Fertil Steril. 2008;89:523-4.
21. Pavone ME, Bulun SE. Aromatase inhibitors for treatment of endometriosis. Fertil Steril. 2012;98(6):1370-9.
22. Fatemi HM, Popovic-Todorovic B, Donoso P, Papanikolau E, Smitz J, Devreoy P. Luteal phase oestradiol suppression by letrozole: a pilot study in oocyte donors. Reprod Biomed Online. 2008;17:307-11.
23. Bentov Y, Burstein E, Esfandiari N, Casper R. Use of letrozole challenge test to adjust gonadotrophin dose in non-downregulated cycles. Fertil Steril. 2011;95(8): 2492-3.
24. Schlegel PN. Aromatase inhibitors for male infertility. Fertil Steril. 2012;98(6):1359-62.
25. Tredway D, Schettz JC, Bock D, Hemsey G, Diamond MP. Anastrazole vs. clomiphene citrate in infertile women with ovulatory dysfunction: a phase II randomized, dose-finding study. Fertil Steril. 2011;95:1720-4.
26. Tredway D, Schettz JC, Bock D, Hemsey G, Diamond MP. Anastrozole single dose protocol in women with oligo- or anovulatory infertility: results of a randomized phase II dose-response study. Fertil Steril. 2011;95:1724-8.
27. Mejia RB, Summers KM, Kresowik JD, Van Voorhis BJ. A randomized controlled trial of combination of letrozole and clomiphene citrate or letrozole alone for ovulation induction in women with PCOS. Fertil Steril. 2019;111(3):571-8.
28. Hajisafi M, Dehgan M, Kiarang N, Sadegh-Asadi N, Shayegh SN, Ghasemi-Rad M. Combined letrozole and clomiphene versus letrozole and clomiphene alone in infertile patients with polycystic ovary syndrome. Drug Des Devel Ther. 2013;7:1427-31.

CHAPTER 5

Gonadotropins

Chaitanya Nagori

INTRODUCTION

Gonadotropins are direct stimulation to ovaries in contrast to clomiphene citrate and letrozole which stimulates hypothalamus and indirectly increases follicle-stimulating hormone (FSH) and luteinizing hormone (LH) simultaneously. Professor Bruno Lunenfeld first reported the use of human menopausal gonadotropin (hMG) followed by pregnancy in 1963. Now purified preparations of gonadotropins are also available. The availability of recombinant FSH (rFSH) has changed the picture for demand of gonadotropins.

PHYSIOLOGY

- Primordial follicles are independent of gonadotropins stimulation and they take 10 weeks to develop into antral follicles.
- Antral follicles can respond to gonadotropin stimulation.
- Under the influence of FSH and LH, antral follicle grows, matures, and ovulates in 2 weeks.
- FSH rise in the late luteal phase of previous cycle decides the dominant follicle.
- For follicular cohort to recruit minimum level of FSH is required and this is called FSH threshold.
- FSH window means number of days the FSH levels are above threshold.
- As the sensitivity of follicle to FSH increases with development, lower amount of FSH is required for further growth of the follicle.
- As the amount of FSH decreases it stops growth of other follicles except the dominant follicle. The process of selection of follicle is completed in 7 days. But when gonadotropins are given from outside, we do not decrease the dose of FSH and so there will be larger number of follicles that grow and ovulate in controlled ovarian stimulation (COS).
- All oocytes are arrested in prophase stage of meiosis in preantral follicles. This inhibition is removed by LH surge and first meiotic division will be complete with extrusion of first polar body. Oocytes should be fertilized within 48–72 hours and second meiotic division occurs otherwise oocyte dies.

FOLLICLE-STIMULATING HORMONE PREPARATIONS AVAILABLE

- *hMG*: 75 IU of FSH and 75 IU of LH activity by human chorionic gonadotropin (hCG) acting as LH surrogate.
- *hMG-HP (highly purified)*: 75 IU of FSH and 75 IU of LH with <5% of urinary proteins.
- *Urinary FSH*: 75 IU of FSH and 1 IU of LH.
- *FSH-HP*: 75 IU of FSH with <0.1 IU of LH and <5% of urinary proteins.
- *Recombinant FSH*: 75 IU of FSH and no LH activity.
- rFSH + rLH combination.

PRINCIPLES OF GONADOTROPIN THERAPY

The basic principles were suggested by Insler and Lunenfeld in 1974.[1]

- *Effective dose*: Ovarian response is seen when certain dose of FSH is given. Below this dose the ovaries do not respond.
- *Latent phase*: This phase lasts for 3–7 days. It starts with onset of stimulation, but there is no estrogen rise or ultrasound demonstrable follicular growth during this phase.
- *Active phase*: This phase starts with ultrasound demonstrable follicle growth to ovulation and it lasts for 4–6 days.

PHYSIOLOGY OF OVULATION

- FSH stimulates the follicle to grow. But continuous stimulation is required for follicle to grow.
- Follicle secretes estrogen which has negative feedback on hypothalamus to secrete less FSH and LH.
- When follicle is mature and estrogen secretion is at its peak, pituitary receives a positive feedback for LH surge by the short loop.
- LH surge causes ovulation to occur.
- Mature follicle is 16–18 mm and estrogen secretion from such a follicle is 150 pgm/mL/follicle.

DIFFERENT REGIMES OF GONADOTROPIN THERAPY

- Step-up protocol (conventional protocol)
- Step-down protocol
- Chronic low-dose protocol

When to use which protocol depends on the baseline scan and has been discussed in the Chapter 16.

Indications of Gonadotropin Therapy

- Hypogonadotropic hypogonadism (substitutional therapy)
- Hypothalamo-pituitary dysfunction:
    - Clomiphene-resistant patients

- Clomiphene failure patients
- Superovulation combined with intrauterine insemination (IUI)
- Gonadotropin as first line of treatment
- Controlled ovarian hyperstimulation (COH) in assisted reproductive technology (ART) cycles

Step-up Protocol

Baseline scan guides to decide the stimulating dose. Conventionally in normal responding ovary, 1 amp, i.e., 75 IU of FSH is started from Day 5 for 5 days. Ultrasound scan is done on Day 6 of stimulation. If this scan shows a follicle of 10–12 mm and/or there is 2–3 mm increase in endometrial thickness, then same dose is continued till follicle and endometrium become mature. If there is no increase in the size of the follicle or not much change in the endometrial thickness, then dose is doubled and scan is repeated after 3 days. If the follicle or endometrium grows, the same dose is continued till follicle and endometrium are mature; otherwise dose is further increased by 75 IU/day. But this is rarely the case now as each patient is assessed on Day 2–3 of period (baseline scan), and this scan diagnosis poorly responding ovaries, and in these patients stimulation is to be started with higher doses.

Step-up protocol has been blamed for higher rates of multiple pregnancies and ovarian hyperstimulation syndrome (OHSS).[2] But I personally do not agree with the statement of higher risk of OHSS as step-up is never used in polycystic ovary syndrome (PCOS) patients. Step-up protocol gives excellent pregnancy rates in normal responding ovary **(Fig. 1)**. We never check estradiol (E2) level before increasing the dose. Good ultrasound monitoring can replace hormonal estimations.

Step-down Protocol (Fig. 2)

This protocol is very useful for the poor responding ovaries or low reserve ovaries. According to this protocol, stimulation is started with higher dose, i.e., 150–225 IU FSH from Day 5 for 5 days. Once the follicle grows to 10–12 mm, the dose is reduced to 75–150 IU FSH; once the follicle size reaches 14 mm, the dose is further reduced, if it was 150 IU, or is continued as 75 IU FSH till follicle and endometrium mature.

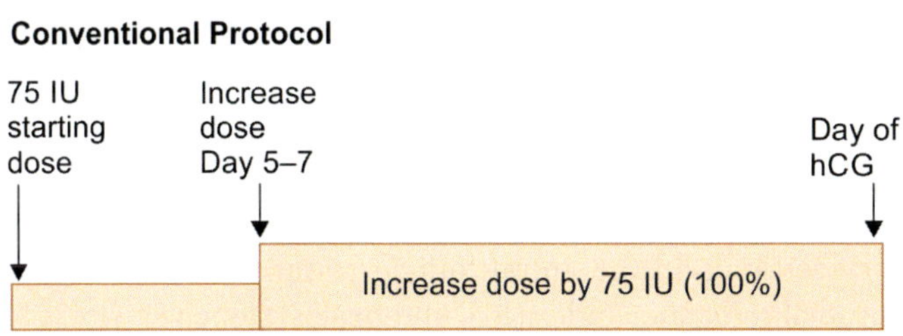

Fig. 1: Conventional protocol (hCG: human chorionic gonadotropin).

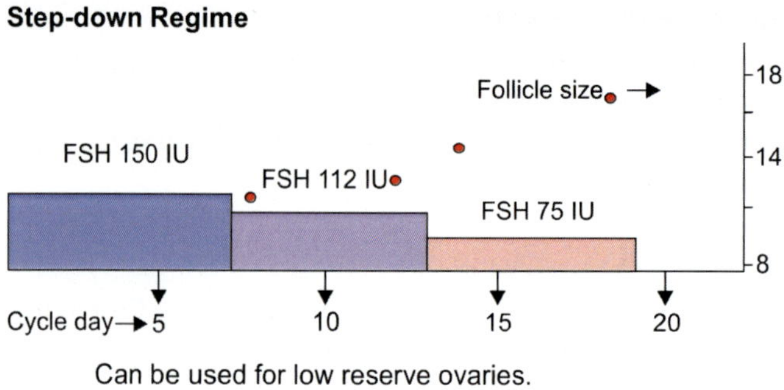

Fig. 2: Step-down protocol (FSH: follicle-stimulating hormone).

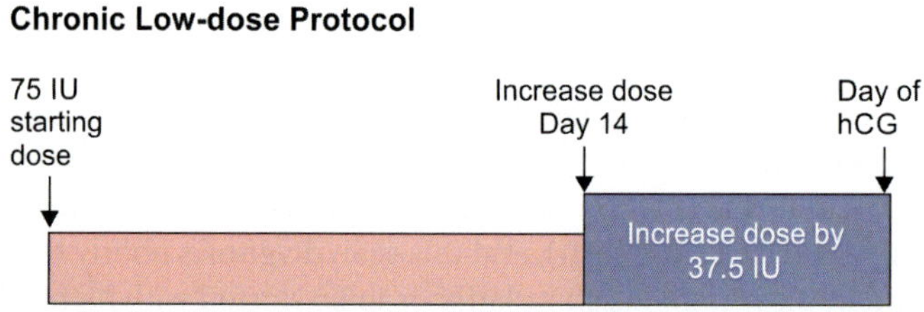

Fig. 3: Chronic low-dose protocol (hCG: human chorionic gonadotropin).

Chronic Low-dose Protocol (Fig. 3)

This protocol is very useful in PCOS patients. Polycystic ovary (PCO) contains twice the number of available FSH sensitive antral follicles in cohort as compared to normal ovaries. This protocol gives good pregnancy rates with very little risk of OHSS or multiple pregnancies. But it is essential that PCOS is confirmed on baseline ultrasound scan. In this protocol, stimulation is started with 37.5/75 IU of FSH and same dose is continued for 14 days. If follicle or endometrium grows, then same dose is continued till mature follicle and endometrium are achieved otherwise the dose is increased by 37.5 IU for other 7 days. Almost all the patients develop good follicle and endometrium and incidence of multiple pregnancy and OHSS is extremely low.[3] Majority of the patients develop good follicle within 14 days, and we should strongly resist ourselves to increase the dose till then. There may be spotting or some bleeding during this period which should be ignored. With chronic low-dose protocol, there is monofollicular development in 70% of cycles, OHSS can be almost totally eliminated and multiple pregnancy rate is <6% with same pregnancy rate as conventional protocol.[4]

Though the stimulation protocols should be tailor made for individual patients, depending on the antral follicle count (AFC), ovarian volume, ovarian stromal resistance index (RI), and peak systolic velocity (PSV). This reduces the risk of OHSS to <1%. According to this study, depending on the

Table 1: Baseline scoring system.

Score	*1*	*2*	*3*	*4*	*5*
Age	>40	35.1–40	30.1–35	25.1–30	≤25
BMI	>30	30–28.1	28–25.1	25–22.1	≤22
AFC	<5	5–10	10–15	15–20	>20
Ovarian volume	≤3	3.1–5	5.1–7	7.1–10	>10
Stromal RI	>0.75	0.75–0.66	0.65–0.56	0.55–0.46	≤0.45
Stromal PSV	≤3	3.1–5	5.1–7	7.1–10	>10

(AFC: antral follicle count; BMI: body mass index; PSV: peak systolic velocity; RI: resistance index)

Table 2: Starting dose of rFSH for IUI and IVF depending on the baseline score.

Score	*IUI starting dose of rFSH*	*IVF starting dose of rFSH*
≥25	25 IU	75 IU
21–24	37.5 IU	150 IU
16–20	75 IU	225 IU
11–15	112.5 IU	300 IU
6–10	150 IU	375 IU

(IUI: intrauterine insemination; IVF: in vitro fertilization; rFSH: recombinant follicle-stimulating hormone)

above-described ultrasound parameters, age and body mass index (BMI), the scoring system is devised, and depending on the initial score of the patient on the baseline scan the starting dose of rFSH can be decided **(Tables 1 and 2)**.[5,6]

RECOMBINANT FOLLICLE-STIMULATING HORMONE

The invention of rFSH has changed the management of infertile patients. In 1990, 6 lacs urine donors were required for 120 million liters of urine for urinary gonadotropin production. This was becoming extremely difficult as with developing techniques in ART, the need for gonadotropins were further increasing. Therefore there was an urgent need for an alternative to produce FSH. It was 1992 that Professor Paul Devroey and Germond reported the clinical utility of rFSH. But it was first made commercially available only in 1995.

How is Recombinant Follicle-stimulating Hormone Produced?

The objective of recombinant deoxyribonucleic acid (rDNA) technology is to insert genes in the cell to produce desired proteins. The gene that is coded for desired protein is isolated enzymatically from DNA chain. The isolated gene is put in vector (a large segment of DNA). This is known as rDNA in host cell. This rDNA produces desired proteins—rFSH. Therefore human DNA genes into a mammalian cell line produces rFSH which is 99.9% pure without LH activity. rFSH has bioactivity of 10,000 IU/mg of protein.

Preparations

Follitropin-alpha is produced by transfection of Chinese hamster ovary cells with genes for the α- and β-subunits of human FSH.

The secretory products of these cells undergo six step purification process to get a final preparation which is highly pure biochemically (>99% FSH).

Properties

- It has highest bioactivity.
- It has no LH or hCG-like activity.
- It has no protein.
- It has high batch-to-batch consistency.
- It does not produce FSH antibodies in patients.
- It has low level of oxidation and/or degradation, i.e., 10% compared to 40% with urinary FSH (uFSH)
- Bioactivity mimics the preovulation FSH in normal cycles.

Comparison of rFSH with uFSH

The study conducted by Hedan B clearly indicates superiority of rFSH **(Table 3)**.[7]

The meta-analysis conducted by Salim Daya and Gunby of 12 randomized controlled trials has proved that rFSH is 20% more likely to achieve pregnancy than uFSH. The amount of FSH used was 400 IU less.[8]

The meta-analysis data was summarized by the author as "The overall conclusion from this meta-analysis is that rFSH is more effective than uFSH because of the higher rates of clinical pregnancy per cycle started and is more

Table 3: Comparison of rFSH with uFSH.

	rFSH	*uFSH*
Higher number of oocytes	10.8	8.9
Lower dose of FSH	2,138 IU	2,385 IU
Shorter period	10.7	11.3
High quality embryos	3.1	2.6
Pregnancy rate with cryopreservation	25.5%	20.4%

(FSH: follicle-stimulating hormone; rFSH: recombinant FSH; uFSH: urinary FSH)

Table 4: Comparison of rFSH with highly purified uFSH.

	rFSH	*uFSH*	*P value*
Number of ampoules	21.9 ± 5.1	31.9 ± 13.4	<0.0001
FSH days	11 ± 1.6	13.5 ± 3.7	<0.001
Oocytes retrieved	12.2 ± 5.5	7.6 ± 4.4	<0.0001
Embryos transferred	2 ± 0.19	1.9 ± 0.4	NS
Pregnancy rates	53/119 (45%)	42/114 (37%)	NS
Implantation	32	31	NS

(FSH: follicle-stimulating hormone; rFSH: recombinant FSH; uFSH: urinary FSH)

efficient because the total dose of gonadotropin required was lower",[8] i.e., 400 IU less.

Prospective meta-analysis has proved that clinical pregnancy rate is 5% higher in rFSH, and if cryopreserved embryos are taken into account, pregnancy rate is 6.4% higher.[9]

Though a recently published Cochrane review has shown no difference in pregnancy outcomes with fresh embryo transfers when rFSH and uFSH were compared. It was concluded that "all available gonadotropins in clinical practice are equally effective and safe" and the choice is based on availability, convenience, and cost.[10]

Comparison of rFSH with uFSH-HP

Recombinant FSH is more effective than highly purified FSH in multiple follicular development according to another study **(Table 4)**.[11]

Frydman and Associates also published the data that rFSH gives more number of oocytes, more embryos with lesser number of injections.[12]

Gearon and Abdalla from Lister hospital, London in an unpublished study have reported for the first time improvement in quality of oocytes in older women treated with rFSH instead of uFSH-HP. Another randomized single blind, multicentric multinational study by Schats et al. also confirmed the same findings.

Recombinant FSH gives more embryos with lesser ampoules **(Table 3)**. More than four embryos in culture have higher chance of achieving pregnancy.[13] The chances of blastocyst transfer is increased, if more than four oocytes are retrieved.[14] But some randomized trials have failed to show the difference in terms of pregnancy rate or miscarriage rate in normal reserve patients as well as PCOS.[15,16]

One another study has also shown that recombinant FSH was associated with higher per cycle pregnancy rate than uFSH-HP, when used at the same dose, where as the pregnancy rates were similar when the dose of rFSH was 50% lower.[17]

Recombinant Follicle-stimulating Hormone versus Human Menopausal Gonadotropin

Meta-analysis of eight randomized controlled trials comparing rFSH with hMG has shown that rFSH has 50% higher pregnancy rates.[18] The FIVNAT (French National Register on In Vitro Fertilization) report 1999 showed that the pregnancy rates were higher with rFSH than hMG.

Prospective analysis of 24,000 ART cycles from Germany also showed higher birth rate and lower dosage with rFSH than hMG.[19] In patients where LH and FSH ratio is high in PCOS, only FSH rather than hMG will improve the results.[20] There is a subgroup of patients like poor responders and elderly patients in whom hMG-HP is given. It has given higher pregnancy rates, so either rLH or hMG-HP is useful in a subgroup of patients.[21,22]

Meta-analysis including 400,000 IVF cycles showed that compared to rFSH, hMG resulted in fewer oocytes and higher doses.[23]

Facts about Highly Purified Human Menopausal Gonadotropin

- The process is partially successful with specific activity of 2,000 IU/mg of protein **(Table 5)**.
- In many cases, LH activity has to be added using hCG which has longer half-life.
- Presence of variable amount of hCG may further increase variation between different batches of product and result in follicular atresia.[24]
- The hMG-HP contains 30% extraneous proteins including leukocyte elastase inhibitor protein C inhibitor and Zn-α2 glycoprotein apart from hCG.

Types of Recombinant Follicle-stimulating Hormone

- Follitropin-α; 1995
- Follitropin-β; 1996
- Follitropin epsilon; new human rFSH

Table 5: Types of gonadotropin and its specific bioactivity.

Product	*Specific bioactivity*
hMG (1950)	8 IU/mg protein
uFSH (1980)	100–150 IU/mg protein
uhMG-HP	2,000 IU/mg protein
uFSH-HP (1990)	9,000 IU/mg protein
rFSH (1995)	10,000 IU/mg protein

(HP: highly purified; hMG: human menopausal gonadotropin; rFSH: recombinant follicle-stimulating hormone; uFSH: urinary follicle-stimulating hormone; uhMG: urinary hMG)

Immunopotency, biopotency, and internal carbohydrate complexity are same for both but follitropin-α contains higher proportion of acidic glycoforms. Follitropin-α has a specific activity of 13,645 IU/mg where as that for follitropin-β is 9,396 IU/mg.

There is a difference in tolerability between rFSH preparations favoring follitropin alpha over beta.[25] Though follitropin alpha has a higher incidence of OHSS as compared to follitropin beta (4.1% as compared to 2.7%).[26]

Fill by Mass Concept

Dose of gonadotropin is expressed in international units (IU). But recent fill by mass (FbM) technique reflects a constant relationship between mass and bioactivity and guarantees consistency of dose from batch to batch. So drawbacks of vivo bioassay can be avoided. Bioassay of FSH preparation is 50 years old. Steelman–Pohley bioassay which is cumbersome and requires large number of animals and variation can be 10–20%. But FbM is by liquid chromatography supported by glycine mapping isoelectric focusing that demonstrates physicochemical consistency of the product.

Duration of stimulation was significantly shorter in FbM group and embryo quality and implantation rates were significantly higher (28.6% in FbM vs. 18.6% in FbIU).[27,28]

Clinical Benefits of Recombinant Follicle-stimulating Hormone[29]

- Improved logistics of pharmaceutical process
- Controlled manufacturing
- Reduced batch-to-batch variability
- Potentially unlimited supply—no shortage
- Not reliant on the urine supply
- No risk of infection
- No risk of contamination with drugs or metabolites
- No seroconversion to antigonadotropin antibodies
- Effective, safe, and less traumatic subcutaneous administration
- Greater purity and specific activity
- Smaller doses required
- More predictable response
- Cost benefit

There are reports also that there is no difference in OHSS rate when rFSH was compared with uFSH or urinary gonadotropins.[30]

PROTOCOLS FOR ASSISTED REPRODUCTIVE TECHNOLOGY

Gonadotropins in Assisted Reproductive Technology

In ART cycles also, stimulation protocol is decided by baseline scan.

Long Agonist Protocol

Downregulation from 21st Day of previous cycle as nasal spray or subcutaneous injections of gonadotropin-releasing hormone (GnRH) agonist (Leuprolide acetate 0.5 mg or decapeptyl 0.1 mg) and is continued till periods. The dose is halved from the day of period. Depot preparations of agonist can be used instead of daily agonist injections on Day 21 of the previous cycle. The most common starting dose for COS with rFSH is 150–225/day. Increasing the dosage in elderly women does not result in increased oocyte yield.[31] It has been found that 150 IU of rFSH is equivalent to 225 IU of uFSH for follicular growth. The dose of 150 IU is optimum,[28] rather than 100 IU that has been mentioned in a comparative study for IVF patients.

Short Protocol

This protocol exploits the flare-up effect of agonist during the ovarian stimulation. Agonist is started with the beginning of the menstrual cycle and flare up provides the surge of gonadotropins secretion. A few days later, exogenous gonadotropins are administrated to supplement the flare. Both agonist and gonadotropins are continued till the day of ovulation trigger. This protocol is preferred for poor responders.

Ultrashort Protocol

Agonist is given on Day 2, 3, and 4 of the stimulation cycle in the dose of 500–1,000 µg per day and then gonadotropins are given subsequently till day of hCG.

Antagonist Protocol

High resistance, low velocity stromal flow, fewer antral follicles, smaller ovarian volume, high BMI and age >35 years are the parameters which decide higher doses for stimulation with antagonist protocol where as low resistance, high velocity stromal flow, polycystic ovaries, low BMI, and age <24 years are the parameters which would be in favor of lower doses of gonadotrophins with antagonist protocol. Antagonist is started from Day 6 and continued till the day of hCG. In these patients, GnRH agonist can be used for ovulation trigger, instead of hCG. This protocol reduces the incidence of OHSS significantly. This is known as fixed antagonist protocol. Antagonist can also be used as flexible protocol, when antagonist is started when at least one follicle is 14 mm in diameter.[32] Antagonist protocol has high cumulative pregnancy rate in both groups, high anti-Müllerian hormone (AMH) (40.1–63.6%) and low AMH (11.1–18.7%).[33] They have also devised a stimulation protocol based on AMH levels **(Table 6)**. A meta-analysis of 45 randomized controlled trials involving 7,511 women comparing GnRH

Table 6: Individualized dose calculation for COS.[33]

AMH level	***Predicted response to COS***	***Treatment strategies***
15 pmol/L	High responders (150 IU)	• GnRH antagonist protocol • Normal oocyte yield, very low excess response, low embryo cryopreservation, high/maintained fresh CPR
5–15 pmol/L	Normal responders (225–300 IU)	*GnRH agonist protocol:* Very low cancellation of oocyte pick-up and OHSS
<5 pmol/L	Poor responders (375 IU)	*High dose FSH:* Long stimulation, high cancellation *Antagonist strategy:* Short stimulation, moderate cancellation

(AMH: anti-Müllerian hormone; CPR: clinical pregnancy rate; COS: controlled ovarian stimulation; FSH: follicle-stimulating hormone; GnRH: gonadotropin-releasing hormone; OHSS: ovarian hyperstimulation syndrome)

antagonist protocol and long agonist protocol for COS in ART has found no significant differences in live birth or ongoing pregnancy rates, but marked decrease in OHSS with antagonist protocols.[34] Another meta-analysis comparing agonist and antagonist protocols for poor responders has shown advantage in terms of FSH stimulation, but no statistically significant difference in terms of oocytes retrieved or clinical pregnancy rates.[35]

Antagonist-agonist Protocol

This protocol is especially used for PCOS patients. It is known as OHSS-free protocol. Fixed antagonist protocol is used for downregulation, and then agonist is used for ovulation trigger.

Antagonist-agonist Protocol with Human Chorionic Gonadotropin as Luteal Support

The above-mentioned protocol is very likely to lead to luteal phase defect. It is therefore recommended to supplement the luteal phase with 1,500 IU of hCG on Day 3-7-10 of ovum pick-up.[36] But this can increase the risk of OHSS.

PREDICTORS OF OVARIAN RESPONSE

- Age
- Body mass index
- Baseline FSH
- Anti-Müllerian hormone (not mentioned in Collin-Howles study)
- Antral follicle count

Table 7: Cost-effectivity of predictors of ovarian response.		
	rFSH	***uFSH***
UK	5,906£	6,060£
USA (Social) (Insurance)	40,688$ 28,481$	47,096$ 32,967$
Spain (Public Insurance)	12,791€	13,007€
Spain (Private)	19,739€	20,467€
Germany	21,686€	22,189€

(rFSH: recombinant follicle-stimulating hormone; uFSH: urinary follicle-stimulating hormone)

A nomogram can be prepared using these predictors. *Howles and colleagues have prepared a manuscript on the same.*[37] The cost-effectivity has been mentioned in the results presented **(Table 7)**.

Newer Developments

- *Long-acting FSH:* Long-acting FSH is corifollitropin alpha. It keeps the FSH above the threshold level for multifollicular growth. It is convenient for the patients for having less number of injections. There is no difference in live births and OHSS rate.[38]
- Sustained release rFSH
- Oral FSH

LUTEINIZING HORMONE SUPPLEMENTATION: FOR WHOM, WHEN, AND WHY?

Two-cell-two gonadotropins Theory

- Both FSH and LH are required for E2 synthesis. LH binds to theca cells to induce androgen synthesis. Androgen diffuses into granulosa cells, where FSH-stimulated aromatization leads to estrogen synthesis.[39]
- Luteinizing hormone in follicular phase helps conversion of progesterone to androgen to reduce follicular phase progesterone, which is detrimental to endometrial receptivity.[40] A combination of rFSH and rLH in a ratio of 2:1 is indicated for women with severe gonadotropin deficiency—hypogonadotropic hypogonadism.[41]

Luteinizing Hormone Threshold

Luteinizing hormone is required for terminal stages of follicular maturation, for meiosis, and ovulation.

Luteinizing Hormone Ceiling Effect

- High LH causes follicular atresia, premature luteinization and oocyte quality may be compromised.[42]
- In patients over responding to FSH, adding 30 µg rLH leads to monofollicular development.[43] This indicates LH ceiling effect.

Current Opinion about LH Supplementation

- Current opinion is that there is no absolute requirement for LH supplementation in unselected patient population.[44]
- However, LH may have benefit in women aged >35 years and those who are poor responders to COS.[45] Though Cochrane review[36] and studies subsequently published have shown that LH supplementation, including for women with advanced age, has no benefit on ongoing pregnancy, with an adjusted odds ratio (OR) of 0.99 [confidence interval (CI) 0.76–1.29).[44]
- Luteinizing hormone supplementation may improve outcomes in patients with suboptimal response to FSH stimulation.[46]
- No LH cutoff value is known to identify a female requiring LH supplementation and LH assessment is therefore of no use.[47]
- In antagonist cycle, LH supplementation is controversial. Though some studies have shown that it improves results in selected groups.
- Luteinizing hormone estimation may not be a reliable guide to decide for LH supplementation because of variable bioactivity and polymorphism.

RECOMBINANT LUTEINIZING HORMONE

Adding LH increases the number of developmentally competent oocytes in woman with endogenous LH suppressed below 1 IU/L at the start of stimulation. However with LH >1 IU/L, adding LH is associated with significant lower embryo quality and implantation rate compared with rFSH alone.[48] Recombinant-human luteinizing hormone (r-hLH) alone can trigger follicular growth arrest in a significant number of patients supporting the existence of LH ceiling during late follicular maturation.[49] rFSH with r-hLH 150 IU from Day 6 might be beneficial in subgroup women in older reproductive age, having LH polymorphism and less sensitivity to LH.

The results of analysis by age showed a trend towards higher implantation rate with rFSH alone in patients aged <35 years. In contrast, the group aged >35 years had numerically higher implantation rate in the rFSH plus r-hLH group.[50,51]

Recombinant-human luteinizing hormone supplementation on Day 8 in patients having E2 <180 pgm/mL and no follicles >10 mm, significantly increases the number of oocytes retrieved and requirement of rFSH was also decreased.[52]

In summary, recombinant human-luteinizing hormone (r-hLH) supplementation, when:

- Age >35 years
- Poor initial response to rFSH.

Carry Home Message

- Gonadotropins give better pregnancy rates than clomiphene citrate.
- Step-up protocol is used for normal responding ovaries.
- Chronic low dose protocol is best for PCO.
- Recombinant FSH requires lower dosage with better efficacy.
- Recombinant FSH is better than all urinary preparations.
- Recombinant LH is used in poor responders and patients of age >35 years.

REFERENCES

1. Lunenfield B, Insler V, Rabau E. The principles of gonadotrophin therapy. Acta Endocrinol Suppl (Copenh). 1970;148:52-101.
2. Westergard LG, Erb K, Laursen SB, Rex S, Rasmussen PE. Human menopausal gonadotropin versus recombinant follicle-stimulating hormone in normogonadotropic women down-regulated with gonadotropin-releasing hormone agonist who were undergoing in vitro fertilization and intracytoplasmic sperm injection: a prospective randomized study. Fertil Steril. 2001;76(3):543-9.
3. Homburg R, Levy T, Ben-Rafael Z. A comparative prospective study of conventional regimen with chronic low dose administration of follicle stimulating hormone for anovulation associated with polycystic ovary syndrome. Fertil Steril. 1995;63(4):729-33.
4. Driebergen R, Baer G. Quantification of follicle stimulating hormone (follitropin alfa): Is in vivo bioassay still relevant in recombinant age? Curr Med Res Opin. 2003;19:41-6.
5. Panchal S, Nagori CB. Ultrasound based decision making on stimulation protocol for superovulated IUI cycles. IJIFM. 2016;7(1):7-13.
6. Panchal S, Nagori CB. Ultrasound based decision making on stimulation protocol in IVF. DSJUOG. 2016;10(3):330-37.
7. Hedon B, Out HJ, Hugues JN, Camier B, Cohen J, Lopes P, et al. Efficacy and safety of recombinant follicle stimulating hormone (Puregon) in infertile women pituitary suppressed with triptorelin undergoing in vitro fertilization: a prospective randomized, assessor-blind, multicentre trial. Hum Reprod. 1995;10:3102-6.
8. Daya S. Updated meta-analysis of recombinant follicle-stimulating hormone (FSH) versus urinary FSH for ovarian stimulation in assisted reproduction. Fertil Steril. 2002;77(4):711-14.
9. Out HJ, Driessen SG, Mannaerts BM, Coelingh Bennink HJ. Recombinant follicle-stimulating hormone (follitropin beta, Puregon) yields higher pregnancy rates in in vitro fertilization than urinary gonadotropins. Fertil Steril. 1997;68:138-42.
10. van Wely M, Kwan I, Burt AL, Thomas J, Vail A, der Veen FV, et al. Recombinant versus urinary gonadotropin for ovarian stimulation in assisted reproductive technology cycles. Cochrane Database Syst Rev. 2011(2):CD005354.
11. Bergh C, Howles CM, Borg K, L Hamberger, B Josefsson, L Nilsson, et al. Recombinant follicle stimulating hormone (r-hFSH; Gonal-F) versus highly purified urinary FSH

(Metrodin HP): results of a randomized comparative study in women undergoing assisted reproductive techniques. Hum Reprod. 1997;12:2133-9.
12. Frydman R, Haverell C, Camier B. A double blind randomized study comparing the efficacy of recombinant human (FSH: Gonal F) versus highly purified urinary FSH (Metrodin-HP) in inducing superovulation in women undergoing assisted reproductive techniques. Hum Reprod. 1998;13:180-5.
13. XV FIGO World Congress of Gynecology and Obstetrics. Copenhagen, Denmark, 3-8 August 1997. Abstract. Part 1. Acta Obstet Gynecol Scand Suppl. 1997;167 Pt 1:1-119.
14. Scholtes MC, Zeilmaker GH. Blastocyst transfer in day-5 embryo transfer depends primarily on the number of oocytes retrieved and not on age. Fertil Steril. 1998;69:78-83.
15. Yaralli H, Bukulmez O, Gurgan T. Urinary follicle-stimulating hormone (FSH) versus recombinant FSH in clomiphene citrate-resistant, normogonadotropic, chronic anovulation: a prospective randomized study. Fertil Steril. 1999;72:276-81.
16. Bayram N, vanWely M, van der Veen F. Recombinant FSH versus urinary gonadotropins or recombinant FSH for ovulation induction in subfertility associated with polycystic ovary syndrome. Cochrane Database Syst Rev. 2002(1):CD002121.
17. Matorras R, Osuna C, Exposito A, Crisol BS, Pijoan JI. Recombinant FSH versus highly purified FSH in intrauterine insemination: systematic review and meta-analysis. Fertil Steril. 2011;95:1937-42.
18. Daya S, Gunby J, Hughes EG, Collins JA, Sagle MA. Follicle-stimulating hormone versus human menopausal gonadotropins for in vitro fertilization cycles: a meta-analysis. Fertil Steril. 1995;27:347-54.
19. Ludwig M, Rabe T, Buhler K. Wirksamkeit von recombinanten humane FSH in Vergleich zu urinarem hMG nach Downregulation im langen Protokoll–eine Analyse von 24.764 ART-Zyklen in Deutschland. J Reprod Med Endocrinol. 1994;4:284-8.
20. Hughes E, Collins J, Vandekerckhove P. Ovulation induction with urinary follicle stimulating hormone vs human menopausal gonadotropin for clomiphene resistant polycystic ovary syndrome. Cochrane Database Syst Rev. 2000;(2):CD000087.
21. Coomarasamy A, Afnan M, Cheema D, der Veen FV, Bossuyt PMM, van Wely M. Urinary hMG versus recombinant FSH for controlled ovarian hyperstimulation following an agonist long down-regulation protocol in IVF or ICSI treatment: a systematic review and meta-analysis. Hum Reprod. 2008;23:310-5.
22. Al-Inany HG, Abou-Setta AM, Aboulghar MA, Mansour RT, Serour GI. Efficacy and safety of human menopausal gonadotropins versus recombinant FSH: a meta-analysis. Reprod Biomed Online. 2008;16:81-8.
23. Lehert P, Schertz JC, Ezcurra D. Recombinant human follicle stimulating hormone produces more oocytes with low total dose per cycle in assisted reproductive technologies compared with highly purified HMG: a meta-analysis. Reprod Biol Endocrinol. 2010;8:112.
24. Filicori M, Cognigni GE, Taraborrelli S, Spettoli D, Ciampaglia W, Tabarelli de Fatis C, et al. Luteinizing hormone activity in menotropins optimizes folliculogenesis and treatment in controlled ovarian stimulation. J Clin Endocrinol Metab. 2001;86:337-43.
25. Brinsden P, Akagbosu F, Gibbons, et al. A comparison of the efficacy and tolerability of two recombinant human follicle-stimulating hormone preparations in patients undergoing in vitro fertilization-embryo transfer. Fertil Steril. 2003;73:114-6.
26. Devroey P, Boostanfar R, Koper NP, Mannerts BM, Ijzerma-Boon PC, Fauser BC. A double blind non-inferiority RCT comparing corifollitropin-alpha and rFSH during first seven days of ovarian stimulation using GnRH antagonist protocol. Hum Reprod. 2009;24(12):3063-72.
27. Balasch J, Fabergues F, Peñarrubia J, Creus M, Manau D, Vidal E, et al. Outcome from consecutive assisted reproduction cycles in patients treated with recombinant

follitropin alfa filled-by-bioassay and those treated with recombinant follitropin alfa filled-by-mass. Reprod Biomed Online. 2004;8:408-13.

28. Hugues JN, Barlow DH, Rosenwaks Z, Cedrin-Durnerin I, Robson S, Pidoux L, et al. Improvement in consistency of response to ovarian stimulation with recombinant human follicle stimulating hormone resulting from a new method for calibrating the therapeutic preparation. Reprod Biomed Online. 2003;6:185-90.
29. Ludwig M, Diedrich K. Evaluation of luteal phase support protocol in IVF. Obstet Gynecol Scand. 2001;80:452-66.
30. van Wely M, Kwan I, van der Veen F. Recombinant FSH versus urinary gonadotropins for ovarian hyperstimulation in IVF and ICSI cycles: a systematic review and meta-analysis. Hum Reprod. 2009;24:S1-34.
31. Out HJ, Braat DD, Linsten BM, Gurgan T, Bukulmez O, Gökmen O, et al. Increasing the daily dose of recombinant follicle stimulating hormone (Puregon) does not compensate for the age-related decline in retrievable oocytes after ovarian stimulation. Hum Reprod. 2000;15:29-35.
32. Ludwig M, Katalinic A, Banz C, Schröder AK, Löning M, Weiss JM, et al. Tailoring the GnRH antagonist cetrorelix acetate to individual patients' needs in ovarian stimulation for IVF: results of a prospective, randomized study. Hum Reprod. 2002;17(11):2842-5.
33. Nelson SM, Yates RW, Lyall H, Jamieson M, Traynor I, Gaudoin M, et al. Anti-Müllerian hormone-based approach to controlled ovarian stimulation for assisted conception. Hum Reprod. 2009;24:867-75.
34. Al-Inany HG, Youssef MA, Aboulghar M. Gonadotropin-releasing hormone antagonists for assisted reproductive technology. Cochrane Database Syst Rev. 2011;5:CD001750.
35. Pu D, Wu J, Liu J. Comparison of GnRH antagonist versus GnRH agonist protocol in poor ovarian responders undergoing IVF. Hum Reprod. 2011;26(10):2742-9.
36. Humadian P, Ejdrup BH, Westergaard LG, Yding AC. 1,500 IU human chorionic gonadotropins administered at oocyte retrieval rescues the luteal phase when gonadotropins-releasing hormone agonist is used for ovulation induction: a prospective randomized controlled study. Fertil Steril. 2010;93:847-54.
37. Howles CM. Predictive factors for ovarian reserve. Reprod Biomed Online. 2008;16(S2):pS-5.
38. Pouwer AW, Farquhar C, Kremer JA. Long acting FSH versus daily FSH for women undergoing assisted reproduction. Cochrane Database Syst Rev. 2012;6:CD009577.
39. Kobayashi M, Nakano R, Ooshima A. Immunohistochemical localization of pituitary gonadotropins and gonadal steroids confirms the 'two cell two gonadotropins, hypothesis of steroidogenesis in the human ovary. J Endocrinol. 1990;126(3):483-8.
40. Fanchin R, Righini C, Olivennes F, Taieb J, de Zeigler, Frydman R. Computerized assessment of endometrial echogenicity: clues to the endometrial effects of premature progesterone elevation. Fertil Steril. 1999;71(1):173-81.
41. Bosch E. Recombinant human FSH and recombinant human LH in a 2:1 ratio combination: a new tool for ovulation induction. Exp Rev Obstet Gynecol. 2009;4(5):491-8.
42. Hillier SG. Current concepts of the roles of follicle stimulating hormone and luteinizing hormone in folliculogenesis. Hum Reprod. 1994;9:188-91.
43. Hughes JN, Soussis J, Calderon I, Balasch J, Anderson RA, Romeu A. Recombinant LH study group 2005. Does the addition of recombinant LH in WHO group II anovulatory women over-responding to FSH treatment reduce the number of developing follicles? A dose-finding study. Hum Reprod. 2005;20:629-35.
44. Mochtar MH, Van der Veen F, Zeich M, van Wely M. Recombinant luteinizing hormone (rLH) for controlled ovarian hyperstimulation in assisted reproductive cycles. Cochrane Database Syst Rev. 2007;2:CD005070.

45. Howles CM. Luteinizing hormone supplementation in ART. In: Kovacs G (Ed). How to Improve your ART Success Rates. Cambridge, UK: Cambridge University Press; 2011. pp. 99-104.
46. Lisi F, Rinaldi L, Fischel S, Lisi R, Pepe G, Picconeri MG, et al. Use of recombinant FSH and recombinant LH in multiple follicular stimulation for IVF: a preliminary study. Reprod Biomed Online. 2001;3(3):190-4.
47. Loumaye E, Engrand P, Howles CM, O'Dea L. Assessment of the role of serum luteinizing hormone an estradiol response to follicle stimulating hormone on in vitro fertilization treatment outcome. Fertil Steril. 1997;67:889-99.
48. Tesarik J, Mendoza C. Effects of exogenous LH administration during ovarian stimulation of pituitary down-regulated young oocyte donors on oocyte yield and developmental competence. Hum Reprod. 2002;17:3129-37.
49. Loumaye E, Engrand P, Shoham Z, Hillier SG, Baird DT. Clinical evidence for an LH 'ceiling' effect induced by administration of recombinant human LH during the late follicular phase of stimulated cycles in World Health Organization type I and type II anovulation. Hum Reprod. 2003;18:314-22.
50. Marrs R, Meldrum D, Muasher S, Schoolcraft W, Werlin L, Kelly E. Randomized trial to compare the effect of recombinant human FSH (follitropin alfa) with or without recombinant human LH in women undergoing assisted reproduction treatment. Reprod Biomed Online. 2004;8:175-82.
51. Humadian P, Bungum M, Bungum L, Yding Andersen C. Effects of recombinant LH supplementation in women undergoing assisted reproduction with GnRH agonist down-regulation and stimulation with recombinant FSH: an opening study. Reprod Biomed Online. 2004;8:635-43.
52. De Placido G, Alviggi C, Mollo A, Strina I, Ranieri A, Alviggi E, et al. Effects of recombinant LH (rLH) supplementation during controlled ovarian hyperstimulation (COH) in normogonadotrophic women with an initial inadequate response to recombinant FSH (rFSH) after pituitary downregulation. Clin Endocrinol. 2004;60:637-43.

CHAPTER 6

Intrauterine Insemination

Chaitanya Nagori, Sonal Panchal

INTRODUCTION

Intrauterine insemination (IUI) has attained a wide popularity in management of infertility. But it is still the least standardized procedure as far as infertility treatment is concerned. Optimal guideline adherence has substantial economic benefits when compared with suboptimal guideline adherence.[1] IUI is blamed for low pregnancy rates but meticulous patient selection, stimulation protocol, good ultrasound (US) monitoring, and good semen preparation if combined with IUI only then gives good results.

In IUI, a bolus of sperms is placed in the uterus directly, bypassing the vaginal acidity and cervical hostility. This allows a safe quick access of the sperms to ova in the ampullary part of the oviduct. IUI must be done with the washed sample and never with nit sample of semen. Using unwashed/nonprocessed semen leads to uterine cramps, infection, and collapse. Primary treatment with IUI is much more cost-effective than in vitro fertilization (IVF).[2]

INDICATIONS OF INTRAUTERINE INSEMINATION

Most Common Indications

- Unexplained infertility.
- *Dysovulatory infertility*: Absolute pregnancy rate is higher with multifollicular compared to monofollicular growth.[3]
- *Male subfertility*: When the total motile sperm count before sperm preparation is >10 million, it is called mild male factor subfertility. Mild ovarian hyperstimulation with IUI is done in these cases.[4]
- *Mild to moderate endometriosis*: These patients must be treated as those with unexplained subfertility and benefit with mild ovarian hyperstimulation with IUI, which results in two to three follicles.

Other Uncommon Indications

- Cervical hostility
- Immunological infertility—IUI is the first choice before IVF/intracytoplasmic sperm injection (ICSI).[5]
- HIV +ve male partner with HIV –ve female partner

- Single patent tube
- Ejaculatory failure
- Failed artificial insemination with donor sperm (AID)
- *Frozen samples*: When husband is absent or on antineoplastic treatment.

STEPS OF INTRAUTERINE INSEMINATION

The success of IUI depends on following steps, each step having equal importance:

- Ovulation stimulation (superovulation)
- Ultrasound monitoring and timing of ovulation trigger
- Timing and method of IUI
- Semen preparation
- Luteal support

Superovulation

Advantages

- To increase the number of oocytes available for fertilization
- More oocytes, more chances of conception
- Increased steroids may improve chances of fertilization and implantation
- Subtle hormonal deficiencies are corrected
- Luteal phase defect (LPD) is corrected
- Increased fertilization window as several oocytes are released over protracted period.

Superovulation with IUI has higher pregnancy rates than after timed intercourse and clomiphene citrate (CC).[6]

This study shows:

- *No stimulation*: Pregnancy rates vary from 2 to 8% per cycle, but it is always lower than the stimulated cycle. As stimulated cycles have higher multiple pregnancy rates, many centers including Bourn Hall clinic, London, offers natural cycle IUI. In couples with cervical factor subfertility, IUI in natural cycles significantly increases the probability of conception.[7]
- *Clomiphene citrate*: It can be given from Day 5 to 9 in dosage of 50–100 mg/day. Cycle fecundability in spontaneous and CC-induced cycle is the same (6–13%) as compared to gonadotropins (14–24%).[8] We do not prefer CC for IUI as pregnancy rates are extremely low.
- *Gonadotropins*: Gonadotropin with IUI is more successful than only gonadotropin or only IUI or CC + IUI. Gonadotropins with IUI have 10–15% chances of pregnancy as compared to 1–2% with natural cycle in idiopathic infertility. The pregnancy rates are far better when IUI is combined with gonadotropins as compared to when IUI is combined with natural cycle, CC or CC + human menopausal gonadotropin (hMG).[9]

Existing treatments such as empirical CC and unstimulated IUI do not offer superior birth rates compared with expectant management of unexplained infertility.[10,11] A UK randomized controlled trial (RCT) (Scottish unexplained infertility trial, SUIT) compared the effectiveness of CC and IUI with that of expectant management and concluded that neither showed superior live birth rates compared with expectant management.[12] Higher pregnancy rates are obtained when IUI is combined with gonadotropins than with antiestrogen agents.[13]

Conventional Protocol (Fig. 1)

Gonadotropins are started from Day 5 in patients with normal ovaries on baseline scan. 75 IU follicle-stimulating hormone (FSH) is given daily from Day 5 to 9. If follicle or endometrium grows, same dose is continued otherwise the dose is doubled for 3 days. US monitoring will help to decide whether to continue the same dose till the follicle matures or to further increase the dose to 225 IU. Gonadotropins are continued till mature follicle and endometrium are achieved.

Step-down Protocol (Fig. 2)

If the baseline scan indicates a poor responding ovary, then we start with higher dose for stimulation, 150–225 IU till a follicle of 10 mm or larger appears. Then the dose is decreased to 75 IU till we get a mature follicle and receptive endometrium.

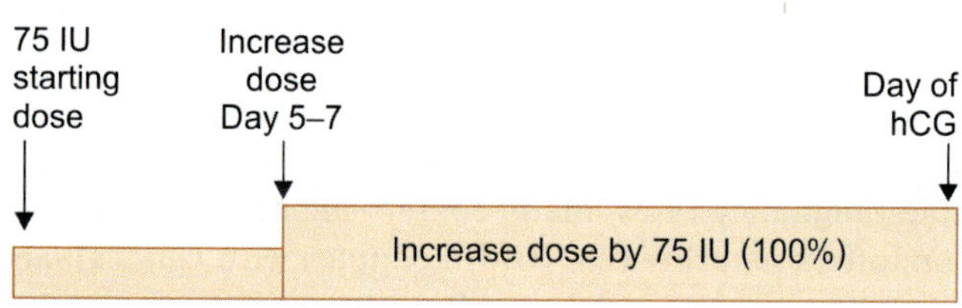

Fig. 1: Conventional protocol (hCG: human chorionic gonadotropin).

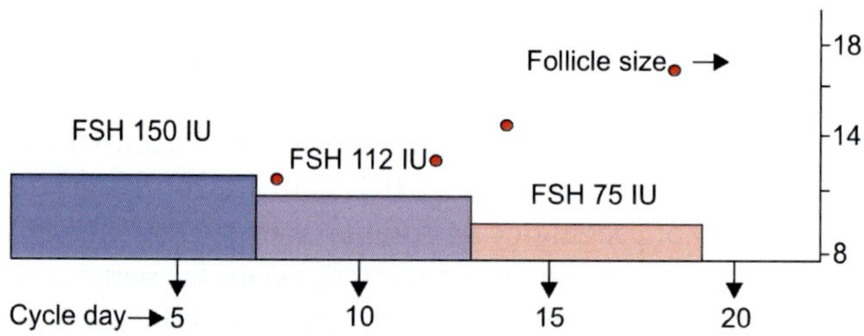

Fig. 2: Step-down protocol (FSH: follicle-stimulating hormone).

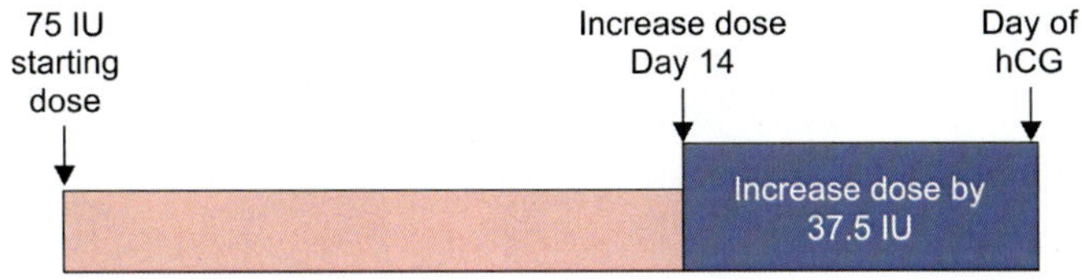

Fig. 3: Chronic low-dose protocol. (hCG: human chorionic gonadotropin)

Chronic Low-dose Protocol (Fig. 3)

In polycystic ovary syndrome (PCOS) patients, stimulation is started with 37.5–75 IU and is continued up to 10–14 days before increasing the dose in spite of no follicular growth documented. This protocol is very effective in PCOS patients to decrease the incidence of ovarian hyperstimulation syndrome (OHSS) and multiple pregnancy.

Letrozole + Gonadotropins

We have found this combination very effective in decreasing the consumption of gonadotropins and incidence of multiple pregnancy rates with equally high conception rates compared with only gonadotropins with IUI.

Letrozole is given from Day 3 to 7. From Day 7, FSH 75 IU is given daily for 5 days. Then according to the findings on US monitoring, the dose is adjusted. This is an excellent combination for poor responders.

Role of Gonadotropin-releasing Hormone Agonist and Antagonist

Gonadotropin-releasing hormone (GnRH) agonist is not used routinely in IUI protocols for down-regulation. It increases the total dose of gonadotropins consumed, increases incidence of OHSS, and multiple pregnancy rates. It has no advantage in IUI protocols and we never use it for IUI cycles.

GnRH antagonist may be used in IUI protocols. Adding GnRH antagonist in cycles with mild ovarian hyperstimulation in an IUI program routinely does not increase live birth rate.[14] Though it is very useful in thin lean PCOS patients in whom luteinizing hormone (LH) is tonically high. Here antagonist is given when follicle size of 14 mm is reached, till the day of trigger. It prevents premature LH surge and improves the quality of ova and embryo, which in turn gives higher pregnancy rates.

Ultrasound Monitoring and Timing of hCG

This has been discussed in the Chapter 16 of this book in detail. It is the key factor for achieving good conception rates with IUI. Good US monitoring may also give information about the hormonal milieu of the patient and

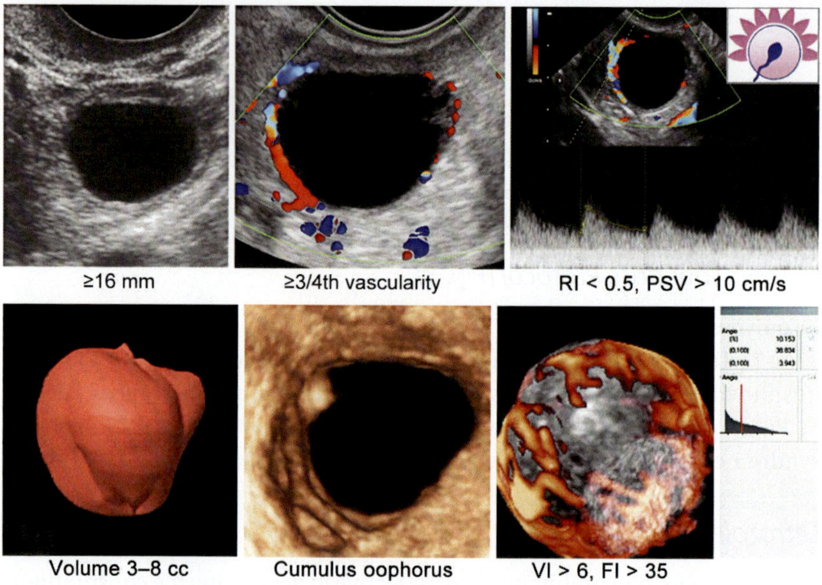

Fig. 4: Pre-hCG follicular parameters (FI: flow index; hCG: human chorionic gonadotropin; PSV: peak systolic velocity; RI: resistance index; VI: vascularization index).

hormonal assays can be omitted. Timing of hCG is the key point for success of IUI cycles.

We decide the timing of IUI based on following factors:[15]

Optimal Pre-hCG Follicular Parameters (Fig. 4)

- Follicular diameter at least 16 mm and 3–7 cc volume. The optimal size of the leading follicle in ovulation induction with CC and letrozole is similar and is closely related to endometrial thickness.[16] The optimal size for the leading follicle has been suggested as 18–22 and 23–27 in different studies[16,17]
- Vascularity covering at least three-fourths of follicular circumference
- Perifollicular resistance index (RI): 0.4–0.48
- Perifollicular peak systolic velocity (PSV) >10 cm/sec
- Follicular vascularization index (VI) >6 and flow index (FI) >35
- Presence of cumulus oophorus.

Optimal Pre-hCG Endometrial Parameters (Fig. 5)

- Endometrial thickness of at least 6 mm preferably 8 mm
- Grade A/B endometrium
- Endometrial vascularity in zone 3–4, covering >5 mm^2 area

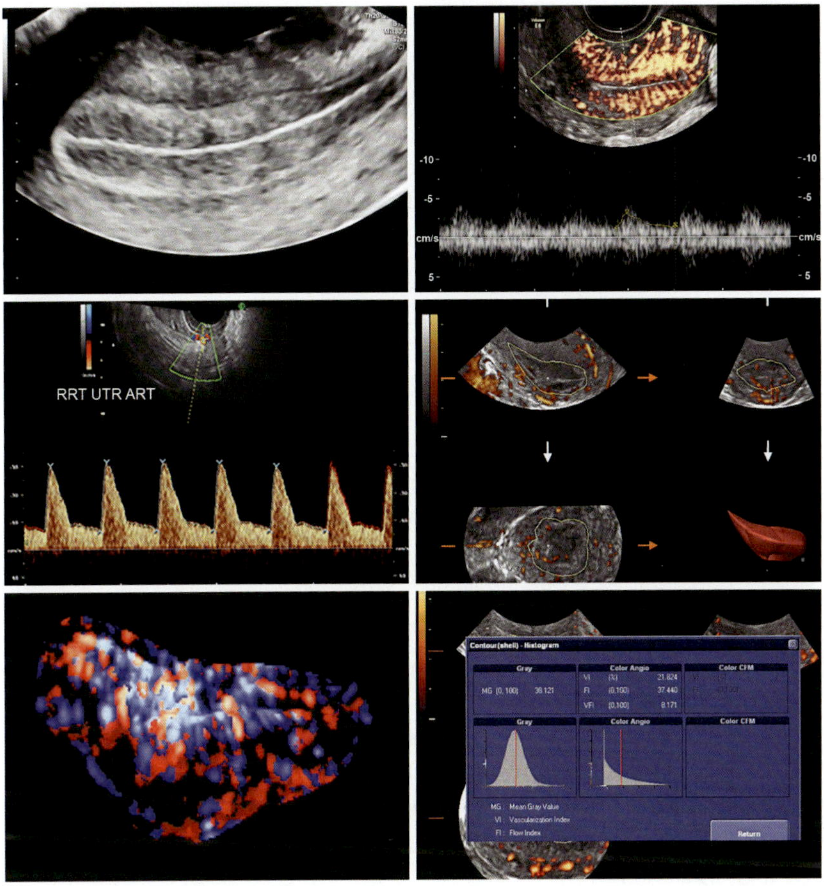

Fig. 5: Pre-human chorionic gonadotropin (hCG) endometrial parameters.

- Endometrial vessels RI: 0.49–0.59 and pulsatility index (PI):1.1–2.3
- Uterine artery PI <3.2
- Endometrial volume >3 cc
- Endometrial FI >40 and vascularization flow index (VFI) >20.

Ovulation Trigger

- Recombinant hCG (rhCG) 250 IU is given when preovulatory follicular and endometrial parameters on ultrasound are satisfied.
- Urinary hCG (uhCG) 10,000 IU.
- *GnRH agonist*: Leuprolide acetate 1 mg. Some advocate 1.5 mg 12 hours apart in two dose and some centers use 2 mg single dose or decapeptyl 1 mg. GnRH agonist is given in PCOS patients when there are multiple follicles and when OHSS is anticipated.

Timing of Insemination

Life span of ovum is about 8–10 hours, maximum. So during that time spermatozoa should be around the ovum. Urinary LH kit is useful to decide the LH surge but we have not found it to be useful. We give trigger by deciding follicle maturity and endometrial receptivity by US and then after 36–38 hours, we do IUI in normal patients. Literature shows following timings of insemination:

- 36–38 hours (between 32 and 38 hours)[18,19]
- 18 hours and 42 hours
- 24 hours and 48 hours
- 38 hours and 24 hours later if rupture is not seen on US.

We have found insemination between 36 and 38 hours as excellent as it has given highest number of pregnancies. A retrospective cohort study by Kucuk showed significantly higher cycle pregnancy rates after follicular rupture, 36–38 hours post-hCG compared with that when follicle rupture was not evident.[20]

Double Intrauterine Insemination

In literature, it has not been quoted when to do double IUI. There are various papers which say that double IUI does not increase the pregnancy rates.[21]

The Cochrane review also suggests that double IUI adds to cost and inconvenience without improving efficacy.[22] Though double IUI may improve pregnancy rates in male factor subfertility.[22]

Physiology of Rupture of Follicle

The LH surge starts when PSV of the follicle is 10 cm/s. It gradually increases and reaches up to 45 cm/s just before the rupture. This means that when PSV of the follicle is higher, follicle is not 36 hours away from rupture but is closer. This means if hCG is given at this time, follicle will not rupture at 36 hours but will rupture earlier and therefore IUI should be done earlier.

Our Experience on Double IUI

We have done a study of 500 superovulation with IUI cycles,[23] with different stimulation protocols, viz., CC, gonadotropins, and letrozole with gonadotropins. We have found that no matter what stimulation protocol is used, if perifollicular PSV is >20 cm/s, double IUI (first one done between 12–14 hours after hCG and second done between 36–38 hours of hCG) gives significantly higher pregnancy rates as compared to single IUI done between 36–38 hours after hCG. This is because higher the PSV earlier is the follicle likely to rupture (Also refer to Chapter 16 of this book).

Semen Preparation

It has been separately discussed in Chapter 7.

Among the factors that may affect the success of IUI:

- The most important is the age of the female. Success rate of IUI sharply decreases after 40 years of age of the female partner.[24] It has been observed that increasing male age seems to be associated with decline in semen volume, sperm motility, and sperm morphology but not with sperm concentration.[25] This has a synergistic adverse effect when female partner is also above 35 years.[26] If the sperm morphology score is >4%, IUI can be performed with an acceptable success rate if the insemination motile count (IMC) is >1 million.[27] Pregnancy rate per cycle is highest in the first three treatment cycles.[28] Couples with mild male subfertility, unexplained fertility or mild endometriosis show acceptable cumulative ongoing pregnancy rates after six cycles of IUI with ovarian hyperstimulation.[29]

Intrauterine insemination: Important points to remember in IUI are as follows:

- Measure uterocervical length (UCL) by US at the time of baseline scan.
- IUI is done with all aseptic preparations.
- There is no need to use antiseptics or saline.
- Do not touch the endometrium with IUI cannula to avoid injury to endometrium.
- We generally use Sims speculum and hold the anterior lip of cervix with Alyce's forceps to straighten the cervicouterine canal. With Cusco's speculum, without using Alyce's forceps, there is often difficulty in negotiating the cannula in many cases. In our more than 12,000 IUI pregnancies, we have used Sims speculum and Alyce's forceps.
- About 0.3–0.7 mL of wash sample is put inside the uterine cavity slowly.
- Allow the patient to rest for 15 minutes. About 10–15 minutes of immobilization after IUI significantly improves cumulative ongoing pregnancy rates and live birth rates.[30] Maximum six cycles of IUI should be tried. But all these six cycles should be with gonadotropins and good US monitoring.
- According to literature, minimum postwash sperm count required for IUI is 2 million with 4% normal spermatozoa. But in our own series highest pregnancy rates have been achieved when postwash count is between 6 and 8 million.
- Advanced maternal age along with low antral follicle count (AFC) and anti-Müllerian hormone (AMH) should be offered ovum donation.
- Success rate with IUI is highest when 14% or more sperms show normal morphology, intermediate when 4–14% are normal and very low when only <4% sperms show normal morphology.

- IUI has replaced intraperitoneal insemination, intratubal insemination, cervical cap, pentoxifylline, and estrogen therapy.

Complications

Complications are very few and very rare. If at all may occur, these are due to superovulation or incorrect semen wash.

- *Those due to superovulation are*: OHSS and multiple pregnancy
- *Those due to incorrect semen wash are*: Infection and pain in abdomen.

Luteal Support

Luteal support is an absolute must when superovulation is done. Protocols for luteal support may be any of the following:

- 200 mg bd, progesterone effervescent tablets
- 300–400 mg bd micronized progesterone vaginal pessaries
- hCG 5,000 IU on Day 5 and Day 9 after IUI
- hCG 2000 IU on Day 3-7-10 after IUI.

Luteal phase support with vaginal progesterone significantly improves the live birth rates in IUI cycles with gonadotropins stimulation.[31] But it does not improve pregnancy rates in normo-ovulatory women stimulated with CC for IUI.[32]

OUR EXPERIENCES

We have so far achieved more than 12,000 pregnancies with IUI. In our experience, superovulation with recombinant FSH (rFSH) is the best. Follicular monitoring by at least color Doppler and preferably three-dimensional (3D) power Doppler is must for precise timing of hCG. Perfect semen wash is equally important.

We have been able to achieve a success rate of 80–90% in six cycles in patients with idiopathic or dysovulatory infertility, when superovulation with rFSH or highly purified urinary FSH (uFSH-HP) is done with IUI and consistent US monitoring is done as described.

Carry Home Message

- IUI is the preferred method for dysovulatory infertility, idiopathic infertility or male subfertility.
- Superovulation must be done by rFSH/uFSH-HP.
- Letrozole + rFSH gives excellent results.
- Ultrasound monitoring by color Doppler and 3D power Doppler improves results dramatically.
- Ultrasound helps to decide the time of IUI and also whether to do single/double IUI.
- Semen preparation should be meticulous.
- Luteal support is must in superovulation with IUI.

REFERENCES

1. Haagen EC, Nelen WLDM, Adang EM, Grol RPTM, Hermens RPMG, Kremer JAM. Guideline adherence is worth the effort: a cost-effectiveness analysis in intrauterine insemination care. Hum Reprod. 2013;28(2):357-66.
2. Goverde AJ, McDonnell J, Vermeiden JP, Schats R, Rutten FF, Schoemaker J. Intrauterine insemination or in vitro fertilization in idiopathic subfertility and male subfertility: a randomised trial and cost-effectiveness analysis. Lancet. 2000;355:13-8.
3. Van Ruste MME, Custers IM, Van der Veen F, van Wely M, Evers JLH, Mol BWJ. The influence of number of follicles on pregnancy rates in intrauterine insemination with ovarian stimulation: A meta-analysis. Hum Reprod Update. 2008;14:563-657.
4. Van Weert JM, Repping S, Van Voorhis BJ, Van der Veen F, Bossyut P, Mol BW. Performance of post wash total motile sperm count as a predictor of pregnancy at the time of intrauterine insemination: a meta-analysis. Fertil Steril. 2004;82(3):612-20.
5. Ombelet W, Vandeput H, Janssen M, Cox A, Vossen C, Pollet H. Treatment of male infertility due to sperm surface antibodies: IUI or IVF? Hum Reprod. 1997;1296:165-70.
6. Hughes EG. Stimulated intra-uterine insemination is not a natural choice for the treatment of unexplained subfertility. Hum Reprod. 1998;18(5):912-4.
7. Steures P, Vander Steeg JW, Hopes PG, Bossyut PM, Habbema JD, Eijkmans MJ, et al. Effectiveness of intrauterine insemination in subfertile couples with an isolated cervical factor: a randomised clinical trial. Fertil Steril. 2007;88(6):1692-6.
8. Guzick DS, Sullivan MW, Adamson GD, Cedars MI, Falk RJ, Peterson EP, et al. Efficacy of treatment for unexplained infertility. Fertil Steril. 1998;70:207.
9. Mahani IM, Afnan M. The pregnancy rates with intrauterine insemination (IUI) in superovulated cycles employing different protocols [Clomiphene citrate (CC), human menopausal gonadotropin (hMG) and hMG+CC] and in natural ovulatory cycle. J Pak Med Asso. 2004;54(10):503-5.
10. Wordsworth S, Buchanan J, Mollison J, Harrild K, Robertson L, Tay C, et al. Clomiphene citrate and intrauterine insemination as first line treatments for unexplained infertility: are they cost-effective? Hum Reprod. 2011;26(2):369-75.
11. Verhulst SM, Cohlen BJ, Hughes E, te Velde E, Heineman MJ. Intrauterine insemination for unexplained subfertility. Cochrane Database Syst Rev. 2006;(4):CD001838.
12. Bhattacharya S, Harrild K, Mollison J, Wordsworth S, Tay C, Harrold A, et al. Clomiphene citrate or unstimulated intrauterine insemination compared with expectant management for unexplained infertility: pragmatic randomised controlled trial. BMJ. 2008;337:a716.
13. Cantineau AE, Cohlen BJ. Ovarian stimulation protocols (anti-oestrogens, gonadotropins with and without agonists/antagonists) for intrauterine insemination in women with subfertility. Cochrane Database Syst Rev. 2007;(2):CD005356.
14. Cantineau AEP, Cohlen BJ, Klip H, Heineman MJ, Dutch IUI study Group Collaborators. The addition of GnRH antagonists in intrauterine insemination cycles with mild ovarian hyperstimulation does not increase live birth rates—a randomised, double-blinded, placebo-controlled trial. Hum Repord. 2011;26(50):1104-11.
15. Kurjak A, Chervenak FK. 3D and 3D PD assessment of pre-hCG follicle and endometrium. Donald Sch J Ultrasound Obstetrics Gynecology. 2008;2(2):35-47.
16. Palatnik A, Strawn E, Szabo A, Robb P. What is the optimal follicular size before triggering ovulation in intrauterine insemination cycles with clomiphene citrate or letrozole? An analysis of 988 cycles. Fertil Steril. 2012;97:1089-94.
17. Farhi J, Orvieto R, Gavish O, Homburg R. The association between follicular size on hCG day and pregnancy rate in clomiphene citrate treated polycystic ovary syndrome patients. Gynecol Endocrinol. 2010;26:546-8.

18. ESHRE Capri Workshop Group. Intrauterine Insemination. Hum Reprod Update. 2009;15:265-77.
19. Ragni G, Somigliana E, Vegetti W. Timing of intrauterine insemination: where are we are? Fertil Steril. 2004;82:25-6.
20. Kucuk T. Intrauterine insemination: is the timing correct? J Assist Reprod Genet. 2008;8:427-30.
21. Bagis T, Haydardedeoglu B, Kilicdag EB, Cok T, Simsek E, Parlakgumus AH. Single versus double intrauterine insemination in multi-follicular ovarian hyperstimulation cycles: a randomised trial. Hum Reprod. 2010;25:1684-90.
22. Cantineau AEP, Heineman MJ, Cohlen BJ. Single versus double intrauterine insemination in stimulated cycles for subfertile couples. Cochrane Database Syst Rev. 2003;(1):CD003854.
23. Nagori C, Panchal S. Role of Double IUI in patients with high perifollicular PSV. London: 16th World Congress on Ultrasound in Obstetrics and Gynecology; 2006.
24. Broekmans FJ, Soules MR, Fauser BC. Ovarian aging: mechanisms and clinical consequences. Endocr Rev. 2009;30(5):465-93.
25. Kidd SA, Eskenazi B, Wyrobak AJ. Effects of male age on semen quality and fertility: a review of literature. Fertil Steril. 2001;75(2):237-48.
26. Mathieu C, Ecochard R, Bied V, Lornage J, Czyba JC. Cumulative conception rate following intrauterine artificial insemination with husband's spermatozoa: influence of husband's age. Hum Reprod. 1995;10(5):1090-7.
27. Ombelet W, Vandeput H, Vande Putte G, Cox A, Janssen M, Jacobs P, et al. Intrauterine insemination after ovarian stimulation with clomiphene citrate: predictive potential of inseminating motile count and sperm morphology? Hum Reprod. 1997;12:1458-63.
28. Aboulghar M, Mansour R, Serour G, Abdrazek A. Controlled ovarian hyperstimulation and intrauterine insemination for treatment of unexplained infertility should be limited to a maximum of three trials. Fertil Steril. 2001;75(1):88-91.
29. Custers IM, Steures P, Hompes P, Flierman P. intrauterine insemination: how many cycles should we perform? Hum Reprod. 2008;23(4):885-8.
30. Saleh A, Tan SL, Biljan MM, Tulandi T. A randomised study of the effect of 10 minutes of bed rest after intrauterine insemination. Fertil Steril. 2000;74:509-11.
31. Erem AA, Erdem M, Atmaca S, Guler I. Impact of luteal phase support on pregnancy rates in intrauterine insemination cycles: a prospective randomised study. Fertil Steril. 2009;91:2508-13.
32. Kyrou D, Fatei HM, Tournaye H, Devroey P. Luteal phase support in normo-ovulatory women stimulated with clomiphene citrate for intrauterine insemination: need or habit? Hum Reprod. 2010;25:2501-6.

CHAPTER 7

Sperm Preparation

Chaitanya Nagori

INTRODUCTION

After assessment of the semen sample, preparation is done. The preparation of the semen sample depends on the count, motile sperms, volume, viscosity, presence of antibodies, white blood cell (WBC), and debris.

The purpose of semen preparation is to concentrate the normal motile sperms with intact functional and genetic properties including normal morphology, with minimal deoxyribonucleic acid (DNA) damage, and intact cell membranes with functional binding properties. It makes sperms hyperactive after removal of seminal plasma. Seminal plasma has prostaglandins, anticapacitation and antifertilization factors, dead sperms, WBC, bacteria, and germ cells.

COLLECTION OF SEMEN SAMPLE

Abstinence is not preferred before intrauterine insemination (IUI) as long abstinence may result in higher sperm volume and concentration but results in lower sperm motility and high sperm DNA fragmentation levels. Though 24 hours of abstinence is advised as abstinence shorter than that may result in poor chromatin packaging. It has been shown that IUI outcomes were optimal after 2 days of ejaculatory abstinence[1] and therefore, ≤2 days of abstinence is advised before IUI.

It is collected by aseptic technique in sterilized jar. Water or wet hands must not touch semen or inner surface of the jar. Ask the patient to clean and dry parts before collection. Possibly collection should be done in the premises, but if not the case, transport time from collection to incubator should not be more than 30 minutes at body temperature. Seminal plasma contains several substances that may reduce the fertilizing capacity of the sperms.[2] During transport, semen should not be exposed to direct sunlight.

Semen is allowed to stand in the incubator at 37°C temperature for liquefaction for 20–30 minutes. Semen preparation should begin as soon as possible after liquefaction. Liquefaction is required for homogeneous population of sperms throughout the semen sample. If liquefaction does not occur needling through 23 gauge needle can be done, though sperm damage is known to occur by this.

As a rule the liquefied sample must be examined under the microscope using Meckler chamber or Neubauer chamber for count, motility and morphology before processing. Motility and morphologically abnormal sperms are counted as percentage against normal sperms. Method of semen wash is decided, based on these parameters.

Split ejaculation is collection of semen twice at a short interval. Split ejaculation collection is now not recommended as the results are the same and spillage can occur with split ejaculation.

When antisperm antibodies are present, semen is collected directly in culture media as it decreases free antibodies and improves chances of fertilization. Similarly semen with high viscosity is also collected in culture media.

Instruments and Equipment Required for Good Sperm Preparation

- Incubator for 37°C temperature
- Laminar airflow
- Microscope
- Centrifuge
- CO_2 incubator
- Neubauer/Mackler chamber
- Semen collection jar
- *Disposables*: Double lock tubes, pipette, tips, slides, and cover slips
- Syringe
- IUI cannula

Sperm preparation laboratory should preferably be in the same set-up where IUI is to be done. Laboratory should be a cool place and should not have windows and should not be in the direction of sunlight for long hours of the day. It should preferably not be the top floor of the building.

Composition of Sperm Preparation Media

- Earle's balance media
- Sodium pyruvate
- Synthetic serum replacement
- HEPES buffer
- Sodium bicarbonate
- Human serum albumin 1%
- Penicillin 50,000 IU/L + streptomycin 50 mg/L
- Phenol red.

Proteins and buffers in media promote sperm capacitation while serum appears to be important for sperm motility. Inclusion of protein is required to prevent sperm adhering to surfaces. Bicarbonate is required for capacitation. Media containing glucose is always better.

Selection of method depends on:

- Motile count
- Volume of semen
- Presence of leukocytes, debris, and other cells
- Viscosity
- Whether it is for IUI, in vitro fertilization (IVF) or intracytoplasmic sperm injection (ICSI). It is important to keep in mind here that sperm preparation time of 40–80 minutes has a positive effect on pregnancy rates.[3]

SPERM PREPARATION METHODS

- Simple washing
- Swim-up
- Density gradient methods.

Other methods such as migration gravity sedimentation and glass-wool columns are rarely used now.

Simple Washing

It is the oldest method and is also known as simple dilution and washing technique. Only seminal plasma is removed by this technique, cellular debris, dead and nonmotile sperms, and bacteria are not removed completely as there is no swim-up. Semen is diluted with a large amount of medium (five to ten times of semen volume). It is then centrifuged at 300 g for 10 minutes with a purpose to wash it. Supernatant medium is removed and pellet is resuspended in medium and again centrifuged at 300–500 g for 5 minutes. Again the supernatant is removed and the pellet is resuspended in medium appropriate for insemination and is incubated till insemination. This method is not used routinely.

Reagents for Swim-up

- *Self-prepared medium*: Earle's balanced salt (EBSS) + streptopenicillin [(penicillin 50,000 IU/L, streptomycin 50 mg/L + Na pyruvate + serum albumin readymade media (available from various companies)]
- Flushing medium, sperm preparation media (SPM) (Medicult Origio)
- Cryoprep (Medline)
- G sperm (Scandinavian)
- FertiCult Flushing medium.

Swim-up Methods

- Swim-up from ejaculate.
- Swim-up from pellet—different culture media have some variation.

Swim-up from ejaculate: This is the ideal method as it does not require centrifugation.

- It is used only for normal semen sample.
- It is based on selection of the sperms based on their capability to swim-up in the media.
- Morphologically abnormal sperms and reactive oxygen species (ROS) are not filtered.
- The total yield of sperms is lower than washing technique. It is therefore, used for samples with high sperm count.
- The time for which the samples are left for swim-up depends on the total sperm count, but allowing to swim-up for a long time allows more abnormal sperms to swim-up.

Method: Aliquots of liquefied semen are placed directly under medium (1 mL) in round bottom tubes and these tubes are placed at 45° angle in a stand to be placed in the incubator for 30–60 minutes. The upper part of the layered medium from each test tube is collected, without disturbing the interface and washed in 2 mL medium by centrifugating at 300–500 g for 10 minutes. Then the supernatant is removed and pellet is resuspended in the amount of medium sufficient for insemination and incubated till insemination.

Swim-up from pellet: This method is used for normal or marginally abnormal sperms, viscous samples, or samples collected in media.

Method:

- Take 2 mL of culture medium in a test tube
- Pipette 1.5 mL of semen and mix it with medium
- Centrifuge at 300–500 g for 10 minutes
- Remove supernatant
- Resuspend the pellet in another 2 mL of medium
- Centrifuge for 5 minutes at 300 g
- Remove supernatant
- Layer the pellet with 1 mL of medium
- Put it in CO_2 incubator for swim-up for 30–60 minutes
- Gently aspirate 0.5–0.7 mL of the solution from upper layers of medium without disturbing the pellet.

Sperm capacitation requires presence of bicarbonate ions. Therefore, if prepared sperms are stored before IUI, sperm buffer is advised, a zwitterions buffered medium (such as HEPES). This will prevent premature capacitation and hyperactivated motility. If IUI is performed soon after sperm processing, bicarbonate buffered medium can be used for entire process.

This technique has advantage of not using other chemicals than culture media. Most of the samples can be prepared by this method with different culture media. But alternative methods are also described. Flushing media is most commonly used for IUI for swim-up.

Method using sperm preparation media (swim-up from ejaculate):

- Layer 1–1.5 mL of semen underneath 1–2 mL of pre-equilibrated SPM.
- The tubes are kept tilted in CO_2 incubator for 30–60 minutes.
- After swim-up, upper 0.5–1 mL is aspirated and put together.

Alternatively:

- Sample is diluted 1 : 3 v/v with media and is allowed to stand for 15 minutes at room temperature (+22°C)
- Centrifuge at 300 g for 10 minutes
- Remove supernatant, resuspend in 4 mL of SPM
- Centrifuge at 200 g for 5 minutes, remove supernatant
- Gently overlay the pellet with 2 mL of SPM and leave in CO_2 incubator for 120 minutes
- Upper 0.1 mL has dead sperms and debris. This is removed
- Then upper 0.7 mL is taken for insemination.

Variations: In non-assisted reproductive technology centers, flushing media is used rather than sperm preparation media. The difference in two media is shown in **Table 1**.

To compensate for albumin content, add 5.62 mL of human albumin solution to 125 mL of bottle of flushing media. It gives equally good results with lower costs.

Method for sperm preparation media (Medicult): Two to four test tubes with culture media are taken and in each tube semen is put underneath the media. After 30 minutes collect upper portion from each tube.

Second alternative is that we can dilute semen three times with media and after 15 minutes centrifugation is done.

First centrifugation is at 300 g/10 minutes. Then resuspend in 4 mL of SPM. Then pellet is suspended with 2 mL in incubator for 60–120 minutes.

G Sperm (Scandinavian Media):

- Take two to four tubes with 1 mL semen
- Overlay with 2 mL media and incubate for 60 minutes
- Aspirate 1 mL from all tubes

Table 1: Difference between flushing media and sperm preparation media (SPM).

Component	*Flushing*	*SPM*
Albumin	0.1%	1.0%
pH	7–7.3	7.2–7.4
Bicarbonate	1.1	2.2

- Add 5 mL media and centrifuge for 10 minutes at 300–600 g
- Discard supernatant
- Repeat centrifugation after adding 5 mL media with 300–600 g for 10 minutes. Resuspend in G Fert and take 0.5–0.7 mL for insemination.

Swim-up from pellet is most widely used method as it separates motile sperms from nonmotile sperms and debris. Here sperms are concentrated prior to swim-up and do not have to escape seminal plasma. So it is advantageous for viscous, moderate density or moderate motility samples. It is suitable for samples collected in media or cryopreserved samples.

The disadvantage of centrifuge is production of ROS, which is harmful for fertilization.

Tips for Better Intrauterine Insemination

- Work under laminar airflow as far as possible and use completely sterile technique.
- Gloves should not touch the inner side of the tubes, rubber is toxic for sperms.
- Work with more tubes rather than a single large tube when semen sample is large or count is too high.
- Leaving for swim-up for a long time may allow the debris to swim-up. Longer time may be required for swim-up of low count or low motility samples, that means an optimum time for swim-up must be modified as per the count and motility of the sample.
- Semen processing is done within 30 minutes after collection and maximally within 1 hour.
- While loading avoid contact of cannula with inner side of the tube.
- Rubber of syringe should not touch the sample that means when the sample is loaded in the cannula with the syringe attached, there should be a small air gap between the sample column and the rubber piston.
- Air should not be injected during IUI.
- No antiseptics are applied in the vagina.
- Equal volume of pentoxifylline solution can be added before centrifugation to improve motility in oligoasthenospermia.
- *For centrifuge machine*: Different companies have different parameters of speed—the conversion formula is; rpm: $\sqrt{[g/(1.118 \times r)]}$.
- Media is kept overnight in CO_2 incubator with loosened cap in a slanted test tube rack for equilibrium **(Fig. 1)**.
- With low count large amount of semen may help.
- Clean the vagina and the vulva with normal saline before wash, but it is not a must.
- Slanting test tube position during swim-up allows larger surface and therefore, larger sperm cohort.

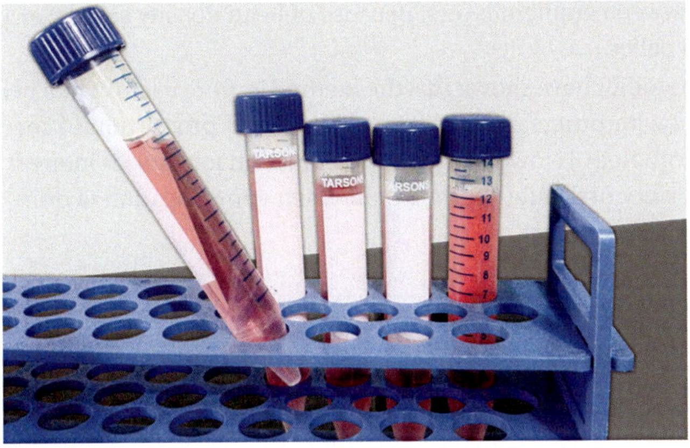

Fig. 1: Test tubes are kept in slanting position in rack.

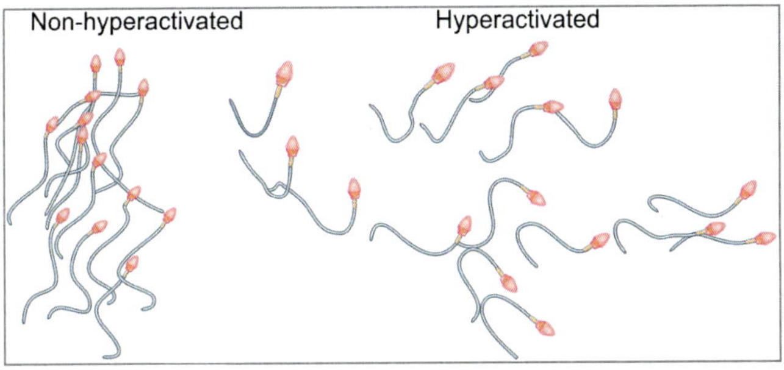

Fig. 2: Hyperactivated post semen wash sperms on right side and non-hyperactivated sperms on left side.

- Proper labeling of tubes is a must.
- A good wash sample is one which has at least 95% actively motile sperms and no debris **(Fig. 2)**.

Density Gradient Methods

This is the method which gives better recovery of sperms for IUI and conversion IVF. This method selects sperms according to their density and gravity (mass per unit volume) and results in cells being dispersed throughout the gradient column according to the gradient that matches their density. Normal spermatozoa have a density of 1.12 g/mL and immature abnormal sperms have density of 1.06–1.09 g/mL. Normal sperms can be isolated in the solution with highest concentration of gradient.

It is suitable for viscous samples as well as sample having more debris and WBCs and low count. Dead and defective sperms and leukocytes produce ROS which cause lipid peroxidation of sperm membrane and decrease motility. These are best removed by gradient method. Debris and immotile sperms are held in between gradient layers. Because of head density sperms swim down and form pellet.

Some studies have shown that the method is more useful when percentage of sperms with progressive motility is lower and proportion of sperms with good morphology is lower. Higher centrifugation for shorter interval will give good recovery of motile sperms, than when centrifugation is done at lower speed for longer time.

Universal Method

- From bottom to top 90% density gradient, then 45% density gradient then semen sample.
- Centrifuge at 1,500 rpm for 15 minutes.
- Remove supernatant.
- Transfer pellet to sterile centrifuge tube (may not be required).
- Add 3–5 mL SPM and mix pellet.
- Centrifuge at 1,000 rpm for 5 minutes.
- Remove supernatant
- Mix pellet with 0.5–0.7 mL washing media.
- Load the catheter for IUI.

Gradient media available are:
- Suprasperm (Medicult)
- IxaPrep (Medicult)
- Puresperm (Nidacon)
- SpermGrad (Shivani Scientific)
- Sil-Select (Microm, UK).

Method for Suprasperm

Suprasperm is a salt solution containing a colloidal suspension of silica particles stabilized with covalently bound hydrophilic saline.
- 2 × 1 mL of semen should be used to run two gradients for each semen sample.
- Dispense 2 mL of 55% suprasperm to a test tube and dispense 2 mL of 80% medium underneath this with a pipette.
- Carefully dispense 1 mL of semen on the top of this and centrifuge at 300 g for 20 minutes.
- Remove the supernatant and resuspend the pellet in 2–3 mL of SPM and centrifuge at 200 g for 10 minutes.
- Remove supernatant, leave pellet and repeat the wash process.
- Finally resuspend the pellet in the desired concentration of SPM.

Final wash with culture medium to remove the gradient solution is the drawback of this method.

Variations with Other Media

- *IxaPrep*: It has two pure cell separating agents. Polysucrose and iodixanol with HEPES buffer. Top layer has SPM + Polysucrose. Bottom layer has SPM + Polysucrose + Iodixanol. Semen preparation is done in the same way.
- *Scandinavian method (SpermGrad)*: Bottom layer has 90% density and upper layer has 45% and washing is done with G Fert.
- *Puresperm (Gradient method)*: It has 90% and 45% solution. First centrifugation is at 500 g for 10 minutes, and the other two centrifugations are at 250 g for 5 minutes.
- *Sil-select gradient method*: It has 80% and 40% solutions and centrifugation is done at 300–600 g for 10–20 minutes.

Gradient media are available as readymade media where two separate media of different densities are available. Media are also available as 100% media. These can be diluted to desired densities using flushing media. For example, 45% gradient medium is to be made, in a syringe of 1 mL, 0.45 mL of 100% gradient medium is taken and to that 0.55 mL of flushing medium is added. If the usage is higher the preparation can also be made in samples of 10 mL.

Tips for a Better Yield of Sperms in Gradient Method

- Longer centrifugation time increases the recovery of both motile and immotile sperms.
- Higher centrifugation speed increases recovery of motile sperms and low density particles, so shorter time is required with higher speeds.
- Because of the low density, debris, round cells, and the abnormal sperms with amorphous heads and cytoplasmic droplets never reach the bottom of the tube.

Density gradient method is generally thought to be superior to other two techniques as it gives more morphologically normal sperms with grade A motility and normal DNA integrity with less chromatin and nuclear DNA anomalies in prepared sample. It also reduces ROS and leukocyte concentration. Though in a Cochrane review by Boomsma et al. showed in a meta-analysis that there was no evidence of a difference in effectiveness of a swim-up versus density gradient method on pregnancy rates per couple. Swim-up technique versus wash and centrifugation also showed no significant difference in pregnancy rates.[4] So no one SPM is better than other in present scenario though it depends on the nature of semen sample.

Recovery rate of sperms after swim-up is lower (<20%) as compared to that with density gradient method which is >20%.[5]

Preparation from the Frozen Sample

Dealing with atypical semen samples:

- Frozen sample
- Retrograde ejaculation
- Human immunodeficiency virus (HIV)-positive sample.

Frozen sample:

- Thaw the specimen 30 minutes before IUI
- Place frozen vials in 37° water bath for 10 minutes
- Shake vials gently to confirm the disappearance of ice crystals
- Then treat as a fresh sample.

Retrograde ejaculation: Patient first empties his bladder. Then alkalizer is given to the patient. After sometime he is asked to masturbate. The urine sample is collected in culture media and is centrifuged at 500 g for 8 minutes. The supernatant is removed and pellet is washed by gradient method.

Human immunodeficiency virus positive sample: HIV viruses are found in plasma. They are not inside the sperm cell. Here semen is prepared by gradient method followed by swim-up. Then the sample can be used for IUI.

Newer methods for sperm preparation like selection based on sperm surface charge and nonapoptotic sperm selection are at present used only for IVF. Selection based on sperm surface charge method is based on electrophoresis-based technology and electronegative charge on the sperm. CD52 (a specific surface protein) is correlated with normal sperm morphology and capacitation.

This technique is used in samples with high DNA damage. Zeta method selects sperms with respect to membrane surface charges or zeta potential. This method has been found to increase fertilization, implantation, and pregnancy rates.[6]

Nonapoptotic sperm selection: This method utilizes magnetic-activated cell sorting using Annex in V microbeads.[6]

Carry Home Message

- For regular IUI, swim-up is a very good method and is much cheaper than density gradient method.
- We have observed that pregnancy rate is very high with 8–10 million post wash count.
- It is very vital that you select a method and modify it to achieve that count.
- We can have our own modification for speed of centrifugation and time of centrifugation according to the count and motility of the sample.

REFERENCES

1. Nijs M. Study of sperm parameters in assisted reproduction outcome. Maastricht, Netherlands: Datawyse Bockproducties; 2009.
2. Bjorndahl L, Mortimer D, Barratt C, Castilla JA, Menkveld R, Kvist U. Practical guide to basic laboratory andrology. Cambridge: Cambridge University Press; 2010.
3. Fauque P, Lehert P, Lamotte M, Bettahar-Lebugle K, Bailly A, Diligent C, et al. Clinical success of intrauterine insemination cycles is affected by the sperm preparation time. Fertil Steril. 2014;101(6):1618-23.e1-3.
4. Boomsma CM, Heineman MJ, Cohlen BJ, Farquhar C. Semen preparation techniques for intrauterine insemination. Cochrane Database Syst Rev. 2012;(6):CD005996.
5. Morshedi M, Duran HE, Taylor S, Oehninger S. Efficacy and pregnancy outcome of two methods of semen preparation for intrauterine insemination: a prospective randomized study. Fertil Steril. 2003;79:1625-32.
6. Said TM, Land JA. Effects of advanced selection methods on sperm quality and ART outcome: a systematic review. Hum Reprod Update. 2011;17(6):719-33.

CHAPTER 8

Luteal Phase Defect

Chaitanya Nagori, Sonal Panchal

INTRODUCTION

Luteal phase starts from ovulation and ends at the onset of menstruation or when the pregnancy is diagnosed. The dominant follicle after ovulation is converted into corpus luteum (CL) and it is one of the most hormonally active glands in the body. Progesterone secretion from CL is the hallmark of luteal phase.

Luteal phase defect (LPD) is defined as inadequate corpus luteal function in the latter half of the ovulatory cycle. It is due to insufficient endogenous progesterone production or suboptimal response of endometrium to normal progesterone level. LPD is also known as luteal phase insufficiency or CL insufficiency or inadequate luteal phase. LPD is associated with infertility, early pregnancy loss, short cycles, and premenstrual spotting.

LUTEAL PHASE PHYSIOLOGY (BOXES 1 AND 2)

Preovulation luteinizing hormone (LH) surge is the stimulus for the luteinization. LH from pituitary continues to act through endocrine feedback

Box 1: Role of progesterone in luteal phase.

- Brings about secretory changes for implantation
- Vasodilatation for improved flow in endometrium
- Downregulates ERs, LIF, and beta-integrin
- Decidualization with pinopode formation
- Upregulation of IGF-1, interleukin, *HOXA* genes, cytokines, EGF, TGF, VEGF, mucin I, integrins, selectins, immunoglobulins, etc.
- Relaxes uterine musculature
- Improves endometrial receptivity

(EGF: epidermal growth factor; IGF-1: insulin-like growth factor 1; LIF: leukemia inhibitory factor; TGF: transforming growth factor; VEGF: vascular endothelial growth factor)

Box 2: Progesterone ensures receptive endometrium by modulating secretory transformation.

- Giant mitochondria
- Subnuclear glycogen deposit
- Pinopodes
- Nuclear channel system

Flowchart 1: Production of progesterone.

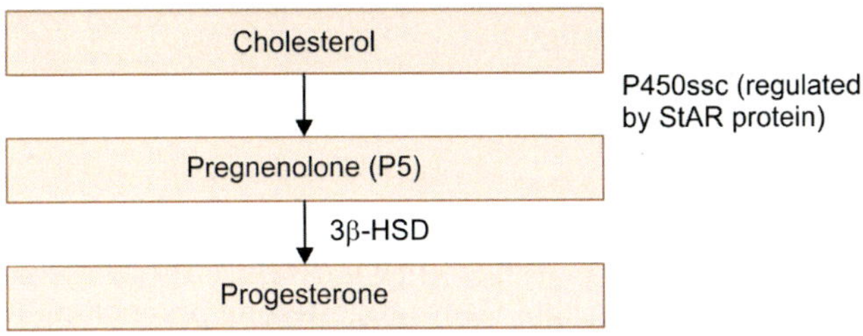

(3β-HSD: 3β-hydroxysteroid dehydrogenase; StAR: steroidogenic acute regulatory)

during entire luteinization process. In patients with luteal phase <10 days, lower levels of follicle-stimulating hormone (FSH) and LH are found in proliferative phase. Long follicular phase cycles do not have short luteal phase in majority of cases. Day 3 high estrone-3-glucuronide (ETT) and pregnanediol-3-alpha-glucuronide (PDG) are predictors of short early luteal phase. Here, LH is increased in about half of the cycles. Luteal phase has three phases. The first phase is a modulated luteinization process whereas second and third phases are relatively less modulated processes of progesterone and luteolysis.

- Duration is 12–14 days.
- Progesterone peak is 6–8 days after ovulation.
- Progesterone is secreted in pulses.
- Luteinizing hormone peak decides the quality of CL.
- Pulsatile LH is necessary for CL function.
- Steroidogenic acute regulatory (StAR) protein governs cholesterol transport for progesterone production.
- Corpus luteum is refractory to LH in later half.
- Human chorionic gonadotropin (hCG) can rescue CL by StAR and vascular endothelial growth factor (VEGF) after implantation.
- Minimum required levels of progesterone are not confirmed.
- Luteal phase estradiol (E2) is LH dependent and not FSH dependent.[1]
- Decline in StAR protein expression decreases steroidogenesis and leuteolysis.[1] This StAR protein is not present in granulosa cells and appears after LH peak only. Before preovulatory period, this protein expression is on the theca cells and converts cholesterol into androgen **(Flowchart 1)**.

PATHOPHYSIOLOGY OF LUTEAL PHASE DEFECT

- Deficient progesterone secretion from CL can be due to abnormal folliculogenesis, leading to unhealthy follicle that secretes low levels of E2, therefore inadequate LH surge. Inadequate LH surge may cause luteinization but ovulation might not occur and produces unhealthy CL, producing low level progesterone.

Box 3: Progesterone does immunomodulation.

- Favoring Th1-Th2 shift toward Th2
- Modulates chemokines transcription factor
- Inhibits tissue rejection
- Protects conceptus

- So, LH surge is must for a healthy CL. It is the most vascular organ. Blood flow to CL is 6–10 mL/g/mt.[2] Daily progesterone production from CL is 25–50 mg and is secreted in pulses, every 90 minutes. Progesterone and E2 secretion from CL correlates with LH pulse. Average E2 production is 0.6 mg/day in luteal phase. CL secretes estrogen under the influence of LH and insulin-like growth factor (IGF-1) and not FSH.
- Corpus luteum has two types of cells. The large cells develop from granulosa cells and secrete progesterone in the first half of luteal phase under the influence of LH pulse. The small cells develop from theca internal and produce progesterone after the stimulation of hCG.[3,4]
- Estrogen induces progesterone receptors.
- Progesterone acts through its own receptors and produces mediator protein known as "progesterone-induced blocking factor (PIBF)". PIBF produces asymmetrical antibodies, i.e., Th2 and natural killer (NK) cells for protection.

If PIBF is inadequate, Th1 and lymphokine-activated killer (LAK) cells are produced which are cytotoxic and reject the embryo.[5] So, the acceptance or rejection depends on the estrogen and progesterone **(Box 3)**.

RESCUE OF CORPUS LUTEUM IN INFERTILE PATIENT

Human chorionic gonadotropin from embryo restores StAR protein expression to late CL and induces progesterone production and production of VEGF that cause angiogenesis.

Implantation occurs between days 8 and 10 after LH surge. Miscarriage rate is very high if implantation is late because unhealthy embryo produces less hCG and inadequate rescue signals in spite of normal CL. So, low progesterone in early pregnancy is because of low hCG produced by unhealthy embryo and progesterone supplementation does not work.[6] Placental steroidogenesis starts at 7 weeks. CL starts reducing after 5 weeks of pregnancy but remains active up to 11 weeks. 17-hydroxyprogesterone (17-OHP) is secreted by CL only which starts regressing after 5 weeks along with regressing vascularity.

After 5 weeks, even hCG does not increase neoangiogenesis and this indicates that hCG-induced rescue for CL is temporary.[7]

DIAGNOSIS OF LUTEAL PHASE DEFECT

- *History*: Short luteal phase of <13 days from the LH surge to menstruation may be indicative of LPD. Patient may have premenstrual spotting, infertility, and early abortions, but history is not conclusive for diagnosis of LPD.
- *Basal body temperature (BBT) chart*: Absence or inadequate thermogenic shift in BBT chart indicates LPD. Its utility is questioned, and presently it has no place in diagnosis of luteal phase abnormality.
- *Endometrial biopsy*: Noyce criteria for dating of endometrium are very popular since 6 decades. Though endometrial histology is an indirect marker of progesterone action. There is interobserver variation and also intercycle variability. There is no consensus whether biopsy should be taken in one or two or three cycles. Biopsy taken in the latter half of the luteal phase indicates total progesterone effect rather than progesterone secretion on that day. The most interesting thing is that out of phase endometrial histology is also seen in fertile patients and patients who conceive.[8] So, endometrial histology is not used as a criteria for diagnosis of LPD.
- *Serum progesterone*: Progesterone secretion starts after 30 minutes of LH surge. In early luteal phase, progesterone secretion is nonpulsatile but in mid and late luteal phases, its secretion becomes pulsatile. Therefore, single assessment does not reflect the actual progesterone secretion. It was reported that three readings between days 5 and 9 postovulatory should be taken and cutoff of 30 ng/mL was thought to have a sensitivity of 100% and specificity of 80%.[9] Normal progesterone level in midluteal phase is 10 ng/mL, but there are no studies to confirm these findings. Histology of the endometrium does not correlate with progesterone level. So, progesterone does not differentiate normal and defective luteal phase. Serum progesterone >3 ng/mL only documents ovulation, but it is not used for diagnosis of LPD.
- *Ultrasound*:
    - Correlation of CL, resistance index (RI), and serum progesterone.
    - Corpus luteum Doppler shows high resistance flow (RI 0.58 ± 0.4) **(Figs. 1A and B)**.
    - Bilateral high resistance intraovarian flow and same in both ovaries, unlike normal luteal phase that shows low resistance in the dominant ovary.
    - Increased resistance in spiral artery (RI 0.72 ± 0.065) **(Figs. 2A and B)**.
- *New promising tests*:
    - Daily salivary progesterone measurement
    - Progesterone-induced blocking factor measurement.

Currently, no tests can stamp the diagnosis of LPD and differentiate fertile from infertile patients.[6]

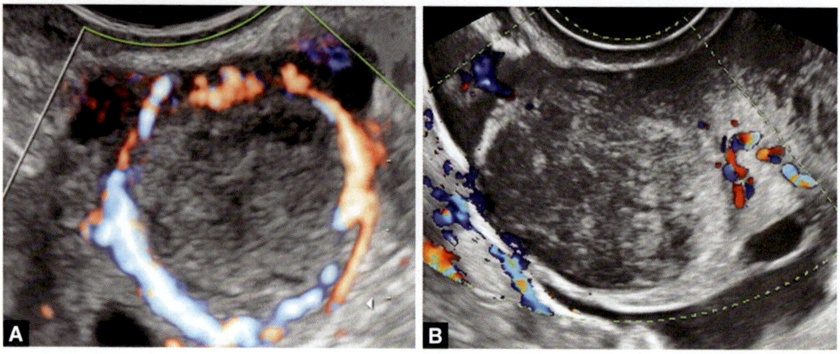

Figs. 1A and B: (A) Normal corpus luteal flow as complete ring of color; and (B) Scanty corpus luteal flow of corpus luteal inadequacy—luteal phase defect (LPD).

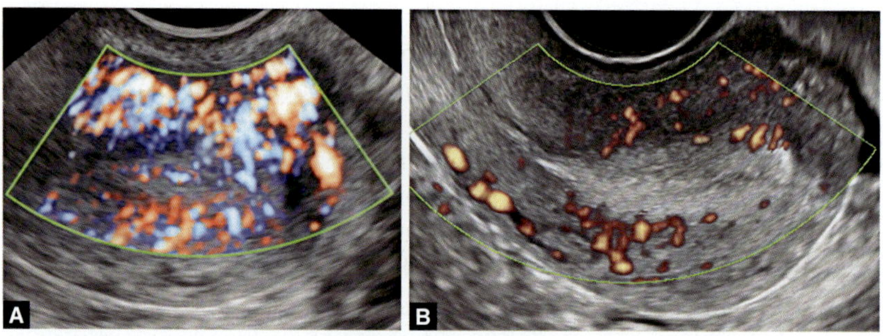

Figs. 2A and B: (A) Normal secretory endometrial flow; and (B) Scanty secretory endometrial flow—luteal phase defect (LPD).

Etiological factor beyond progesterone may be pinopodes development, insulin-like growth factor-binding protein (IGFBP), integrins, cytokines, etc. Tests to detect, these abnormalities are experimental and are not useful in clinical practice.

CONTROVERSIES IN DIAGNOSIS

- Luteal phase defect can exist with normal progesterone levels.[10]
- There may be no correlation of endometrial histology and serum progesterone.
- Pregnancy can continue with lower serum progesterone levels.
- Serum progesterone and estradiol benzoate (EB) are not related tests.
- Some papers say that E2 : Progesterone ratio is more important than only progesterone levels.[11]
- No tests can stamp the diagnosis.

The timing of embryo transfer depends on the duration of exposure rather than blood levels.[12]

LUTEAL PHASE SUPPORT

There are two dilemmas:
1. What to use for luteal support?
2. When to use luteal support?

What to Use for Luteal Support?

A. Progesterone
B. Human chorionic gonadotropin

A. Progesterone: Different progesterone preparations
- ***Natural progesterones*:**
  - *Not commonly used routes*:
    - Intranasal
    - Sublingual
    - Rectal.
  - *Commonly used routes*:
    - Oral
    - Injectable
    - Vaginal routes.
  - *Oral progesterones*:
    - It is available as soft gelatin capsules or tablet form and as sustained-release tablets.
    - It causes drowsiness, flushing, and nausea and it has selective and hypnotic effect because of metabolites.
    - It causes fluid retention.
    - Efficacy changes with food particle size and its vehicle. Bioavailability is only 10% when taken orally.
    - Extensive first-pass hepatic metabolism and therefore multiple doses are required. It has poor intestinal absorption.
    - It is ineffective in inducing an in-phase secretory endometrium.[13]
    - It has lower pregnancy rate.

      Oral sustained-release tablets: Slow-release (SR) EROMAT is a new technology. The drug is released gradually in a controlled manner over a span of 16–24 hours in the distal part of the gastrointestinal (GI) tract allowing lymphatic absorption of intact drug into systematic circulation and direct entry of the drug through the mucosal lining of colon into systemic circulation. The dose of sustained-release progesterone capsule is 200–400 mg daily. This has less side effects compared to conventional oral preparation. Only 20% of the drug is released in first 4 hours and minimize hepatic and prehepatic metabolism. Rest of the drug is released in distal GI tract. The serum progesterone level should be >14 ng/mL for threatened abortion and LPD. Oral SR preparations 400/300/200 mg/day give blood levels up to 46.2/36.2/20.6 ng/mL, respectively.

The drug at present is available in very few countries and there are not many international trials available to prove its role. The sole application of this drug is not recommended by majority of the assisted reproductive technology (ART) clinics. It is always used in combination of other progesterones. This drug still requires further studies in spite of its wide availability.

- *Injectable progesterones*:
  - *Intramuscular progesterone*: It gives high serum concentrations, adequate endometrial secretory features, and satisfactory pregnancy rates, comparable to vaginal progesterone.
    - Daily injections are uncomfortable and are very painful and may result in inferior secretory endometrial histology.
    - It can cause inflammation at injection site leading to redness, pain, and even sterile abscess at injection site because of the preservative (benzyl alcohol) used.
    - Rarely, it may also cause acute eosinophilic pneumonia.
    - It is not preferred in favor of vaginal progesterone or subcutaneous progesterone injection.
  - Subcutaneous aqueous progesterone preparations are also available now, in which progesterone is combined with cyclodextrin, a starch residue and is given as 25 mg or 50 mg doses a day and has shown results compatible with intramuscular progesterone.[14] Lockwood et al. have proved that subcutaneous injection of water-soluble progesterone 25 mg is safe and as effective as vaginal progesterone gel and remains an option for those who do not want vaginal progesterone on cultural, personal, or medical reasons.[15]

    Transdermal progesterone is not the option because the skin is rich in 5α-reductase, which will inactivate progesterone. Another reason is that daily E2 production is 0.5 mg/24 h while that of progesterone is 25 mg/24 h. Such large doses are difficult to deliver by transdermal patches.
- *Vaginal progesterones*:
  - *Vaginal suppositories*: Vaginal application is the most accepted route for progesterone administration **(Box 4)**. It has several advantages:
    - It avoids all GI side effects, sedative and hypnotic effect.
    - The first uterine pass effect (FUPE) **(Fig. 3)** is another major advantage: From the vagina, the drug is directly transported to

Box 4: Natural micronized progesterone.

- Reduced size
- Enhances dissolution
- Maximum serum concentration
- Reduced destruction
- Increases half-life

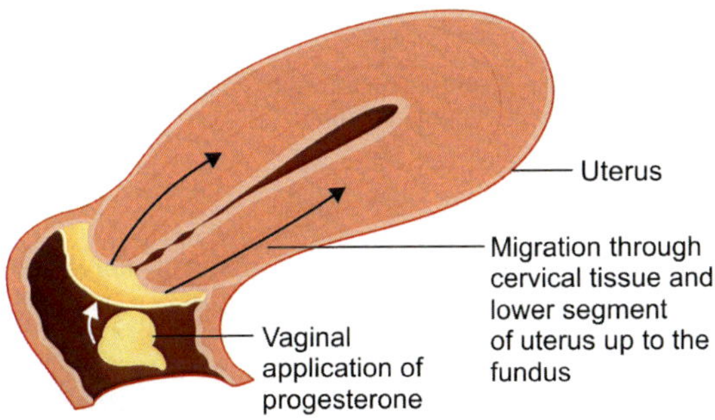

Fig. 3: Diagrammatic representation of first uterine pass effect.

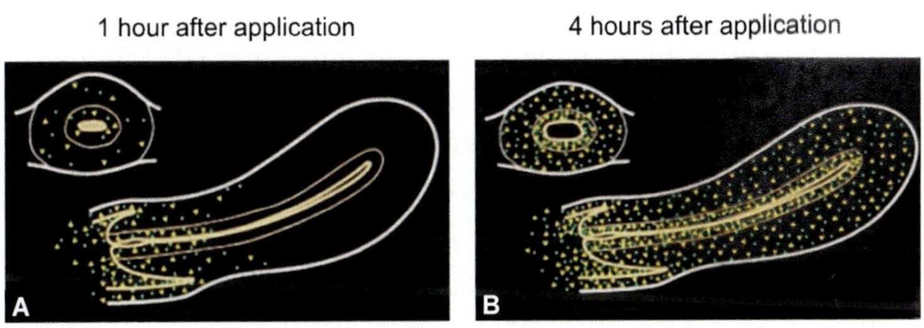

Figs. 4A and B: Progressive diffusion of progesterone from the cervix to the fundus of the uterus.

the uterus. So, in spite of low blood levels of progesterone, its level in uterus is high. Migration of the drug occurs from cervix and lower segment of uterus to the fundus of the uterus.[16] A countercurrent exchange **(Figs. 4A and B)** also occurs in the upper third of the vagina. The drug is absorbed in the veins of the vagina and from there directly goes to the arteries of the uterus, without entering into the general circulation. This leads to low serum level but high concentration in the uterus.[17-19]

These mechanisms lead to consistent tissue level of progesterone with vaginal application.[16] In spite of low blood levels, this improves implantation rates and decreases early pregnancy loss.[20]

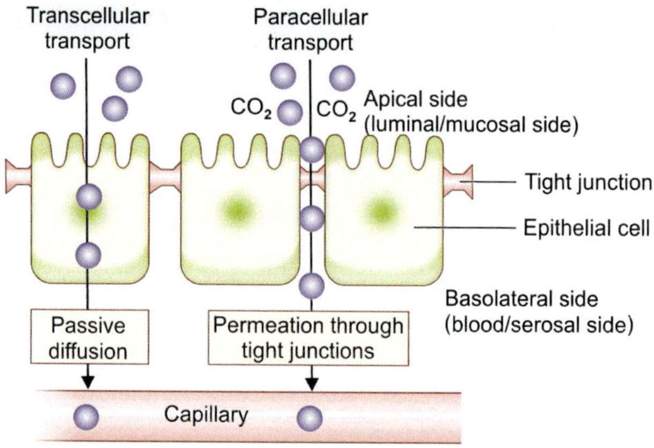

Fig. 5: Diagrammatic explanation of the vaginal absorption of effervescent progesterone vaginal tablets (from monogram Susten VT).

Czajkowski et al. proved that vaginal progesterone 300 mg is effective in reducing spiral artery pulsatility, pulsatility index (PI), and S/D ratio as compared to 30 mg of oral dydrogesterone.[21] Abdelhakim AM et al. have found in their study that vaginal versus intramuscular (IM) progesterone for luteal support in ART in systematic review and meta-analysis of randomized controlled trial (RCT) that vaginal progesterone has same results as IM progesterone in ART and is more satisfactory.[22]

- *Progesterone vaginal effervescent tablets*: This is a new delivery system of progesterone. Disintegration of tablet occurs in 7–10 minutes. It increases absorption. Twice a day dosage can achieve higher concentration of progesterone and reach steady state within 24–32 hours and maintain mean concentration above 10 ng/mL.[23]

As explained in **Figure 5**, the absorption of progesterone occurs by passive diffusion as well as paracellular transport which results in greater concentration and prolonged blood levels. Carbon dioxide (CO_2) opens up tight junctions of the cells and so paracervical absorption is increased.

Advantages of effervescent tablet:

- Greater bioavailability
- Effective systemic absorption
- Avoids hepatic first-pass metabolism
- Higher concentration in endometrium
- Lower doses are required
- Less fluctuation in serum levels

  - Healthy vaginal environment because of acidic pH
  - As efficient as other vaginal progesterone
  - Less irritation and discharge.
- *Vaginal progesterone rings* are also available now. These rings once inserted would release 10–20 nmol/L for 90 days. Compared to 50 mg/day IM progesterone, this product has shown comparable or better implantation rate.[24]
- *Progesterone gel*: It contains 90 mg (8%) of progesterone. It contains micronized progesterone in emulsion system which also contains water-insoluble polymer, "polycarbophil", having mucin-like actions. It is as effective as vaginal tablets. There is no substantial difference in ongoing pregnancy rate between vaginal progesterone gel and vaginal micronized progesterone tablets.[25] But vaginal gel has given higher pregnancy rates than intramuscular progesterone below the age of 35 years in IVF patients and after the age of 35 years, pregnancy rates were same for both the gel and the intramuscular progesterone group.[26] Its dosage schedule is once a day, so acceptance is very good. Only disadvantage of this preparation is its high cost. Gel preparation is always used in the morning and the patient is advised not to rest after that. Because of the movements, friction occurs between the vaginal walls and that helps to separate progesterone and facilitate its absorption. Absorption will be poor if it is applied at night. If it is to be applied twice a day, the evening application should be at least 3–4 hours before bedtime.

  Progesterone combinations:
  - *Progesterone + E2*: No role except in long protocol where it may improve implantation.[27]
  - *Progesterone + Ascorbic acid*: No role.[28]
  - *Progesterone + Prednisolone*: No role.[29]
  - *Progesterone + Aspirin*: No role.[30]
  - Prednisolone and aspirin might have role in recurrent IVF failures.

- ***Synthetic progesterones:*** Dydrogesterone is the drug which is available since 60 years. In spite of that much, RCTs are not available in literature. Formerly drug was marketed for its use in recurrent pregnancy loss (RPL) and early pregnancy loss. But since last few years, few workers have tried and documented it for luteal phase support.

Former studies by Fatemi et al.[31] documented that all oral progesterones including dydrogesterone do not give "in phase" endometrium, when used as luteal phase support. Other trials also advocated vaginal progesterone for better pregnancy rates, when compared with oral progesterones.

But recently LOTUS I and LOTUS II trial compared dydrogesterone 30 mg with 600 mg vaginal progesterone or 8% micronized vaginal progesterone (MVP) gel. In these studies, the pregnancy rates and the live birth rates were the same.[32,33]

Infant safety data are similar in these studies and maternal safety profile is also normal with both the drugs. It is recommended as the drug can be taken orally.

LOTUS are the only trials available at present and are supported by the pharma.[32,33] Though this drug is available since many years, very few studies are available. More RCTs are required for further research that can give the correct idea about the role of this drug in luteal support. As mentioned earlier, these studies have compared the effect of dydrogesterone with 600 mg of MVP, but in most ART clinics, the dose of MVP used is 800–1,200 mg/day. So, studies with higher dose of MVP are recommended. Most centers do not use dydrogesterone alone as luteal support in ART cycles. It is used in combination with other progesterone supplement. Therefore, its efficacy cannot be clearly established. There better planned and larger studies are required to evaluate the effect of dydrogesterone as luteal phase support.

Two Indian studies compared 20 mg and 30 mg of dydrogesterone with 600 mg of MVP and claimed superiority of dydrogesterone in 2005 and 2007.[34,35] But these were single-center studies and to prove the efficacy of the drug, larger multicentric studies are required.

Study by Fatemi et al.[36] concluded that dydrogesterone has not proved its efficacy in absence of endogenous progesterone and therefore in presence of endogenous progesterone (as in natural cycle), the efficacy of dydrogesterone is difficult to establish. In frozen embryo transfer (FET) cycles, effect of dydrogesterone is not much studied. As mentioned earlier also, in these cases, dydrogesterone is used with other progesterone also since endogenous progesterone is absent.

The European Society for Human Reproduction and Embryology (ESHRE) 2017 guidelines also are for RPL and not for lipopolysaccharide (LPS). So, though LOTUS trial shows promising results for dydrogesterone for LPS, further larger and independent trials are required.

B. **Human chorionic gonadotropin supplementation:** In a normo-ovulatory female, in unstimulated cycle, administration of hCG in luteal phase does not downregulate LH secretion in luteal phase.[37] It stimulates theca lutein cells to produce more progesterone and other steroids that are required for the maintenance of normal pregnancy. hCG also increases the placental protein 4 and relaxin that are required for implantation. It is administered every 3–4 days. It is given in the dosage of 2,000 IU on days 3, 7, and 10 or 5,000 IU on days 5–9 postovulatory. It is an excellent drug in non-in vitro fertilization (IVF) patients and in poor responders in IVF also. But if the pretrigger E2 is >1,600 IU in intrauterine insemination (IUI) cycle and >4,000 IU in IVF cycle, hCG is not given as a trigger for the risk of ovarian hyperstimulation syndrome (OHSS). In these cases, agonist is given as a trigger. In these cases, hCG 1,500 IU is given at the time of IUI or at the time of ovum pick-up (OPU) to rescue the CL, if the number of follicles are not >25 and >11 mm in diameter. It gives equal pregnancy rates as hCG triggers and avoids OHSS.[38,39]

It can be used safely even in IVF cycles, especially in poor responders. But now since antagonist can be used to suppress LH surge and agonist can be used for ovulation trigger, hCG in these patients can be used in the dose of 1,500 IU every fourth day as a luteal phase support.

Disadvantages of human chorionic gonadotropin: It should not be given when E2 is >1,600 pg/mL in IUI cycles and >4,000 pg/mL in IVF cycles because of development of OHSS and multiple pregnancies. When there are more follicles, it will increase E2 and may change E2:Progesterone which may decrease implantation but this is only theoretical assumption. Even the low dose of hCG as 1,500 IU is given, every 3 days after agonist trigger, can cause OHSS.[38]

Prolonged hCG exposure in proliferative phase may affect endometrial receptivity.[40] During natural menstrual cycle, LH in luteal phase seldom exceeds 5–10 IU/mL, which is capable of eliciting progesterone level in excess of 25–35 nmol/L. So, supraphysiological levels of LH/hCG are not required in luteal phase. Endogenous progesterone is very high due to multiple corpus lutea and exogenous progesterone results in concentration of <75 nmol/L only.

Microdose supplement 100–150 IU/day of hCG throughout the luteal phase without using any exogenous progesterone is sufficient. The progesterone level, thus, achieved is similar to that achieved when ovulation trigger is given by 6,500 IU hCG and progesterone support. When this microdose hCG is used with agonist trigger, hCG levels remains within physiological limits, i.e., 5–10 IU/mL. The only difficulty is the delivery of microdose.[41]

When to Use Luteal Support?

- Natural cycle
- Clomiphene citrate (CC)

- Letrozole
- Gonadotropin stimulation
- Human chorionic gonadotropin trigger
- Gonadotropin-releasing hormone antagonist protocol
- Gonadotropin-releasing hormone agonist trigger.

These are the clinical situations when luteal support is used. Let us now evaluate the role of luteal support in each particular situation and also understand why this support is required.

- *Luteal support in natural cycle:* In natural cycle when follicle develops, E2 is >150 pgm/mL/follicle. This E2 is sufficient to develop progesterone receptors and to cause positive feedback for LH release. This high LH lasts for >48 hours and is enough to rescue the corpus luteal function. These FSH and LH surge last for about 48 hours. The LH surge has short ascending phase of 14 hours, a peak plateau of 20 hours, and descending phase of 20 hours. This LH surge is sufficient to maintain luteal phase and so routine use of progesterone in luteal phase is not justified in natural unstimulated cycles.[1] So, routine use of progesterone is not justified in natural cycle. Progesterone is, therefore, not routinely started after spontaneous rupture of the follicle.

  The cause of LPD in natural non-ART cycles is abnormal folliculogenesis. Unhealthy follicle that produces less E2, leading to less progesterone receptors and lower peak of LH. This lower LH peak will give unhealthy CL and low progesterone levels. LH surge has short ascending limb of 14 hours, a peak plateau of 20 years, and descending phase of 20 hours. This LH surge is sufficient to maintain luteal phase and so routine use of progesterone is not justified in natural cycle.[1] The clinical situations when LH surge is inadequate:

  - Hypoprolactinemia
  - Extremes of age
  - Stress
  - Polycystic ovary syndrome (PCOS)
  - Endometriosis
  - Obesity
  - Anorexia
  - Athletes
  - Postpartum
  - Infections.

  Hypothalamic-pituitary dysfunction disturbs GnRH pulsatility, which in turn disturbs FSH and LH secretion which leads to abnormal folliculogenesis and LPD. So, all these patients require ovulation induction to improve quality of the follicle.

- *Luteal phase support with CC:* CC acts on hypothalamus and pituitary to secrete FSH and LH that leads to development of follicles and secretes more estrogen. High estrogen causes upregulation of LH and progesterone receptors. Therefore, in clomiphene-stimulated cycles, LPD is not common. In spite of estrogen receptors being occupied by CC, multiple follicles develop and there is no abnormality of LH or progesterone secretion because of high E2 level. LPD found in CC cycle is due to high LH, particularly in PCOS patients, that is detrimental to ovum leading to abnormal folliculogenesis and is responsible for LPD. Adding estrogen to CC is not proved to improve the pregnancy rate. So, luteal phase support is not justified in CC cycles.
- *Luteal phase support in letrozole-stimulated cycle:* Letrozole prevents aromatization of androgen to estrogen leading to estrogen deficiency. This E2 deficiency has negative feedback to pituitary causing release of FSH and LH which develops follicle. E2 from developed follicle goes to pituitary and decreases FSH and LH to give monofollicular development. This decrease in LH may cause LPD and decrease in E2 may lead to poor development of progesterone receptors. Therefore, when letrozole is used for ovulation induction, luteal phase support is indicated, though sufficient literature on the same is still not available. Luteal phase support with vaginal progesterone increases clinical pregnancy rate in women with PCOS using letrozole for ovulation induction.[42]
- *Luteal phase support in gonadotropin-stimulated cycles:* Exogenous gonadotropins affect the ovaries to produce more E2. This leads to negative feedback to hypothalamic-pituitary-ovarian (HPO) axis and may lead to abnormal LH pulsatility and abnormal progesterone secretion from CL.[43] Though progesterone is important for pregnancy, elevated progesterone level, on the day of trigger, affects pregnancy rates adversely. Progesterone level of 1.5 ng/mL is a threshold for poor ovarian responders, >1.75 ng/mL is associated with low ongoing pregnancy rates for intermediate responders and 2.25 ng/mL can be applied for high responders.[44] This progesterone level is elevated in superovulated cycles as each mature follicle secretes a trace of progesterone. Endometrium is exposed to progesterone before hCG injection leads to decreased endometrial receptivity.[45] A systematic review and meta-analysis suggest that luteal phase support improved the likelihood of clinical pregnancy and live birth in gonadotropin-stimulated IUI cycles.[46]

It is an established fact that luteal phase is defective in all stimulated cycles.[38] In controlled ovarian stimulation, there are multiple follicles which grow giving supraphysiological levels of E2 and progesterone which inhibit LH secretion by the pituitary by negative feedback at hypothalamic-pituitary axis level for LH release which causes early demise of CL and fall in progesterone level.[47] Moreover, antagonist has already suppressed LH in follicular phase and therefore endogenous LH is very low. Adequate LH is important for maintenance of CL. So, luteal phase support is required in all the patients when antagonist is used. Endogenous LH is also important for secretion of other growth factors and cytokines and leukemia inhibitory factor (LIF) for implantation. Exogenous hCG helps to rescue CL. In gonadotropin stimulation, there is advancement of histology in late proliferative phase, earlier shift into implantation window, and asynchrony if the maturation of mid- and late luteal phase due to high E2, i.e., altered E2/P ratio.[48] So, in all gonadotropin-stimulated cycles, luteal phase support is mandatory.

- *Luteal phase support with human chorionic gonadotropin trigger:* In follicular phase, LH is low because of agonist or antagonist as well as high E2 and progesterone giving negative feedback to pituitary for LH. However, early luteal phase function of LH is covered by bolus of hCG (5,000–10,000 IU), which is routinely used for trigger. Normally, 500 IU of hCG is required for completion of meiosis and 9,500 IU of hCG is required for follicular rupture. Therefore, in IUI cycles, usually 10,000 IU of hCG is given. But this dose may be too large for ART cycles. But this large dose takes care of the CL in the early luteal phase and maintains progesterone secretion from CL. hCG also secures growth factors and cytokines for implantation. The hCG supports CL only for 5 days and the embryo starts producing hCG after 8th day after ovulation that will again support the CL. So, from 5th till 8th day, CL is not supported and there is progesterone deficiency and is known as "luteal gap" and leads to implantation failure or early abortions.[49]

  After Day 5, endogenous LH levels are also low due to high surrogate LH and high progesterone.[50] It is crucial to have certain amplitude and frequency of LH during the luteal phase. Progesterone supplement is, therefore, essential for the luteal phase support when hCG trigger is given.[51]
- *Luteal phase support when using antagonist:* Antagonist in IUI cycles is started from the day when the lead follicle reaches 14 mm. It suppresses the LH level temporarily before ovulation trigger.

  It was formerly believed that antagonist cycles do not require luteal phase support and so lots of pregnancies were wasted. But then it was understood that suppression of LH by antagonist also continues in the luteal phase and it reduces luteal phase length and compromises pregnancy rate.

  Antagonist downregulation decreases the risk of OHSS and does allow the use of agonist as a trigger, thus almost abolishing the risk of OHSS.
- *Gonadotropin-releasing hormone agonist trigger and luteal phase support:* GnRHa trigger is preferred to hCG trigger when:
  - There is a risk of OHSS
  - When preimplantation genetic diagnosis (PGD)/preimplantation genetic screening (PGS) is to be done

- In donor cycles
- When fresh transfers are not to be done.

Gonadotropin-releasing hormone agonist causes FSH and LH surge while hCG causes only LH surge. FSH surge is a must in animals for completion of meiosis of the ovum and rupture of the follicle, but its role in human being is yet fully understood. LH surge that occurs after GnRHa trigger completes meiosis but is inadequate for the luteal support and thus leads to LPD. LH surge that occurs after GnRHa has only 4 hours of ascending limb and 14 hours of descending limb whereas the natural LH surge has an ascending limb of 14 hours, plateau of 20 hours, and descending limb of 20 hours. This gap between the two cannot be bridged by increasing the dose of GnRHa as the defect is because of low LH. The normal progesterone level on ovulation + Day 5 of 11 ng/mL was only achieved after 600 mg/day of exogenous progesterone which indicates complete luteal phase insufficiency after agonist trigger.

Strategies for supporting luteal phase after GnRHa trigger:

1. Exogenous E2 + Progesterone support with close monitoring
2. *Dual trigger*: Agonist + hCG (1,000–2,500 IU)
3. Low-dose hCG in luteal phase
4. Luteal phase LH administration.

1. *Intensive luteal support*: Intramuscular (IM) progesterone 25–75 mg/day or micronized progesterone 800 mg/day vaginally with E2 patch 0.1 mg, 3–4 mg, on alternate days, or 2–8 mg with oral E2 valerate is given. Adjust the dose to keep serum E2 level above 2,000 pgm/mL and progesterone level 20 ng/mL by frequent testing. The results are similar to those of hCG trigger and progesterone support.[52]
2. *Dual trigger: Agonist + hCG (1,000–2,500 IU)*: Along with GnRHa trigger, hCG 1,000–2,500 IU is added for rescuing CL by providing additional signal for adequate luteinization. It has given pregnancy rate up to 53% with one case of OHSS.[53] If serum E2 is <4,000 pgm/mL, GnRHa trigger with 1,000–2,500 IU of hCG gives pregnancy rates as high as 53% with almost no risk of OHSS.

   So, hCG at the time of ovulation trigger gives excellent pregnancy rates with very low OHSS risk. The other advantage of dual trigger is that sometimes LH peak may not be sufficient with agonist trigger and if it is <9 IU/mL, meiosis may not occur and an ovum pick-up no ova will be retrieved, as it may occur in empty follicle syndrome. Adding low-dose hCG with agonist assures meiosis and is, therefore, preferred compared to low-dose hCG at the time of ovum pick-up.
3. *Human chorionic gonadotropin at the time of IUI*: When pretrigger E2 is <1,600 pgm/mL or when there are <25 follicles of >11 mm in diameter, hCG 1,500 IU is given at the time of IUI to rescue the CL and

achieve comparable pregnancy rates to hCG trigger. Second bolus is not given as it may increase the risk of OHSS.[38]

So, modified luteal phase support may be GnRHa trigger, hCG 1,500 IU after IUI, vaginal micronized progesterone 400 mg BD, and E2 2 mg BD supplementation. This regimen reduces OHSS, gives equal live birth rates.[38]

4. *Low-dose beta-hCG*: 100–150 IU hCG as luteal support is enough to rescue the CL and produces sufficient progesterone for adequate luteal support.[54] In the same paper, it has also been mentioned that it causes blood levels of progesterone as high as 10–15 IU/L, which is sufficient for mid-luteal phase and is similar to 6,500 IU of hCG for ovulation trigger and vaginal progesterone, but delivery of this small dose of hCG is difficult at present. This might prove to be a choice of luteal phase support if hCG becomes available in pen device.

   Recombinant LH: It is very useful as it lowers the incidence of OHSS for fresh cycle transfer, but it is very expensive and therefore its usage is not accepted in clinical practice.

PROGESTERONE RESISTANCE

- Endometriosis
- Polycystic ovary syndrome with androgen elevation.

Progesterone resistance is because of inhibitor progesterone receptor A (PRA) isoform and the absence of the stimulation isoform progesterone receptor B (PRB).[55] There is pituitary ovarian dysfunction.[56] This is because of impaired follicular growth giving low FSH and LH because of low E2 and causing LPD. It causes abnormal expression of endometrial biomarkers of implantation,[57] but this is a controversial issue. In case of progesterone resistance, luteal support will not be efficient until the resistance is removed. So, before initiating the treatment, progesterone resistance must be corrected. In endometriosis, ART outcome was improved by 3–6 months of ovarian suppression by GnRHa.[58] Recently, it has been shown that 6–8 weeks with oral contraceptive (OC) pills normalized implantation and pregnancy rates in women suffering from endometriosis.[59] It is doubtful if similar treatment is helpful in PCOS. This is because of androgen excess. OC pills lower the LH and in turn androgen. Whether higher levels of progesterone can counter progesterone resistance or not, it is also not proved.

ONSET OF LUTEAL SUPPORT

Progesterone started on the day of IUI decreases uterine contractility rather than started late. Uterine contractility was higher 4 days after hCG administration than the natural cycle LH surge. Higher E2 level increases uterine contractility and this high E2 causes uterine resistance to the uterine relaxing property of progesterone.[60] The vaginal progesterone causes selective tissue concentration in the uterus through direct transport. Increased E2 is because of high androgen secreted from theca cells, where granulosa cells convert it into estrogen. So, progesterone being an intermediate product, it is always high whenever E2 is high in proliferative phase. So, even normal progesterone level will appear early and initiate premature secretory changes. This leads to advancement of endometrium.

Vaginal progesterone, if it is delayed for a day or two, gives good results as compared to IM progesterone which is given on the day of IUI. So, the route of administration is also important along with the starting day of the luteal support.[26]

DURATION OF LUTEAL SUPPORT

Prospective RCT[61] indicated that prolongation of progesterone supplementation in early pregnancy had no influence on miscarriage rate. Theoretically, we can stop progesterone support once beta-hCG is positive, but most of the practitioners continue till 10–12 weeks of pregnancy. Caspo et al. have shown that continuation of pregnancy is independent of CL function as early as 8–10 weeks of pregnancy.[62] The function is taken over by placenta.[63] The study by Kohls G et al. has shown that vaginal progesterone supplementation after IUI can be safely withdrawn at 5 weeks of gestation because cycle outcome was similar to conventional luteal support that is given till 8 weeks of gestation. At 5 weeks, hCG level is >1,000 IU/L and that is sufficient to support CL beyond doubt. The circulating level of progesterone is >8 ng/mL at 5 weeks of pregnancy. But in FET cycle, it is continued till the luteo-placental shift, i.e., 9–10 weeks of pregnancy.

Carry Home Message

- Luteal phase defect is because of low progesterone or suboptimal response with normal progesterone.
- Low progesterone may be due to abnormal folliculogenesis in non-IVF patients.
- Low LH is mainly responsible for LPD in IVF cycles.
- No laboratory tests are reliable for diagnosis of LPD.
- Corpus luteum rescue is because of hCG.
- Low progesterone is because of low hCG in unhealthy embryo.
- Duration of exposure of progesterone is important than blood levels.
- Ovulation induction is a very useful luteal support.
- Human chorionic gonadotropin is also an effective luteal support. About 100–150 IU of hCG may prove to be good alternative to luteal support.
- Micronized progesterone is the best.

Contd...

Contd...

- Vaginal route is the best route.
- Subcutaneous route has replaced IM route.
- Luteal support in natural cycle is not justified.
- Progesterone support in CC cycle is not of much benefit.
- Progesterone support is required in letrozole-stimulated cycle.
- Dydrogesterone and SR tablets are under trial and have shown good results.
- All superovulated cycles require luteal support.
- Antagonist cycles cause LPD.
- With GnRHa trigger, luteal support is always required.
- Judicious use of E2 + Progesterone, dual trigger or 1,500 IU of hCG at the time of IUI are remedies to avoid OHSS.
- Estradiol supplementation is given for LPS in agonist trigger.
- Endometriosis and PCOS have progesterone resistance.
- Luteal support should not be started later than 3 days after IUI.
- Duration of progesterone after positive beta-hCG is controversial.

REFERENCES

1. Speroff L, Fritz MA. Clinical Gynecologic Endocrinology and Infertility, 7th edition. Philadelphia: Lippincott Williams and Wilkins; 2005. pp. 199-242.
2. Niswender GD, Juengel JL, Silva PJ, Rollyson MK, McIntush EW. Mechanisms controlling the function and lifespan of the corpus luteum. Physiol Rev. 2000;80:1-29.
3. Hinney B, Henze C, Kuhn W, Wuttke W. The corpus luteum insufficiency: a multifactorial disease. J Clin Endocrinol Metab. 1996;81:565-70.
4. Kiriakidou M, McAllister JM, Sugawara T, Strauss JF. Expression of steroidogenic acute regulatory protein (StAR) in the human ovary. J Clin Endocrinol Metab. 1996;814:122-8.
5. Daya S. Habitual abortion. In: Copeland LJ (Ed). Textbook of Gynecology. Philadelphia: Saunders; 2000.
6. Practice Committee of the American Society for Reproductive Medicine. The clinical relevance of luteal phase deficiency: a committee opinion. Fertil Steril. 2012;98:1112-7.
7. Jarvela IY, Ruokonen A, Tekay A. Effect of rising hCG levels in the human corpus luteum during early pregnancy. Hum Reprod. 2008;23:2275-81.
8. Balasch J, Vanrell JA. Corpus luteum insufficiency and fertility: a matter of controversy. Hum Reprod. 1987;2:557-67.
9. Jordan J, Craig K, Clifton D, Soules MR. Luteal phase defect: the sensitivity and specificity of diagnostic methods in common clinical use. Fertil Steril. 1994;62:54-62.
10. Check JH, Levin E, Bollendorf A, Locuniak J. Miscarriage in the first trimester according to the presence or absence of the progesterone-induced blocking factor at three to five weeks from conception in progesterone supplemented women. Clin Exp Obstet Gynecol. 2005;32:13-4.
11. Maclin VM, Radwanska E, Binor Z, Dmowski WP. Progesterone: estradiol ratios at implantation in ongoing pregnancies, abortions, and nonconception cycles resulting from ovulation induction. Fertil Steril. 1990;54:238-44.
12. De Ziegher D. Hormonal control of endometrial receptivity. Hum Reprod. 1995;10:4-7.
13. Devroey P, Braeckmans P, Camus M, Khan I, Smitz J, Staessen C, et al. Embryo donation in patients with primary ovarian failure. Hum Reprod. 1988;3:85-7.

14. De Zeigler D, Sator M, Binelli D, Leuratti C, Cometti B, Bourgain C, et al. A randomized trial comparing the endometrial effects of daily subcutaneous administration of 25 mg and 50 mg progesterone on aqueous preparation. Fertil Steril. 2013;100:860-6.
15. Lockwood G, Griesinger G, Cometti B, 13 European Centers. Subcutaneous progesterone versus vaginal progesterone gel for luteal phase support in in vitro fertilization: a noninferiority randomized controlled study. Fertil Steril. 2014;101:112-9.
16. Balasch J, Fabregues F, Ordi J, Creus M, Peñarrubia J, Casamitjana R, et al. Further data favoring the hypothesis of the uterine first-pass effect of vaginally administered micronized progesterone. Gynecol Endocrinol. 1996;10:421-6.
17. Cicinelli E, de Ziegler D. Transvaginal progesterone: evidence for a new functional 'portal system' flowing from vaginal to the uterus. Hum Reprod Update. 1999;5:365-72.
18. Cicinelli E, de Ziegler D, Morgese S, Bulletti C, Luisi D, Schonauer LM. "First uterine pass effect" is observed when estradiol is placed in the upper but not lower third of the vagina. Fertil Steril. 2004;81:1414-6.
19. Artini PG, Volpe A, Angioni S, Galassi MC, Battaglia C, Genazzani AR. A comparative, randomized study of three different progesterone support of the luteal phase following IVF/ET program. J Endocrinol Invest. 1995;18:51-6.
20. Miles R, Paulson R, Lobo R, Press MF, Dahmoush L, Sauer MV. Pharmacokinetics and endometrial tissue levels of progesterone after administration by intramuscular and vaginal routes: a comparative study. Fertil Steril. 1994;62:485-90.
21. Czajkowski K, Seinko J, Mogilinski M, Bros M, Szczenia R, Czajkowski A. Uteroplacental circulation in early pregnancy complicated by threatened abortion supplemented with vaginal micronized progesterone or oral dydrogesterone. Fertil Steril. 2007;87:613-8.
22. Abdelhakim AM, Abd-ElGawad M, Hussein RS, Abbas AM. Vaginal versus intramuscular progesterone for luteal phase support in assisted reproductive techniques: a systematic review and meta-analysis of randomized controlled trials. Gynecol Endocrinol. 2020;36:389-97.
23. Fanchin R, Righini C, Olivennes F, Taylor S, de Ziegler D, Frydman R. Uterine contractions at the time of embryo transfer alter pregnancy rates after in-vitro fertilization. Hum Reprod. 1998;13:1968-74.
24. Zegers-Hochschild F, Balmaceda JP, Fabres C, Alam V, Mackenna A, Fernández E, et al. Prospective randomized trial to evaluate the efficacy of a vaginal ring releasing progesterone for IVF and oocyte donation. Hum Reprod. 2000;15:2093-7.
25. Bergh C, Lindenberg S, Nordic Crinone Study Group. A prospective randomized, multicenter study comparing vaginal progesterone gel and vaginal micronized progesterone tablets for luteal phase support after IVF/ICSI. Hum Reprod. 2012;27:3467-73.
26. Silverberg KM, Vaughn TC, Hansard LJ, Burger NZ, Minter T. Vaginal (Crinone 8%) gel vs. intramuscular progesterone in oil for luteal phase support in in vitro fertilization: a large prospective trial. Fertil Steril. 2012;97:344-8.
27. Farhi J, Weissman A, Steinfeld Z, Shorer M, Nahum H, Levran D. Estradiol supplementation during the luteal phase may improve the pregnancy rate in patients undergoing in vitro fertilization-embryo transfer cycles. Fertil Steril. 2000;73:761-6.
28. Griesinger G, Franke K, Kinast C, Kutzelnigg A, Riedinger S, Kulin S, et al. Ascorbic acid supplement during luteal phase in IVF. J Assist Reprod Genet. 2002;19:164-8.
29. Ubaldi F, Reinzi L, Ferrero S, Anniballo R, Iacobelli M, Cobellis L, et al. Low dose prednisolone administration in routine ICSI patients does not improve pregnancy and implantation rates. Hum Reprod. 2002;17:1544-7.
30. Urman B, Mercan R, Alatas C, Balaban B, Isiklar A, Nuhoglu A. Low-dose aspirin does not increase implantation rates in patients undergoing intracytoplasmic sperm injection: a prospective randomized study. J Assist Reprod Genet. 2000;17:586-90.

31. Fatemi HM, Bourgain C, Donoso P, Blockeel C, Papanikolaou EG, Popovic-Todorovic B, et al. Effect of oral administration of dydrogestrone versus vaginal administration of natural micronized progesterone on the secretory transformation of endometrium and luteal endocrine profile in patients with premature ovarian failure: a proof of concept. Hum Reprod. 2007;22:1260-3.
32. Tournaye H, Sukhikh GT, Kahler E, Griesinger G. A Phase III randomized controlled trial comparing the efficacy, safety and tolerability of oral dydrogesterone versus micronized vaginal progesterone for luteal support in in vitro fertilization. Hum Reprod. 2017;32:1019-27.
33. Griesinger G, Blockeel C, Sukhikh GT, Patki A, Dhorepatil B, Yang DZ, et al. Oral dydrogesterone versus intravaginal micronized progesterone gel for luteal phase support in IVF: a randomized clinical trial. Hum Reprod. 2018;33:2212-21.
34. Chakravarti BN, Shirazee HH, Dam P, Goswami SK, Chatterjee R, Ghosh S. Oral dydrogesterone versus intravaginal micronized progesterone as luteal phase support in assisted reproductive technology (ART) cycles: results of randomized study. J Steroid Biochem Mol Biol. 2005;97:416-20.
35. Patki A, Pawar VC. Modulating fertility outcome in assisted reproductive technologies by the use of dydrogesterone. Gynecol Endocrinol. 2007;23:68-72.
36. Fatemi HM, Popovic-Todorovic B, Papanikolaou E, Donoso P, Devroey P. An update of luteal phase support in stimulated IVF cycles. Hum Reprod Update. 2007;13:581-90.
37. Tavaniotou A, Devroey P. Effect of human chorionic gonadotropins on luteal luteinizing hormone concentrations in natural cycles. Fertil Steril. 2003;80:654-5.
38. Humaidan P, Bredkjaer HE, Westergaard LG, Andersen CY. 1,500 IU human chorionic gonadotropin administered at oocyte retrieval rescues the luteal phase when gonadotropin-releasing hormone agonist is used for ovulation induction: a prospective, randomized, controlled study. Fertil Steril. 2010;93:847-54.
39. Kummer N, Benadiva C, Feinn R, Mann J, Nulsen J, Engmann L. Factors that predict the probability of successful clinical outcome after induction of oocyte maturation with gonadotropin-releasing hormone agonist. Fertil Steril. 2011;96:63-8.
40. Evans J, Salamonsen LA. Too much of a good thing? Experimental evidence suggests prolonged exposure to hCG is detrimental to endometrial receptivity. Hum Reprod. 2013;28:1610-9.
41. Andersen CY, Fischer R, Giorgione V, Kelsey TW. Micro-dose hCG as luteal phase support without exogenous progesterone administration: mathematical modelling of the hCG concentration in circulation and initial clinical experience. J Assist Reprod Genet. 2016;33:1311-8.
42. Montville CP, Khabba M, Aubuchon M, Williams DB, Thomas MA. Luteal support with intravaginal progesterone increases clinical pregnancy rates in women with polycystic ovary syndrome using letrozole for ovulation induction. Fertil Steril. 2010;94:678-83.
43. Tavaniotou A, Albano C, Smitz J, Devroey P. Impact of ovarian stimulation on corpus luteum function and embryonic implantation. J Reprod Immunol. 2002;55:123-30.
44. Xu B, Li Z, Zhang H, Jin L, Li Y, Ai J, et al. Serum progesterone level effects on the outcome of in vitro fertilization in patients with different ovarian response: an analysis of more than 10,000 cycles. Fertil Steril. 2012;97:1321-7.
45. Doldi N, Marsiglio E, Destefani A, Gessi A, Merati G, Ferrari A. Elevated serum progesterone on the day of HCG administration in IVF is associated with a higher pregnancy rate in polycystic ovary syndrome. Hum Reprod. 1999;14:1601-5.
46. Hill MJ, Whitcomb BW, Lewis TD, Wu M, Terry N, DeCherney AH, et al. Progesterone luteal support after ovulation induction and intrauterine insemination: a systematic review and meta-analysis. Fertil Steril. 2013;100:1373-80.
47. Fatemi HM. The luteal phase after 3 decades of IVF: what do we know? Reprod Biomed Online. 2009;19:4331.

48. Devroey P, Bourgain C, Macklon NS, Fauser BC. Reproductive biology and IVF: ovarian stimulation and endometrial receptivity. Trends Endocrinol Metab. 2004;15:84-90.
49. Humaidan P, Papanikolaou EG, Kyrou D, Alsbjerg B, Polyzos NP, Devroey P, et al. The luteal phase after GnRH-agonist triggering of ovulation: present and future perspectives. Reprod Biomed Online. 2012;24:134-41.
50. Miyake A, Aono T, Kinugasa T, Tanizawa O, Kurachi K. Suppression of serum levels of luteinizing hormone by short- and long-loop negative feedback in ovariectomized women. J Endocrinol. 1979;80:353-6.
51. van der Linden M, Buckingham K, Farquhar C, Kremer JA, Metwally M. Luteal phase support for assisted reproduction cycles. Cochrane Database Syst Rev. 2011;10:CD009154.
52. Papanikolaou EG, Verpoest W, Fatemi H, Tarlatzis B, Devroey P, Tournaye H. A novel method of luteal supplementation with recombinant luteinizing hormone when a gonadotropin-releasing hormone agonist is used instead of human chorionic gonadotropin for ovulation triggering: a randomized prospective proof of concept study. Fertil Steril. 2011;95:1174-7.
53. Fatemi HM, Kolibianakis EM, Camus M, Tournaye H, Donoso P, Papanikolaou E, et al. Addition of estradiol to progesterone for luteal supplementation in patients stimulated with GnRH antagonists/rFSH for IVF: a randomized controlled trial. Hum Reprod. 2006;21:2628-32.
54. Anderson CY, Elbaek HO, Alsbjerg B, Laursen RJ, Povisen BB, Thomsen L, et al. Daily low-dose hCG stimulation during the luteal phase combined with GnRHa combined cycles without exogenous progesterone: a proof of concept trial Hum Reprod. 2015;30:2387-95.
55. Attia GR, Zeitoun K, Edwards D, Johns A, Carr BR, Bulun SE. Progesterone receptor isoform A but not B is expressed in endometriosis. J Clin Endocrinol Metab. 2000;85:2897-902.
56. Cahill DJ, Hull MG. Pituitary-ovarian dysfunction and endometriosis. Hum Reprod Update. 2000;6:56-66.
57. Donaghay M, Lessey BA. Uterine receptivity: alterations associated with benign gynecological disease. Semin Reprod Med. 2007;25:461-75.
58. Surrey ES, Silverberg KM, Surrey MW, Schoolcraft WB. Effect of prolonged gonadotropin-releasing hormone agonist therapy on the outcome of in vitro fertilization-embryo transfer in patients with endometriosis. Fertil Steril. 2002;78:699-704.
59. de Ziegler D, Gayet V, Aubriot FX, Fauque P, Streuli I, Wolf JP, et al. Use of oral contraceptives in women with endometriosis before assisted reproduction treatment improves outcomes. Fertil Steril. 2010;94:2796-9.
60. Ayoubi JM, Epiney M, Brioschi PA, Fanchin R, Chardonnens D, de Ziegler D. Comparison of changes in uterine contraction frequency after ovulation in the menstrual cycle and in in vitro fertilization cycles. Fertil Steril. 2003;79:1101-5.
61. Andersen AN, Popovic-Todorovic B, Schmidt KT, Loft A, Lindhard A, Højgaard A, et al. Progesterone supplementation during early gestations after IVF and ICSI has no effect on the delivery rates: a randomized controlled trial. Hum Reprod. 2002;17:357-61.
62. Caspo AI, Pulkkinen MO, Wiest WG. Effects of lutectomy and progesterone replacement therapy in early pregnant patients. Am J Obstet Gynecol. 1973;115:759-65.
63. Schmidt KL, Ziebe S, Popovic B, Lindhard A, Loft A, Andersen AN. Progesterone supplementation during early gestation after in vitro fertilization has no effect on delivery rate. Fertil Steril. 2001;75:337-41.

CHAPTER 9

Ovulation Induction in PCOS

Chaitanya Nagori

INTRODUCTION

Polycystic ovarian syndrome (PCOS) is a common cause of dysovulatory infertility. Ovulation induction is the treatment of choice for dysovulatory infertility. But ovulation induction in patients with PCOS is very different and tricky. Low doses of gonadotropins often do not work and higher doses carries a very high risk of ovarian hyperstimulation syndrome (OHSS). The tact of dealing with this problem, what drugs to be used, what doses can be safe and effective to get success in infertility treatment for these patients are discussed in this chapter.

PRINCIPLES OF TREATMENT

Ovulation induction in polycystic ovary syndrome (PCOS) requires careful assessment of patient and specific therapy to induce ovulation and decrease luteinizing hormone (LH) that is detrimental to ova. Reduction in circulating insulin is also required in some patients to get better ovulation.

TREATMENT MODALITIES IN POLYCYSTIC OVARY SYNDROME

- Weight loss
- Clomiphene citrate
- Letrozole
- Insulin-lowering drugs
- Glucocorticoids
- Gonadotropins
- Gonadotropin-releasing hormone (GnRH) antagonist
- GnRH agonist
- Ovarian drilling
- In vitro fertilization/in vitro maturation (IVF/IVM)

Weight Loss

It is always the first line of treatment. Central obesity is more common to cause metabolic changes. In PCOS, waist : hip ratio is 0.7–0.8 (android type).

- *Body mass index (BMI)*:
    - *Normal:* 20–24.9 kg/m^2

- *Overweight:* 25–29 kg/m^2
- *Obese:* >30 kg/m^2

Loss of intra-abdominal fat is required for improvement of insulin resistance, decrease in androgen levels, and resumption of ovulation. During the initial period of calorie restriction, preferential loss of intra-abdominal fat occurs due to increased lipolysis and its high metabolic activity.[1,2]

About 5–10% of weight loss is important to induce ovulation. It reduces 30% of visceral fat; this regains reproductive functions in 60–100% of cases. The treatment for weight loss includes diet, exercise, group therapy, behavioral counseling, pharmacological treatment, and bariatric surgery. So it is a team work that is required to help the patient to lose weight.

European Society of Human Reproduction and Embryology-American Society for Reproductive Medicine (ESHRE-ASRM) recommendation 2018:

- Antiobesity agents are only under experiment for improving fertility.
- Bariatric surgery should also be considered as experimental.

Clomiphene Citrate

Clomiphene citrate (CC) induces ovulation in 70–80% of cases with 30–40% pregnancy rate and gives 30% cumulative live birth rate. The main advantage is that 70–80% of patients conceive in three cycles. Pregnancy rates are the same whether CC is started on day 2-3-4-5. The dose of >150 mg has only 10% pregnancy rates. Clomiphene citrate acts on hypothalamus to secrete GnRH, which in turn gives follicle-stimulating hormone (FSH) and LH. In PCOS patients, LH is otherwise also high. Therefore CC is continued after first cycle only if on Day 8–9 of the cycle, LH is <10 IU in the first CC cycle. This is because high LH reduces the conception rate and increases the abortion rate.

The ESHRE-ASRM recommendation 2018:

- CC has a lower pregnancy rate than letrozole. CC is not on the list of ovulation induction drugs of choice for PCOS patients.
- Gonadotropins have significantly higher pregnancy rate than CC.
- Two randomized controlled trials (RCTs) concluded that CC+ gonadotropins do not have higher pregnancy rate than either alone.
- CC can be used in obese patients (BMI >30 kg/m^2) with anovulatory infertility.
- Metformin can be added in CC resistant cases.

Letrozole

This is a very good alternative to CC. It causes hypoestrinism and hyperandrogenism. Because of fall in estrogen levels, it leads to rise in FSH and LH levels that stimulates follicular development. The resultant rise in estrogen has negative feedback mechanism, and it reduces FSH and LH thus allowing monofollicular development. Hyperandrogenism caused by letrozole increases the sensitivity of the follicle to FSH. Therefore letrozole with gonadotropins is a synergistic combination.

There are several reports which indicate that letrozole is better than CC for ovulation induction in PCOS,[3,4] and some reports that have shown that letrozole is at least as effective as CC for ovulation induction.[5,6]

All-in-all, the advantages of letrozole are monofollicular development, lesser incidence of multiple pregnancy, lesser risk of ovarian hyperstimulation syndrome (OHSS), and lower abortion rates due to fall in LH levels.

The ESHRE-ASRM recommendation 2018:

- Letrozole should be considered as the first-line treatment for ovulation induction in women with PCOS with anovulatory infertility alone to improve ovulation rate, conception rate, and live-birth rate.
- Likelihood of live birth is increased by 40–60% with letrozole compared to clomiphene.
- Letrozole resistance is less than CC resistance.

Insulin Lowering Drugs

Insulin resistance in PCOS patients causes hyperinsulinemia, which in turn stimulates theca cells of the ovary to secret more androgen. Hyperinsulinemia in women with obesity contributes to anovulation by increased ovarian androgen secretion.[7] More than 50–80% of PCOS patients have insulin resistance.

Earlier metformin was thought to be a useful drug for ovulation induction in PCOS patients. But recent reports indicate that when metformin is used as the only drug for ovulation induction in PCOS patients the live birth rate is only 7.2% as compared to that with CC which is 22.5%.[8] So metformin is as good as placebo in terms of pregnancy rates and abortion rates as a drug for ovulation induction.

It has also been proved that metformin does not lower the dose of CC required when it is used in combination with CC. It is interesting to know that efficacy of metformin is not dose dependent, but side effects are. Therefore metformin should be preferred in lowest possible doses.[9]

Findings of two RCTs indicated that metformin does not increase live birth rates above those observed with CC alone.[10]

The ESHRE-ASRM recommendations 2018:

- Metformin alone does not give good pregnancy rates.
- It is added in CC resistant cases.
- It reduces the risk of OHSS.

The ESHRE/ASRM 2007 consensus:

- There is no clear evidence that addition of metformin to CC as a primary therapy for induction of ovulation has a beneficial effect.[11]
- Use of metformin in PCOS should be restricted to women with glucose intolerance and frank type II diabetes.[12]

Metformin + Gonadotropins

Addition of metformin to gonadotropins has no advantage in improving ovulation rates, pregnancy rates, live birth rates, multiple pregnancy rates or incidence of OHSS.[13,14] But recommendations favor addition of metformin for improving clinical pregnancy rate but not live birth rates.

Metformin in IVF: There are several papers that indicate no difference in metformin and non-metformin group in pregnancy rate in IVF patients.[14,15] In patients with PCOS and poor ovarian reserve, metformin worsened the response to gonadotropins, and it should be stopped before starting controlled ovarian hyperstimulation for IVF.[16]

In a meta-analysis that evaluated the effectiveness of metformin as a cotreatment during IVF cycles in women with PCOS, metformin reduced the risk of OHSS by approximately 75%.[17] Another study also confirms that in patients with PCOS, who are at a high risk for OHSS and who have been stimulated with gonadotropins for IVF cycles, metformin reduces the risk of OHSS by modulating the ovarian response to stimulation.[18] A study by Kjotrod et al. concludes that metformin treatment for 12 weeks before and during IVF or intracytoplasmic sperm injection (ICSI) in nonobese women with PCOS significantly increases pregnancy and live birth rates compared to placebo.[19]

Metformin after conception: Safety of metformin in pregnancy has not been established. A large prospective RCT has shown that when metformin is continued in early pregnancy, it does not decrease the miscarriage rate.[6] Indirect data from a recent meta-analysis has shown no significant benefit of pregestational metformin administration on abortion risk in patients with PCOS, when either used as monotherapy or in combination with other fertility drugs.[20] Metformin crosses the placenta and significant level is found in fetal serum. Therefore metformin should be stopped after the pregnancy test until more consistent data are available.

Metformin for young patients with PCOS have a long timeline to achieve pregnancy. It is a drug of choice in PCOS patients who do not want to conceive immediately. Its action is gradual and within 6 months it establishes ovulatory cycles by decreasing insulin and androgen level. Other advantage of metformin is that it decreases the incidence of multiple pregnancies with ovulation induction drugs. If the patient does not conceive when on metformin, option of CC remains open for her. A recent meta-analysis revealed that metformin does not result in weight loss among overweight and obese PCOS patients.[12]

Metformin alternatives: Insulin sensitizers, pioglitazone and rosiglitazone and other drugs such as acarbose or D-chiroinositol have not found to be superior over metformin and so their routine use for infertile patient has not been established for ovulation induction and is considered as experimental according to ASRM recommendations.

Addition of metformin to lifestyle had no significant benefit on ovulation and circulating androgen levels.[21]

Clomiphene Citrate + Glucocorticoids

About 50% of PCOS patients have adrenal component in hyperandrogenism and evidence by increased dehydroepiandrosterone sulfate (DHEAS) which is entirely from zona reticularis of adrenal cortex. These are the patients who are resistant to 150 mg of CC and require higher doses of gonadotropins. They respond well to dexamethasone 0.5 mg daily for 3–6 months along with CC. Water logging because of the drug can be reduced by adding diuretics once a week or decreasing the dose of dexamethasone to 0.25 mg or one may also discontinue the drug after ovulation. Serious complications are extremely rare and so this drug must be tried in obese PCOS.

Gonadotropins

Gonadotropins are indicated in patients with CC failure with high LH and having antiestrogenic effect of CC.

Specific Bioactivity of Gonadotropins (Table 1)

The bioactivity of highly purified urinary FSH (uFSH-HP) and recombinant FSH (rFSH) is always higher than other preparations, and dose required will be also less of these preparations. rFSH has advantages over uFSH. These are as follows:

- FSH inhibiting substances are absent in rFSH
- rFSH has more basic isoforms
- rFSH has higher consistency
- rFSH has only 10% degenerated forms
- rFSH has less batch-to-batch variations
- rFSH will be released on basis of mass

Table 1: Specific bioactivity of gonadotropins.

hMG (1950)	8 IU/mg of protein
uFSH (1980)	100–150 IU/mg of protein
uhMG-HP	2,000 IU/mg of protein
uFSH-HP (1982)	9,000 IU/mg of protein
rFSH (1995)	10,000 IU/mg of protein

(hMG: human menopausal gonadotropin; HP: highly purified; rFSH: recombinant follicle-stimulating hormone; uFSH: urinary follicle-stimulating hormone; uhMG: urinary hMG)

- rFSH needs lower dosage
- rFSH gives more embryos and allows cryopreservation which increases the cumulative pregnancy rate
- rFSH can be self-administered subcutaneously.

Recombinant Follicle-stimulating Hormone versus Human Menopausal Gonadotropin

Meta-analysis of eight RCTs conforming rFSH with hMG has shown that rFSH has 50% higher pregnancy rates.[22]

The FINVAT report 1999 also showed that the pregnancy rates were higher with rFSH than with hMG. The prospective study of 24,000 assisted reproductive technology (ART) cycles from Germany also showed higher birth rate and lower dosage with rFSH than hMG.[23]

Chronic Low-dose Protocol

Chronic low-dose protocol is the preferred one in PCOS patients. The incidence of OHSS is reduced from 4.6 to 1% and multiple pregnancy rate is reduced to 5.7% as compared to 22–34%. Monoovulatory cycle rate of 70% is achieved with rFSH with chronic low dose protocol.[24]

In chronic low-dose protocol from fifth day 37.5–75 IU of rFSH is started from Day 5 of the cycle, though what should be the initial dose can be better decided by baseline scan as discussed in the Chapter 16. The same dose is continued for 14 days. Though ovulation monitoring is done during this period and in most of the cases a mature follicle develops within these 14 days. If it does not, then the dose of gonadotropin is increased by half of the initial dose for another 7 days. If after that the follicle does not develop again half of the original initial dose is increased. Remember each increment in dose is half the initial dose and one has to wait for 7 days for the follicle to develop with the same dose. This protocol gives monofollicular development and therefore higher pregnancy rates.

Professor Roy Homburg and Collin Howles published a study in 2005 that showed a clear superiority of low-dose FSH over CC for treating anovulatory patients with PCOS. In first cycle, pregnancy rates are 30% with rFSH as compared to 14% with CC, and in second cycle it is 50% with rFSH as compared to 32% with CC.[25]

We have found a combination of Letrozole with rFSH very useful. It is cost-effective as it reduced the consumption of rFSH and also gives monofollicular development. Letrozole is given from Day 3-7 and rFSH is started from Day 8. This regimen decreases the incidence of OHSS and multiple pregnancies with comparable results as those of rFSH alone.

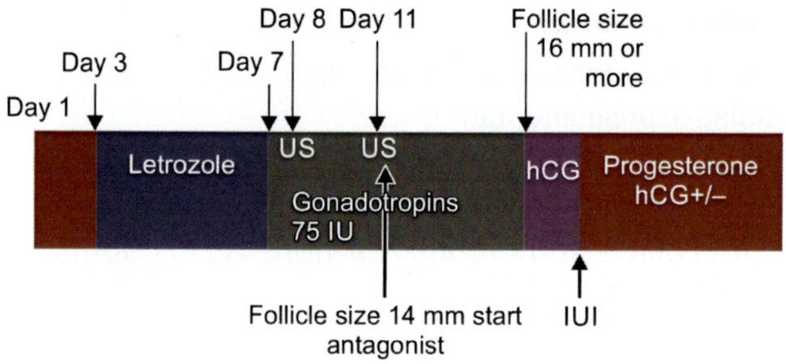

Fig. 1: Antagonist protocol for PCOS (hCG: human chorionic gonadotropin; IUI: intrauterine insemination; PCOS: polycystic ovary syndrome; US: ultrasound).

The ESHRE-ASRM recommendations:

- Gonadotropins are second line of treatment in PCOS after letrozole.
- Gonadotropins can be considered as first line of treatment after counseling as it has very high pregnancy rates.
- These are better than CC + metformin for improving ovulation rate, pregnancy rate, and live birth rate.
- Metformin can be added to gonadotropins to improve ovulation.
- Ovarian drilling should be offered as an alternative before starting gonadotropins after proper counseling of benefits and risks.
- Low dose gonadotropins give monofollicular development.

Gonadotropin Antagonist Protocol (Fig. 1)

Gonadotropin antagonist has a definite place in PCOS patients. In PCOS patients, there is a tonic rise of LH, particularly in thin lean PCOS patients. There is always a possibility of premature LH surge because of high estrogen levels. Therefore antagonist is started when at least one follicle has grown to 14 mm, to prevent LH surge and is continued till follicle matures, i.e., the day of ovulation trigger. Antagonist also helps in correct timing of intrauterine insemination (IUI). But remember antagonist is not to be added when not required, it then causes damage rather than improvement of the developing follicle.

Case Study

- A case of 8 years infertility
- 24 IUI and two IVF failures elsewhere
- Two cycles of rFSH + IUI failure at our center
- Third cycle

Day	*Drug*	*Follicle*	*Endometrium*
09	rFSH	11.5, 11.8	4.5
11	rFSH + anta	14.5, 13.8	6.0B
13	Anta + hCG	18.3, 17.5	7.5B

Gonadotropin Agonist

Gonadotropin is very useful as ovulation trigger in PCOS patients. The main advantage is that the duration of action is shorter than hCG, and therefore leads to lesser rise in estradiol (E2) and progesterone levels and therefore gives better implantation rates and chances of OHSS is also reduced. But whenever agonist is used as trigger, luteal support is mandatory. Luteal support with 1,500 IU hCG, every third day can be used[26] along with progesterone if number of follicles grown are not more than 2–3 on both the sides.

Antagonist + Agonist Protocol

- In PCOS patients, GnRH antagonist is used to prevent LH surge and agonist for final oocyte maturation by triggering LH instead of using hCG.
- But agonist has 24–36 hours duration of action. It leads to lower FSH and LH resulting in luteal phase deficiency. We know that endogenous LH plays a crucial role during luteal phase.
- Therefore, luteal support with 1,500 IU hCG, every third day can be used[27] along with progesterone. If number of grown up follicles are not too many.
- The advantage of agonist as trigger is that it causes FSH and LH surge. The role of FSH surge is not known in human being but in animals it causes nuclear maturation and cumulus expansion.
- If there are multiple follicles, all embryos can be freezed and can be used next month in natural cycle.

Now in soft protocols for IVF, majority of centers use this antagonist + agonist protocol.

Ovarian Drilling

The advantage of ovarian drilling over IVF is that it induces unifollicular development without the risk of OHSS or high order multiple pregnancies[27] and its beneficial effects can last for up to 9 years.[28] Cochrane review shows that 12 months pregnancy rate after drilling and 6 months gonadotropin stimulation both have similar pregnancy rates.

It has also been quoted by Professor Roy Homburg, that spontaneous pregnancy can occur after several years of drilling. Ovarian drilling gives 70–80% of ovulation rate and 60% of pregnancy rates.

According to Neil Johnson, evidence-based medicine has proved drilling to be better than gonadotropins for PCOS patients.

Indications of Ovarian Drilling

- CC resistant cases
- Before starting gonadotropins

- Thin lean PCOS with high LH
- Recurrent pregnancy loss due to PCOS
- Alternative to gonadotropins when cost is prohibiting factor

Mechanism of Action

Ovarian drilling leads to destruction of the stromal cells which in turn reduces androgen production, decrease in stromal blood flow, leading to fall in serum levels of vascular endothelial growth factor (VEGF) and insulin-like growth factor 1 (IGF-1). On drilling along with the stroma, small follicles are also destroyed, which leads to fall in anti-Müllerian hormone (AMH) levels and therefore increases the sensitivity of follicles to FSH.[28,29] Failure of ovarian drilling in women with relatively high power Doppler indices along with high levels of AMH may be due to severity of PCOS in these women. It is possible that the extent of follicle destruction by laparoscopic ovarian drilling (LOD) in these women was not enough to reduce intraovarian AMH to a level consistent with resumption of ovulation.[30] Another study has also shown that adjusted diathermy dose based on ovarian volume for LOD of PCOS has better reproductive outcome compared with fixed thermal dosage.[31]

Advantages

- Onetime procedure
- No follow-up required
- No monitoring required
- Cheaper than gonadotropins

The mean treatment costs per live birth within 8–12 years after initial treatment are significantly lower per live birth when treatment is started with laparoscopic electrocautery compared with when started with ovulation induction with rFSH, and electrocautery is a rational treatment for clomiphene-resistant PCOS. Laparoscopic electrocautery of the ovaries is as effective as ovulation induction with FSH treatment in terms of live births, but reduces the need for ovulation induction or ART in a significantly higher proportion of women and increases the chance for second child.

Method: It should be done with unipolar cautery and has excellent results similar to laser therapy. Various other methods have been described in literature without added advantage. The only one contraindication to ovarian drilling is "polycystic-like ovaries". What does this mean? Many a times, drilling is done by looking at it at the time of laparoscopy. This is a wrong practice. Prior to laparoscopy, baseline ultrasound scan must be done and diagnosis of PCO is mandatory. We have not come across a single case of ovarian failure after drilling because we always confirm PCO on baseline scan before doing drilling.

Newer methods for ovarian drilling—under trials:

- Transvaginal hydrolaparoscopic drilling
- Ultrasound-guided transvaginal ovarian drilling
- Laparoscopic ovarian multi-needle intervention

Unilateral drilling has been suggested by some workers, with an argument that it has an advantage of a short procedure time, minimized adhesions and ovarian tissue damage, but still induces activity in both ovaries.[32] Though according to other authors this requires further evaluation.[33] In a latest study, Sunj et al. have shown that unilateral ovarian drilling using thermal doses adjusted to the ovarian volume(60 J/cc) was more effective than bilateral drilling done with constant thermal doses for both ovaries.[34]

Number of Punctures

- *According to Adem Balen and Armer's technique:* 4 punctures for 4 seconds at 40 W
- *According to Naether and colleagues:* 5–20 punctures for 1 second at 400 W
- *According to Gjoumas:* 5–8 punctures for 5–6 seconds at 300–400 W

Numbers of punctures depend on the stromal volume and ratio of stromal volume to ovarian volume and have results as follows.

The study was conducted from 2002–2009 and total number of patients with PCOS enrolled were 2,733. Out of these, 134 patients did not turn up after initial investigations and 2,699 patients were taken for study. Out of these 2,699 patients, 1,566 patients had come after taking treatment for subfertility for more than a year. Study results are shown in **Table 2** and **Figure 2**.

It is clearly seen that the number of cycles for conception are fewer when ovarian drilling was done and the total conception rate is also high. We have

Table 2: Study results of conception rates with no drilling and with drilling.

	No drilling	***With drilling***
conceived	882 (55.68%)	828 (74.26%)
Not conceived	702	287
Total	1584	1115

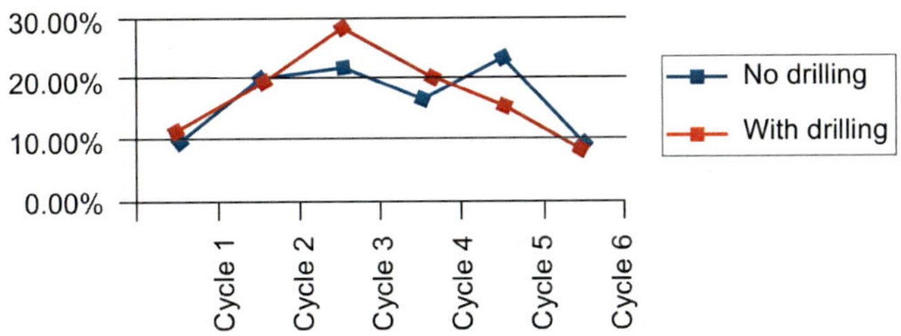

Fig. 2: Conception rates no drilling and with drilling.

done drilling only after confirming insulin resistance and stromal area as well as stromal volume.

But I would like to emphasize that we have not come across a single case of ovarian failure. Api et al. have concluded in their study that there was no concrete evidence of a decreased ovarian reserve nor premature ovarian failure associated with LOD in women with PCOS.[35-39]

The ESHRE-ASRM recommendations 2018:

- It is second line of therapy like gonadotropins in letrozole-resistant cases.
- If laparoscopy is indicated for some other reason, then it can be considered as the first treatment option.
- IVF is the third line of therapy after first and second line fail.
- IVF is effective and single embryo transfer (SET) can minimize multiple pregnancy rate.
- Risks, costs, and benefits should be discussed with the patient.
- Antagonist protocol and agonist trigger with freeze all can avoid OHSS completely.
- Exogenous LH is not required in PCOS.
- All FSH preparations have given good results.

In vitro Maturation

In vitro maturation is a new advance in ART, especially for patients with PCOS as it is 100% OHSS-free treatment. The treatment cost is low as consumption of gonadotropins is very low.

For this technique, stimulation is stopped as the follicle size reaches 10–11 mm. hCG 10,000 IU is given to the patient for final maturation and ovum pick-up is done after 34–36 hours. Period for IVM is 24–48 hours. Thereafter, ICSI is done on these mature oocytes.

Carry Home Message

- Weight loss is the first line of treatment.
- Clomiphene is not preferred treatment for PCOS.
- Letrozole is the drug of choice and first line of treatment.
- Adding metformin has no advantage, CC + metformin can be given in CC-resistant cases.
- Glucocorticoids may be useful in a subgroup.
- Chronic low dose FSH protocol is ultimate and is the second line of treatment.
- Agonist may be used for ovulation trigger.
- Antagonists are very useful in thin lean PCOS.
- Ovarian drilling has excellent results in best hands.
- IVM is the future.

REFERENCES

1. Park HS, Lee K. Greater beneficial effects of visceral fat reduction compared with subcutaneous fat reduction on parameters of the metabolic syndrome: a study of weight reduction programs in subjects with visceral and subcutaneous obesity. Diabet Med. 2005;22:266-72.
2. Smith SR, Zachwieja JJ. Visceral adipose tissue: a critical review of intervention strategies. Int J Obes Relat Metab Disrd. 1999;23:329-35.
3. Begum MR, Ferdous J, Begum A, Quadir E. Comparison of efficacy of aromatase inhibitor and clomiphene citrate in induction of ovulation in polycystic ovarian syndrome. Fertil Steril. 2009;92:853-7.
4. Badawy A, Elnashar A, El-Ashry M, Shahat M. Gonadotropin-releasing hormone agonists for prevention of chemotherapy-induced damage: a prospective randomized study. Fertil Steril. 2009;92:860-3.
5. Badawy A. Clomiphene citrate or letrozole for ovulation induction in women with polycystic ovarian syndrome: a prospective randomized trial. Fertil Steril. 2009;92:849-52.
6. Casper RF. Letrozole versus clomiphene citrate. Fertil Steril. 2009;92(3):858-9.
7. Bohler H Jr, Mokshagundam S, Winters SJ. Adipose tissue and reproduction in women. Fertil Steril. 2010;94:795-825.
8. Creanga AA, Bradley HM, McCormick C, Witkop CT. Use of metformin in polycystic ovary syndrome: a meta-analysis. Obstet Gynecol. 2008;111(4):959-68.
9. Stadtmauer LA, Toma SK, Riehl RM, Talbert LM. Metformin treatment of patients with polycystic ovary syndrome undergoing in vitro fertilization improves outcomes and is associated with modulation of the insulin-like growth factors. Fertil Steril. 2001;75:505-9.
10. Falghesu AM, Romualdi C, Di Florio C, Sanna S, Tagliaferri A, Gambineri A, et al. Is there a dose-response relationship of metformin treatment in patients with polycystic ovary syndrome? Results from a multicentric study. Hum Reprod. 2012;27(10):3057-66.
11. Legro RS, Barnhart HX, Schlaff WD, Carr BR, Diamond MP, Carson SA, et al. Clomiphene, metformin, or both for infertility in polycystic ovary syndrome. N Engl J Med. 2007;356:551-66.
12. Moll E, Bossuyt Patrick MM, Korevaar JC, Lambalk CB, van der Veen F. Effect of clomifene citrate plus metformin and clomiphene citrate plus placebo on induction of ovulation in women with newly diagnosed polycystic ovary syndrome: randomized double blind clinical trial. BMJ. 2006;332(7556):1485.
13. Nestler JE. Metformin in the treatment of infertility in polycystic ovarian syndrome: an alternative perspective. Fertil Steril. 2008;90(1):14-6.
14. Palomba S, Orio F Jr, Falbo A, Manguso F, Russo T, Cascella T, et al. Prospective parallel randomised double-blind, double-dummy controlled clinical trial comparing clomiphene citrate to metformin as the first line of treatment for ovulation induction in nonobese anovulatory women with polycystic ovary syndrome. J Clin Endocrinol Metab. 2005;90:4068-74.
15. Costello MF, Chapman M, Conway U. A systematic review and meta-analysis of randomized controlled trials on metformin co-administration during gonadotropin ovulation induction or IVF in women with polycystic ovary syndrome. Hum Reprod. 2006;21:1387-99.
16. Kjotrod SB, von During V, Carlsen SM. Metformin treatment before IVF/ICSI in women with polycystic ovary syndrome: a prospective, randomized, double blind study. Hum Reprod. 2004;19:1315-22.
17. Palomba S, Falbo A, Cello AD, Cappiello F, Tolino A, Zullo F. Does metformin affect the ovarian response to gonadotrophins for in vitro fertilization treatment in

patients with polycystic ovary syndrome and reduced ovarian reserve: a randomised controlled trial. Fertil Steril. 2011;96(5):1128-33.

18. Tso LO, Costello MF, Albuquerque LE, Freitas V. Metformin treatment before and during IVF or ICSI in women with polycystic ovary syndrome. Cochrane Database Syst Rev. 2009;2:CD006105.
19. Palomba S, Falbo A, Carrillo L, Villani MT, Orio F, Russo T, et al. Metformin reduces the risk of ovarian hyperstimulation syndrome in patients with polycystic ovary syndrome during gonadotropins-stimulated in vitro fertilization cycles: a randomized controlled trial. Fertil Steril. 2011;96(6):1384-90.
20. Kjotrod SB, Carlsen SM, Rasmussen PE, Holst-Larsen T, Mellembakken J, Thurin-Kjellberg K, et al. Use of metformin before and during assisted reproductive technology in non-obese young infertile women with polycystic ovary syndrome: a prospective, randomized, double blind multicentre study. Hum Reprod. 2011;26(8):2045-53.
21. Palomba S, Falbo A, Orio F, Zullo F. Effect of preconceptional metformin on abortion risk in polycystic ovary syndrome: a systematic review and meta-analysis of randomized controlled trials. Fertil Steril. 2009;92:1646-58.
22. Ladson G, Dodson WC, Sweet SD, Archibong AE, Kunselman AR, Demers LM, et al. The effects of metformin with lifestyle therapy in polycystic ovary syndrome: a randomized double-blind study. Fertil Steril. 2011;95(3):1059-66.
23. Daya S, Gunby J, Hughes EG, Collins JA, Sagle MA. Follicle-stimulating hormone versus human menopausal gonadotropin for in vitro fertilization cycles: a meta-analysis. Fertil Steril. 1995;64:347-54.
24. Ludwig M, Rabe T, Buhler K. Wirksamkeit von recombinantem humane FSH in Vergleigh zu urinarem hMG nach Downregulation im langen Protokoll-eine Analyse von 24,764 ART-Zyklen in Deutschland. J Reproduction Med Endocrinol. 1994;4:284-8.
25. Homburg R, Howles CM. Low-dose FSH therapy for anovulatory infertility associated with polycystic ovarian syndrome: rationale, results, reflections and refinements. Hum Reprod Update. 1999;15(5);493-9.
26. Homborg R, Hendriks ML, Konig TE, Anderson RA, Balen AH, Brincat M, et al. Clomifene citrate or low dose FSH for the first-line treatment of infertile women with anovulation associated with polycystic ovary syndrome: a prospective randomised multinational study. Hum Reprod. 2011;27(2):468-73.
27. Humaidan P, Ejdrup BH, Westergaard LG, Andersen CY. 1,500 IU human chorionic gonadotropin administered at oocyte retrieval rescues the luteal phase when gonadotropin-releasing hormone agonist is used for ovulation induction: a prospective, randomized, controlled study. Fertil Steril. 2010;93:847-54.
28. Balen A. Surgical treatment of polycystic ovarian syndrome. Best Pract Res Clin Endocrinol Metab. 2006;20:271-80.
29. Amer SA, Banu Z, Li TC, Cooke ID. Long-term follow-up of patients with polycystic ovary syndrome after laparoscopic ovarian drilling: endocrine and ultrasonographic outcomes. Hum Reprod. 2002;17:2851-7.
30. Amer S, Li TC, Leder WL. The value of measuring anti-Müllerian hormone in women with anovulatory polycystic ovary syndrome undergoing laparoscopic ovarian diathermy. Hum Reprod. 2009;92:1586-93.
31. Nardo LG, Gelbaya TA, Wilkinson H, Roberts SA, Yates A, Pemberton P, et al. Circulating basal anti-Müllerian hormone levels as predictor of ovarian response in women undergoing ovarian stimulation for in vitro fertilization. Fertil Steril. 2009;92:1586-93.
32. Mahmoud S, Kamal MM, Hamed MD. Laparoscopic ovarian drilling in polycystic ovary syndrome: efficacy of adjusted thermal dose based on ovarian volume. Fertil Steril. 2011;95:1115-8.

33. Elmashad AI. Impact of laparoscopic ovarian drilling on anti-Müllerian hormone levels and ovarian stromal blood flow using three-dimensional power Doppler in women with anovulatory polycystic ovarian syndrome. Fertil Steril. 2011;95(7):2342-6.
34. Nahuis MJ, Lohuis EO, Bayram N, Hompes P, Oosterhuis GJE, Kaaijk EM, et al. Long-term follow-up of laparoscopic electrocautery of the ovaries versus ovulation induction with recombinant FSH in clomiphene citrate resistant women with polycystic ovary syndrome: an economic evaluation. Hum Reprod. 2012;27(12):3577-82.
35. Balen AS, Jacobs HS. A prospective study comparing unilateral and bilateral laparoscopic ovarian diathermy in women with polycystic ovary syndrome. Fertil Steril. 1994;62:921-25.
36. Fernandez H, Morin-Surruca M, Torre A, Faivre E, Deffieux X, Gervais A. Ovarian drilling for surgical treatment of polycystic ovary syndrome: a comprehensive review. Reprod Biomed Online. 2011;22:556-68.
37. Sunj M, Canic T, Baldani DP, Tandara M, Jeroncic A, Paplada I. Does unilateral laparoscopic diathermy adjusted to ovarian volume increase the chances of ovulation in women with polycystic ovary syndrome? Hum Reprod. 2011;28(9):2417-24.
38. Api M. Is ovarian reserve diminished after laparoscopic ovarian drilling? Gynecol Endocrinol. 2009;25:159-65.
39. Tulandi T, Watkin K, Tan SL. Reproductive performance and three-dimensional ultrasound volume determination of polycystic ovaries following laparoscopic ovarian drilling. Int J Fertil Womens Med. 1997;42:436-40.

CHAPTER 10

Medical Management of Male Infertility

Chaitanya Nagori

INTRODUCTION

Male factor is partially or completely responsible for infertility in at least 40–50% of all infertility cases. But in today's era of in vitro fertilization (IVF) and intracytoplasmic sperm injection (ICSI), very little importance is given to its medical management. In India, majority of our patients cannot afford multiple attempts of IVF. They may with all difficulties manage one cycle, the success rate of which is barely 25–35%. If the amount that costs for one IVF/ICSI cycle is instead used for medical management of oligozoospermia, it will improve the sperm count permanently. This can give better pregnancy rates than a single IVF/ICSI cycle, moreover can also give spontaneous pregnancies in future also. This is the reason why we insist on medical management of male subfertility as an important treatment option for couples with male factor infertility.

PREVENTIVE MEASURES

Preventive measures must be discussed with the patients before starting the treatment.

Smoking, Caffeine, and Alcohol

Bad effects of smoking and alcohol are person specific and affect a lot who have abnormal sperm parameters. Smoking causes much more damage to patients with varicocele rather than in a normal male. It is essential, therefore, to advice patients to stop smoking and alcohol.

Occupational and Environmental Hazards

Many chemicals and particularly heavy metals damage spermatogenesis. Lead toxicity is well-known. Environmental toxins and pesticides also play a major role in decreasing sperm count. Increased scrotal temperature also alters sperm parameters.

Drugs

Many drugs also reduce the sperm count.

Mobiles and Computers

Because of high frequency shortwave and generation of heat, these equipment can decrease the sperm count and motility.

CRITERIA FOR MEDICAL MANAGEMENT IN MALE INFERTILITY

Semen analysis is still the gold standard for further evaluation and management of infertile male.

Tables 1 and 2 clearly show that the parameters for normal semen analysis have changed and with only 15 million/mL count, 30% motility, and >4% normal sperms, spontaneous conceptions can occur. The whole motto of medical management of a subfertile male is not to increase the sperm count 5–10 times or to achieve excellent semen parameters. The motto is to increase the count by a few million, so that ICSI can be converted to IVF, IVF to intrauterine insemination (IUI), and perhaps IUI into natural conception.

I would like you to look into this case study which is an eye opener. It shows the importance and success of medical treatment of an infertile male and must be thought of before using high-end techniques for conception or after having failures with high-end assisted reproductive technology (ART)—IVF-ICSI.

Table 1: World Health Organization (WHO) 2010 Normal Semen Parameters.

Seminal parameters	*Lower reference value*
Volume	1.5 mL
pH	7.2
Concentration	15 million/mL
Total number of sperms	39 million/ejaculate
Motility	40% total, 32% progressive
Vitality	58% sperms alive/ejaculate
Morphology	4% normal shape

Table 2: Comparison of normal semen parameters according to the WHO 1999 and WHO 2010.

Seminal parameters	*WHO 1999*	*WHO 2010*
Volume	2 mL	1.5 mL
Concentration	20×10^6/mL	15×10^6/mL
Progressive motility	50%	32%
Morphology	15%	4%
Millions of progressive motility	20	7.2 (12)

Case Study

- An industrialist—9 years infertility
- Semen count—3 million
- Seven IVF-ICSI failures
- Husband treated medically [follicle-stimulating hormone (FSH) + human chorionic gonadotropin (hCG)] (Professor Ishidori's regimen)
- Count increased to 22 million
- Conceived naturally—baby boy
- Spontaneously conceived delivered after 2.5 years.

TREATMENT OPTIONS

- Specific therapy
- Empiric therapy

Specific Therapy

There is a definite cause of infertility and specific therapy should be given, which will be highly effective. This means that the treatment is based on the cause of infertility.

Hypogonadotropic Hypogonadism

Estrogen is low because of low follicle-stimulating hormone (FSH) and luteinizing hormone (LH). This is common in congenital Kallmann syndrome associated with anosmia, deafness, renal abnormalities, and cleft palate.

It may also be associated with trauma, tumor, panhypopituitarism, isolated gonadotropin deficiency, etc.

This can be treated by:

- Clomiphene citrate (CC)
- Gonadotropins.

Clomiphene citrate: It was a customary teaching that CC does not work in hypogonadotropic hypogonadism (HH), but here are several recent papers that suggest that CC is very useful for spermatogenesis.[1] It is useful in nonobstructive azoospermia (NOA) and HH.

The recommended dose is 25–75 mg on alternate days. The dose titration is done by morning serum testosterone estimation which should be between 6,000 and 8,000 ng/dL. This treatment is given for 3–9 months. In the same study, 64.3% patients showed sperms in ejaculate with mean density of 3.8 million/mL. In rest of the patients, sperms could be retrieved from testis.[1]

Gonadotropins: In these patients, FSH and LH are very low and have to be supplied from outside. For initiation of spermatogenesis, testosterone is very useful. So, hCG in a dose of 2,000–3,000 IU twice a week or 5,000 IU every fifth day is given for 6–8 weeks till testosterone level comes to normal. Then, human menopausal gonadotropin (hMG)/urinary follicle-stimulating hormone (uFSH)/recombinant follicle-stimulating hormone (rFSH) 75 IU is added thrice a week. hCG is continued once a week, but the dose may be adjusted if gynecomastia occurs.[2] We have found excellent results with this regimen like other studies.[3] Gonadotropin-releasing hormone (GnRH) is not available in our country, but it is a good alternative to hCG-hMG/FSH regimen in HH. It is of no use in patients with disturbed spermatogenesis and high FSH. In about 40% of the patients, spermatogenesis starts. Normally, it takes 6–9 months[4] after FSH/hCG treatment for the sperm parameters to improve.

Hyperprolactinemia

In male, the most common cause of increased prolactin is macroadenoma and it is to be surgically removed. Diagnosis is suspected with the history of loss of libido and pressure effects on optic chiasma and is confirmed by MRI.[5] Macroadenoma is usually >1 cm and serum prolactin level is >200 ng/mL.

But surgery should not be done for microadenoma. Prolactin level is between 100 and 200 μg/mL in these cases and bromocriptine or cabergoline is the treatment. Cabergoline is given 0.5–2 mg in doses divided twice a week to maintain prolactin levels between 10 and 15 μg/mL. Cabergoline is found to be better than bromocriptine.

Genital Tract Infections

Chlamydia is the most common infection and should be treated with doxycycline. In resistant cases, semen culture is done and treated accordingly. If there is prostatic infection, quinolone group of drugs are given.

Disorders of Ejaculation

This is not been elaborated here as these are best to be managed by andrologist.

Immunological Causes

Nowadays, immunological causes in abnormal semen parameters are treated with IUI only. No steroids are given.

Isolated Testosterone Deficiency

It is treated with hCG 2,000 IU twice a week.

Congenital Adrenal Hyperplasia

This is treated with glucocorticoids-dexamethasone 0.5 mg at bedtime.

Empiric Therapy

Empiric therapy is the treatment prior to final diagnosis, based on clinical concepts or theories without proven efficacy. About 25% of cases of male infertility are having idiopathic infertility. Empiric therapy is the only available form of treatment for them.[6,7] All proven drugs used now have been tried earlier as empiric drugs because when a new drug is tried, there is no evidence base. Clinical trials are ahead of all evidence-based medicine and this explains the place of empiric therapy in male infertility.

Clomiphene Citrate (CC)

This is the cheapest available drug. It has been mentioned in the *Textbook on Infertility* written by Insler; that only a subgroup of patients are improved by CC therapy, but we do not know who all are in this subgroup and therefore this cheap, fairly safe drug can be tried in all patients. It is given 25–50 mg for 25 days for 3–6 months.[8] This could achieve a pregnancy rate of 40% in a group of 32 subfertile men. The men with partial androgen resistance and mild HH are the best candidates to respond to this therapy.[9] Follow-up is done every month. The dose setting should be such that it should increase FSH and testosterone should be normal with drug.

A study by Hussein et al. suggested considering a course of CC prior to sperm retrieval in patients with NOA.[1]

Human Chorionic Gonadotropin

Human chorionic gonadotropin (hCG) in a dose of 2,500–5,000 IU twice a week is a very useful regimen in a patient of idiopathic oligozoospermia. This increases the testosterone level. Intratesticular testosterone is 100 times higher than serum level. So, exogenous hCG should be given rather than testosterone. The Leydig cells of the testis can respond positively to exogenous hCG and produces more amount of testosterone even under hypogonadotropic conditions. This suppresses endogenous gonadotropin level by negative feedback. hCG-based hormonal therapy prior to a second micro-testicular sperm extraction (TESE) attempt is effective in men with hypospermatogenesis.[10] Even before the era of ICSI, we have very often used this drug with excellent results. We still use this drug for mild-to-moderate oligozoospermia **(Box 1)**.

Box 1: Mild, moderate, and severe oligozoospermia.

- *Normal count*: >15 million/mL or 30 million/ejaculate
- *Mild oligozoospermia*: 10–15 million/mL
- *Moderate oligozoospermia*: 5–10 million/mL
- *Severe oligozoospermia*: <5 million/mL.

This drug is very useful after varicocele ligation. The first reported studies showed 60% improvement in semen parameters.[11,12] Patients with relative androgen deficiency are more benefited.[13]

Follicle-stimulating Hormone + Human Chorionic Gonadotropin

This is a very useful combination for idiopathic normogonadotropic oligozoospermia.[14] The argument in favor of this therapy by Professor Ishidori (Sweden) is that these are the patients who have inadequate gonadotropin activity. Here, radioimmunoassay (RIA) results are normal but the bioactivity is low. This bioactivity can be assessed by monoclonal antibody testing, but is not easily available. To compensate for this deficient bioactivity, exogenous FSH and hCG are given for 3-6 months.[15] I have found this regimen very useful for idiopathic oligozoospermia. The case report described earlier in this chapter indicates efficacy of this regimen.

Treatment protocol is:
- Human menopausal gonadotropin/rFSH 75-150 IU thrice a week
- Human chorionic gonadotropin 5,000 IU once a week.

For maturation arrest at spermatid level, only FSH can be given for completion of spermatogenesis.[16] FSH therapy improves fertilization after ICSI.

A significant reduction in sperm aneuploidy levels has been detected after varicocele repair[17] and in men treated with rFSH.[18]

Androgen

Testosterone has no role in improving spermatogenesis. Formerly, rebound therapy was given which is discarded because it causes permanent azoospermia in some patients. Testosterone is not a useful drug.[19,20]

Tamoxifen + Testosterone Undecanoate

The World Health Organization (WHO) recommends treatment with antiestrogens—tamoxifen for idiopathic oligozoospermia when motility and morphology are not significantly affected.[21] When serum FSH is not elevated, tamoxifen is given 20 mg/day.

When testosterone undecanoate 120 mg is combined with 20 mg tamoxifen, there is significant improvement in semen quality and increase in pregnancy rate. Pregnancy rates increased from 10.3 to 33% as described in one study.[22]

Zinc

Zinc is very useful in low testosterone levels with zinc deficiency. Recommended dose is 120-220 mg twice a day for 3 months. It improves accessory glands function. It helps in exploration of immature cells. It helps in improving oligozoospermia as well as motility and maturation of spermatozoa.[23,24]

Ketotifen

It inhibits histamine release from mast cells. It helps in blood-testis barrier dysfunction. The dose is 1 mg BD for 3-6 months.[25] It has incompatibility with alchohol.[26] Pregnancy rate in one study was 28.6% versus 0%.[27]

Antiserotonin Agents

Cyproheptadine hydrochloric acid (HCl) 4 mg TDS for 90 days can be given in two courses. It improves sperm count and motility in 33-50% of cases. Mechanism of action is that it reduces uptake of serotonin which reduces testicular damage.[28]

Captopril

It is an angiotensin-converting enzyme (ACE) inhibitor. It inhibits kininase II and prevents degradation of kininogens to kinins. It is given in a dose of 50 mg/day for 3 months. It is contraindicated in presence of inflammation.[29]

Tissue Hormones

Pancreatic kallikrein converts kininogens to kinins which helps in cell proliferation. It helps in oligoasthenoteratozoospermia (OAT). It is given in a dose of 600 mg/day for 3-12 months,[30] but cumulative results are not promising.[31]

Anti-inflammatory Drugs

Chlamydia infection is very common in patients having male factor as a cause of infertility. It is extremely difficult to diagnose infection in genital tract and is very expensive also. Instead one course of doxycycline 100 mg BD for 14 days is cost-effective as the incidence of infection has been quoted between 28 and 91%. It prevents occlusion of passage and local immunity is improved. Tetracycline and metronidazole are very effective, but antibiotic therapy does not necessarily improve conception rates.[32]

Indomethacin

Prostaglandins have inhibitory effect on testicular steroidogenesis. Indomethacin and ketoprofen raise FSH, LH, and testosterone. Indomethacin 25 mg TDS increases sperm count and motility.[33] It is inexpensive and nontoxic and should be tried. Diclofenac 50 mg is recommended for 3-6 months.[32]

Aromatase Inhibitors

Teslac (testolactone) is tried for improving sperm count and motility. It is given 50–100 mg twice daily. It prevents aromatization to estrogen. So, patients having low testosterone/estradiol (E2) are potential candidates to improve with this drug. It should be considered for obese patients and those with elevated E2 levels. Anastrozole is a very potent drug and is used in a dose of 1 mg/day.[34-36]

Autocrine-paracrine Mechanism

Insulin-like growth factor 1 (IGF-1), IGF-2, epidermal growth factor (EGF), and transforming growth factor (TGF) are potent stimulants for spermatogenesis. So, FSH + growth factors can improve spermatogenesis. Corticotropin-releasing factor-β (CRF-β) endorphins are inhibitors of spermatogenesis. Naltrexone is the drug which prevents CRF-β endorphin system. So, FSH + Naltrexone can improve spermatogenesis.

Antioxidants

The definitive role of reactive oxygen species (ROS) testing in the diagnostic situation remains to be established, although detrimental effects of ROS on male reproductive system are now well-established.[37,38]

Therefore, systematic treatment of men with antioxidants has received great interest in recent years and it seems to have some clinical benefit, though the story remains somewhat confused.[39]

8-hydroxy-2'-deoxyguanosine, a biomarker of oxidative deoxyribonucleic acid (DNA) damage highly correlated with sperm DNA fragmentation, in human sperm DNA. It has significant value in predicting the chance of a clinical pregnancy after IUI but not ICSI in ART.[40] Supplementing antioxidants (vitamins C, E and folate) and micronutrients (zinc) can also be helpful in producing sperms with less DNA damage in older man also.[41]

Antioxidants are more useful as follow-up or complimentary treatment to conventional treatment of varicocele, antibiotic treatment for infection, or antiestrogenic treatment for idiopathic oligozoospermia.[21] It has also been suggested that patients with asthenozoospermia should be advised to adhere to a diet rich in fruits, vegetables, poultry, skim milk, and sea foods and low in processed meat and sweets.[42]

According to Lipshultz, high doses of antioxidants have theoretical adverse effects and should be used in low or moderate doses. With exception of patients with specific vitamin deficiency, efficacy of any vitamin therapy in normal men is questionable.

Table 3: Antioxidants used for oligoasthenospermia.	
Tocopherol (vitamin E)	Glutathione
Ascorbic acid (vitamin C)	Arginine
Vitamin B_{12}	Carnitines
Folic acid	Coenzyme Q
Pentoxifylline	Vitamin D
Selenium	Lycopene

ANTIOXIDANTS

Antioxidants reduce sperms' oxidative stress and increase motility in asthenozoospermic patients, but it is yet unclear whether this improvement translates to higher full-term pregnancy rates.[43] Protective effects on DNA damage is most pronounced in elderly people **(Table 3)**.

Vitamin E

It has protective effect on lipid peroxidation in sperm membrane by ROS. It increases sperm motility and increases fertilization rate in IVF.[44] Vitamin E improves motility of spermatozoa. The recommended dose is 300–600 mg daily for 6–12 weeks. Vitamin E improves sperm-oocyte fusion. So, it is included in certain media preparations. Addition of vitamin E in media reduces the damaging effect of configuration during sperm preparation.[45] Astaxanthin is a carotenoid extracted from the algae *Haematococcus pluvialis*. The potency of this antioxidant is much higher as a singlet molecular oxygen quencher compared with vitamin E.[46] A positive effect of astaxanthin on sperm parameters and fertility is seen in a study by Comhaire et al.[47] Pregnancy rate of 23% was achieved as compared to 3.6% in control group because of better fusion and increase in linear progression motility.

Vitamin C

Low levels of vitamin C lead to infertility due to disturbed sperm functions. Vitamin C improves sperm quality. The dose is 1,000 mg daily.[48]

Vitamin B_{12}

This is very useful for synthesis of DNA and ribonucleic acid (RNA). It is useful for oligospermia and asthenospermia. Recommended dose is 1,000–1,500 μg/day for 6 months.[49]

Folic Acid

This is an additive drug and along with other drugs, it helps to improve sperm functions. The dose required is 5 mg/day.[50]

Pentoxifylline

It improves microcirculation. The dose required is 1.2 mg/day for 3–6 months. It improves sperm count and motility.[31,51]

But there are various reports that indicate that pentoxifylline, sildenafil, and other methylxanthines when administered systematically give no response.[52] Sildenafil prior to semen collection may result in increased motility.[53]

Selenium

It is an antioxidant as well as an anti-inflammatory agent. It is concentrated in male reproductive tract. Its highest concentration is in prostate and improves motility. The dose required is 225 µg/day. It is found that only 50% of patients improve as far as motility is concerned.[54]

Glutathione

It has positive effect on sperm motility and is given in a dose of 600 mg intramuscular (IM) daily. Daily injections are cumbersome and therefore this treatment has not gained popularity.[55]

Arginine

It improves sperm motility and recommended dose is 4 g/day.

L-carnitine and L-acetylcarnitine

L-carnitine (LC) brings acetyl-CoA into mitochondria. So, its role is important in sperm cell metabolism. Concentration of LC is highest in epididymal fluid (2,000 times higher) which is available to sperm cells. LC protects cell membrane and DNA against damage by ROS. Combination of LC and L-acetylcarnitine (LAC) are more effective in improving sperm motility than individual one in patients with lower baseline levels.[56] LC and LAC are useful in idiopathic OAT and low-grade varicoceles. It is also useful in patients with prostate-vesiculo-epididymitis after treatment with nonsteroidal anti-inflammatory drug (NSAID).[57,58]

L-carnitine 1 g BD + LAC 500 mg BD + cinnoxicam 30 mg every 4 days showed significant reduction in aneuploid sperms and improved ICSI pregnancies and live births in severe OAT patients.[59] The fact is that LC is not essential as it is synthesized in body. The exogenous source is nonvegetarian food. Deficiency occurs in patients with hemodialysis, but there are several papers giving controversial opinion regarding its role as antioxidant. It has selective role in oligoasthenozoospermia.[60]

We must remember that positive effect of the drug does not last for a long time after therapy. So, during the treatment for fertility, the drug is to be continued. We cannot prescribe the drug and wait for the results. Simultaneous superovulation with IUI or ART is a must.

Total oxyradical scavenging capacity (TOSC) assays differentiate different forms of ROS and its role for specific antioxidants. So, in future, we will be able to decide which antioxidant is required for a particular patient.

Coenzyme Q10

It is the component of mitochondrial respiratory chain. It has very important role in energy metabolism. It is biosynthesized in testis and has protective role as antioxidant for cell membranes and lipoprotein. The natural source of coenzyme Q10 (CoQ10) is broccoli, spinach, soyabean oil, palm oil, vitamins, and minerals that act as cofactors for producing CoQ10.

It is available as 50–100 mg soft gel capsules that have almost 100% absorption. Therapeutic application of CoQ10 for 6 months increases its reduced form ubiquinol which improves kinetic property of sperm cells.[61]

Reduced CoQ10 level is found in seminal plasma and sperm cells in infertile man with idiopathic oligospermia and varicocele associated with oligoasthenospermia.

There is strong support as antioxidant by indirect medium, but there is no conclusion for improved pregnancy rates by this therapy. Like LC, its beneficial effect also does not last long.

Vitamin D

Lately, Vitamin D receptors are found in testis with vitamin D metabolizing enzymes also. These enzymes are also found in epididymis and mature sperms.[62] Vitamin D can also be positively associated with testosterone and free androgen index and negatively with sex hormone-binding globulin (SHBG).[63] Still another study has shown that 1,25-dihydroxyvitamin D3 [1,25$(OH)_2$D3] increases intracellular calcium concentration, sperm motility, and induced the acrosome reaction in mature spermatozoa and vitamin D levels in serum were positively associated with sperm motility.[64] Combined treatment with taurine, cysteine, and glutathione statistically significantly ameliorated the reduction in sperm motility during in vitro manipulation of human sperm.[65] Though other studies do not show that low vitamin D is a risk factor for poor semen quality in a population of young healthy men.[66]

Note: We must remember that we should prescribe the drug only in full therapeutic dose, otherwise it will not be useful. The combinations of drugs available in market should be fully studied well and should be prescribed to appropriate patients. Haphazard prescriptions simply add cost to the patients. Select the combo preparation that has three to four drugs in therapeutic dose.

Lycopene and Carotenoids

Improvement in sperm motility has been found with higher intake of carotenoids, beta-carotene, and lutein and improved sperm morphology is found with high intake of lycopene.

- Lycopene—tomatoes
- Beta-carotene—carrots, lettuce, and spinach
- Lutein—spinach and lettuce

Omega-3 Fatty Acids

Positive effect on spermatogenesis is seen with increased intake of omega-3 fatty acids in the form of diet and supplements rich in nuts and fish. It protects against environmental toxins and slows down the aging process.

Miscellaneous Methods

- *Acupuncture*: Though some workers have tried and documented improvement in males with oligozoospermia and azoospermia with acupuncture therapy. Large and reliable studies are yet to be documented.
- *Traditional Chinese herbal medicine*:
  - Ginseng—improves testosterone and sperm count
  - Astragalus
  - Sarsaparilla

  These drugs do not have research defining risks and benefits so they should be used with caution.
- *Diet*: The higher intake of processed meat and sweets is associated with risk of asthenospermia while high intake of fruits, vegetables, poultry, skim milk, and sea food is associated with low risk. Preconceptional counseling for diet should be done, with the couple wishing conception.

DOSAGE OF DRUGS

- Clomiphene citrate 25–50 mg/day
- Human chorionic gonadotropin 2,000–5,000 IU twice a week
- Follicle-stimulating hormone 75 IU thrice a week + hCG 5,000 IU twice a week
- Tamoxifen 40 mg + testosterone undecanoate 120 mg daily
- Zinc 100–2,000 mg BD
- Ketotifen 1 mg BD
- Cyproheptadine HCl 4 mg TDS
- Captopril 50 mg daily
- Pancreatic kallikrein 600 mg daily
- Indomethacin 25 mg TDS

- Anastrozole 1 mg daily—this is especially useful in patients with low testosterone levels. By preventing aromatization, it increases the testosterone and sperm production.[67]

DOSAGE OF ANTIOXIDANTS

- *Vitamin E*: 300-600 mg daily
- *Vitamin C*: 1,000 mg daily
- *Vitamin B_{12}*: 1,000-1,500 μg daily
- *Folic acid*: 5 mg daily
- *Pentoxifylline*: 1-2 mg daily
- *Selenium*: 225 μg daily
- *Glutathione*: 600 mg IM daily
- *Arginine*: 4 g daily
- *L-carnitine + LAC*: 3 g daily
- *Coenzyme Q10*: 100 mg BD.

Varicocele correction is to be offered to patients with palpable lesion with one or more abnormal semen parameters.[68] Though some workers have tried a documented improvement in males with oligozoospermia and azoospermia with acupuncture therapy, large and reliable studies are yet to be documented.[69]

Carry Home Message

- Hypogonadotropic hypogonadism can be successfully treated with hCG + FSH.
- Clomiphene, letrozole, hCG and gonadotropins given for 3 months to oligospermic patients can give very good results in idiopathic infertility.
- Tamoxifen with testosterone undecanoate gives good results in male infertility.
- Zinc and vitamin E are useful to improve sperm motility.
- Antioxidants should be given in therapeutic doses only.
- By improving the count, IVF can be converted into IUI and IUI can be converted to natural cycle conception.

REFERENCES

1. Hussein A, Ozgok Y, Ross L, Niederberger C. Clomiphene administration for cases of nonobstructive azoospermia: a multicentre study. J Androl. 2005;26:787-91.
2. Sigman M, Jarow JP. Male infertility. In: Walsh PC, Retik AB, Vaughan ED, Wein AJ (Eds). Campbell's Urology, 8th edition. St. Louis: Saunders; 2002. pp. 1475-531.
3. Whitcomb RW, Crowley WF. Male hypogonadotropic hypogonadism. Endocrinol Metab Clin North Am. 1993;22:125-43.
4. Büchter D, Behre HM, Kliesch S, Nieschlag E. Pulsatile GnRH or human chorionic gonadotropin/human menopausal gonadotropin as effective treatment for men with hypogonadotropic hypogonadism: a review of 42 cases. Eur J Endocrinol. 1998;139:298-303.

5. Gillam MP, Molitch ME, Lombardi G, Coloa A. Advances in the treatment of prolactinoma. Endocr Rev. 2006;27:485-534.
6. Dubin L, Amelar RD. Etiologic factors in 1294 consecutive cases of male infertility. Fertil Steril. 1971;22:469-74.
7. Greenberg SH, Lipshultz LI, Wein AJ. Experience with 425 subfertile male patients. J Urol. 1978;119:507-10.
8. Paulson DF, Hammond CB, de Vere White R, Wiebe RH. Clomiphene citrate: pharmacologic treatment of hypofertile male. Urology. 1977;9:419-21.
9. Akin JW. The use of clomiphene citrate in the treatment of azoospermia secondary to incomplete androgen resistance. Fertil Steril. 1993;59:223-7.
10. Shiraishi K, Ohmi C, Shimabukuro T, Matsuyama H. Human chorionic gonadotropin treatment prior to micro-dissection testicular sperm extraction in non-obstructive azoospermia. Hum Reprod. 2012;27:331-9.
11. Glass SJ, Holland HM. Treatment of oligospermia with large doses of human chorionic gonadotropin. Fertil Steril. 1963;14:500-6.
12. Mehan DJ, Chehval MJ. Human chorionic gonadotropin in the treatment of the infertile man. J Urol. 1982;128:60-3.
13. Lunenfield B, Mor A, Mani M. Treatment of male infertility. I. Human gonadotropins. Fertil Steril. 1967;18:581-92.
14. Glezerman M, Lunenfield B. Hormontherapie mannlicher Fertilitäts storingen. In: Kaden R, Lubke F, Schirren C (Eds). Fortschritte der Fertilitats forschung III. Berlin: Grosse; 2007. p. 17.
15. Acosta AA, Khalifa E, Oehninger S. Pure human follicle-stimulating hormone has a role in the treatment of severe male infertility by assisted reproduction: Norfolk's total experience. Hum Reprod. 1992;7:1067-72.
16. Schwarzstein L, Aparicio NJ, Schally AV. D-tryptophan-6-leutinizing hormone-releasing hormone in the treatment of normogonadotropic oligoasthenozoospermia. Int J Androl. 1982;5:172-8.
17. Baccetti BM, Bruni E, Capitani S, Collodel G, Mancini S, Piomboni P, et al. Studies on varicocele III: ultrastructural sperm evaluation and 18, X and Y aneuploidies. J Androl. 2006;27:94-101.
18. Piomboni P, Serafini F, Gambera L, Musacchio C, Collodel G, Morgante G, et al. Sperm aneuploidies after human recombinant follicle stimulating hormone therapy in infertile males. Reprod Biomed Online. 2009;18:622-9.
19. Charny CW. The use of androgens for human spermatogenesis. Fertil Steril. 1959;10:557-70.
20. Charny CW, Gordon JA. Testosterone rebound therapy: a neglected modality. Fertil Steril. 1978;29:64-8.
21. Rowe PJ, Comhaire FH, Hargreave TB, Mahmoud AM, World Health Organization. WHO Manual for the Standardized Investigation, Diagnosis and Management of the Infertile Male. Cambridge: Cambridge University Press; 2000. p. 91.
22. Adamopoules DA, Pappa A, Billa E, Nicopoulou S, Koukkou E, Michopoulos J. Effectiveness of combined tamoxifen citrate and testosterone undeconate treatment in men with idiopathic oligozoospermia. Fertil Steril. 2003;80:914-20.
23. Ebisch IM, Pierik FH, De Jong FH, Thomas CM, Steegers-Theunissen RP. Does folic acid and zinc sulphate intervention affect endocrine parameters and sperm characteristics in men? Int J Androl. 2006;29:339-45.
24. Wong WY, Merkus HM, Thomas CM, Menkveld R, Zielhuis GA, Steegers-Theunissen RP. Effects of folic acid and zinc sulphate in male factor subfertility: a double-blind, randomized, placebo-controlled trial. Fertil Steril. 2002;77:491-3.

25. Matsuki S, Sasagawa I, Suzuki Y, Yazawa H, Tateno T, Hashimoto T, et al. The use of ebastine, a mast cell blocker, for treatment of oligozoospermia. Arch Androl. 2000;44:129-32.
26. Schill WB, Schneider J, Ring J. The use of ketotifen, a mast cell blocker, for treatment of oligo- and asthenozoospermia. Andrologia. 1986;18:570-3.
27. Yamamoto M, Hibi H, Miyake K. New treatment of idiopathic severe oligozoospermia with mast cell blocker: results of single-blind study. Fertil Steril. 1995;64:1221-3.
28. Schill WB, Michalopoulos M. Treatment of male fertility disturbances. Current concepts. Drugs. 1984;28:263-80.
29. Schill WB, Parsch EM, Miska W. Inhibition of angiotensin-converting enzyme: a new concept of medical treatment of male infertility? Fertil Steril. 1994;61:1123-28.
30. Kamidono S, Hazama M, Matsumoto O, Takasa KI, Tomioka O, Ishigami J. Kallikrein and male subfertility: usefulness of high-unit kallikrein tablet. Andrologia. 1981;13:108-20.
31. Keck C, Behre HM, Jockenhovel F, Nieschlag E. Ineffectiveness of kallikrein in treatment of idiopathic male infertility: a double-blind, randomized, placebo-controlled trial. Hum Reprod. 1994;9:325-9.
32. Haidl G. Management strategies for male factor infertility. Drugs. 2002;62:1741-53.
33. Barkay J, Harpaz-Kerpel S, Ben-Ezra S, Gordon S, Zuckerman H. The prostaglandin inhibitor effect of anti-inflammatory drugs in the therapy of male infertility. Fertil Steril. 1984;42:406-11.
34. Schlegel PN, Raman JD. Aromatase inhibitors for male infertility. J Urol. 2002;167:624-9.
35. Pavlovich CP, King P, Goldstein M, Schlegel PN. Evidence of a treatable endocrinopathy in infertile men. J Urol. 2001;165:837-41.
36. Raman JD, Schlegel PN. Aromatase inhibitors for male infertility. J Urol. 2002;167:624-9.
37. Saleh RA, Agarwal A. Oxidative stress and male infertility: from research bench to clinical practice. J Androl. 2002;23:737-52.
38. Agarwal A, Saleh RA, Bedaiwy MA. Role of reactive oxygen species in the pathophysiology of human reproduction. Fertil Steril. 2003;79:829-43.
39. Agarwal A. Role of antioxidants in treatment of male infertility: an overview of the literature. Reprod Biomed Online. 2004;8:616-27.
40. Thomson LK, Zieschang JA, Clark AM. Oxidative DNA damage in sperm has a negative impact on clinical pregnancy rate in intrauterine insemination but not in intracytoplasmic sperm injection cycles. Fertil Steril. 2011;96:843-7.
41. Schmid TE, Eskenazi B, Marchetti F, Young S, Weldon RH, Baumgartner A, et al. Micronutrients intake is associated with improved sperm DNA quality in older men. Fertil Steril. 2012;98:1130-7.
42. Elsamian G, Amirjannati N, Rashidkhani B, Sadeghi MR, Hekmatdoost A. Intake of food groups and idiopathic asthenozoospermia: a case-control study. Hum Reprod. 2012;27:3328-36.
43. Gharagozloo P, Aitken RJ. The role of sperm oxidative stress in male infertility and the significance of oral antioxidant therapy. Hum Reprod. 2011;26:1628-40.
44. Geva E, Bartoov B, Zabludovsky N, Lessing JB, Geva LL, Amit A. The effect of antioxidant treatment on human spermatozoa and fertilization rate in an in vitro fertilization program. Fertil Steril. 1996;66:430-4.
45. Keskes-Ammar L, Feki-Chakroun N, Rebai T, Sahnoun Z, Ghozzi H, Hammami S, et al. Sperm oxidative stress and the effect of an oral vitamin E and selenium supplement on semen quality in infertile male. Arch Androl. 2003;49:83-94.
46. Di Mascio P, Devasagayam TP, Kaiser S, Sies H. Carotenoids, tocopherols and thiols as biological singlet molecular oxygen quenchers. Biochem Soc Trans. 1990;18:1054-6.

47. Comhaire FH, Garem YE, Mahmoud A, Eertmans F, Schoonjans F. Combined conventional/antioxidant "astaxanthin" treatment for male infertility: a double-blind randomized trial. Asian J Androl. 2005;7:257-62.
48. Dawson EB, Harris WA, Teter MC, Powell LC. Effect of ascorbic acid supplementation on the sperm quality of smokers. Fertil Steril. 1992;58:1034-9.
49. Sandler B, Faragher N. Treatment of oligozoospermia with vitamin B12. Infertility. 1984;7:133-2.
50. Ebisch IMW, van Heerde WL, Thomas CMG, van der Put N, Wong WY, Steegers-Theunissen RPM. C677T methylenetetrahydrofolate reductase polymorphism interferes with the effects of folic acid and zinc sulphate on sperm concentration. Fertil Steril. 2003;80:1190-4.
51. Schill WB. Therapy of idiopathic astheno- and oligozoospermia with pentoxifylline. Fortschr Med. 1982;100:696-700.
52. Burger M, Sikka SC, Bivalacqua TJ, Lamb DJ, Hellstrom WJ. The effect of sildenafil on human sperm motion and function from normal and infertile men. Int J Impot Res. 2000;12:229-34.
53. du Plessis SS, de Jongh PS, Franken DR. Effect of acute in vivo sildenafil and in vitro 8-bromo-cGMP treatments on semen parameters and sperm function. Fertil Steril. 2004;81:1026-33.
54. Scott R, MacPherson A, Yates RW, Hussain B, Dixon J. The effect of oral selenium supplementation on human sperm motility. Br J Urol. 1998;82:76-80.
55. Lenzi A, Culasso F, Gandini L, Lombardo F, Dondero F. Placebo-controlled, double-blind, cross-over trial of glutathione therapy in male infertility. Hum Reprod. 1993;8:1657-62.
56. Lenzi A, Sgrò P, Salacone P, Paoli D, Gilio B, Lombardo F, et al. A placebo-controlled double-blind randomized trial of the use of combined L-carnitine and L-acetyl-carnitine treatment in men with asthenozoospermia. Fertil Steril. 2004;6:1578-84.
57. Cavallini G, Ferraretti AP, Gianaroli L, Biagiotti G, Vitali G. Cinnoxicam and L-carnitine/acetyl-L-carnitine treatment for idiopathic and varicocele-associated oligoasthenospermia. J Androl. 2004;25:761-70.
58. Vicari E, La Vignera S, Calogero AE. Antioxidant treatment with carnitines is effective in infertile patients with prostatovesiculoepididymitis and elevated seminal leukocyte concentrations after treatment with nonsteroidal anti-inflammatory compounds. Fertil Steril. 2002;78:1203-8.
59. Cavallini G, Magli MC, Crippa A, Ferraretti AP, Gianaroli L. Reduction in sperm aneuploidy levels in severe oligoasthenoteratospermic patients after medical therapy: a preliminary report. Asian J Androl. 2012;14:591-8.
60. Lenzi A, Lombardo F, Sgrò P, Salacone P, Caponecchia L, Dondero F, et al. Use of carnitine therapy in selected cases of male factor infertility: a double-blind crossover trial. Fertil Steril. 2003;79:292-300.
61. Balercia G, Buldreghini E, Vignini A, Tiano L, Paggi F, Amoroso S, et al. Coenzyme Q10 treatment in infertile men with idiopathic asthenozoospermia: a placebo-controlled, double-blind randomized trial. Fertil Steril. 2009;91:1785-92.
62. Jensen MB, Nielsen JE, Jørgensen A, Rajpert-De Meyts E, Kristensen DM, Jørgensen N, et al. Vitamin D receptor and vitamin D metabolizing enzymes are expressed in the human male reproductive tract. Hum Reprod. 2010;25:1303-11.
63. Wehr E, Pilz S, Boehm BO, Marz W, Obermayer-Pietsch B. Association of vitamin D status with serum androgen levels in men. Clin Endocrinol (Oxf). 2010;73:243-8.
64. Bloomberg JM, Bjerrum PJ, Jessen TE, Nielson JE, Joenson UN, Oleson IA, et al. Vitamin D is positively associated with sperm motility and increases intracellular calcium in human spermatozoa. Hum Reprod. 2011;26:1307-17.

65. Yun JI, Gong SP, Song YH, Lee ST. Effects of combined antioxidant supplementation on human sperm motility and morphology during sperm manipulation in vitro. Fertil Steril. 2013;100:373-8.
66. Ramlau-Hansen CH, Moeller UK, Bonde JP, Oslen J, Thulstrup AM. Are serum levels of vitamin D associated with semen quality? Results from a cross-sectional study in young healthy men. Fertil Steril. 2011;95:1000-4.
67. Schlegel PN. Aromatase inhibitors for male infertility. Fertil Steril. 2012;98:1359-62.
68. Sharlip ID, Jarow JP, Belkar AM, Lipshultz LI, Sigman M, Thomas AJ, et al. Best practice policies for male infertility. Fertil Steril. 2002;77:873-82.
69. Senior K. Acupuncture: can it take the pain away? Mol Med Today. 1996;2:150-3.

CHAPTER 11

Recurrent Pregnancy Loss

Chaitanya Nagori

INTRODUCTION

Recurrent pregnancy loss (RPL) is a social stigma and the couple has a tremendous stress, frustration, and uncertainty regarding future reproductive outcome. According to the Royal College of Obstetricians and Gynecologists (RCOG) and European Society of Human Reproduction and Embryology (ESHRE) guidelines, RPL is defined as three or more consecutive pregnancy losses. But according to the American College of Obstetricians and Gynecologists (ACOG), RPL is two or more pregnancy losses. About 80% of these losses occur in first 12 weeks of pregnancy, but only 20% of pregnancy losses in RPL occur after cardiac activity has established. Incidence of RPL is 1–2% in fertile population.

Detailed history must be taken which in majority of cases give a clue to diagnosis and correct diagnosis is the basis for successful treatment.

Counseling plays a very important role in treating these couples. Narrating the fact that chances of a successful full-term pregnancy after three abortions are 55–60% that give considerable mental relief and psychological support to the patient. About 50% of cases of RPL will not have a clearly defined etiology.[1] Bed rest does not help in improving the reproductive outcome. Patient should be allowed to do her regular work and exercise program.

CAUSES OF RECURRENT PREGNANCY LOSS

- Anatomical
- Autoimmune
- Thrombophilia
- Genetic
- Alloimmunity
- Infections
- Environmental
- Endometriosis
- Psychological
- Endocrinal
- Male factor

Anatomical Causes

Incidence is 1–4% and in RPL 15–25%.

a. Congenital Causes

- Failure of one or more Müllerian duct to develop
- Failure of the ducts to canalize
- Failure to fuse or abnormal fusion of Müllerian ducts
- Failure of resorption of midline uterine septum.

These are also called as Müllerian duct abnormalities. These were classified earlier by the American Fertility Society (AFS) as unicornuate, bicornuate, didelphys, septate, and arcuate uterus. This was named as AFS classification (2003).[2] But in 2013, a new classification—ESHRE-European Society for Gynecological Endoscopy (ESGE) classification[3] was published and was claimed to be more practical and treatment oriented, so since then the new classification is used **(Table 1)**. According to this classification, Müllerian duct abnormalities are divided into seven classes and cervical and vaginal shape is also divided into classes.

Investigations

- *Ultrasonography—Volume ultrasound (US)*: Three-dimensional (3D) and four-dimensional (4D) have a major role to play in the diagnosis of uterine anomaly. It is known as virtual hysteroscopy. Sensitivity and specificity of volume US for detection of congenital uterine abnormality is almost 100% and therefore is considered to be a gold standard for diagnosis of these abnormalities **(Figs. 1A to C)**.
- *Hysterosalpingography (HSG)*: It has a very limited role for differential diagnosis of congenital uterine abnormalities such as bicornuate, septate, and arcuate uterus.
- *Sonohysterography (SHG)*: SHG along with 3D is very useful.
- *MRI*: It is not required most of the times as 3D US is sufficient except when visibility of uterus is poor or there is a rudimentary horn. Moreover, it is much more inconvenient and expensive for the patient.
- *Diagnostic laparoscopy and hysteroscopy*: Diagnostic laparoscopy and hysteroscopy are not required as these are invasive and same diagnostic accuracy is achieved by volume US. These procedures are used only for operative corrections of these abnormalities.
- *Intravenous pyelography (IVP)*: It is used for renal abnormalities.
    - Class U0 is the normal uterus.
    - Class U1—dysmorphic uterus is divided into two subclasses: (1) T-shaped uterus and (2) uterus infantilis. The later was earlier named as hypoplastic uterus.

Table 1: ESHRE/ESGE classification of female genital tract anomalies.

	Uterine anomaly		*Cervical/Vaginal anomaly*	
	Main class	***Subclass***	***Coexistent class***	
U0	Normal uterus		*C0*	Normal cervix
U1	Dysmorphic uterus	a. T-shaped b. Infantilis c. Others	*C1* *C2*	Septate cervix Double "normal" cervix
U2	Septate uterus	a. Partial b. Complete	*C3* *C4*	Unilateral cervical aplasia Cervical aplasia
U3	Bicorporeal uterus	a. Partial b. Complete c. Bicorporeal septate	*V0*	Normal vagina
U4	Hemi-uterus	a. With rudimentary cavity (communicating or not horn) b. Without rudimentary cavity (horn without cavity/no horn)	*V1* *V2*	Longitudinal nonobstructing vaginal septum Longitudinal obstructing vaginal septum
U5	Aplastlc	a. With rudimentary cavity (bi- or unilateral horn) b. Without rudimentary cavity (bi- or unilateral uterine remnants/ aplasia)	*V3* *V4*	Transverse vaginal septum and/or imperforate hymen Vaginal aplasia
U6	Unclassified malformations			
U			*C*	*V*

(ESGE: European Society for Gynecological Endoscopy; ESHRE: European Society of Human Reproduction and Embryology)
Source: Grimbizis GF, Gordts Stephan, Compo R. The ESHRE-ESGE consensus on the classification of female genital tract congenital anomalies. Hum Reprod. 2013;28(8):2032-44.

Class U1—Dysmorphic uterus:
US findings: The US findings of Class U1 are described in **Table 2**.

Management: In these cases, delivery at term is extremely rare. About 50% abort by 2nd trimester end. Hysteroscopic metroplasty followed by cervical encerclage during pregnancy can be very useful.

Clinical significance of diethylstilbestrol (DES)-exposed (T-shaped) uterus is rapidly decreasing as population of women exposed to DES now has crossed the active reproductive age. DES was used from 1948 to 1971. Since then it is banned and the women who might have taken it in 1971 also now must be 50-year-old. But correct identification of T-shaped uterus is still important because narrow uterine cavity is often diagnosed as T-shaped uterus. These may be Koch's affected uterus.

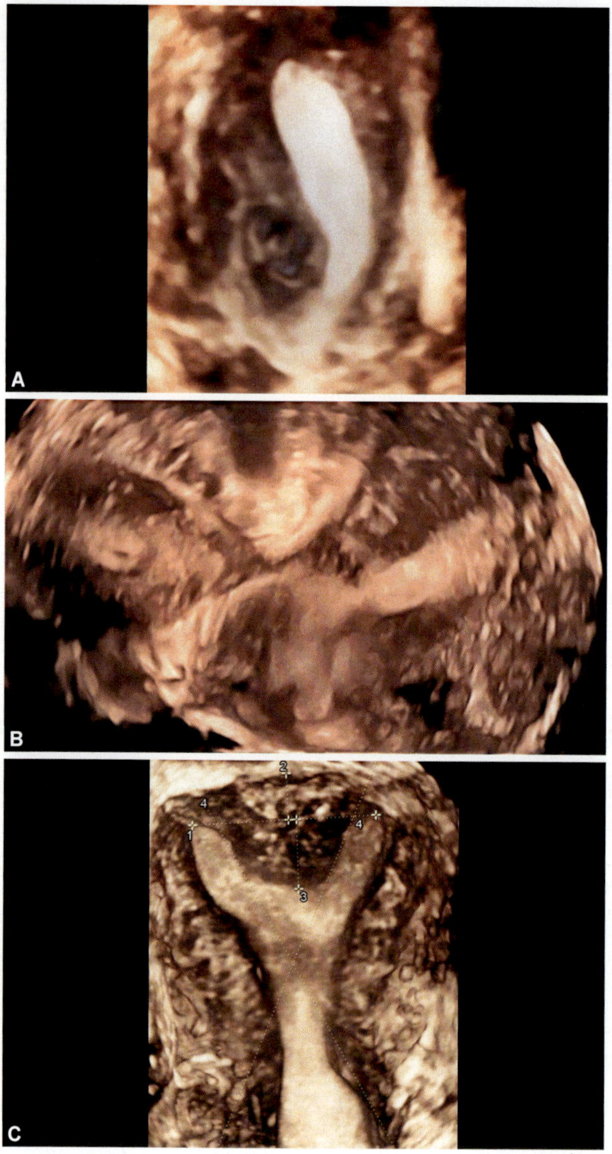

Figs. 1A to C: Three-dimensional ultrasound images: (A) Unicornuate uterus; (B) Bicorporeal uterus; (C) Septate uterus.

Table 2: Ultrasound findings of Class U1—dysmorphic uterus.

T-shaped uterus (Class U1a)	*Uterus infantilis (Class U1b)*
• Narrow cavity • Normal uterocervical ratio • Thick lateral wall	• Narrow cavity • Reverse uterocervical ratio • Normal wall

Class U2—Septate uterus: This is subclassified into:

- Partial septum
- Complete septum

With normal outer fundal contour, there is septum dividing the endometrial cavity. If this septum reaches the internal os, it is complete septum and short of that it is partial septum.

It is important to note here that the indentation of the endometrial fundus should be >50% of the total myometrial wall thickness to name the deformity as septum.

This is the most common uterine anomaly among the patients presenting with RPL. Causes postulated for abortion in septate uterus are:

- Septum has less connective tissue resulting in poor decidualization and placentation.
- Increased muscle mass in septum causes local uncoordinated myometrial contractility.
- High-resistance vascularity in septum leads to poor blood supply to endometrium overlying the septum.
- When there is high septal length to uterine cavity ratio, chances of abortion are higher.[4]
- Cervical incompetence.

Management:

- Operative hysteroscopy for septum resection has good outcome, but there is no definite data to justify its widespread use.[5,6]
- No pre- or postsurgical treatment is required if surgery is planned.
- Surgery should be deferred before pregnancy loss.[5,6]
- Chances of uterine rupture are increased in subsequent pregnancy after surgery.[7]
- Cervical encerclage is beneficial along with progesterone.

Class U3—Bicorporeal uterus: Class U3 is bicorporeal uterus with two corpora (body).

This class is further subclassified into:

- Partial bicorporeal
- Complete bicorporeal
- Bicorporeal septate.

The anomalies included in this class were earlier named as bicornuate and uterus didelphys, though this differentiation was based on the shape of the cervix also. Uteri in this class are placed when the uterine outer contour shows indentation, >50% of the myometrial wall thickness along with the division of the endometrial cavity also. When this indentation divides corpus of the uterus till internal os, it is complete bicorporeal and if it is short of that it is partial bicorporeal. But if in spite of indentation of the fundus, the dividing wall between the two endometrial cavities, its thickness is 1.5 times the myometrial wall thickness, this is named as bicorporeal septate uterus. If complete bicorporeal uterus also has double cervix, it is uterus didelphys according to the AFS classification.

For this shape of the uterus, pregnancy prognosis is the best (64%) among all congenital uterine abnormalities as far as pregnancy outcome is concerned. Unification of uterus by surgery is rarely required. Particularly in this era of good neonatal care, late trimester babies can be well-managed in neonatal intensive care units.

Abortion rate quoted in literature for bicorporeal uterus is 20–40%. These patients have cervical incompetence in up to 40% of patients. Cervical encerclage is primary line of treatment and results are similar to metroplasty (Strassman's operation).

One more so called abnormality, arcuate uterus, is no more considered as abnormal because when indentation in the endometrial cavity is <50% of the myometrial wall thickness, it is considered as normal uterus. Evidently, it does not require any treatment.

Class U4—hemi-uterus (unicornuate uterus): Its subclasses are: (a) with rudimentary horn and (b) without rudimentary horn.

It is seen in 6–20% of all congenital uterine malformations. In 90% of patients having hemi-uterus, rudimentary horn is present. Rudimentary horn should be removed in case of hematometra, ectopic pregnancy, or severe dysmenorrhea. In 40% of cases, it is associated with renal anomalies.

It has the worst outcome among all congenital uterine malformations.[2] Fetal loss can be up to 40–45% before completion of 2nd trimester. Preterm deliveries are extremely common. Abortions are due to abnormal vasculature, decreased muscle mass, and reduced space.

Prophylactic cervical encerclage is extremely useful. Vaginal micronized progesterone is useful to prevent uterine contractions.

b. Acquired Causes (Figs. 2A to C)

- Myomas
- Polyps
- Intrauterine adhesions
- Cervical incompetence

Myomas: Submucous myomas >2 cm in size can cause pregnancy loss and should be removed. Intramural myomas > 4 cm in size can cause abortions as these interfere with endometrial vascularization. Any myoma touching the endometrium can cause abortion because of interference with vascular supply and distortion of endometrial cavity. Saravelos et al. have shown in their study that myomas are more commonly associated with midtrimester

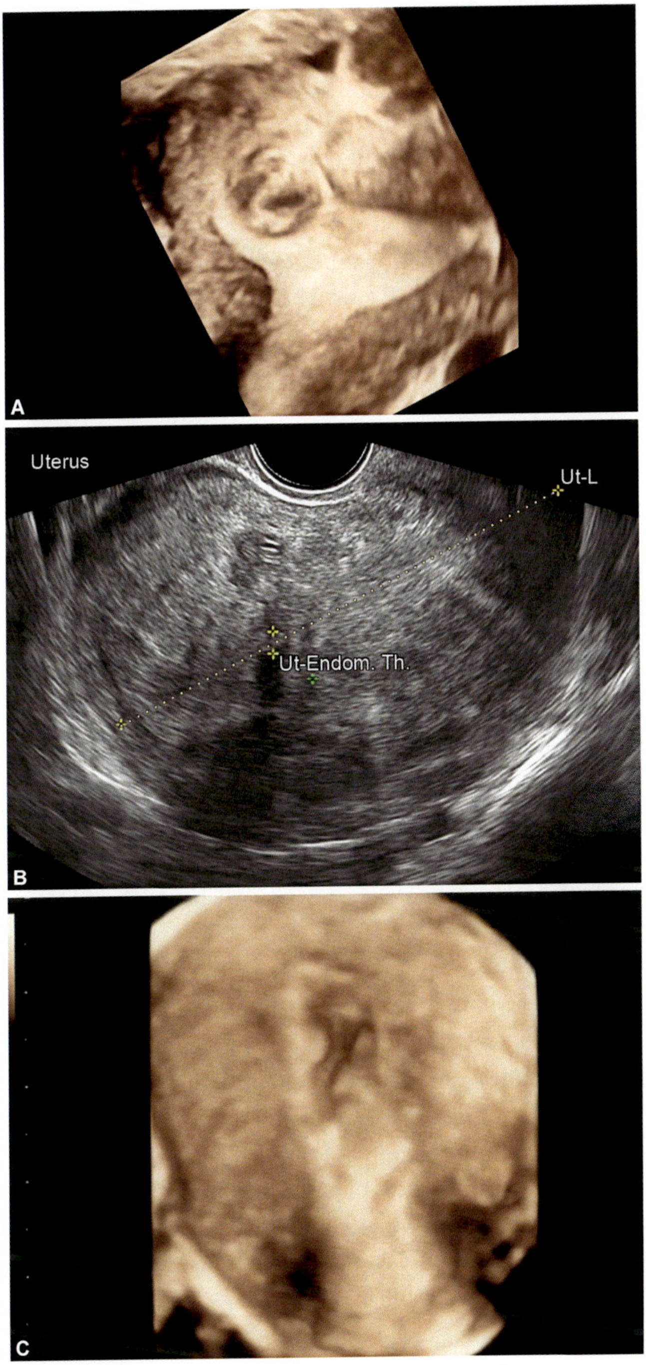

Figs. 2A to C: (A) Three-dimensional ultrasound of a fibroid; (B) B-mode of adenomyosis; (C) Three-dimensional ultrasound showing endometrial synechiea.

losses and resecting the fibroids that distort the endometrial cavity which can double the live birth rate in subsequent pregnancies.[8]

Myomectomy should be done by endoscopy. Laparoscopic-assisted myomectomy (LAM) is very popular. Myomectomy is preferred over uterine artery embolization if fertility is to be preserved. This is so because embolization can cause transient ovarian failure, endometrial atrophy, and amenorrhea.

MRI-guided focused high-frequency ultrasound ablation has been approved by the United States–Food and Drug Administration (US-FDA).

Polyps: Polyp is usually not a cause of RPL. But when RPL is present and no other cause than polyp is found for the same, polyp should be removed. If polypectomy is done with resectoscope, the recurrence rate is 0% and if done with polyp forceps, the recurrence rate is 17%. Bipolar forceps can also be used.

Chronic inflammation and polyp may act as foreign body and therefore lead to abortion.

Intrauterine adhesions: Intrauterine adhesions are expected to be more common among patients with RPL. About 21% of patients had intrauterine adhesions who otherwise had no cause for three abortions.[9] Hysteroscopic surgery may be beneficial.

Cervical incompetence: Congenital cervical incompetence is more common as compared to iatrogenic as surgeries on cervix such as Manchester's operation, cone biopsy of cervix, etc., are done very rarely.

Diagnosis: History of ruptured membranes without pain and setting of labor are the most common presentations. Easy passage of no. 8 Hegar's dilator is diagnostic of cervical incompetence, but now US has replaced Hegar's test as well as HSG.

Ultrasound findings are:

- Cervical length <3 cm
- Internal os diameter >1.5 cm in 1st trimester and >2 cm in 2nd trimester
- Bulging membranes into cervical canal through internal os
- Thinning of anterior part of lower segment
- *Cervical index*: Funnel length + 1/Endocervical length; if the value is >0.52, it increases the chances of preterm labor
- *Elastography*: This is a new modality assessing the elasticity or firmness of tissues. Soft cervix on elastography increases the risk of opening of cervical canal with increasing fetal weight.

Management: Dr Shirodkar was the first person to suggest a surgery for cervical incompetence in 1955. He recommended fascia lata for os tightening, but now mersilene is used in its place.

As Shirodkar's operation is technically difficult, majority of the surgeons use McDonald's operation, in which silk is tied at the lower level without opening the vaginal wall. There are more than 10 different surgeries suggested, but are not used routinely.

Antiphospholipid Syndrome (APS)

Definition

It is a triad of:

- Arterial/venous thrombosis
- Recurrent pregnancy loss
- Thrombocytopenia with elevated levels of antiphospholipid (APL) antibodies, i.e., lupus anticoagulant (LA) and/or anticardiolipin antibody (ACA).

  This syndrome is systemic and affects all tissues and organs of the body.

Etiology

- It has genetic susceptibility.
- Antiphospholipid binds with β2-glycoprotein I (β2GPI) antigen. This complex has affinity for membrane phospholipids.
- Skin infections, human immunodeficiency virus (HIV), pneumonia, hepatitis C, urinary tract infection (UTI), and *Helicobacter pylori* are associated with APS. Molecular mimicry between β2GPI and bacterial and viral epitopes is the principal mechanism that links infection to APS.
- In false-positive tests for syphilis, only APL antibody is raised but in APS, β2GPI is recognized by raised antibody titer.

Mechanism of Reproductive Failure in APS

- *Thrombosis*:
  - There is altered activity of platelets, fibrinolysis, coagulation cascade, and tissue factor.
  - Complement activation has been recently proved.
  - Thromboxane A2 (TXA2)/Prostaglandin I2 (PGI2) ratio is changed because of activation of platelets. APL inhibits arachidonic acid release and so PGI2 production is reduced.
- *Anticytokine effect*: Anti-inflammation cytokine interleukin 3 (IL-3) is decreased and leads to fetal loss. Aspirin and ciprofloxacin can revert this.
- *Induction of placental apoptosis*: APL affects adhesion molecules between elements of syncytiotrophoblasts and damages the trophoblasts. This effect is unrelated to thrombosis. So, there is role of steroid in early pregnancy loss. Cell adhesion molecule 1 (CAM-1) and vascular cell

adhesion molecule 1 (VCAM-1) levels are increased and there is no protection to trophoblast.

- Antiphospholipid decreases human chorionic gonadotropin (hCG) production and therefore supplementation of hCG is useful.
- Production of autoantibodies and so there is a role of immunoglobulins and steroids.
  - Autoantibodies to proteins C and S
  - Autoantibodies to plasmin and plasminogen
  - Autoantibodies to annexin V, which otherwise protects phospholipids
- Antiphospholipid antibodies can be directly toxic to the fetus.

Diagnosis of antiphospholipid antibodies:

- *Detection of APL antibodies*:
  - *Not prolonging clotting*:
    - Anticardiolipin (aCL), antiphosphatidylethanolamine (aPE), antiphosphatidylserine (aPS), antiphosphatidylcholine (aPC), antiphosphatidylglycerol (aPG), antiphosphatidylinositol (aPI), antiphosphatidic acid (aPA), and aβ2GPI.
    - 1 APL unit = 1 μg/mL phospholipid binding capacity.
    - Antibody may be immunoglobulin G (IgG), immunoglobulin M (IgM), and immunoglobulin A (IgA) and called GPL, MPL, and APL.
  - *Prolonging clotting assays*: Lupus anticoagulant (LA). These include:
    - Activated partial thromboplastin time (APTT)
    - Dilute Russell's viper venom test (dRVVT)
    - Kaolin clotting time (KCT).
  - *One laboratory feature:*
    - Lupus anticoagulant
    - Anticardiolipin antibody

    Laboratory results must be assessed twice at least 6 weeks apart.
    - One clinical feature
    - Arterial, venous, or small vessel thrombosis
    - *Pregnancy complications*:
      - Three abortions before 10 weeks
      - One abortion after 10 weeks
      - Intrauterine growth restriction (IUGR) with pregnancy at <34 weeks because of thrombosis.

      Early losses are due to noninvading blood vessels and direct action on trophoblast.
- *Types of APL antibodies*: LA and ACA independently increase the pregnancy loss. In reproductive autoimmune failure syndrome (RAFS), full APL panel should be measured. This includes LA, aCL, aPE, aPS, aPC, aPG, aPI, aPA, and aβ2GPI.

aPS and aPE are responsible for early loss as these affect trophoblastic functions. Here, in isotype, high IgM may be due to infection and drugs. High IgG >40 GPL is diagnostic and patient will benefit from drug prophylaxis. Both IgM and IgG should be measured. Low levels lower than 40 GPL have doubtful significance.

Time of testing:

- The test should be performed during pregnancy or close to pregnancy loss.
- Increased titers of APL must be present in serum in two measurements at interval of 6 weeks.
- Occasionally, aCL may be high outside.
- β2 glycoprotein, aPS, and annexin do not provide additional information and are not done routinely.
- Antinuclear antibody (ANA) and antithyroid antibody (ATA) are not required in RPL because there is no logic or proven treatment and it has uncertain relevance.
- Lupus anticoagulant is more responsible for adverse outcome than aCL.
- Anticardiolipin is for late complications.

Treatment

- Aspirin 75 mg
- Heparin 20,000 IU
- Prednisolone 40–60 mg
- Immunoglobulins

Aspirin: Aspirin in a dose of 75 mg daily should be started as soon as the diagnosis of pregnancy is done. Majority of papers believe that it is very useful, but several papers indicate that it has no role.[10,11]

Heparin: Low-molecular-weight heparin (LMWH) is extremely useful and a standard treatment for APS. It should be started after cardiac activity has appeared and it improved live birth rate by 80%. Dose of LMWH in RPL without history of thrombosis is 1 mg/kg/day but when thrombosis is present, the dose is doubled to 1 mg/kg/bd. This same dose is given when there is a history of previous loss after 10 weeks.

Combination of heparin and aspirin gives better pregnancy rates than one of the two alone.[12]

Side effects: LMWH has generally no side effects, but occasionally it may cause hemorrhage, osteopenia, and thrombocytopenia. LMWH does not cause overlap between anticoagulant and antithrombotic effect and so there is no bleeding and therefore there is a little need of monitoring. LMWH does not prolong PTT and so is monitored by factor Xa.

Mechanism of action of heparin:

- Anticoagulant effect
- It binds directly to APL
- Heparin inhibits complement activation.

Dose of heparin:

- APS with history of thrombosis—full dose of heparin is given (1 mg/kg/bd).
- APS with history of fetal loss after 10 weeks—full dose of heparin is given (1 mg/kg/bd).
- APS with early pregnancy losses (three or more)—lower doses 1 mg/kg/day is used.

Glucocorticoids:

- Glucocorticoid is very useful in patients having APS secondary to systemic lupus erythematosus (SLE).
- It is found to be very useful in early pregnancy loss but should be stopped after 10 weeks.
- It also prevents complement activation which is proinflammatory and procoagulant.

Intravenous immunoglobulin (IVIG): It improves thrombogenicity in experimental APS. However, clinical trials have found that it is not more effective in preventing pregnancy loss than heparin with aspirin. IVIG is found to be more effective in late pregnancy complication such as pregnancy-induced hypertension (PIH) or IUGR. Now it seems that IVIG may have a place as a second line of treatment in patients who are refractory to heparin who suffer from late obstetric complication.

Antinuclear antibody causes inflammation around placenta and corticosteroids are useful.

Antithyroid antibodies increase natural killer (NK) cells and are treated by IVIG, thyroid replacement therapy, and steroids.

When ANA and ATA are positive:

- Increase in peripheral CD19+ and CD5+
- Immunoglobulin M antibodies are against estrogen, progesterone, hCG, endorphin, and serotonin leading to insufficient decidualization and abortion.

Thrombophilia

In a normal pregnancy with hemostatic pathway, there is equilibrium between **(Table 3)**:

- *Procoagulant factors*: Factors V, VII, VIII and fibrinogen.
- *Anticoagulant factors*: Protein C, protein S, and antithrombin III.

Table 3: Factors with procoagulant effect and anticoagulant effect.

Procoagulant effect	*Anticoagulant effect*
• Factor XIII • Homocysteine • Fibrinogen • High thrombin generation • Factor V Leiden • Factor II prothrombin gene mutation *G20210A* • Cytokines, IL-6/4/10, and TNF-α • Microparticles	• Protein C • Protein S • Antithrombin • TFPI • FS fibrinolytic factor

(IL-6: interleukin 6; TFPI: tissue factor pathway inhibitor; TNF-α: tumor necrosis factor-α)

- *Fibrinolytic factors*: High plasminogen activator inhibitor (PAI) 1 and 2 genes.

These are all shifted in favor of procoagulant state during pregnancy.

Hereditary/congenital thrombophilia can be classified as:

- Antithrombin III deficiency
- Protein C deficiency
- Protein S deficiency

These are less common but more thrombogenic and others which are more common but weak thrombogenic factors are:

- *Factor V Leiden (FVL)*: Mutations/APCR (Northern Europe) (G1691A) common
- Prothrombin (G20210A) mutations (Southern Europe)
- Methylenetetrahydrofolate reductase (MTHFR) (C677T)
- *Antithrombin III deficiency*: It is inhibitor of thrombin and prevents conversion of fibrinogen to fibrin. Antithrombin III has thrombin binding site and a heparin binding site. The later of the two has 100 folds higher antithrombin activity. As large number of mutations are seen in *antithrombin III* gene, its deficiency can be assessed by functional clot-based assay such as thromboelastography.

  What is thromboelastography?

  Hemostasis is a dynamic process of interaction between prothrombotic and antithrombotic cellular and plasma components. Measurement of any single factor is, therefore, not useful, but the net result of the process must be studied. Elastography assesses the whole process and decides if it is hypo- or hypercoagulation state and so is a dynamic information.
- *Protein C deficiency*: Protein C is activated by thrombin to exert anticoagulant effect. It inactivates factor Va and VIII. Protein C deficiency also can be diagnosed by clot-based assay.
- *Protein S deficiency*: Protein S is a cofactor for protein C and is vitamin K dependent. It inactivates factor V and factor VII and requires clot-based assay for diagnosis.

- *Factor V Leiden mutations*: Substitution of glutamine from arginine at amino acid 506 in factor V protein abolishes the cleavage site that activates protein C and so factor V is resistant to activated protein C. It is seen in 10–15% of people of Northern Europe origin. It is a single point mutation. It has a weak thrombogenic potential but if it is a heterogeneous mutation, it is three to eight-fold more thrombogenic and if it is homogeneous mutations, it is 80-folds more thrombogenic.
- *Hereditary factor XIII deficiency—Autosomal recessive trait*: Its concentration decreases to 50% in normal pregnancy and only 0.5–2% is required for normal hemostasis. This is important for implantation and attachment of placenta to uterus. Its deficiency affects fibrin-fibronectin cross-linking adversely. Recombinant factor XIII is available with a half-life of 10–12 days and is to be given in a dose of 20 IU/kg once in every 4 weeks.
- *Fibrinogen deficiency*: This may present as afibrinogenemia, hypofibrinogenemia, or dysfibrinogenemia. Normal fibrinogen level to maintain pregnancy is 60 mg/100 mL. Its half-life is 4 days and its infusion in case of deficiency is given twice a week. It may lead to catastrophic thrombosis and therefore heparin is advocated.

Acquired Thrombophilia

Hyperhomocysteinemia: Homocysteine is an intermediate byproduct formed during metabolism of methionine. It generates hydrogen peroxide (H_2O_2) through its effect on endothelium and impairs endothelial cell thrombomodulation. Its modest elevation is described in association with inherited polymorphism of MTHFR with vitamin B_{12} and folic acid deficiency. C to T mutations at nucleotide 677 in gene coding of MTHFR enzyme leave only 30% of functionally active enzyme. This results in increased homocysteine levels and increases thrombogenicity by two- to threefold.

Currently, identified thrombophilia is less common in African and Asian population. Meta-analysis from 31 studies found that thrombophilias are commonly associated with 2nd and 3rd trimester losses. Evidence says that thrombophilias predispose to a high risk of both early and late pregnancy loss, but reproductive performance is normal with thrombophilia in some patients. It is not possible to establish as to which patient with RPL has increased risk with thrombophilia.

Pathophysiology of Pregnancy Loss in Thrombophilia

- Thrombosis in placental vessels in 2nd and 3rd trimester causes fetal loss.
- Placental contact of spiral artery and placental intervillous space starts developing only after 8 weeks and therefore pregnancy loss before 10 weeks may not be related to hemostasis. Early pregnancy loss in patients with thrombophilia, therefore, cannot be explained.

- Fetal thrombophilia can cause thrombosis in fetal vessels. Paternal thrombophilia can also cause fetal vessels thrombosis when fetus is homozygous or there is a combined maternal and paternal defect. Genetic mutation, therefore, increases the risk of pregnancy loss in subsequent pregnancies.
- Only a minority of patients with thrombophilia experience RPL. It is a combination of genetic and acquired risk factors usually.
- Though several studies have found no correlation of thrombophilia to pregnancy loss.
- Factor V Leiden deficiency is usually responsible for 3rd trimester loss.
- Prothrombin 20210A mutation may lead to late trimester but nonrecurrent fetal loss.
- Protein S deficiency also causes late trimester fetal loss.
- Methylenetetrahydrofolate reductase, protein C, and antithrombin III deficiency are not associated with fetal loss.

It has been shown in a meta-analysis by Rey et al.[13] that:

- Thrombophilia increases fetal loss.
- But not all thrombophilias are associated with fetal loss.
- First trimester losses are associated with FVL deficiency, protein C deficiency, and prothrombin mutation.
- Late trimester losses are associated with FVL deficiency and prothrombin mutation.

To conclude, thrombophilia increases the risk of pregnancy loss by three- to eightfold. FVL deficiency may be the cause for early and late trimester losses. Activated protein C resistance may lead to early trimester losses in patients with RPL. Prothrombin gene mutation increases the risk of pregnancy loss by two- to threefold. But it has been found in this same meta-analysis that protein C and protein S deficiency and hyperhomocysteinemia have a doubtful and conflicting role as a cause of RPL whereas MTHFR mutation does not show any association with RPL.

Screening for thrombophilia is done in patients with three or more 1st trimester losses after 8 weeks or in patients with two or more 2nd trimester losses or with past history or family history of RPL. Patients with unexplained stillbirth must also be screened, but patient should be counseled for the clinical uncertainty of the results and should be referred to a hematologist.

Treatment

- *Prophylactic LMWH*: It is safe and has minimal risk of allergic reaction. It has a high bioavailability and a long half-life with predictable therapeutic response. It is given in a dose of 40 mg daily. Rarely, it may cause thrombocytopenia or osteoporosis. Low-molecular-weight heparin therapy should be monitored by:

- Baseline assessment of platelets repeated after 1 week and repeated every month during therapy.
- Antifactor Xa levels are assessed for assessment of the drug response, but the results are not very consistent and so are less suitable to follow.
- Tissue factor pathway inhibitor (TFPI) can also be used for monitoring LMWH therapy.
- If patient requires a regional anesthesia, the dose of LMWH is omitted for a day to prevent spinal hematoma.

- Aspirin is still an optional treatment. It is given in a dose of 100 g/day.
- Progesterone produces IL-4 cytotoxins, therefore increases Th2 response.
- Human chorionic gonadotropin helps in cytokine production of endometrium (TNF-α and IL-4).

But heparin is preferred in patients with pregnancy loss after 10 weeks. Most times, both heparin and aspirin are combined. Heparin also has an anti-inflammatory effect. Its anti-inflammatory effect is by increasing serum TNF-α binding protein. Heparin inhibits TNF-α production. It has a direct effect on trophoblast and increases hCG production.

More research is required to find out why only few women get pregnancy loss. There are some other factors that play role in coagulation such as protein Z and vitamin K. These factors need further study. There are some more mutations that have been found to be responsible such as thrombomodulation gene, plasminogen activation gene, and factor V Cambridge mutation. These mutations also need further research to know their exact role.

Genetic Causes

Genetic factors are common cause for sporadic abortions (50–80%) while single gene defects are common cause of birth defects. A Japanese study has shown that abnormal karyotype is the most common cause of recurrent miscarriage and only in 24.5% of patients with RPL, the cause was unexplained. In 41.1%, the cause is abnormal embryonic karyotype.[14] Comparative genomic hybridization (CGH) microassays [or multiplex fluorescence in situ hybridization (M-FISH)] also find anomalies in abortus not found in karyotype.

Chromosomal abnormalities may be autosomal trisomy, double trisomy, polyploidy, tetraploidy, monosomy X, and sex chromosomal polysomy.

The question is that does recurrent aneuploidy exist? Recurrent aneuploidy can be seen in certain families. So if the first abortus is abnormal, chances of abnormal abortus are increased. Maternal age plays a major role. Higher the age, recurrent aneuploidy may be more possible.

The structural chromosomal rearrangements include translocations and inversions which play a major role in repeated losses.

Balanced translocation is higher in females. There may be history of stillborn or abnormal live born. There are two types of translocations: (1) Robertsonian and (2) Reciprocal. They have higher likelihood of abortions and abnormal live born. In a couple having balanced translocation with RPL, they should be offered preimplantation genetic diagnosis (PGD).

Other rare causes may be Mendelian and polygenic or multifactorial etiology. There may be uniparental disomy (UPD) where sole contribution is from single parent.

It has been shown in a very interesting study that cumulative chance of a healthy child is the same for carrier couples as for noncarrier couples and therefore selective karyotyping is advised instead of offering karyotyping to all couples with RPL.[15]

Place of Fetal Karyotyping in Recurrent Pregnancy Loss

In favor: Karyotyping of abortus allows the patient to be given prognostic information regarding subsequent outcome. Aneuploidy report can save further investigations and treatment. It assures to have better chance of normal embryo. If repeated abnormal karyotype abortuses are found, PGD is offered. Parental karyotyping does not provide diagnosis or prognosis for future outcome and treatment.

Against:

- About 60–70% of women with unexplained RPL will have a successful subsequent pregnancy.
- As the number of miscarriage increases, the possibility of chromosomal abnormality decreases.
- Current laboratory techniques are obstacles in making the diagnosis because of contamination and growth of maternal cells, cytogenic analysis is expensive. Histological features are not useful.
- More than 86% of chromosomally abnormal abortuses have numerical abnormality which occurs randomly and incidentally.
- The ACOG, RCOG, Royal College of Pathologists (RCPath), and International Workshop (Denmark, 2002) do not advise karyotyping of abortus as a routine procedure.

Role of Preimplantation Genetic Diagnosis

- It is very expensive as patient has to take in vitro fertilization (IVF)/ intracytoplasmic sperm injection (ICSI) cycles only.
- Preimplantation genetic diagnosis does not perform better than expectant management.
- Even in couples who are carriers of structural chromosomal rearrangements, PGD does not improve pregnancy rates as compared to expectant management.

So, routine use of PGD is not justified in RPL.

Alloimmunity

Normal pregnancy requires maternal immunological recognition and response to paternally-derived antigens on embryonic tissue and abnormality in this response may lead to RPL. Large proportions of unexplained RPL (80%) may be due to immunological causes. In alloimmune abortions, the maternal immune system reacts against the embryo and damages trophoblasts through allogeneic rejection type reactions.

When no other presentation except reproduction failure is present, it is known as RAFS. Apart from APL antibodies, ANA and antibodies against deoxyribonucleic acid (DNA) [single-stranded DNA (ssDNA), double-stranded DNA (dsDNA)], antibodies against histone or non-DNA components [Sm, ribonucleoprotein (RNP), single-strand annealing (SSA), single-stranded binding (SSB), and Scl-70], and ATA may be present.

The presence of these antibodies explains the role of IVIG to neutralize antibody-modulated immune response.

Apart from ANA and ATA, there is an increase in CD19+ and CD5+ cells which produce antibodies against estradiol (E2), progesterone, hCG, and neurotransmitters such as endorphins and serotonins. These cause insufficient decidualization and decreased blood supply to endometrium.

Genetic background of HLA-DQA1*0505 sharing is found in patients with RPL. Th2 type reaction favors implantation while Th1 type causes reaction. Increased NK cell activity favors abortion.

Immune Response in Normal Pregnancy

There is immunological paradox of pregnancy because embryo is not rejected even though it has genes inherited from father. This is because facilitation reaction prevails over the rejection reaction.

This is because of:

- *Th2 type immune response instead of Th1 type immune response*: Th2 type cytokines (IL-4, IL-5, and IL-10) predominate over Th1 type cytokines [IL-2 and interferon γ (INF-γ)—cerebrospinal fluid interferon-γ (CIFN-γ)] and prevent antitrophoblast cytotoxic reaction. Granulocyte-macrophage colony-stimulating factor (GM-CSF), IL-3 and transforming growth factor-β (TGF-β) also favor implantation. Progesterone influences Th2 type response by inducing production of IL-4 by γδT lymphocytes.
- *Role of NK cells in monitoring pregnancy*: Uterine NK cells are characteristically CD56 antigen. Peripheral NK cells have CD16 and CD3 antigens. Uterine NK cells participate in alternative defense system against microbiological and malignant invasion called innate immune system. These are increased in luteal phase, may be due to

progesterone, but they do not express progesterone receptors. They have prolactin, estrogen, and progesterone receptors. Uterine NK cells help in decidualization of endometrial stroma and control trophoblast invasion. Uterine NK cells become active and play major role for the production of INF-γ and Th2 type reaction. A function of uterine NK cells is to regulate endometrial angiogenesis important for implantation.[16] It helps in placental augmentation and local immunosuppression and immunomodulation. Uterine NK cells cause production of array of cytokines such as TNF-α, INF-α, leukemia inhibitory factor (LIF), and GM-CSF. Direct antigen-receptor interactions between uterine NK cells and extravillous trophoblast occur[17] and polymorphism of uterine NK cell receptor and trophoblast antigen have been associated with RPL.[18] Defective decidualization correlates with high uterine NK cell density >5% and a lack of 11β-hydroxysteroid dehydrogenase type 1 in stromal cells.[19] 11β-hydroxysteroid dehydrogenase type 1 activates cortisol, hence administration of glucocorticoid prednisolone may overcome this deficit and also reduce endometrial uterine NK cell density, production of angiogenic cytokines to help endometrial angiogenesis.[16] There is interaction with human leukocyte antigen-G (HLA-G) molecule which is in placenta only. NK cells of conventional CD3–, CD56+, and CD16+ type are increased in abortion. They are also increased in blood. Uterine NK cells do not express classical HLA antigens—HLA-C, HLA-G, and HLA-E.

To summarize the role of uterine NK cells:
- It is hostile to invading trophoblast
- It may facilitate abnormal blastocysts
- More uterine NK cells—poor pregnancy outcome.

Diagnostic Tests

- Antipaternal lymphocytic antibodies
- Maternal blocking antibody
- Human leukocyte antigen sharing
- Maternal immune suppression
- Mixed lymphocyte culture reactivity
- Peripheral blood NK cells

But these tests have no clinical utility.

The prognostic value of measuring peripheral NK or uterine NK cell parameters in women with RPL remains uncertain as a predictive test for screening women who may benefit from immunotherapy.[20]

Treatment

- Active immunization of woman using paternal or third-party lymphocytes. The Cochrane review 2006 does not support this therapy. This therapy has only marginal benefit. According to the American Society for Reproductive Medicine (ASRM), it has higher rate of side effects. Progesterone and hCG favor Th2 > Th1.

- Passive immunization by IVIG. It is very useful in increasing NK cells in peripheral blood. IVIG shifts to Th2 type response.
- IVIG appears to include CD200-dependent activity that results in suppression of NK cells. The dose is 0.5 g/kg at 5 weeks, followed by 0.35 g/kg every 3 weeks till 24 weeks. This treatment is very useful in very early abortions when NK cells are raised as it decreases NK cells and enhances CD8+ cell activity. The Cochrane review does not support this therapy. Cytokines such as GM-CSF and TGF-β are the future.

  Though several trials and meta-analysis concluded that IVIG is ineffective for primary RPL.[21]

  How IVIG acts?
  - It decreases the killing action of NK cells
  - Increases the activity of suppressor T-cells
  - Suppresses B-cell production of autoantibodies
  - It has antibodies to idiopathic antibodies
  - Binds with Fc component of IgG
- Preconceptional prednisolone or intrauterine prednisolone 20 mg/day from days 1–2 of the cycle for 4 weeks, prior to embryo transfer has been recommended.
- High proportions of women with RPL have vitamin D deficiency and this have immunological implications in RPL. Vitamin D is associated with B and NK cell immunity and Th1/Th2 balance. Women with low vitamin D have a tendency to develop APA and other autoantibodies related to autoimmune disorders and poor reproductive outcome.[22]
- Cytokines such as GM-CSF and TGF-β are likely to replace parental leukocytes and IVIG.

Points against Parental Lymphocyte Immunization

- A meta-analysis of trials on paternal leukocytes immunization concluded that it had no beneficial effect.[23]
- Increased sharing of HLA class I alleles between partners has been refuted in recent meta-analysis.[24]
- The hypothesis of blocking antibodies is not validated.
- Miscarriage occurs despite blocking antibody.
- Patient without blocking antibody has successful pregnancy.

Points against IVIG

- Relation between peripheral blood NK cells and reproduction failure is most controversial.

- It is unclear regarding number of NK cells which is abnormal.
- Rise in NK cells are mostly transient and not chronic.
- Beneficial effect is not observed and it is difficult to define who will be benefitted with IVIG.

Infections and Recurrent Pregnancy Loss

The role of infection in recurrent pregnancy loss (RPL) is unclear. Various infections quoted in literature are:

- Tuberculous
- Listerioses
- TORCH
- *Chlamydia*
- Syphilis
- Bacterial vaginosis
- Mycoplasmas

Infections are not the cause of RPL.

Environmental Factors

- Smoking
- Alcohol
- Heavy coffee
- Anesthetic gases
- Heavy metals
- Herbicide
- Radiation
- Electromagnetic field
- Wilson's disease
- Chemicals

Role of these factors in causing RPL is not proved; these factors may have a supporting role for pregnancy loss.

Endometriosis

Milder cases of endometriosis have highest risk for causing pregnancy loss as these are functionally more active. Spontaneous abortion rate decreases after treatment, but sufficient data is not yet available for considering it as a cause of RPL.

Endometriosis can act through:

- *Local factors*:
  - Endometrial stromal cell proliferation
  - High macrophage cytotoxicity

    - High cytokine
    - Low NK cell activity
- *Systemic factors*:
    - Raised immunoglobulin production
    - More T1 helper cells
    - Embryotoxicity
    - Suppression of NK cells
    - Low cell immunity
    - Abnormal autoimmune function

Psychological Causes

Role of Stress

- Stress-related hormones have endocrine role and affect placental hormones.
- It has autocrine and paracrine role.
- Hypothalamic-pituitary-ovarian axis reacts to anxiety and depression.
- Secretion of catecholamines play vital role in steroidogenesis.

Role of Tender Loving Care

- Limbic system is the seat of emotional activity.
- There is link between limbic system and immune system.
- Immune system prevents implantation.
- Tender loving care (TLC) creates lifelong bond and helps in preventing pregnancy loss.

The "ESHRE" special interest group concluded that only interventions that do not require more randomized controlled trials are TLC and health advice.[25]

Endocrine Causes

- Hypo-hyperthyroidism
- Diabetes mellitus
- Luteal phase defect (LPD)
- Polycystic ovarian syndrome (PCOS)

Thyroid

There is no direct evidence that subclinical hypo-hyperthyroidism causes RPL.[26] ATAs may be high due to autoimmune cause, though it has been shown that a transient impairment of thyroid function in early pregnancy may cause inadequate adaptation to the increased thyroid requirement and may be implicated in RPL.[27]

Recently upper limit of thyroid-stimulating hormone (TSH) is 2.5 IU/L for subclinical hypothyroidism. Clinical practice guidelines by the American Association of Clinical Endocrinologists and the American Thyroid Association (ATA) state that antithyroid peroxidase (anti-TPO) and antithyroglobulin (anti-TG) measurements should be considered during evaluation of RPL. They suggest that in patients of normal TSH with presence of anti-TPO, L-thyroxine should be given if there is history of miscarriage. But in few studies, there is no statistical difference in RPL.

Diabetes Mellitus

- High glycosylated hemoglobin in 1st trimester can cause abortion or malformation.
- In uncontrolled group, pregnancy loss is high and it can cause infertility.
- Hemoglobin A1c (HbA1c) assessment should be done for patients with RPL (ASRM guidelines).
- It is recommended to maintain at ≤7.5.

Luteal Phase Defect

Diagnosis and management have been discussed at length in the chapter dedicated to LPD. It has been shown that increased uterine artery resistance may be a contributing factor to some causes of RPL.[28,29] Here, we shall discuss LPD in relation to RPL only. Literature quotes incidence of LPD between 23% and 60%.

Why progesterone should be used?

Progesterone-induced blocking factor (PIBF) expression was less in patients who aborted than the healthy pregnant women. For donor-oocyte programs also, progesterone is given for 8 weeks.

As the diagnosis of LPD is very difficult to establish, progesterone should be given in suspected cases or on empirical basis. The argument in favor of empirical therapy is that it prevents 33% miscarriage rate when it is given to 100% of patients.

Follicular maturing drugs may not correct the luteal phase abnormality and so progesterone supplementation reduced miscarriage rate from 28 to 6%.[30,31] Progesterone is started after ovulation that is preconceptional stage.

Whenever serum progesterone is <8 ng/mL, progesterone supplementation will salvage 60% of pregnancies.[32] Therefore, it is very convincing that it is better to give benign treatment that may be later found not effective rather than not to treat her.

My personal opinion is to give progesterone to all patients of RPL, particularly when ovulation-inducing drugs are used or in patients of RPL when loss occurs very early in pregnancy.

Human chorionic gonadotropin supplementation: Patients with LPD are more likely to have early pregnancy losses before appearance of fetal cardiac activity. Human chorionic gonadotropin supplementation is particularly useful in patients with oligomenorrhea.[33,34] Majority of these women have PCOS. LPD is common in PCOS patients and so hCG supplementation is justified. Majority of studies have proved a benefit of 30% in patients with RPL, especially early pregnancy losses and history of oligomenorrhea. If we stick to early pregnancy loss and oligomenorrhea, 30% of patients with RPL are in this group and hCG supplementation gives favorable results in 85% of these patients.[35]

I use hCG for LPD since last 20 years and combination of progesterone and hCG since last 12 years as progesterone was introduced in India only 12 years back.

Low-dose aspirin and omega-3 fatty acids are effective in improving uterine artery blood flow velocity in women with recurrent miscarriage due to abnormal uterine perfusion.[36]

Hyperprolactinemia and pregnancy loss: High prolactin level interferes with corpus luteum function. High prolactin level in follicular phase interferes with progesterone secretion in luteal phase. Patients with hyperprolactinemia, treated with bromocriptine, have better chances of successful pregnancy. Therefore, normal level of prolactin may play important role in the growth and implantation of early embryo.

Polycystic Ovarian Syndrome

Diagnosis and management of PCOS are discussed in Chapter 16. Here, we shall discuss the role of PCOS in RPL.

Pregnancy loss in RPL is because of high luteinizing hormone (LH) that in turn causes high androgen and high insulin levels. These are detrimental to ova and embryo and lead to poor implantation rate and high early miscarriage rate.

Ovarian drilling is very useful in reducing pregnancy loss as it decreases LH levels. Antagonist can be used in thin lean PCOS to prevent early pregnancy loss or infertility. Role of metformin is debatable at present. Majority of the studies have shown that metformin has no role for ovulation induction or to prevent pregnancy loss. Metformin actually should be stopped during pregnancy as it crosses placenta. Metformin does not decrease early pregnancy loss.

Male Factors

Significant DNA fragmentation, abnormal sperm morphology, and decreased scores of sperm function tests are found in the male partners of patients with

RPL. Sperms do not have power of endogenous DNA repair. Damaged DNA is a major source of embryonic mortality.

There are two tests required:

1. DNA fragmentation index (DFI)
2. Fluorescence in situ hybridization for evaluating sperm aneuploidy.

About 40% of men with RPL have sperm aneuploidy. In these patients, IVF with preimplantation genetic screening (PGS) is recommended. Counts <10 million have higher aneuploidy rate. But despite 50 years of innovation and progress, we are no closer to understanding the mechanisms of contribution of male factor to pregnancy loss. So, routine testing of DFI and FISH is not recommended according to practice committee of the ASRM, 2012.

INVESTIGATIONS FOR RECURRENT PREGNANCY LOSS

- *Anatomical*: Three-dimensional of uterus
- *Antiphospholipid syndrome*:
  - Lupus antigen
  - Activated partial thromboplastin time
  - Dilute Russell viper venom test
  - Kaolin clotting time
  - Anticardiolipin antibody
  - Antinuclear antibody
  - β_2 glycoprotein
  - Antiphospholipid
- *Karyotyping*:
  - Male
  - Female
  - Fetus
- *Endocrine*:
  - Baseline scan days 2–3
  - Mid-luteal scan
  - Triiodothyronine (T3), T4, and TSH
  - Insulin
  - Blood sugar
  - Minor preoperative profile
- *Alloimmunity*:
  - Anti-HLA antibody
  - Natural killer cell activity
  - Human leukocyte antigen sharing
  - Homocysteine

- *Thrombophilia*:
    - Protein C
    - Protein S
    - Antithrombin
    - Factor V Leiden
    - Factor IL

Carry Home Message

- *Anatomical:*
    - *Congenital:*
        - Expectant management
        - Cervical encerclage
        - Septum resection
    - *Acquired:*
        - Removal of fibroid or polyp
        - Cervical encerclage
        - Intrauterine adhesiolysis
- *Antiphospholipid syndrome:*
    - Ecosprin 75 mg/day
    - Low-molecular-weight heparin 60 mg/day
    - Prednisolone 10 mg QDS in selected patients
    - Human chorionic gonadotropin 5,000 IU twice a week
    - Intravenous immunoglobulin 0.35 g/kg every 3 weeks (in resistant patients)
- *Genetic causes:*
    - Fetal karyotyping is not required
    - Parental karyotyping
    - Chorion biopsy or preimplantation genetic diagnosis (PGD) for translocations
- *Alloimmunity:*
    - Micronized vaginal progesterone 400 mg TDS
    - Parenteral or third-party lymphocytes are not recommended because of only marginal benefit.
    - Human chorionic gonadotropin 5,000 IU twice a week
    - Intravenous immunoglobulin 0.5 g/kg followed by 0.35 g/kg every 3 weeks in very early losses
- *Infections:* Not a cause of RPL
- *Environmental:* Not a cause of RPL
- *Endometriosis:* Not a cause of RPL
- *Psychological:*
    - Tender loving care
    - Health advice
- *Endocrine:*
    - *Luteal phase defect:*
        - Micronized vaginal progesterone
        - Human chorionic gonadotropin 5,000 IU twice a week

Contd...

Contd...

- *Polycystic ovarian syndrome:*
  - Ovarian drilling
  - Antagonist and/or chronic low-dose follicle-stimulating hormone (FSH) stimulation protocol
  - Micronized vaginal progesterone
  - Human chorionic gonadotropin 5,000 IU twice a week.
- *Hereditary—thrombophilia:* Low-molecular-weight heparin 40–80 mg/day

REFERENCES

1. Practice Committee of the American Society for Reproductive Medicine. Evaluation and treatment of recurrent pregnancy loss: a committee opinion. Fertil Steril. 2012;98:1103-11.
2. The American Fertility Society Classifications of Adnexal Adhesions, Distal Tubal Occlusion, Tubal Occlusion Secondary to Tubal Ligation, Tubal Pregnancies, Müllerian anomalies and Intrauterine Adhesions. Fertil Steril. 1998;49:944-55.
3. Grimbizis GF, Gordts S, Di Spiezio Sardo A, Brucker S, De Angelis C, Gergolet M, et al. The ESHRE/ESGE consensus on the classification of female genital tract congenital anomalies. Hum Reprod. 2013;28:2032-44.
4. Salim R, Regan L, Woelfer B, Backos M, Jurkovic D. A comparative study of the morphology of congenital uterine anomalies in women with and without a history recurrent first trimester miscarriage. Hum Reprod. 2003;18:162-6.
5. Homer HA, Li TC, Cooke ID. The septate uterus: a review of management and reproductive outcome. Fertil Steril. 2000;73:1-14.
6. Heinonen PK. Complete septate uterus with longitudinal vaginal septum. Fertil Steril. 2006;85:700-5.
7. Sentilhes L, Sergent F, Roman H, Verspyck E, Marpeau L. Late complications of operative hysteroscopy: predicting patients at risk of uterine rupture during subsequent pregnancy. Eur J Obstet Gynecol Reprod Biol. 2005;120:134-8.
8. Saravelos SH, Yan J, Hassan R, Tin-Chiu Li. The prevalence and impact of fibroids and their treatment on the outcome of pregnancy in women with recurrent miscarriage. Hum Reprod. 2011;26:3274-79.
9. Ventolini G, Zhang M, Gruber J. Hysteroscopy in the evaluation of patients with recurrent pregnancy loss: a cohort study in a primary care population. Surg Endosc. 2004;18:1782-4.
10. Pattison NS, Chamley LW, Birdsall M, Zanderigo AM, Liddell HS, McDougall J. Does aspirin have a role in improving pregnancy outcome for women with the antiphospholipid syndrome? A randomized controlled trial. Am J Obstet Gynecol. 2000;183:1008-12.
11. Cowchock S, Reece EA. Do low-risk pregnant women with antiphospholipid antibodies need to be treated? Organizing Group of the Antiphospholipid Treatment Trial. Am J Obstet Gynecol. 1997;176:1099-100.
12. Kutteh WH. Antiphospholipid antibody-associated recurrent pregnancy loss: treatment with heparin and low-dose aspirin is superior to low-dose aspirin alone. Am J Obstet Gynecol. 1996;174:1584-9.
13. Rey E, Kahn SR, David M, Shrier I. Thrombophilic defect and fetal loss: A meta-analysis. Lancet. 2003;361:901-8.

14. Sugira-Ogasawara M, Ozaki Y, Katano K, Suzumori N, Kitaori T, Mizutani E. Abnormal embryonic karyotype is the most frequent cause of recurrent miscarriage. Hum Reprod. 2012;27:2297-303.
15. van den Boogaard E, Hermens RP, Verhoeve HR, Kremer JA, van der Veen F, Knegt AC, et al. Selective karyotyping in recurrent miscarriage: are recommended guidelines adopted in daily clinical practice? Hum Reprod. 2011;26:1965-70.
16. Quenby S, Nik H, Innes B, Lash G, Turner M, Drury J, et al. Uterine natural killer cells and angiogenesis in recurrent reproductive failure. Hum Reprod. 2009;24:45-54.
17. Moffett-King A. Natural killer cells and pregnancy. Nat Rev Immunol. 2002;2:656-63.
18. Hiby SE, Regan L, Lo W, Farrel L, Carrington M, Moffett A. Association of maternal killer-cell immunoglobulin-like receptors and parental HLA-C genotypes with recurrent miscarriage. Hum Reprod. 2008;23:972-6.
19. Kuroda K, Venkatakrishnan R, Salker MS, Lucas ES, Shaheen F, Kuroda M, et al. Induction of 11β-HSD 1 and activation of distinct mineralocorticoid receptor and glucocorticoid receptor-dependent gene networks in decidualizing human endometrial stromal cells. Mol Endocrinol. 2012;27:192-202.
20. Tang AW, Alfirevic Z, Quenby S. Natural killer cells and pregnancy outcomes in women with recurrent miscarriage and infertility: a systematic review. Hum Reprod. 2011;26:1971-80.
21. Ata B, Tan SL, Shehata F, Holzer H, Buckett W. A systematic review of intravenous immunoglobulin for treatment of unexplained recurrent miscarriage. Fertil Steril. 2011;95:1080-5.
22. Ota K, Dambaeva S, Han AR, Beaman K, Gilman-Sachs A, Kwak-Kim J. Vitamin D deficiency may be a risk factor for recurrent pregnancy loss by increasing cellular immunity and autoimmunity. Hum Reprod. 2014;29:208-19.
23. Porter TF, LaCoursiere Y, Scott JR. Immunotherapy for recurrent miscarriage. Cochrane Database Syst Rev. 2006;2:CD000112.
24. Beydoun H, Saftlas AF. Association of human leukocyte antigen sharing with recurrent spontaneous abortions. Tissue Antigens. 2005;65:123-35.
25. Jauniaux E, Farquharson RG, Christiansen OB, Exalto N. Evidence-based guidelines for the investigation and medical treatment of recurrent miscarriage. Hum Reprod. 2006;21:2216-22.
26. Bernardi LA, Cohen RN, Stephenson MD. Impact of subclinical hypothyroidism in women with recurrent early pregnancy loss. Fertil Steril. 2013;100:1326-31.
27. Lago AD, Vaquero E, Pasqualetti P, Lazzarin N, Carolis CD, Perricone R, et al. Prediction of early pregnancy maternal thyroid impairment in women affected with unexplained recurrent miscarriage. Hum Reprod. 2011;26:1324-30.
28. Lazzarin N, Vaquero E, Exacoustos C, Romanini E, Amadio A, Arduini D. Midluteal phase Doppler assessment of uterine artery blood flow in nonpregnant women having a history of recurrent spontaneous abortions: correlation to different etiologies. Fertil Steril. 2007;87:1383-7.
29. Habara T, Nakatsuka M, Konishi H, Asagiri K, Noguchi S, Kudo T. Elevated blood flow resistance in uterine arteries of women with unexplained recurrent pregnancy loss. Hum Reprod. 2002;17:190-4.
30. Check JH, Nowroozi K, Wu CH, Adelson HG, Lauer C. Ovulation-inducing drugs versus progesterone therapy for infertility in patients with luteal phase defects. Int J Fertil. 1988;33:252-6.
31. Check JH, Chase JS, Wu CH, Adelson HG, Teichman M, Rankin A. The efficacy of progesterone in achieving successful pregnancy: I. Prophylactic use during luteal phase in anovulatory women. Int J Fertil. 1987;32:135-8.

32. Choe JK, Check JH, Nowroozi K, Benveniste R, Barnea ER. Serum progesterone and 17-hydroxyprogesterone in the diagnosis of ectopic pregnancies and the value of progesterone replacement in intrauterine pregnancies when serum progesterone levels are low. Gynecol Obstet Invest. 1992;34:133-8.
33. Quenby S, Farquharson RG. Human chorionic gonadotropin supplementation in recurring pregnancy loss: a controlled trial. Fertil Steril. 1994;62:708-10.
34. Scott JR, Pattison N. Human chorionic gonadotropin for recurrent miscarriage. Cochrane Database Syst Rev. 2000;2:CD000101.
35. El-Zibdeh MY. Dydrogesterone in the reduction of recurrent spontaneous abortion. J Steroid Biochem Mol Biol. 2005;97:431-4.
36. Lazzarin N, Vaquero E, Exacoustos C, Bertonotti E, Romanini ME, Arduini D. Low-dose aspirin and omega-3 fatty acids improve uterine artery blood flow velocity in women with recurrent miscarriage due to impaired uterine perfusion. Fertil Steril. 2009;92:296-300.

CHAPTER 12

Practical Tips for Infertility Management

Chaitanya Nagori

INTRODUCTION

The practical tips for infertility practice presented here is the essence of my experience of 25 years as an infertility consultant that has resulted in about 12,000+ pregnancies.

DRUGS

- Clomiphene should be given maximum for 3 months with ultrasound (US) monitoring.
- Dose of clomiphene citrate (CC) should be up to 100 mg for 5 days. Extended regimens are not useful in clinical practice.
- Human chorionic gonadotropin (hCG) should be combined with CC only when intrauterine insemination (IUI) is to be done or delayed luteinizing hormone (LH) surge is suspected.
- CC + estrogen has no role.
- CC + bromocriptine is used for spikers and galactorrhea. Empirical use of bromocriptine has no role.
- CC + dexamethasone is used in CC-resistant chronic anovulatory patients and resistant polycystic ovary syndrome (PCOS).
- Metformin is given only to CC-resistant cases. CC is better than metformin for ovulation induction in PCOS patients.
- Ovarian drilling has excellent results. Number of punctures should depend on stromal volume.
- CC + gonadotropin reduces the requirement of gonadotropins but does not increase the pregnancy rate because of high LH due to CC.
- Letrozole is very useful in CC-resistant cases and PCOS, when baseline estradiol (E2) is >35 pgm/mL. Letrozole has replaced CC in PCOS patients and in poor responders.
- Letrozole + gonadotropins give excellent pregnancy rates with less number of gonadotropins used and lower multiple pregnancy rates.
- Low dose follicle-stimulating hormone (FSH) should be used as a first-line treatment for anovulatory PCOS patients.

- Recombinant FSH (rFSH) and recombinant hCG (rhCG) are superior over the urinary products and give very high pregnancy rates.
- Gonadotropins + antagonist + IUI. This regimen has given excellent results in patients with thin lean PCOS.
- Medical management of male infertility helps to improve the count and motility and in vitro fertilization (IVF) and intracytoplasmic sperm injection (ICSI) may be converted into IUI cycles.
- Gonadotropins by Ishidori's regimen helps to improve count in idiopathic oligozoospermia.
- Antioxidants are only supportive treatment in male subfertility and their effect vanishes once the drug is stopped.
- Aspirin + corticosteroids are very useful in patients with early pregnancy loss due to antiphospholipid syndrome in our series. Corticosteroids are not continued after 3 months of pregnancy. Heparin can be used after positive pregnancy test.

INVESTIGATIONS

- Investigations should not be asked for without provisional diagnosis.
- Packages and profiles for infertility are useless.
- FSH/LH is generally not required for diagnosis of PCOS and does not add anything to your management.
- Serum dehydroepiandrosterone sulfate (DHEAS) should not be assessed routinely for all the patients of PCOS.
- Fluctuating prolactin levels between 25 and 50 ng/mL are not of much clinical significance and bromocriptine is usually not required. Mostly it is because of PCOS.
- Serum estrogen and serum progesterone levels during follicular monitoring are not required now with good US monitoring.
- Antisperm antibodies testing in serum of male or females has no value.
- Normal postcoital test (PCT) more or less rules out the male infertility and is very satisfying for the couple.
- Anti-Müllerian hormone (AMH) is not useful for non-assisted reproductive technology (ART) patients. Antral follicle count (AFC) is equally reliable.
- 2 hours glucose tolerance and insulin response tests can be used to decide for ovarian drilling and treatment of PCOS.
- Ovarian reserve testing is not required before IUI.
- Ultrasound can replace serum FSH, serum LH, E2, progesterone, androgen, and AMH.
- Only tests required in any female presenting with infertility are serum prolactin, serum thyroid-stimulating hormone (TSH), and 2 hours glucose and insulin tolerance test.

PROCEDURES

- Superovulation with gonadotropins with IUI is a treatment of choice in cases of idiopathic infertility and has very high success rate of up to 80% in six cycles.
- Only IUI does not improve pregnancy rate unless it is backed by good stimulation protocol, good US monitoring, proper semen preparation, and good luteal support.
- Good semen preparation means 6–8 million count with >95% motile sperms.
- IUI should be done at 36–38 hours post-hCG routinely but double IUI (additional earlier IUI) is done when peak systolic velocity (PSV) >20–25 cm/s, i.e., first IUI after 12 hours of trigger and second after 36–38 hours.
- CO_2 incubator is must for good IUI preparation.
- *Ovarian drilling*: It gives excellent results in CC-resistant cases. Four punctures are not much beneficial and number of punctures should depend on the ovarian volume. Mostly all PCOS ovaries require at least 15–20 punctures or even more for duration of 1 second with 400 watts.
- After ovarian drilling superovulation with IUI should be done without wasting any cycle.
- All laparoscopies must be combined with hysteroscopies and continuous recording should be given to the patient for all future references. This will save the patient from unnecessary repeat laparoscopy.
- Tubal recanalization is useful only in patients with blocked tubes due to tubal ligation; otherwise IVF is a better option.
- Dilatation and curettage (D&C) has no role in modern infertility except for diagnosis of genital tuberculosis. Hysteroscopy must be preferred to hysterosalpingography (HSG) and combined with laparoscopy.
- Unnecessary removal of fibroids during routine endoscopy for infertility should be avoided to prevent iatrogenic infertility due to tubo-ovarian adhesions with uterus.
- All septa in uterus do not require resection unless there is history of abortion. Results are comparable with or without surgery.
- In patients with risk of ovarian hyperstimulation syndrome (OHSS), (cut-off E2 4,000 pgm/mL), IV albumin at the time of pick up and cabergoline 0.5 mg daily for 8 days have avoided OHSS in most cases in long protocol IVF cases.
- Transvaginal removal of fluid in OHSS is the treatment of choice to improve renal parameters and clinical improvement rather than the last resort as mentioned in previous textbooks.

IN VITRO FERTILIZATION AND INTRACYTOPLASMIC SPERM INJECTION

- Counseling for the procedure is a must.
- Counseling for the total expenditure and the results—pregnancy rate—can avoid all litigations and disharmony.
- IVF is done after 6–9 IUI failures in idiopathic fertility.
- Intracytoplasmic sperm injection is done for low count, which is not improved by medical management.
- Many patients conceive spontaneously or by IUI after IVF/ICSI failure.
- Endometriosis of grade III or IV requires ART.
- Embryo donation should be discussed with all the patients above 42 years or poor responders, even if younger, because results of ovum donation are always better for these patients.
- Antagonist protocol + agonist trigger + freeze all can completely avoid OHSS.

ULTRASONOGRAPHY

- Use only transvaginal scan (TVS) for monitoring of infertility patients.
- Baseline scan on Day 2–3 is a must to assess uterocervical length for IUI as well as to decide the starting dose of stimulation protocol. The baselines can determine polycystic ovaries (PCO), normally responding and poor responding ovaries.
- Human chorionic gonadotropin timing should be determined by two-dimensional (2D), color Doppler, pulse Doppler, and three-dimensional (3D) power Doppler of follicle and endometrium. This is the secret of success for IUI.
- Always do US at 5 weeks from last menstrual period (LMP) for confirmation of intrauterine pregnancy and 6 weeks for cardiac activity.
- We do nuchal scan with nasal bone assessment, ductus venosus flow, tricuspid flow, and intracranial translucency with early fetal echocardiography for all pregnant patients between 11 and 14 weeks.
- Detailed structural scan including fetal echocardiography is done between 18 and 20 weeks.
- We evaluate all pregnancies by color Doppler at 30–32 weeks for future prognosis and management.
- Complete documentation of all scans in detail is a must.

PRESCRIPTION

- Prescription is your image, a doctor is evaluated by his prescription, not by his face.
- Length of prescription is inversely proportional to your knowledge.

- Many times prescription indicates the year of passing.
- Do not write because you have to write something.
- Avoid writing drugs to help the pharmaceutical companies. Save patients' money for better indicated costly drugs.
- Usually indicated drugs are cheap and nonspecific drugs are very expensive.

FOR BEGINNERS

- Be transparent and honest with patients.
- There is no option to hard work.
- Wise persons learn from other's mistakes.
- Do not be afraid of criticism.
- It is very easy to criticize, but very difficult to appreciate your colleague.
- Keep away from short-term gains.
- Try to see the roots rather than fruits on the tree.
- Keep updating your knowledge and equipment with latest technology.
- Books and journals help us like God in crisis, so keep them with you.

Be an Infertility Consultant, not an IVF Consultant.

Section 2

Ultrasound

- **Optimizing the Image and Basic Transvaginal Sonography**
  Sonal Panchal
- **Ultrasound in Uterine Diseases**
  Sonal Panchal
- **Ultrasound in Gynecology: Adnexal Diseases**
  Sonal Panchal
- **Cycle Assessment for Infertility Treatment by Ultrasound**
  Sonal Panchal
- **Normal and Abnormal First-trimester Pregnancy**
  Sonal Panchal
- **Normal Fetal Anatomy in Second Trimester**
  Sonal Panchal
- **Fetal Screening for Chromosomal Anomalies**
  Sonal Panchal
- **Systematic Examination of Fetal Central Nervous System: How Much Should an Obstetrician Know?**
  Sonal Panchal
- **Fetal Echocardiography for Obstetrician**
  Sonal Panchal
- **Role of Ultrasound in Diagnosis and Management of Fetal Growth Restriction**
  Sonal Panchal
- **Ultrasonography in Male Infertility**
  Sonal Panchal
- **3D and 4D Ultrasound in Obstetrics and Gynecology**
  Sonal Panchal

CHAPTER 13

Optimizing the Image and Basic Transvaginal Sonography

Sonal Panchal

EQUIPMENT SETTINGS

Usually, there are presets on all the equipment for different scans and there is one for each scan and there is one for gynec scans also. The advantage of using correct preset is that one does not have to manipulate multiple knobs with every scan. The probes now available are multifrequency probes and the frequency setting changes with the depth of scanning selected. The transvaginal probe, if a multifrequency probe, either 5–9 MHz or 6–12 MHz, is preferred.

OPTIMIZING THE IMAGE

The basis of correct diagnosis on B-mode and Doppler study and three-dimensional (3D) image is a good quality B-mode image. Good image quality on B-mode or two-dimensional (2D) ultrasound means better resolution and higher frame rate. Resolution is assessed by number of pixels in a unit area. More the pixels, better is the resolution. Since the 2D scan that is done is a live real-time scan, it can be truly real time if there are more 2D still frames coming one after the other. Number of frames being changed in a unit time is frame rate. Higher the frame rate, better is the quality of the scan. The basic settings to be made with each scan and several times in each scan. The understanding of the settings and optimization of the image equally applies to any route of the scan, may it be transvaginal, transabdominal, transrectal and which ever probe one uses.

- *Scanning angle*: The scanning angle decides the width of scanning area. The scanning angle is kept open, to its full limits when the probe is introduced into the vagina, so that a pilot view of all pelvic organs and their relationship can be studied. The maximum scanning angle for different transvaginal probes vary from 120° to 180°. Once the general anatomy is understood and one needs to concentrate on a particular organ, e.g., uterus or ovary, then the scanning angle is narrowed to accommodate a particular structure and marginal surroundings. This improves the frame rate and in turn resolution of the image **(Figs. 1A and B)**.
- *Scanning depth*: Same as for scanning angle, the scanning depth also is set at least 8–10 cm in the preset. But after the overview of the general

anatomy, when one concentrates on a particular organ or lesion, the scanning depth is also decreased like angle, so that the region of interest fills two-thirds of the image. This also increases the frame rate and improves resolution **(Figs. 2A and B)**.

- *Zoom*: After the overview scanning, decreasing the scanning angle and depth, image should be zoomed large enough to fill up at least three-fourths of the screen. One may zoom the whole image (Pan zoom) or may use a zoom box to define which part of the image needs to be zoomed (HD zoom). This improves resolution of the image **(Figs. 3A and B)**. But it is important here to mention that Pan zoom just increases the distance between the pixels and does not improve the image quality, though it may improve the visibility of smaller details due to magnification. So, Pan zoom is not to be used while doing live scans. When used on a frozen image, it does not damage the image quality. For live scan, therefore, it is best to use HD zoom.

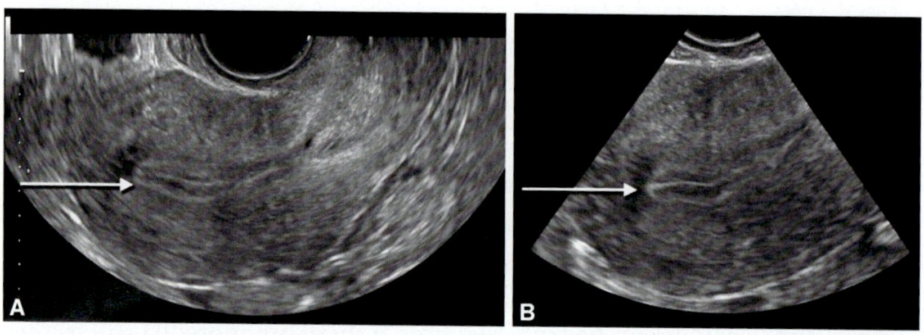

Figs. 1A and B: Change in resolution by changing scanning angle.

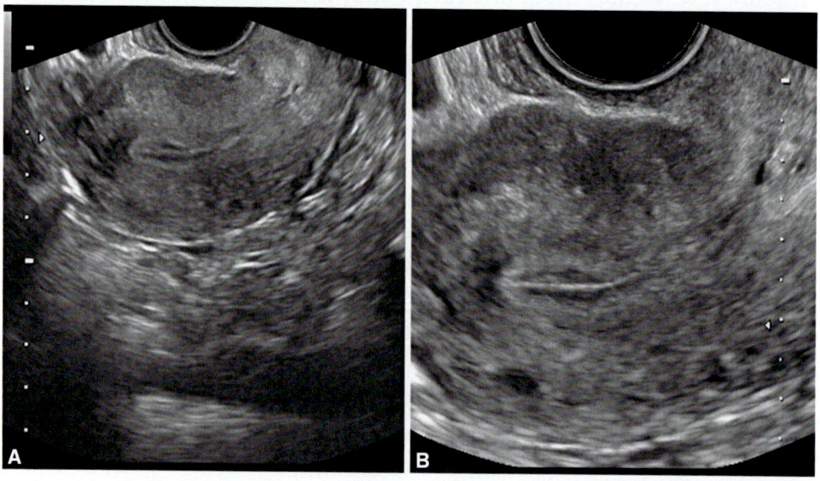

Figs. 2A and B: Change in resolution by changing scanning depth.

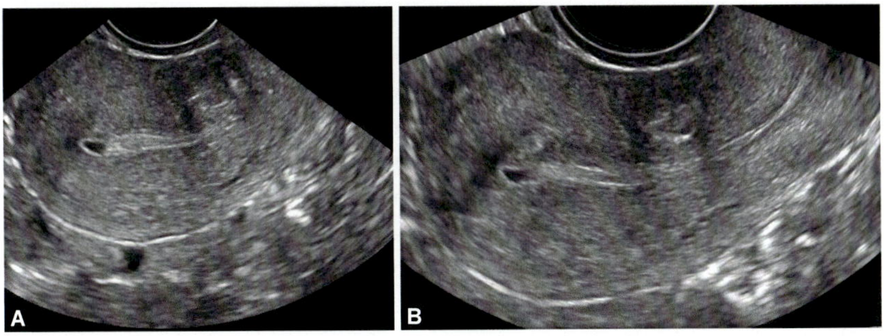

Figs. 3A and B: Change in image quality by zooming the image.

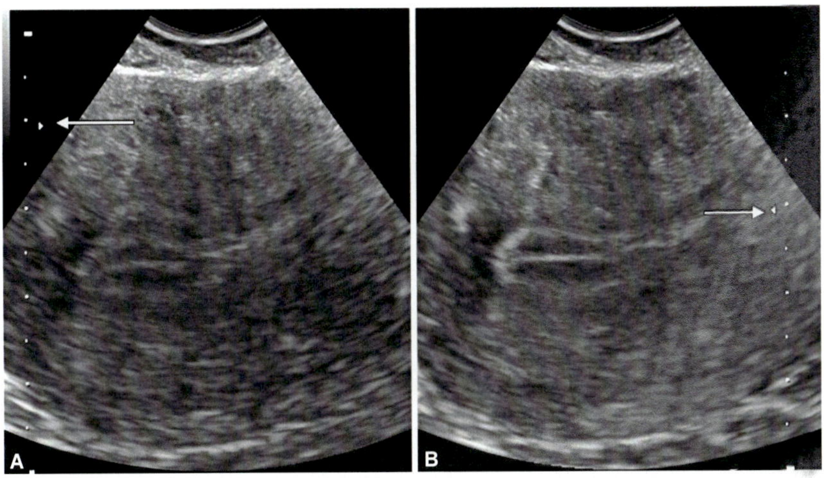

Figs. 4A and B: Change in image quality by changing the level of focal zone.

- *Setting the focal zone*: The arrowhead on right side of the image indicates the focal zone. Focal zone is the level at which the ultrasound beam converges to become narrowest and therefore, the image is the sharpest. So, focal zone is always set at the level of area of interest. There is also an option of having more than one focal zone, when there are multiple levels at which the image needs to be sharp. But increasing the number of focal zones decreases the frame rate, and therefore usually single focal zone is selected except when large lesions are scanned or anatomical relationship of pelvic organs is required **(Figs. 4A and B)**.
- *Gains*: It is known that structures far from the probe appear hypoechoic (darker) than what they are. This is because as the ultrasound beam traverses through the tissues, it loses its intensity and this may cause an error of diagnosis and decreased visibility. When the image is too dark or unclear, the examiner may be tempted to change the gains of the image, but changing gains inadvertently may lead to erroneous diagnosis. With

increased gains, even the anechoic structures may appear echogenic. Therefore, the gains are set in such a way that the urinary bladder appears anechoic, but its walls do not lose thickness **(Figs. 5A and B)**.

- *Contrast/Dynamic range*: Contrast or dynamic range indicates the number of gray shades displayed in the image. Higher the contrast, less number of gray shades are seen and with lower contrast, more number of gray shades are seen. This means that when contrast is high, soft tissue details will be obliterated and when contrast is low, there are so many shades of gray that it is virtually difficult to differentiate one from the other.

Harmonics, speckle reduction imaging (SRI), and compound resolution imaging (CRI) are more advanced tools used to further enhance the image quality.

- *Harmonics*: This is selective regulation of chosen frequency of sound waves from the returning signals. This reduces artifacts and enhances image quality **(Figs. 6A and B)**.

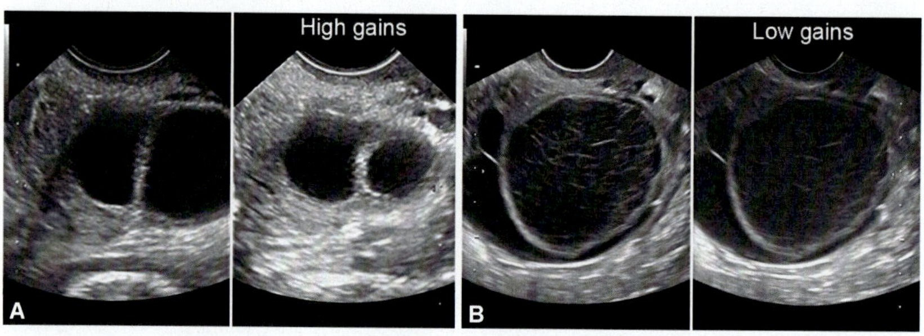

Figs. 5A and B: Change in image quality by changing gains.

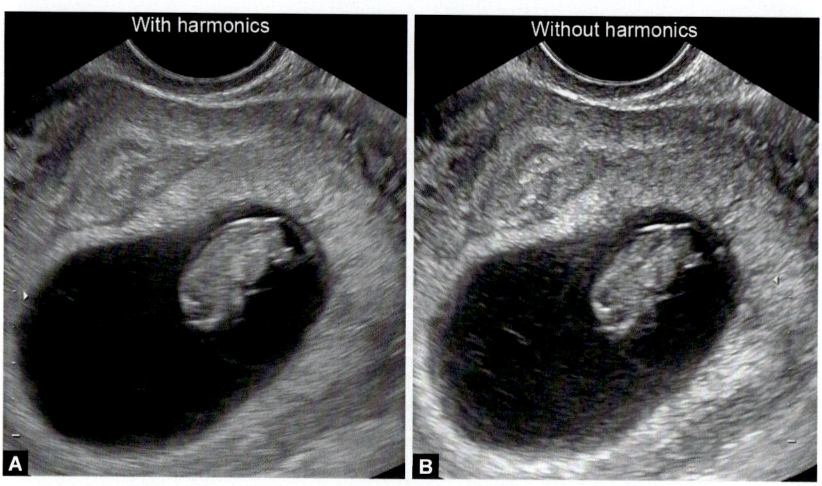

Figs. 6A and B: Better image quality is seen in Figure A with harmonics.

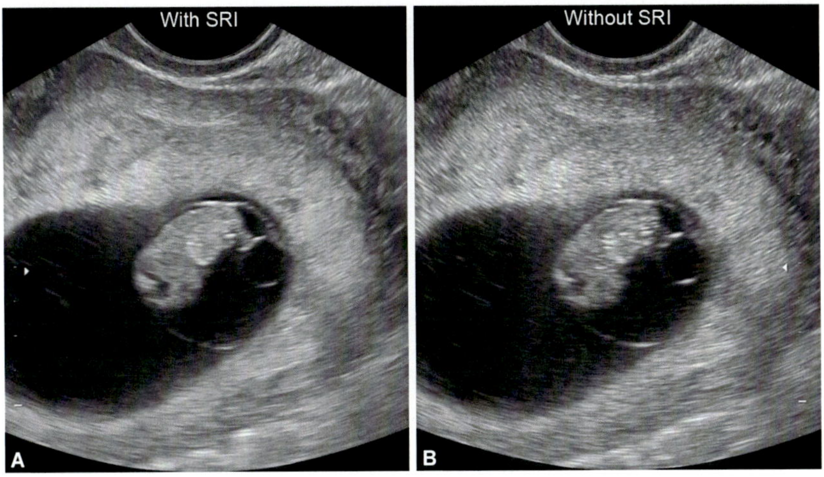

Figs. 7A and B: Figure A with speckle reduction imaging (SRI) shows better tissue plane differentiation.

- *Speckle reduction imaging*: *Speckles* are inherent artifacts to ultrasound imaging and are created by refracted sound waves from any solid particle that the sound beam hits. SRI—cuts off this undesired refracted sound beam information and improves edge definition **(Figs. 7A and B)**.
- *Compound resolution imaging (CRI)*: CRI is a result of multiple coplanar images from different angles combined into a single image in real time. Though the borders for each steering angle are the same, the noise and speckle position change for each frame and average out noise and smoothen borders **(Figs. 8A to C)**. It is especially of use for definition of margins of cystic structures. It is also of use to visualization of the tissue details across hyperechoic structures such as bones.

DOPPLER SETTINGS

Like B-mode image settings, certain settings are also required for Doppler mode—for color or power Doppler and for spectral Doppler. Though discussion of physics of Doppler is out of the scope of this chapter, an insight into the basic adjustments required, is a must. Before discussing the Doppler settings, recapitulating the basic facts about the color, power, and spectral Doppler.

Color Doppler

- It shows the direction of the flow.
- Red color is the flow towards the probe and blue color is the flow away from the probe as a default (though it must be remembered that it can be inverted of required).

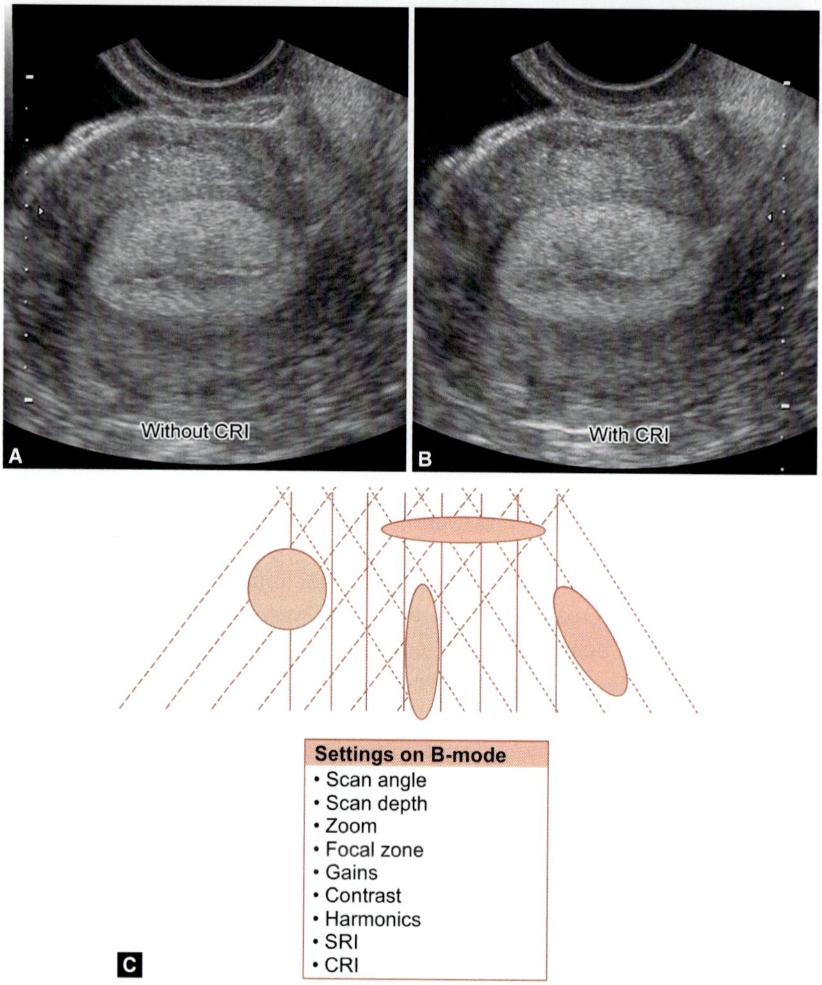

Figs. 8A to C: Better image quality by compound resolution imaging (CRI) is seen in Figure B. Diagrammatic explanation (C) of how CRI improves margin definition (SRI: speckle reduction imaging).

- Brighter color indicates higher velocity.
- Flow at right angle to the sound beam cannot be documented.
- Pulsatile flow is arterial and nonpulsatile flow is venous.

Power Doppler

- It shows flow in unicolor and so does not indicate the direction of the flow.
- It shows flow perpendicular to the sound beam also.
- Higher velocity shows brighter color.

Pulsed Wave Doppler

- It shows as a spectrum on the baseline.
- Flow towards the probe is seen above the line and flow away from the probe is seen below the line.
- Spiky flow is arterial and flat flow is venous.

Making the Correct Doppler Settings

- *Region of interest (ROI)*: This is the color box size in color or power Doppler and sample volume size in spectral Doppler. Smaller the size of ROI, better is the frame rate and so better color pick up. Therefore, the color box or ROI should be set just large enough to cover the area in which the blood flows are to be studied whereas for pulse Doppler, the size of sample volume should be as much as the diameter of the vessel being interrogated. A sample size larger than the vessel diameter may show noise artifacts because of signals from vessel wall and surrounding tissues and if the sample volume is smaller than the vessel diameter, it will assess only of a part of the total flow through the vessel **(Figs. 9A and B)**. This is important because the flow velocity in any vessel is high in the central stream as compared to close to the walls. The slower velocity in the peripheral stream is due to friction of the flowing fluid with the wall of the vessel.
- *Pulse repetition frequency (PRF)*: PRF decides the maximum velocity assessable by the Doppler. The physics is fairly complicated but it is enough to remember that for high velocity flow, high PRF is required and for low velocity flow, low PRF is required. Low PRF for high velocity flow leads to aliasing and high PRF for low velocity flow leads to nondetection of the flow signals **(Figs. 10A and B)**. Aliasing on color Doppler appears as mixing of red and blue colors and on pulsed wave Doppler, it appears as overshooting of the systolic peak on the opposite side of the baseline.

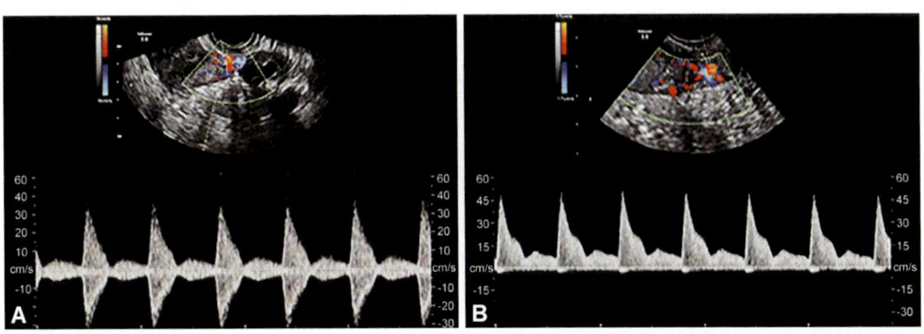

Figs. 9A and B: (A) Large sample volume leading to spectrum on both sides of baseline as it is recording the flow from two vessels carrying flow in opposite direction; and (B) Sample volume of the size of the vessel shows spectral trace from only one and the desired vessel.

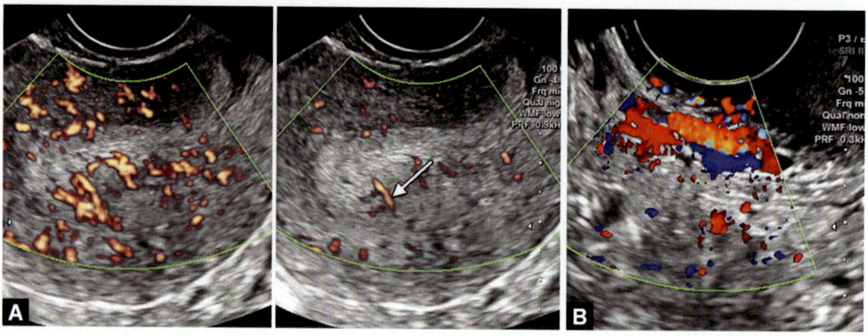

Figs. 10A and B: (A) Higher pulse repetition frequency (PRF) for low velocity flow obscures the blood flow that is present as shown by arrow; and (B) Low PRF for high velocity flow leads to turbulence-color mixing and spilling of color outside blood vessels.

- *Gains*: Gain adjustment in Doppler is as important as in B-mode. The gains on color/power Doppler should be so adjusted that the color fills up the whole vessel lumen, but does not spill out of the vessel. On spectral Doppler, spectrum should appear bold and no signals should be seen other than the actual flow spectrum **(Figs. 11A and B)**.
- *Filters*: It is known that Doppler signals are produced by the signals received from any moving object, including bowel and vessel wall. Signals from high velocities are more intense as compared to signals from the low velocities. These signals do not contribute to any fruitful information; on the contrary, it causes a lot of artifact. These signals can be filtered out by using filter. Filter is useful for eliminating the signals coming from structures moving at very low velocity. Filter can be set at different levels. In slow flow areas (e.g., veins), use low wall filter setting and vice versa. Higher wall filters may obliterate the diastolic or low velocity flows and thus may give erroneous information as absent diastolic flow.
  When interrogating high velocity blood flows, (e.g., arteries), use higher wall filter setting **(Figs. 12A and B)**.
- *Balance*: When Doppler is switched on, the scanner has to simultaneously work for two modalities: (1) grayscale and (2) color. It has to balance between the importance of both during the scans. By setting the balance, the operator can order the scanner to show B-mode or color predominantly during the scan. Evidently, this cannot be set continuously during the entire scan, so it is to be set at particular level during the scan depending on the echogenicity of the part being scanned. When Doppler is initiated on the scanner, on the screen, on the right upper corner of the screen, a gray bar and a color bar are seen. A green line is seen on the gray bar. If the whiteness of the image on the screen matches the gray tone below the line, the color pickup is smooth but if the gray tone matches to the gray tone above the green line on the gray bar, the B-mode details predominate and

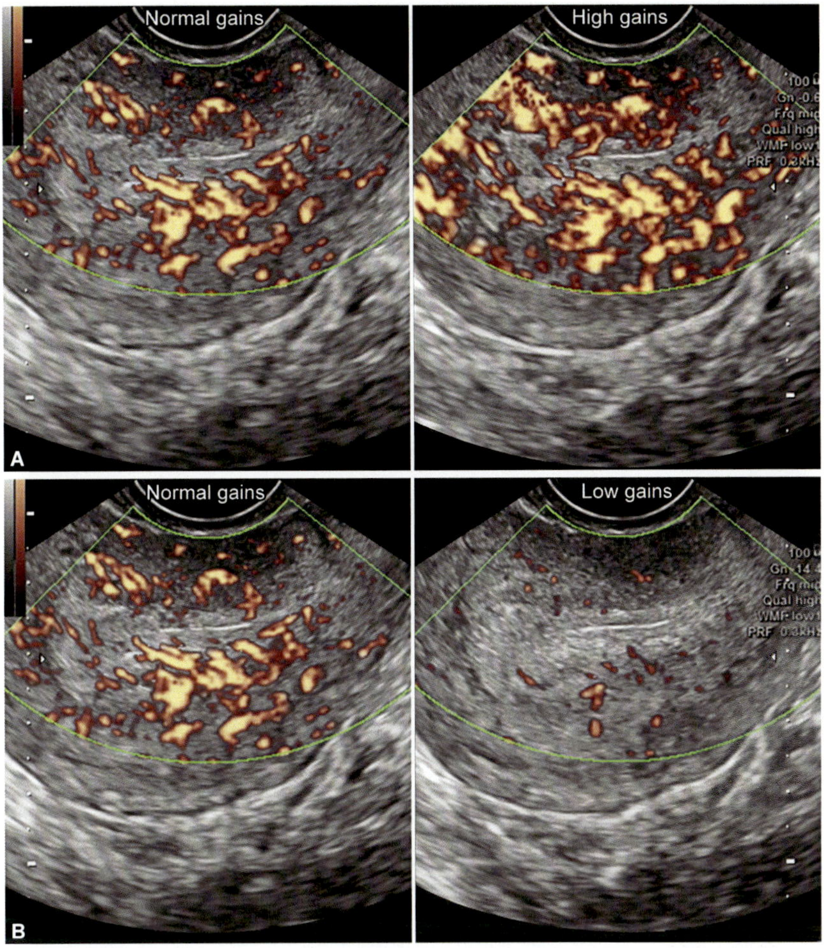

Figs. 11A and B: (A) Spill of color outside blood vessels in the image on right side due to high gains; and (B) No color filling in the image on right side due to low color gains.

therefore, it appears like snow on the color and the color pickup becomes patchy. The balance is, therefore, set to a level where the details of the B-mode and color are optimally appreciated **(Figs. 13A and B)**.

- *Doppler angle*: This is a setting for pulsed wave Doppler or spectral Doppler only. Angle adjustment for pulse Doppler has an important bearing on the flow velocity calculations. This is so because the velocity is calculated by the equation that has three other variables—frequency of the incident beam, frequency of the received beam, and cos of the angle at which the sound beam hits the moving object. Since the value of cos 0° is 1, absolutely correct velocity values can be calculated of the direction of the moving object is parallel to the sound beam. But value of cos 90° is 0 and so if

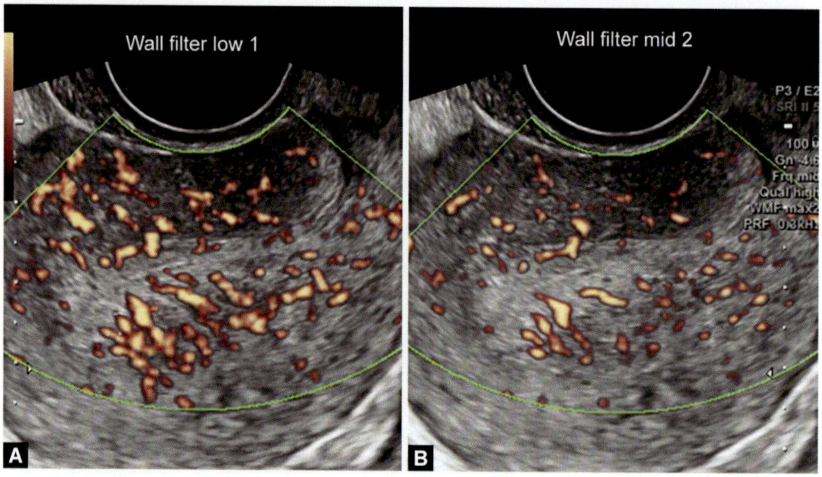

Figs. 12A and B: Higher wall filter in Figure B leads to less filling of blood vessels, especially with low velocities.

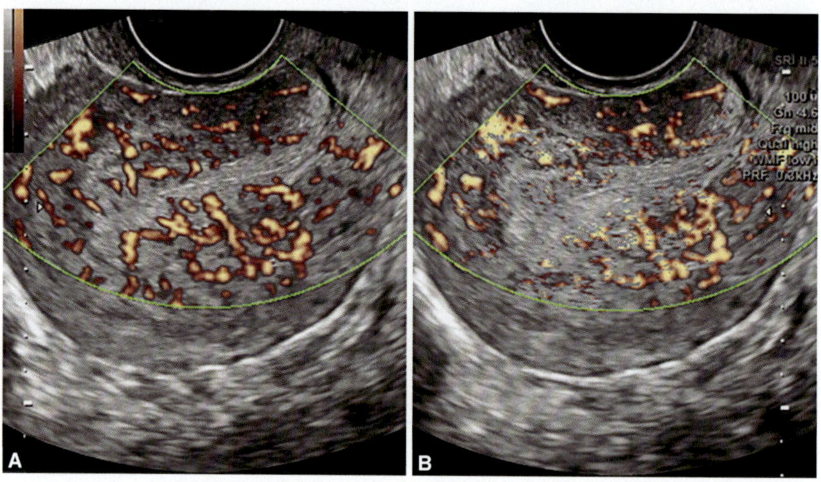

Figs. 13A and B: Figure B shows patchy filling of color due to low balance, but higher balance in Figure A shows solid filling of blood vessels.

the direction of the moving object is perpendicular to the sound beam, the flow cannot be documented at all. Value of cos keeps on decreasing fast as the angle increases. Doppler angle should, therefore, always be adjusted to <60°, preferably <30° to get correct velocity calculations. If therefore the operator is seeing the vessel on the screen that has an angle of >60°, first manipulation of the probe is required to decrease this angle to the minimum and after that angle correction is required to minimize the angle between the vessel and the sound beam. Direction of the sound beam for Doppler is shown by dashed line on the screen. Though when it comes to calculating ratios-resistance indices, angle corrections are not required as systolic and diastolic velocities are equally affected.

Artifacts

The most common of the artifacts in Doppler studies are aliasing and mirror image artifacts.

Aliasing in color Doppler is mixing of red and blue color. This is seen when there is turbulence in the flow, but it also occurs when the velocity of blood is more than half the PRF. This means that aliasing occurs when low PRF is selected for assessing high velocity flows. Aliasing in spectral Doppler indicates overshooting of the systolic peak on to the other side of the baseline as discussed earlier **(Fig. 14)**.

Mirror image artifact is seen on pulse Doppler tracing, when sample volume is placed on the curved vessels and show artifactual bidirectional flow or when two vessels placed very close to each other and having flows in opposite directions are insonated together **(Fig. 9A)**.

Tips for good Doppler settings.

- Optimum PRF for the vessel to be sampled
- Appropriate color box size for color Doppler or sample volume for vessel size for pulse Doppler
- Sample volume is placed in the center of the large vessels as close to the walls of the vessels, the flow is slow
- Choose proper wall filters—high for large vessels/heart, low for smaller vessels/low flow
- Use optimum gains
- Adjust the optimum balance settings
- Never use a Doppler angle >60°

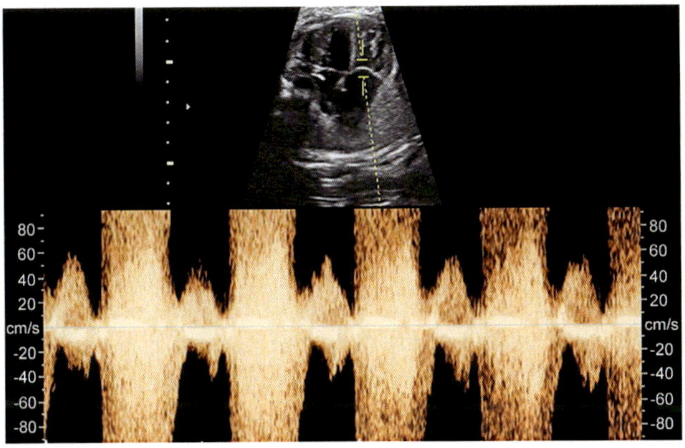

Fig. 14: Overshooting of spectral signals due to high velocity flow recorded in low pulse repetition frequency (PRF) settings—aliasing.

Sonography is one of the most useful and indispensable investigations for the assessment of the female pelvis.

Pelvic organs can be scanned by:

- Transabdominal route
- Transvaginal route
- Transrectal route

The scan for pelvic organs must start as abdominal scan. An abdominal approach to the pelvic organs gives an overall idea about the pelvic organs and surrounding anatomy before the detailed study of uterus and ovaries individually. This scan is done on full bladder. Low ultrasound frequencies are preferred, 3–5 MHz probe, to allow visualization of the uterus and ovaries from the acoustic window of full bladder **(Figs. 15 and 16)**. Patient is placed in supine position and is asked to relax and not to blow up her abdomen. At times, pressure with the probe may be required and probe may have to be angulated toward the pelvic cavity. Sonography of the pelvic organs—uterus, ovaries, and adnexa is preferred by transvaginal route for better visibility and accuracy of diagnosis. This advantage is because of close placement of the probe. Because of less distance that the sound waves have to travel, these probes are high frequency (6–12 MHz) and so give better resolution.

Transvaginal route cannot be used in virgins or in patients with vaginal infections and in these patients, transabdominal ultrasound with full bladder may be done, but this route has a disadvantage of poor resolution because of low frequency (3–5 MHz) probe which has lower resolution. Moreover, the pelvic organs are far from the probe leading to less visibility and low accuracy of image. Approximately 42% of ovarian details are missed by transabdominal scan.[1]

Transrectal sonography in such cases is preferable and informative as compared to transabdominal approach. The probe used is transvaginal or endocavitary probe, a high-resolution probe so resolution is very similar to that of a transvaginal scan (TVS) but the disadvantage is that rectal placement is much more painful than transvaginal placement and needs bowel preparation. Moreover, the orientation of pelvic organs that appear on the image created by transrectal scan is different than that of a TVS and so interpretation may be a little difficult. Therefore, the approach of choice is transvaginal.

METHOD

For TVSs, at least a verbal consent of the patient is essential. Patient is asked to empty the bladder. Patient is placed in lithotomy-like position on the gynecological couch in the same way as for per speculum or per vaginal examination. Gynecological couch is preferred to a simple bed as it allows free mobility of the probe. Ultrasound gel is placed on the head of the transvaginal probe and then the probe is covered with condom, not to allow any air between the probe and the condom. A small amount of gel is then placed over the condom on the probe head and the probe is gently slided into the patient's vagina. Counseling the patient before examination and explaining the whole procedure and adequate privacy help eliminate the anxiety and resistance. In case of difficulty in introduction of probe or patient's resistance to introduction, she is advised to take deep long breaths with open mouth, i.e., deep inspirations and long complete expirations. In spite of that if introduction of probe needs any force, the pressure should be exerted posteriorly toward the rectum which will make introduction of the probe into the vagina easier. Probe is introduced in the longitudinal position, i.e., the position in which the indicators on the probe remain up, facing the roof of the room that correlates with the anterior aspect of the patient **(Fig. 15)**.

This indicator on the probe matches the indicator (logo of the company) on the screen **(Fig. 16)**.

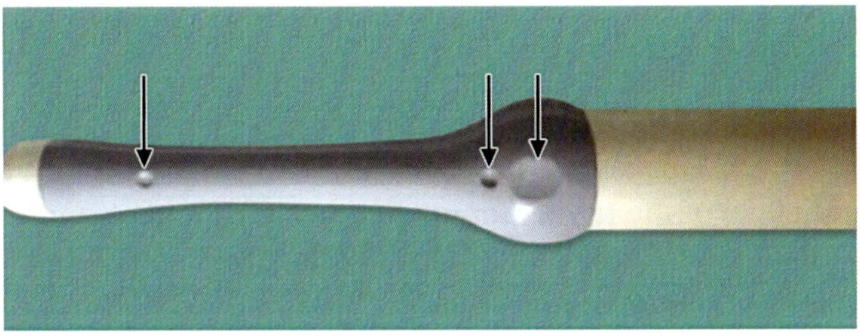

Fig. 15: A volume transvaginal probe with arrows showing pits for biopsy attachment. The same act as markers and correspond with the company logo on ultrasound image.

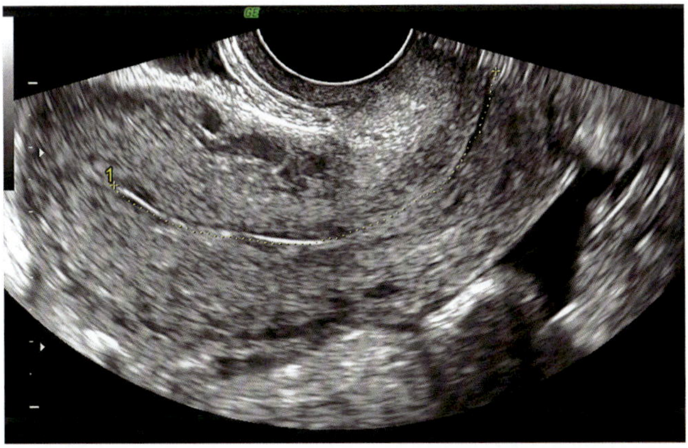

Fig. 16: Longitudinal section scan of the uterus showing company logo, as marked by the arrow. This corresponds to the indicators on the probe as shown in Figure 17.

This means that if the indicator on the screen is on the right side of the screen, the structures anteriorly placed are on the right side of the screen and vice versa.

Pre-scan protocol.

- Patient is explained about the procedure
- Patient's consent is taken for the procedure: Written/verbal
- Patient is asked to undress and lie down on gynecological couch in lithotomy-like position
- The couch is covered with a disposable sheet
- She is adequately covered
- Adequate privacy is maintained in the examination room
- Ultrasound gel is placed on probe head
- The probe is covered with condom or a probe cover

Tips for easy probe introduction.

- Patient counseling and explanation of the procedure
- Maintain adequate privacy
- Ask the patient to take deep inspiration followed by long complete expiration
- Press the probe toward the rectum to overcome resistance

BASIC PROBE MOVEMENTS

There are four basic types of probe movements:

1. *In and out movement* **(Fig. 17)**: This movement is done for introduction or withdrawal of the probe from patient's vagina and also to assess the mobility of tissue planes (to exclude adhesions).
2. *Side-to-side or spanning movement* **(Fig. 18)**: This movement can be done with probe rotated at any degree. It is done for survey of pelvic anatomy or for anatomical survey of a particular organ.
3. *Rotation movement or screwing movement* **(Fig. 19)**: This movement is done to align the organ of interest in desired axis—longitudinal or transverse.
4. *Up and down or anteroposterior movement* **(Fig. 20)**: This movement is done usually to bring the organ or lesion of interest in alignment with the

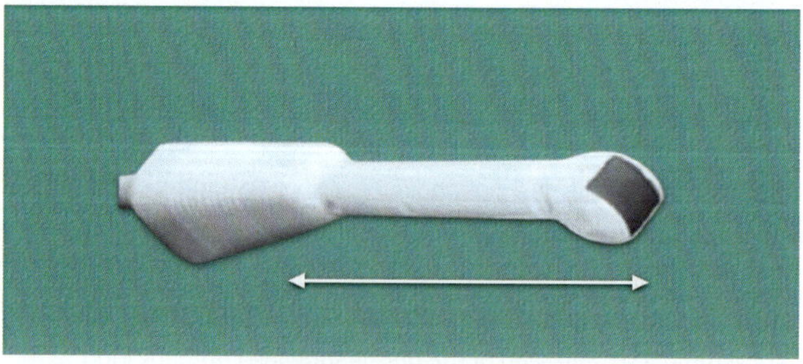

Fig. 17: In and out movement.

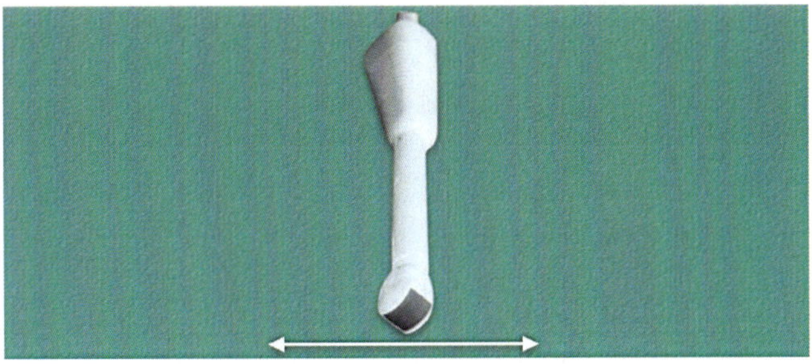

Fig. 18: Side-to-side movement.

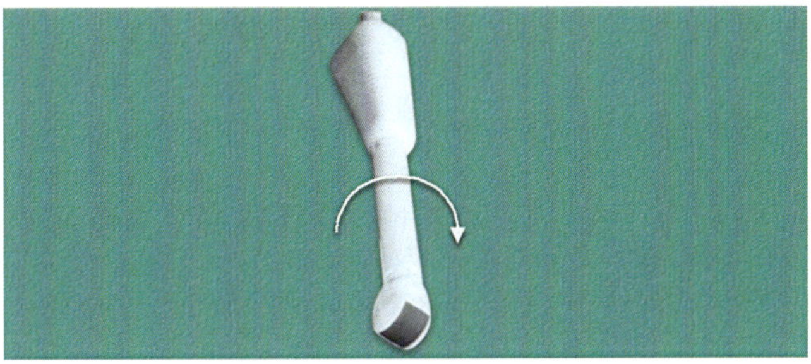

Fig. 19: Rotation movement.

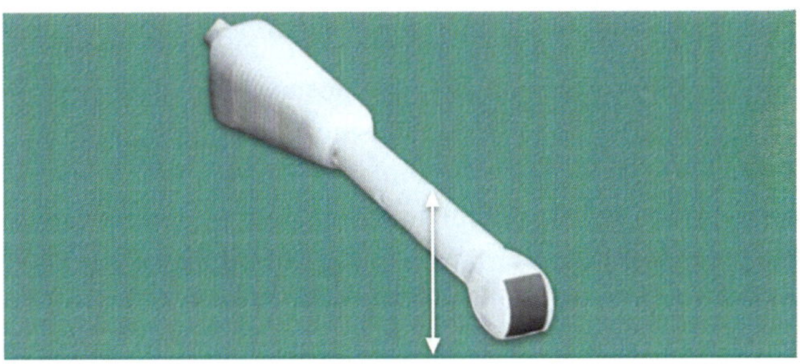

Fig. 20: Up and down movement.

probe. When the structure of interest is seen on the right side of the screen with the probe in the longitudinal position, this means that the structure is anteriorly placed then the probe handle should be moved down so that its distal end angulates up. This movement is also done for survey of the uterus in transverse axis.

ORIENTATION, OBSERVATION, AND INTERPRETATION OF TRANSVAGINAL SCAN

Orientation

When the probe is introduced through the introitus with the markers facing the anterior aspect of the patient **(Fig. 21)**, it normally shows the long axis of

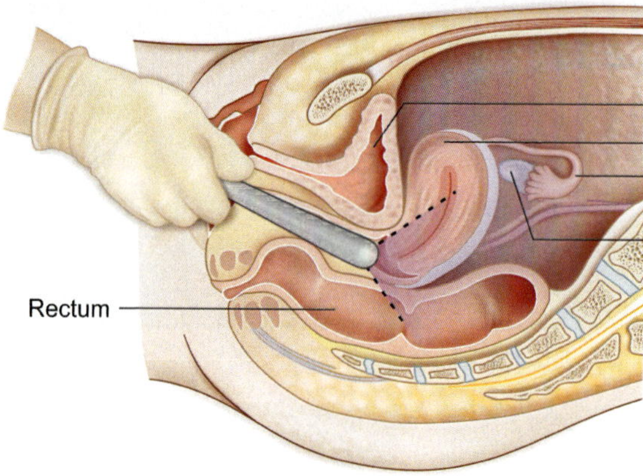

Fig. 21: Probe position in a transvaginal scan.

the uterus. It may be anteverted or retroverted and anteflexed or retroflexed. Version indicates the direction of cervix whereas flexion indicates the direction of fundus of the uterus. Anteversion is when the cervix from external os to internal os is directed from posterior to anterior and retroversion is when cervix from external os to internal os traverses from front to back. When anteflexed, the uterine fundus will be directed toward the indicator on the screen and urinary bladder is also seen on the same side of the screen, when retroflexed fundus will be on the opposite side of the indicator and the urinary bladder **(Figs. 22A to D)**. But it is important here to understand that one can change the image orientation also. Though in this book, we shall always discuss keeping in mind the image orientation just describes, i.e., on longitudinal imaging plane, the image shows the footprint of the image up and the logo of the scanner which correlates with the markers of the probe on the right side. But one can also work with the image turned upside down, which means the footprint of the probe faces down and the logo of the scanner is on the left side of the screen. In this case, the entire orientation can change. This can be done by the two reversed and inverted "R" switch on the scanner. But it is always essential that you use the same orientation of the image always to avoid all confusions. It is also essential that one should never insert the probe through the introitus with the markers on the probe facing down.

If the uterus is not seen in midline, it means that the uterus is deviated toward one side. When it is deviated, it would indicate that either it is pulled on the side of the pathology-like adhesions or is pushed away by the pathology which is on the opposite side: an ovarian or tubo-ovarian mass or uterine fibroid or any other pelvic mass. The second possibility is congenital abnormality of the uterus such as hemiuterus or bicorporeal uterus. We shall discuss the uterine abnormalities in the chapter dedicated to it.

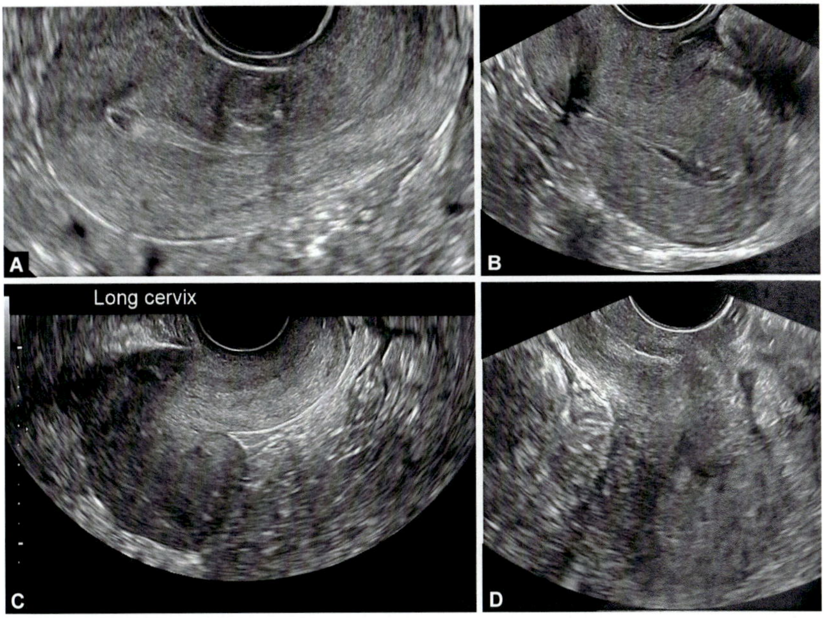

Figs. 22A to D: (A) Anteverted anteflexed uterus; (B) Retroverted retroflexed uterus; (C) Anteverted retroflexed uterus; and (D) Retroverted anteflexed uterus.

Now having located the uterus in the midline and decided whether it is anteverted or retroverted, its structure is evaluated systematically. The probe is spanned from right to left side of the patient, without rotating it, to scan the uterus in long axis from one side to other.

Systematic Assessment of the Uterus

Endometrium

- Symmetry of the endometrial shape (pear-shaped)
- Contour and continuity of central endometrial line (cavity)
- Intraendometrial lesions such as polyp, adhesions, etc.
- Endometriomyometrial junction
- Endometrial morphology corresponding with the phase of the cycle.

Endometrium is broadest at the fundus and narrows down smoothly toward cervix. The central line of the multilayered endometrium which indicates the endometrial cavity is smooth and runs in the center of the endometrium. Any bulge or irregularity of this line would indicate an intraendometrial lesion. Any echogenic solid lesion in between the lines of endometrium is suggestive of pathologies such as polyps, synechiae, etc. In all the phases, there is a thin hypoechoic zone seen surrounding the echogenic outline of endometrium, which is known as endometriomyometrial junction or junctional zone. This actually is the innermost layer of myometrium, but is an important landmark of endometrial health and so is considered along with the endometrium. Breach in this zone is suggestive of inflammatory or invasive pathology of endometrium, either endometritis, adenomyosis, or neoplasm **(Figs. 23A and B)**. Depending on the phase of the cycle, endometrium is expected to change the morphology. It is thin linear in early follicular phase, multilayered in preovulatory phase, and thick and hyperechoic in secretory phase.

Myometrium

- Homogenicity of the myometrium
- Mass lesions
- Scar tissues

Myometrium is homogeneously echogenic normally. Any generalized heterogenicity or localized hypo-/hyperechogenicity is suggestive of a pathology. The most common ones are fibroid and adenomyosis **(Figs. 24A and B)**. Scars due to any surgeries, such as myomectomy or cesarean sections may be seen traversing across the myometrial thickness **(Fig. 25)**.

Serosa

- Smoothness of contour
- Continuity
- Maintenance of tissue interface

Outer layer of uterus is covered by peritoneum and is the serosal layer. It defines the margins of uterus and therefore its integrity confirms that the uterus is normal **(Fig. 26)**. Any mass lesion in the uterus changes the contour of the uterus and therefore, the smooth pear shape is distorted. In and out movement of the probe confirms the mobility of the uterus and rules out adhesions.

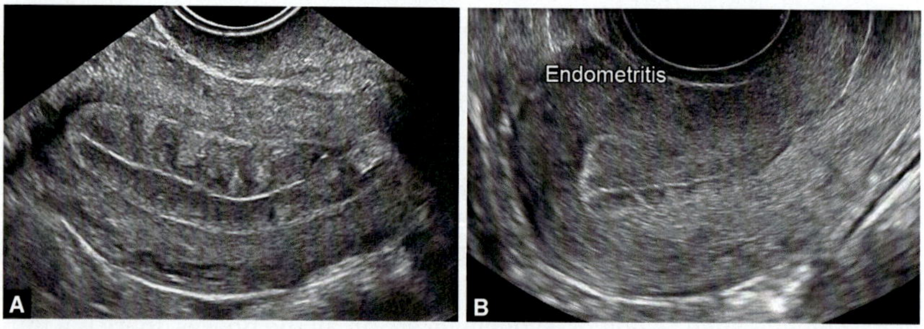

Figs. 23A and B: (A) Normal multilayered endometrium with smooth contour, uniformly curved central line, and intact hypoechoic endometriomyometrial junction; and (B) Obliterated endometriomyometrial junction makes definition of endometrium difficult, this is pathological.

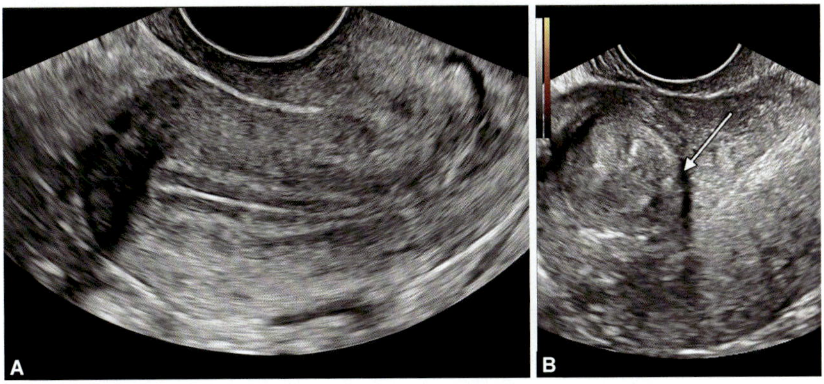

Figs. 24A and B: (A) B-mode ultrasound image of normal uterus showing homogeneous myometrium of equal thickness anteriorly and posteriorly; (B) A rounded well-defined isoechoic mass lesion (fibroid) seen in the thickened anterior myometrial wall, displacing endometrium posteriorly.

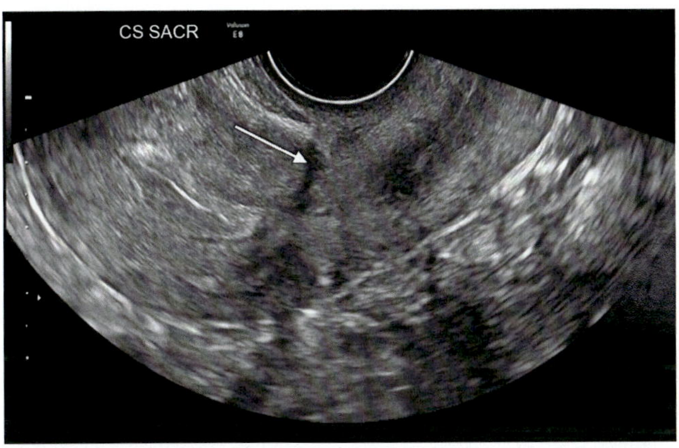

Fig. 25: A linear hypoechoic shadow (scar) is seen traversing the anterior myometrial wall just above the internal os.

Cervix

Length, mucous: The cervical length is assessed by identifying the internal os and the external os. Internal os can be identified by two landmarks: (1) The entry of uterine vessels on transverse section and (2) Cervical glands surrounding the cervical mucosa on longitudinal section. Thickness of endometriomyometrial junction is narrowest at the internal os and beyond that toward cervix is a hypoechoic area that is seen widening toward the external os. Because of these cervical glands forming triangular zone, apex of this triangle is internal os **(Figs. 27A and B)**. Cervical glands are seen as hypoechoic area in all other phases of the menstrual cycle, except periovulatory when it appears mildly hyperechoic, due to engorgement of the cervical glands with secretions.

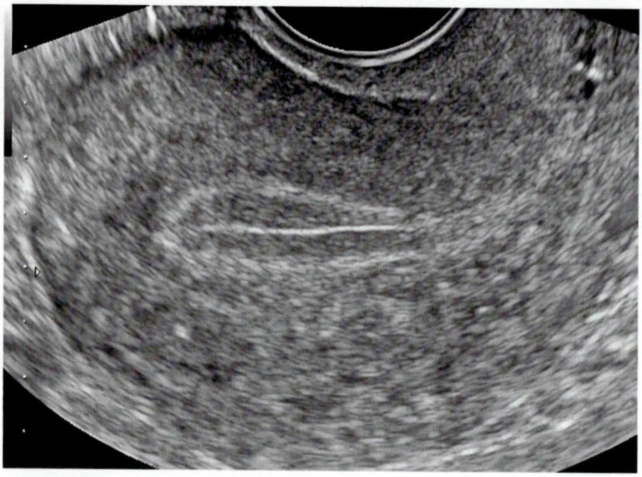

Fig. 26: Smooth pear-shaped outer contour of the uterus with well-defined margins.

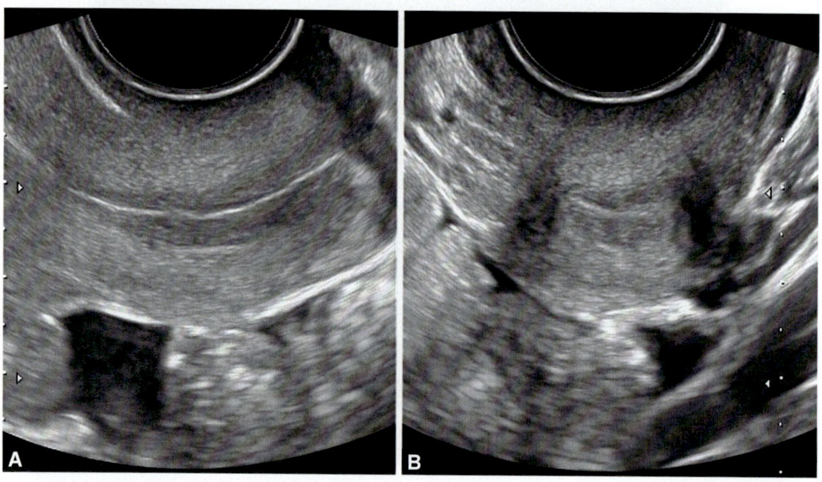

Figs. 27A and B: B-mode image of cervix in longitudinal (A) and transverse (B) sections. Long section shows hypoechoic cervical glands, central echogenic line—cervical canal.

Presence of fluid (mucus) in the cervical canal may also define the cervical canal. Cervical lesions like polyps are seen as solid lesions protruding in the cervical canal. Homogenicity of the cervical wall indicates the absence of any mass lesion-like fibroids or nabothian cysts in cervix. Serosal integrity of the uterus is also essential for the cervix.

Measurements

Physiological uterocervical length is measured in longitudinal section of the uterus. A true longitudinal section of the uterus is the one in which the endometrial cavity in fundus and body of the uterus are seen in continuity with the cervical canal. Physiological uterocervical length or endometrial trace is measured as a continuous tracing from the fundal endometrial tip to the external os. This length must be used for intrauterine insemination (IUI) and embryo transfer as reference. The actual anatomical uterocervical length can be measured from the fundal serosa to the external os as a trace and never as a straight line. Visual assessment of symmetry of thickness of anterior and posterior myometrium is done and if in doubt actual measurements may be taken. Myometrium is measured from outer margin of outer hyperechoic line of endometrium to the serosa, perpendicular to central line of endometrium. Though the endometrium fairly clearly is seen in this image, it is best not to measure the endometrial thickness in this plane. Once the entire long axis of the uterus is assessed, the probe is angulated up or down depending on the uterine orientation anteverted or retroverted, respectively, to bring the uterus fundus in the center of the image and decrease the scanning angle. This makes the margins of the endometrium very clear as in this position, the endometrium becomes almost perpendicular to the sound beam. On this image, endometrial thickness is measured as the distance from the outer margin of the hyperechoic line of one endometrial outline to the outer margin of the hyperechoic line of the other endometrial outline perpendicular to the central endometrial line. It is best to measure the myometrial thickness also in this plane. The anteroposterior thickness of the uterus is also measured on this plane as maximum distance from anterior serosa to posterior serosa is perpendicular to the central line of endometrium **(Fig. 28)**.

Now probe is rotated 90° anticlockwise. This maneuver will give transverse view of the uterus with the right side of the patient on right side of the

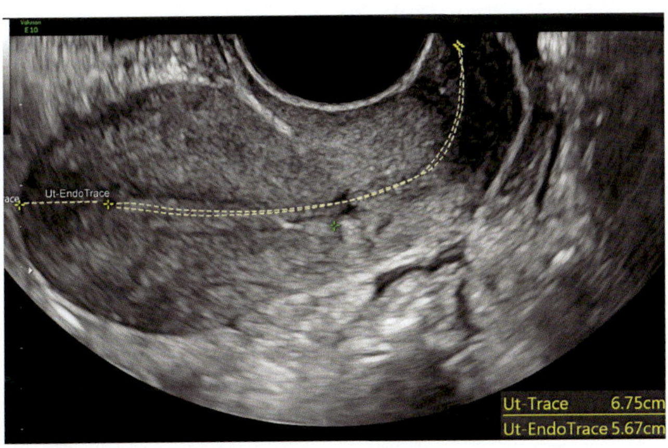

Fig. 28: Midline longitudinal section of the uterus with three different cursor sets showing anatomical uterocervical length, physiological uterocervical length, and endometrial thickness.

screen. In this transverse position, also the whole uterus is evaluated from the fundus to the cervix by angulating the probe up and down in the vagina. This survey should give a complete idea about the anatomy of the uterus and the exact location of any lesion in the uterus **(Figs. 29A and B)**. On this section, measure the transverse diameter of the uterus, as longest side-to-side diameter, at the level where the central endometrial shadow appears as the widest.

Now span the probe toward right side and in transverse position at the level of uterine cornu, gradually look at the adnexal soft tissue band and follow it to the ovary. Extend the movement up to the lateral pelvic wall, if ovary is not located. Most reliable landmark to locate the ovary is the internal iliac vessels. These are seen as thick anechoic band running obliquely across the image on longitudinal parasagittal scan. Ovaries are located superomedial to these vessels. Locate the ovary and rotate the probe to find true long axis of the ovary, the largest longitudinal diameter. On the same plane, measure the longest distance perpendicular to the longest diameter and this is the anteroposterior (AP) diameter of the ovary. Then rotate the probe 90° with no other movement and on this image, the longest side-to-side diameter is the transverse diameter of the ovary. The largest longitudinal, transverse, and AP diameters of the ovary will help calculate the ovarian volume **(Figs. 30A and B)**. Assess the ovaries for any pathological mass. Then span the probe, come back to the midline, and follow the same procedure for the opposite adnexa and ovary. In and out movement of the probe with the ovary in

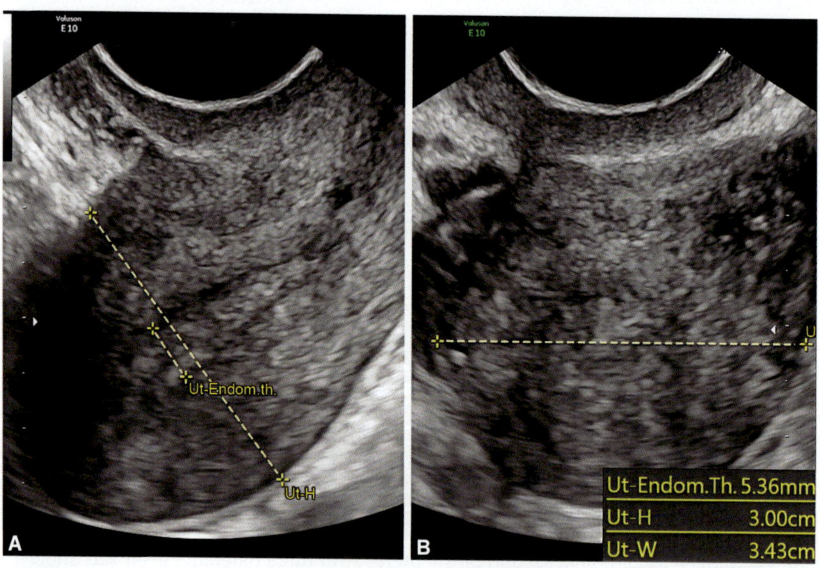

Figs. 29A and B: Transverse section of the uterus showing width and anteroposterior diameter of the uterus.

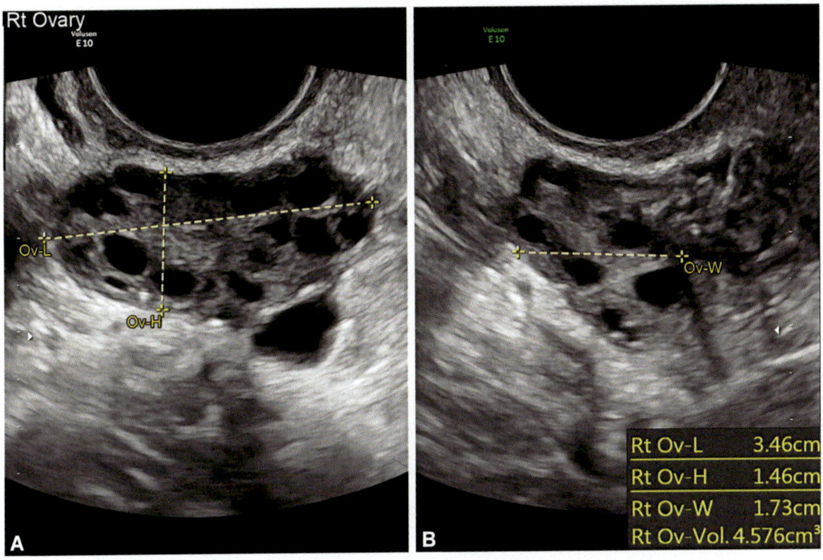

Figs. 30A and B: Transverse (A) and longitudinal (B) section of the ovary showing longitudinal, transverse, and anteroposterior diameters.

view or pressing from the abdomen when probe is looking at the ovary and checking the sliding of the organs against each other confirms mobility of the ovaries and rules out adhesions. This is also known as "Timor-Tritsch sign" or a "sliding organ sign". The same maneuver is also done to check the adhesions around the uterus and cervix.

Adnexa

- Look for mass lesion
- Localized fluid collection
- Thickening of the adnexa

Come back to the midline and angulate the probe head posteriorly and look for fluid in pouch of Douglas. The probe is then gently withdrawn from the introitus. This completes the B-mode routine TVS.

For color Doppler of the uterine artery, the probe is brought back in the midline in longitudinal plane and then again moving laterally, serpiginous tubular structure is seen at the level of internal os, which is the uterine artery. It can also be traced in transverse axis of the uterus, moving the probe to the level of internal os, when arteries will be seen on both the sides **(Figs. 31A and B)**. On transabdominal scan, the uterine arteries are found by moving from midline at the level of pubic symphysis laterally till the iliac vessels are seen as large prominent vessels running mediolaterally, superoinferiorly. After tracing these vessels, the probe, if angled slightly medially, shows a vessel perpendicularly crossing them, this is uterine artery **(Figs. 32A and B)**.

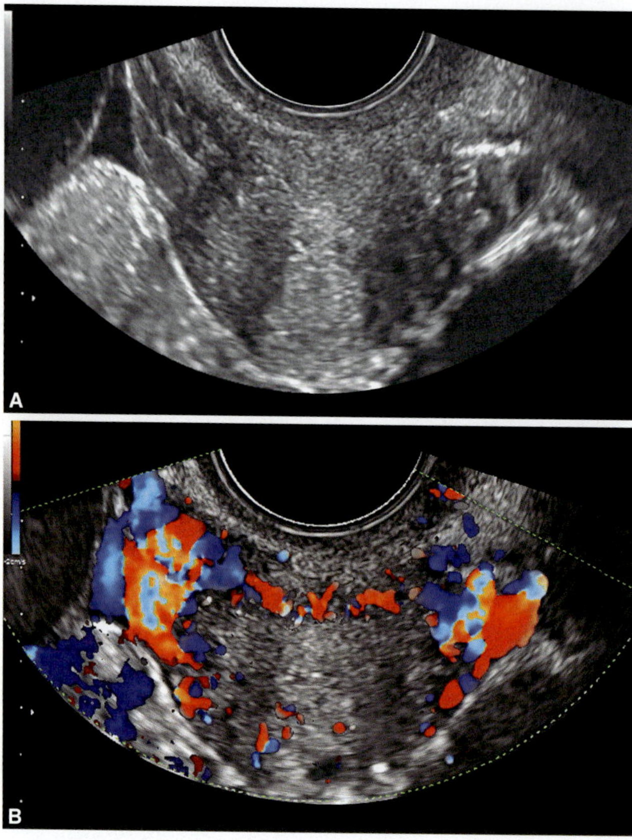

Figs. 31A and B: (A) B-mode ultrasound of uterus at the level of internal os showing longish anechoic serpiginous areas (vessels) on both sides; and (B) Color Doppler at the same level shows uterine vessels on both sides.

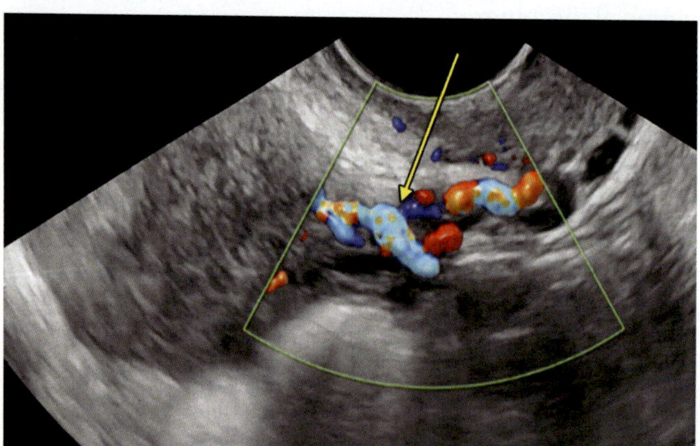

Fig. 32A

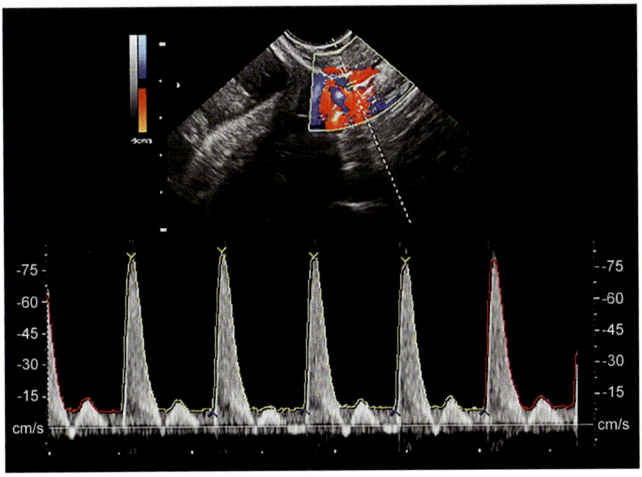

Fig. 32B

Figs. 32A and B: (A) Off midline longitudinal section of the uterus showing color-filled uterine artery; and (B) Spectral Doppler of the uterine artery showing high velocity, high resistance flow.

Color Doppler is also used to evaluate the endometrial flow. The blood vessels entering the endometrium are spiral artery and are seen as vessels perpendicular to the endometrium. The ovarian stromal vessels are studied for baseline scan. These are the vessels that are lying in the ovarian stroma and not close to the follicles. This finishes the basic TVS.

Carry Home Message

- Optimization of the image is the basic need for correct diagnosis.
- Transvaginal scan should be done in a systematic manner.
- Understanding of orientation of image and organs are important.
- Analysis of every image in the systematic way and correct standarized interpretation are basics to correct diagnosis.

REFERENCE

1. Hull MGR. Polycystic ovarian disease: clinical aspects and prevalence. Res Clin Forums. 1989;11:21-34.

CHAPTER 14

Ultrasound in Uterine Diseases

Sonal Panchal

INTRODUCTION

Uterine abnormality is the cause of majority of the gynecological complaints and ultrasound (US) is now considered a first-line investigation for its assessment. Uterus can be visualized on US by transabdominal route as well as transvaginal route. Though the assessment by transvaginal ultrasound (TVS) is the best choice, transabdominal scan is usually preferred before the transvaginal scan if the patient is being assessed for a particular complaint for the first time. Doppler is very essential for differential diagnosis of various uterine pathologies. Volume US [three-dimensional–four-dimensional (3D–4D) US] can significantly add to the details available and is considered essential for the diagnosis of Müllerian abnormalities and endometrial pathologies of the uterus. Saline infusion sonohysterography (SIS) is also a useful modality for evaluation of the endometrial pathologies.

Uterine abnormalities can be divided into Müllerian duct abnormalities and acquired pathologies.

MÜLLERIAN DUCT ABNORMALITIES

Uterus is formed by the fusion of the two paramesonephric (Müllerian) ducts at 10 weeks of gestation followed by resorption of fused midline tissues occurring by 20th week by apoptosis. Arrest of these processes at different stages may result into various Müllerian duct abnormalities.

- Failure of one or both Müllerian duct to develop
- Failure of the ducts to canalize
- Failure to fuse or abnormal fusion of Müllerian ducts
- Failure of resorption of midline uterine septum.

Incidence of Müllerian duct abnormalities is 0.1–3.8% in normal fertile females but reaches 6.7% in infertile patients.[1] These abnormalities were classified in 2003 by American Fertility Society (AFS) **(Fig. 1).**[2]

But in 2013, European Society of Human Reproduction and Embryology (ESHRE) and European Society of Gynecological Endoscopy (ESGE) joined together and devised a new classification system named ESHRE-ESGE classification for Müllerian abnormalities **(Figs. 2A and B)**. This was thought to be required because there were lot of confusions and overlapping of classes

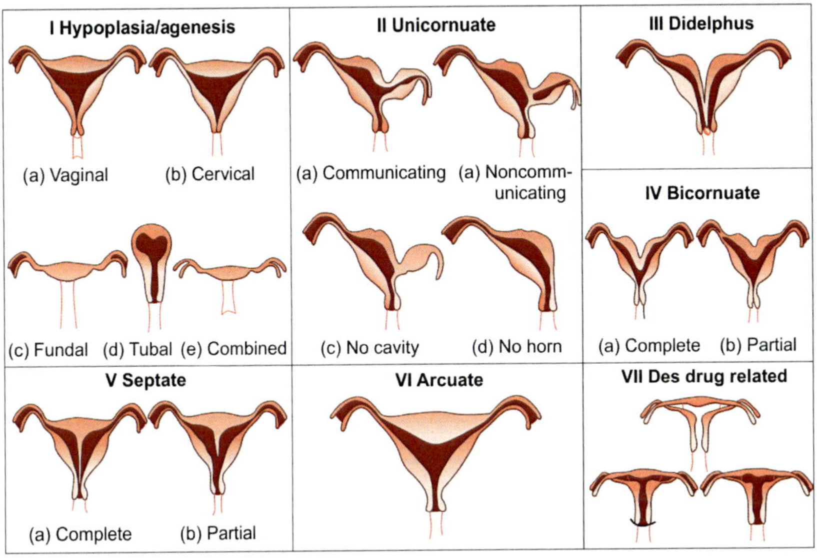

Fig. 1: *Uterine abnormalities:* American Fertility Society Classification (DES: diethylstilbestrol).

in the AFS system. The new classification is claimed to be more accurate clear and is correlated with clinical management. Cervical and vaginal anomalies are classified independently. It is thought to be more practical also because according to this system, the uterus own myometrial wall thickness measurement is used as a standard to evaluate the abnormalities of the shape, unlike absolute measurements.[3,4]

This classification system can be explained as follows.

Class U0

It is a normal uterus **(Fig. 3)**. It shows a straight or convex contour of the uterine fundus and endometrium. But even when the endometrial contour is concave, if the depth of the indentation at the fundal midline does not exceed 50% of the myometrial wall thickness; it is still considered a normal uterus. When the uterus is seen in the mid coronal plane, the vertical distance between the highest point on the endometrium and the highest point on the fundus is defined as myometrial wall thickness. This means arcuate uterus is considered as normal uterus and it is not a separate entity.

Class U1—Dysmorphic Uterus

Dysmorphic uterus is small with normal uterine fundal shape.

Class U1a—T-shaped uterus: Narrow uterine cavity due to thickened lateral walls with normal uterocervical ratio (2:1). It is measured as a perpendicular

ESHRE/ESGE Classification
Female Genital Tract Anomalies

Uterine anomaly	
Main class	*Subclass*
U0 Normal uterus	
U1 Dysmorphic uterus	a. T-shaped b. Infantilis c. Others
U2 Septate uterus	a. Partial b. Complete
U3 Bicorporeal uterus	a. Partial b. Complete c. Bicorporeal septate
U4 Hemiuterus	a. With rudimentary cavity (communicating or not horn) b. Without rudimentary cavity (horn without cavity/no horn)
U5 Aplastic uterus	a. With rudimentary cavity (bi- or unilateral horn) b. Without rudimentary cavity (bi- or unilateral uterine remnants/Aplasia)
U6 Unclassified malformations	
U	

Cervical/Vaginal anomaly	
Coexistent class	
C0	Normal cervix
C1	Septate cervix
C2	Double "Normal" cervix
C3	Unilateral cervical aplasia
C4	Cervical aplasia
V0	Normal vagina
V1	Longitudinal non-obstructing vaginal septum
V2	Longitudinal obstructing vaginal septum
V3	Transverse vaginal septum and/or imperforate hymen
V4	Vaginal aplasia
C	*V*

A

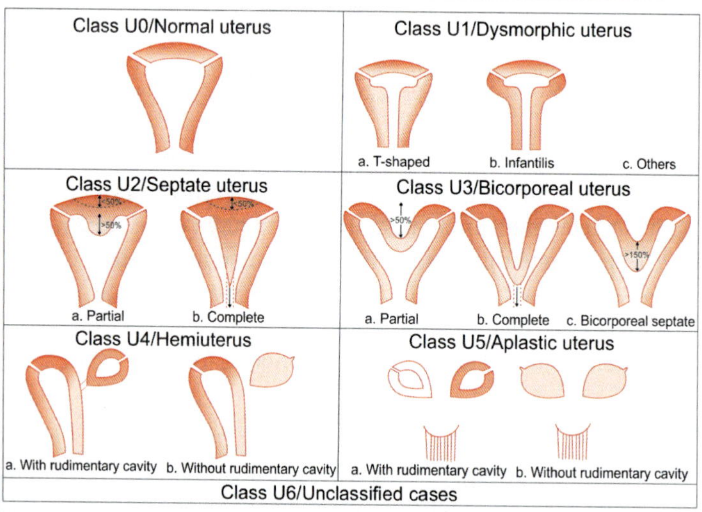

B

Figs. 2A and B: (A) Tabulated presentation of European Society of Human Reproduction and Embryology-European Society of Gynecological Endoscopy (ESHRE-ESGE) classification of Müllerian abnormalities;[5] (B) Diagrammatic presentation of ESHRE-ESGE classification of Müllerian abnormalities.[5]

distance between the cornu-internal os line to lateral wall and it is considered thick when it is ≥1.4 times the myometrial wall thickness **(Fig. 4A)**.

Class U1b—Uterus infantalis: Narrow uterine cavity without lateral wall thickening and an inverse utero-cervical ratio **(Figs. 4B)**.

Class U1c—Others: Minor deformities of the uterine cavity including those with an inner indentation at the fundal midline level of <50% of the uterine wall thickness **(Fig. 4C)**.

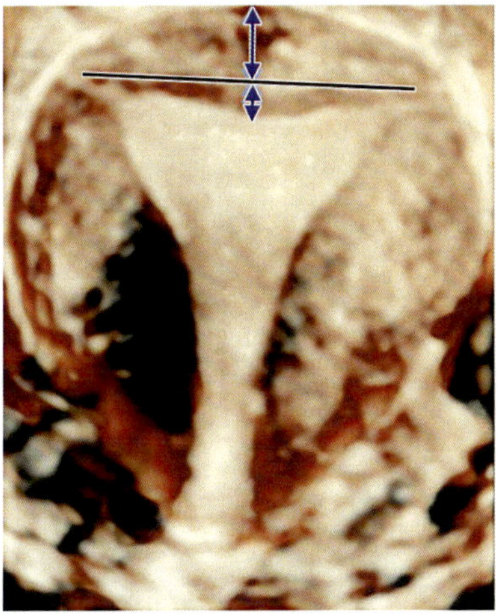

Fig. 3: Three-dimensional ultrasound of the normal uterus showing interostial line (black line) and the two blue arrows, the longer one indicating uterine wall thickness.

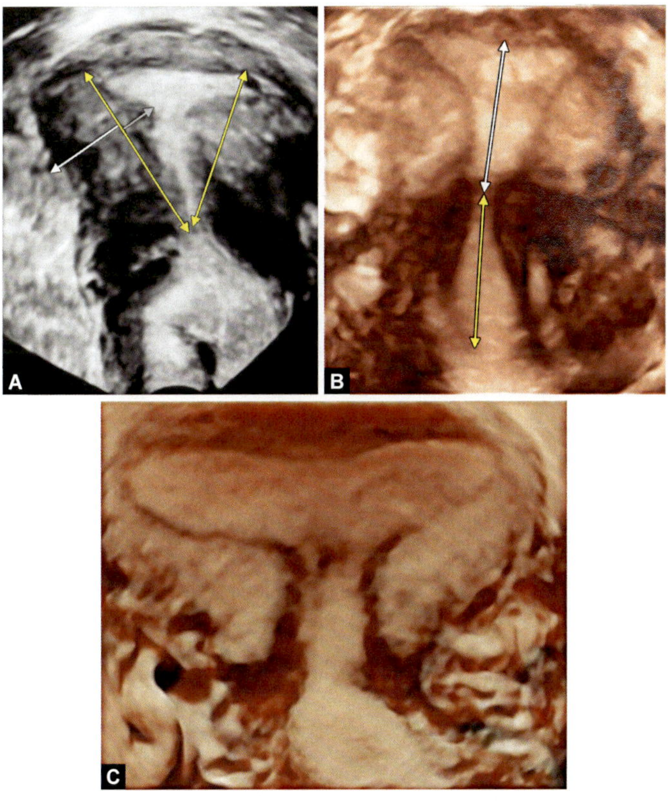

Figs. 4A to C: (A) Class U1a—T-shaped uterus; (B) Class U1b—hypoplastic uterus; (C) Class U1c—dysmorphic uterus.

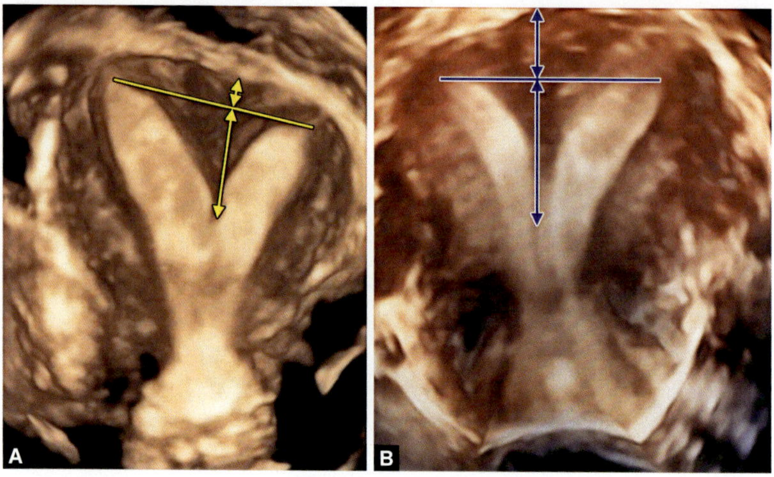

Figs. 5A and B: (A) Class U2a—partial septum; (B) Class U2b—complete septum.

Class U2—Septate Uterus

Normal fusion of Müllerian ducts but abnormal absorption of the midline septum leads to septate uterus. Outer contour of the fundus is normal. Endometrial contour shows indentation on coronal plane exceeding 50% of the myometrial wall thickness. If indentation ends short of internal os, it is a partial septum-subseptate uterus (class U2a) **(Fig. 5A)**, but if it extends up to internal os it is complete septum (class U2b) **(Fig. 5B)**. The later entity may sometimes be associated with cervical septum.

Septate uterus is one of the most common amongst the Müllerian duct abnormalities and it has the most clinical impact as it may the cause of recurrent abortions, premature labor, abnormal fetal lie, and even infertility. It was thought that if the septum divides at least two-thirds of the uterine cavity **(Figs. 6A and B)**, it was more likely to cause abortion but studies have shown that there is no correlation between the septal length and thickness and the incidence of abortions.[6] But other studies show that in case of septum, the length of remaining uterine was significantly shorter and distortion ratio was significantly higher in patients with recurrent miscarriage.[7] There are controversial opinions about the results after surgical correction of the septum also.[8] The current consensus therefore is that if there is a septum and there is a history of infertility or recurrent abortions and all other causes are ruled out then operate the septum.

Class U3—Bicorporeal Uterus

When there is indentation on the external contour of the uterus exceeding 50% of the myometrial wall thickness with division of the endometrial cavity

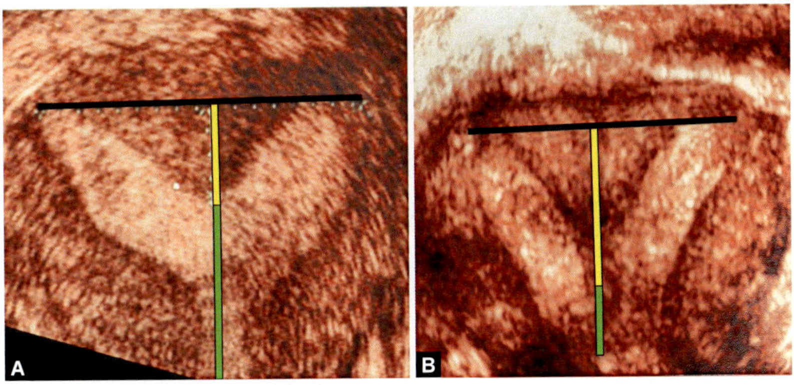

Figs. 6A and B: (A) Septum dividing one-third endometrial cavity; (B) Septum dividing two-thirds endometrial cavity.

also it is bicorporeal uterus. If the outer indentation divides the two corpora partially it is partial bicorporeal uterus (class U3a) **(Fig. 7A)** but if it extends till the internal os, it is complete bicorporeal uterus (class U3b) **(Fig. 7B)**. The later may be associated with duplication of cervix, septum in the cervix or single cervix and then it can be compared with uterus didelphys (two totally separate cornu), bicornuate bicollis uterus or uterus bicornuate unicollis respectively of AFS classification.

There used to be confusion for nomenclature of those uteri that had fundal indentation but otherwise looked like septum. When there is a fundal indentation of more than 50% of the myometrial wall thickness, but there is a thick long (1.5 times the myometrial wall thickness) septum between the two endometrial cavities, it is bicorporeal septate uterus (class U3c) **(Fig. 7C)**.

On B-mode US, it is suspected when midsagittal plane of the uterus is not seen in the midline and on spanning from one side to the in longitudinal plane, two well-developed uterus shadows are seen. These may be at variable distance from midline. On transverse section two separate horns are seen **(Fig. 8)**. Two horns may show symmetrical or asymmetrical development.

Ovaries are seen close to the respective horns. Abdominal scan to exclude renal abnormalities is essential in these cases. 3D is diagnostic. For these patients it is best to scan in the transverse section to acquire a 3D volume as the two horns may be far and it may be difficult to acquire both the horns completely, if volume is acquired in longitudinal plane. In these cases separate volume is acquired for cervix.

The criteria used earlier for differentiating between septate and bicornuate uterus-like angle between the two cavities and distance between the intercornual line and the deepest point on the fundus are no longer considered valid when this classification is used but still in cases of confusion

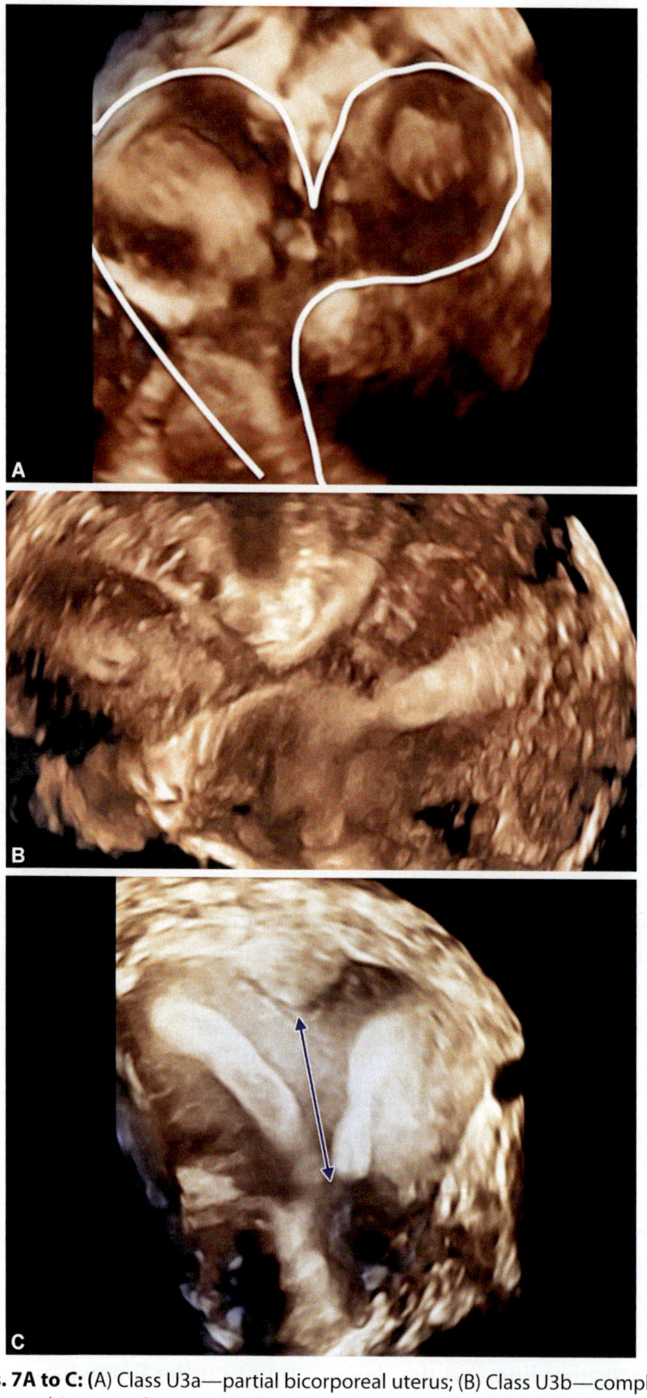

Figs. 7A to C: (A) Class U3a—partial bicorporeal uterus; (B) Class U3b—complete bicorporeal uterus; (C) Class U3c—bicorporeal septate uterus.

the angle between the two endometrial cavities may be taken as an additional criteria.

Bicorporeal uterus has best pregnancy prognosis of all Müllerian malformations, though premature deliveries are common.

Class U4—Hemiuterus

When only one of the two Müllerian ducts develops fully, it is hemiuterus **(Fig. 9A)**. The contralateral part could be incompletely formed but functional

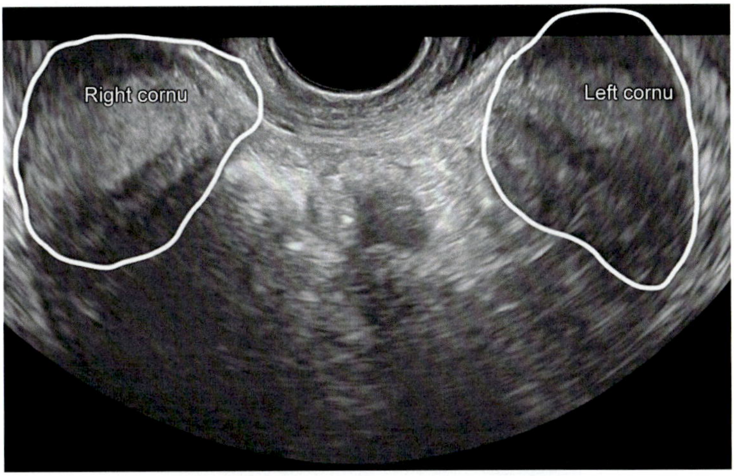

Fig. 8: B-mode ultrasound showing transverse section image of pelvis with two cornu of bicorporeal uterus.

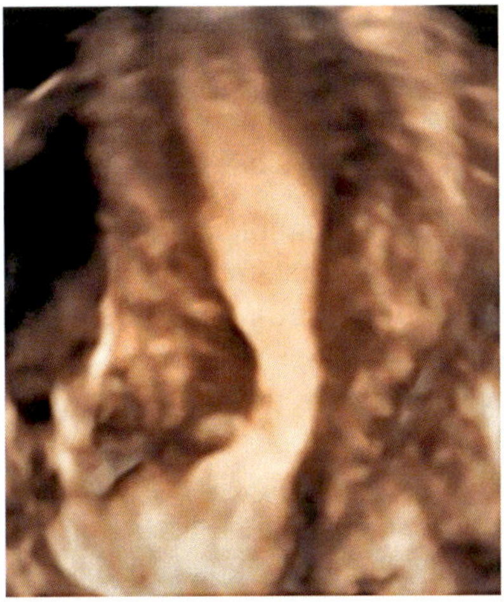

Fig. 9A

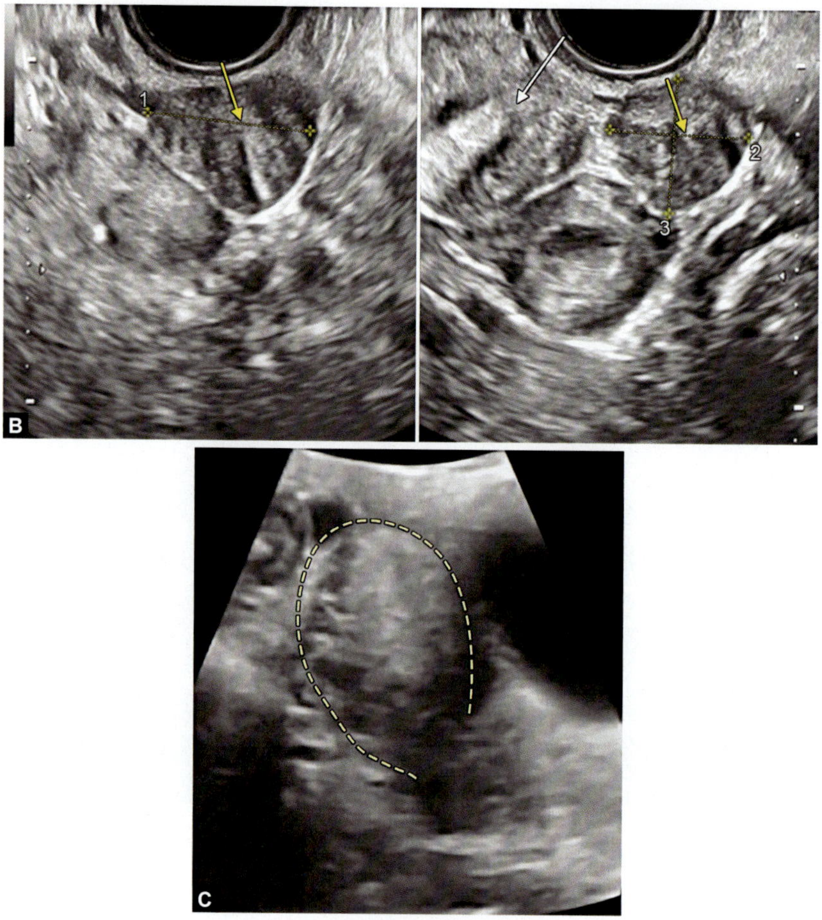

Figs. 9B and C

Figs. 9A to C: (A) Class U4—hemiuterus on three-dimensional ultrasound; (B) Class U4a—hemiuterus (white arrow) with functional rudimentary horn (yellow arrow) on B-mode; (C) B-mode image of the rudimentary horn of uterus with absent central hyperechoic line of endometrium.

and communicating or noncommunicating developed horn (class U4a) **(Fig. 9B)** or nonfunctional contralateral uterine horn or aplasia of the contralateral part (class U4b) **(Fig. 9C)**.

On US it is diagnosed when uterus is not seen in midline but is deviated on one side and is seen on spanning the probe towards lateral pelvic wall. No uterine shadow or a rudimentary horn is seen on other side. Ovary is seen near the respective horn. On transverse scan at the level of uterine fundus a beak like projection from the endometrial shadow, cornu is seen only on one side. 3D US is ultimate and clearly shows a banana-shaped uterine cavity **(Fig. 9A)**.

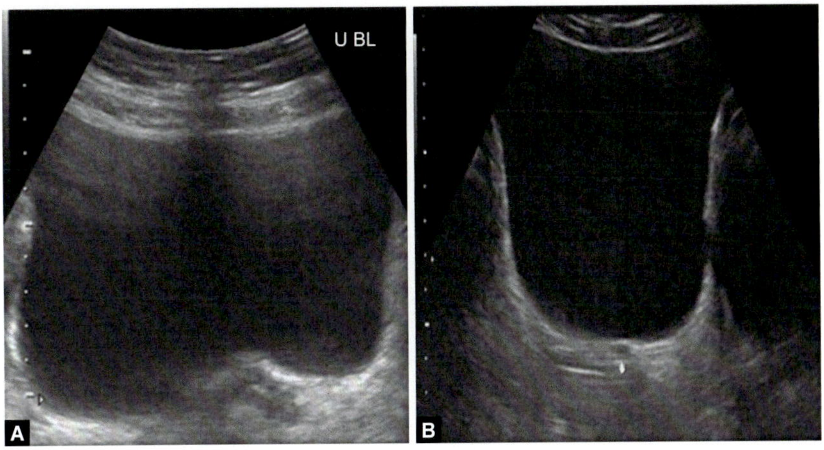

Figs. 10A and B: Bladder with dimple: Normal, bladder with convex base—uterine aplasia.

Class U5—Aplastic Uterus–Uterus Aplasia

No evidence of fully developed uterus or hemiuterus is seen with or without presence of rudimentary horn on one side or both the sides. Coexistent defects (e.g., vaginal aplasia/Mayer-Rokitansky-Küster-Hauser syndrome) are common with this group of abnormalities. The subclasses in this class are:

- *Class U5a* is aplastic uterus with rudimentary (functional) bilateral or unilateral functional horn.
- *Class U5b* is aplastic uterus without rudimentary (functional) cavity.

These patients present typical with the history of primary amenorrhea and on abdominal scan absence of dimple on the posterior fundal contour, indicates aplasia of the uterus **(Figs. 10A and B)**. Presence of rudimentary horns may be difficult to confirm. In these cases MRI is recommended.

Class U6—Unclassified Cases

Infrequent anomalies, subtle changes or combined pathologies of the uterus that could not be allocated correctly to one of the six classes are placed into this class.

The exact description of the anatomy of uterus, cervix, and vagina is possible using classification of cervical canal anomalies and vaginal anomalies also.

C0-normal cervix **(Fig. 11A)**, C1-septate cervix **(Fig. 11B)**, and C2-double normal cervix can be confidently diagnosed by 3D US **(Fig. 11C)**.

Though unilateral cervical aplasia which constitutes C3 class cannot be easily diagnosed on US. Cervical aplasia is rare.

For duplication abnormalities of the uterus, 3D US is the method of choice and has shown accuracy comparable to MRI. Volume US has >98% sensitivity

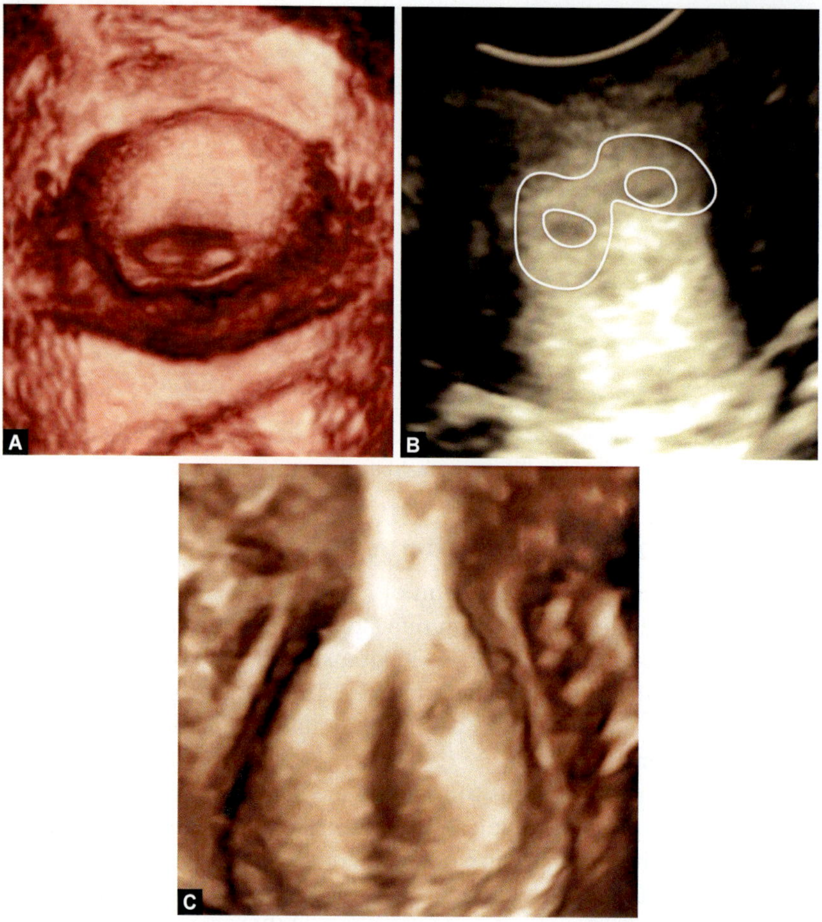

Figs. 11A to C: (A) Single normal cervix—C0; (B) Cervix with septum—C1; (C) Normal double cervix—C2.

and 100% specificity for these lesions.[9] With 3D US for septate uteri, the sensitivity was 100%, specificity was 88.9%, PPV was 95.5%, NPV was 100%, and kappa was 0.918.[10] And for bicorporeal uteri, the sensitivity was 83.3%, specificity was 100%, PPV was 100%, NPV was 98.2%, and kappa was 0.900.[10] Though MRI is suggested in all cases with poor visibility on US and in cases where there is doubt about presence or absence of the rudimentary horn.

ACQUIRED UTERINE ABNORMALITIES

These abnormalities can be divided as:
- Myometrial lesions
- Endometrial lesions
- Cervical lesions

Myometrium is normally homogeneously echogenic and serosal surface is smooth and regular. Heterogeneity of the myometrium or abnormality of the serosal contour suggests abnormality of the myometrium. Common myometrial lesions are fibroids, adenomyosis, adenomyomas, and leiomyosarcomas.

Fibroid

These are found in 20–40% of women from age 30 years onwards and are more common in nulliparous. These are mostly an incidental finding, but may sometimes present with dysmenorrhea and menorrhagia. It may also lead to infertility, early abortions, abnormal fetal lie, and adherent placenta.

On US fibroid appears as well defined, hypoechoic, homogeneous, round/oval, solid lesions, with peripheral hypoechoic rim due to displacement of myometrial fibers **(Fig. 12A)**. Edge shadows are seen in fibroid **(Fig. 12B)**.

Degeneration in fibroids causes heterogeneity of texture **(Fig. 12C)**. Echogenicity increases with amount of fibrous tissue and vascularity. Cystic degeneration may show anechoic areas in the fibroid **(Fig. 12D)**. Fibroids show peripheral vascularity usually but when degenerated it also shows intralesional vascularity **(Fig. 12E)**. Calcification may be seen sometimes **(Fig. 12F)**.

Fibroids occur in various locations and according to their location these are classified submucosal, intramural, and subserosal grossly. But according to the International Federation of Gynecology and Obstetrics (FIGO) classification or the PALM-COEIN classification[11] the fibroids are classified into eight types depending on their penetration in the uterine wall **(Fig. 13)**.

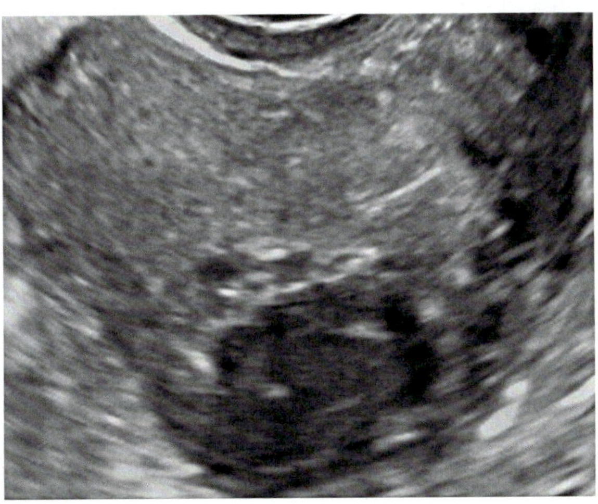

Fig. 12A

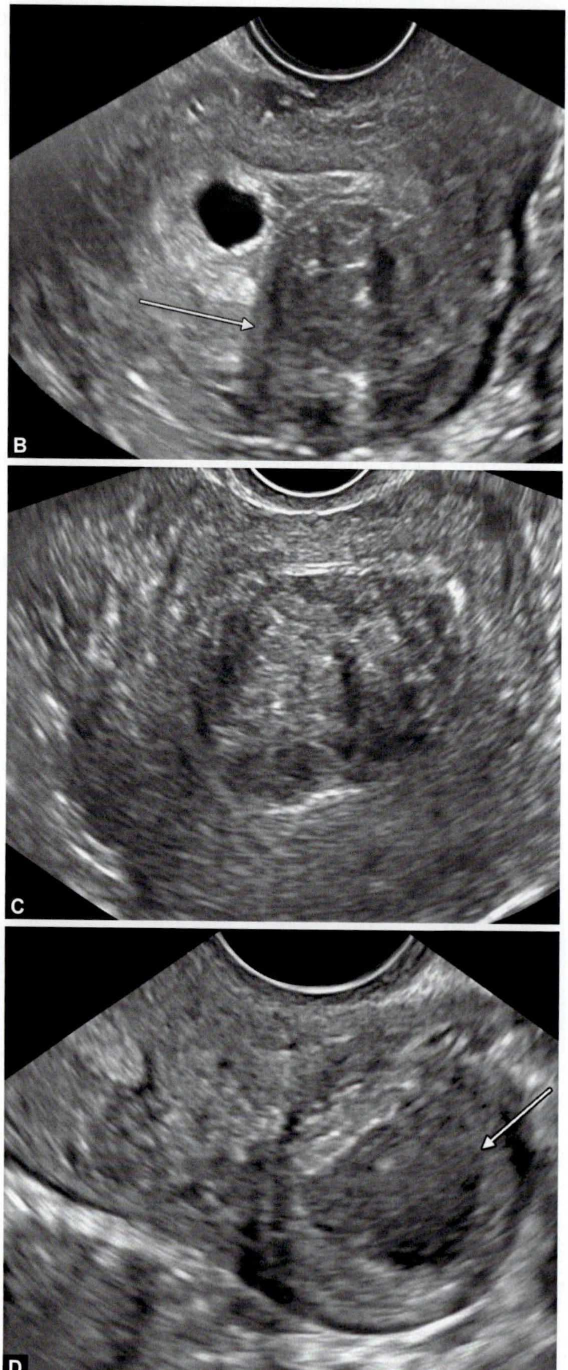

Figs. 12B to D

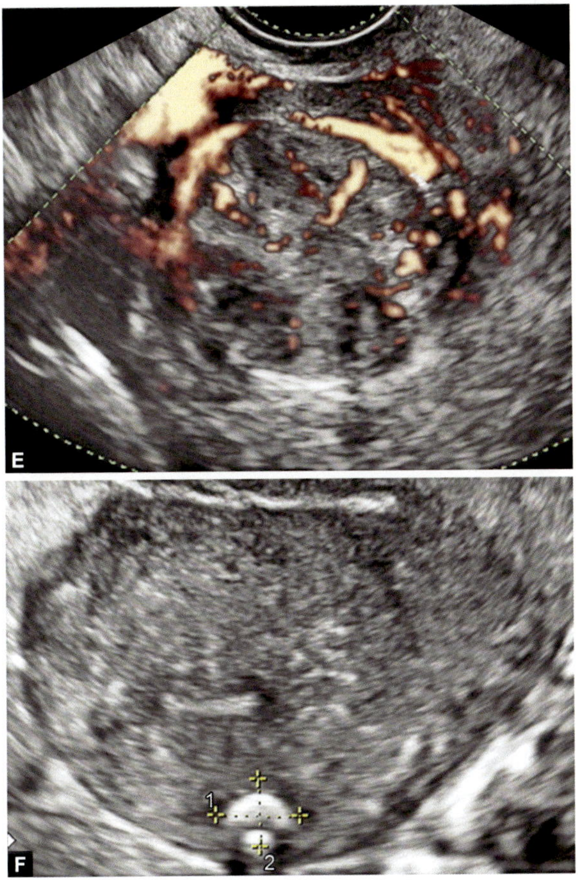

Figs. 12E and F

Figs. 12A to F: (A) Fibroid on B-mode; (B) Edge shadow (arrow) on B-mode; (C) Degenerated heterogeneous fibroid; (D) Cystic degeneration of fibroid; (E) Doppler of degenerated fibroid with peripheral and intralesional vascularity; (F) Calcification in fibroid.

The FIGO has also provided a classification of the fibroids, depending on their relation to the uterine wall.

- *Class 0*: Intraendometrial pedunculated
- *Class 1*: Subendometrial with <50% of the fibroid intramural
- *Class 2*: Subendometrial with >50% of the fibroid intramural
- *Class 3*: 100% intramural fibroid, touching the endometrium
- *Class 4*: Intramural
- *Class 5*: Subserosal ≥50% intramural
- *Class 6*: Subserosal ≤50% intramural
- *Class 7*: Exophytic pedunculated subserosal fibroid
- *Class 8*: Others (cervical/parasitic, etc.)

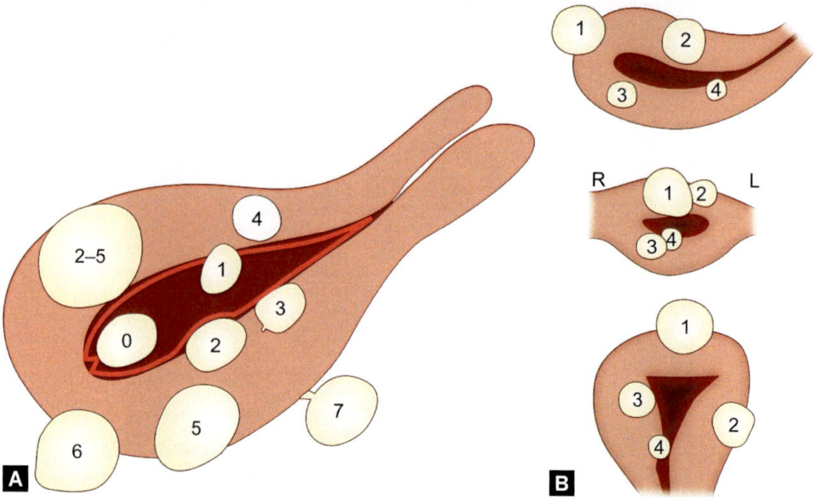

Figs. 13A and B: (A) Diagrammatic demonstration of the International Federation of Gynecology and Obstetrics (FIGO) classification of fibroids (the numbers here show the FIGO type of fibroid); (B) Hand-drawn diagram showing exact location of fibroids in sagittal, axial and coronal planes for fibroid mapping. The numbers in this figure shows the identification of fibroid.

Exact location of the fibroid need to be reported for proper planning of the treatment. The details to be included in the report therefore are the location of the fibroid—upper middle or lower third of the uterus, penetration (type) of the fibroid, size of the fibroid (as three orthogonal diameters) and its minimum distance from the endometrium and from the serosa. It is also important to mention the echogenicity of the fibroid, regularity of its margins, echogenicity of the margins, and vascularity. These details can be gathered by longitudinal and transverse survey of the uterus. And the report is to be given along with the line diagram **(Fig. 13B)**. Fibroids are also seen arising from the cervix and show similar appearances as fibroid in the uterus.

On Color Doppler

Peripheral vascularity is typical of a fibroid **(Fig. 12E)**. When degenerated the fibroids show intralesional vascularity with lower resistance in addition to the peripheral vascularity. Amount of vascularity decides the activity or growth potential of fibroid. Malignant change leading to leiomyosarcoma shows a resistance as low as 0.37 ± 0.03 resistance index (RI), with rapid growth in size and disruption of well-defined margins. But resistance indices of vessels cannot be used as only evidence for malignant change as resistance can be low in degenerated fibroids also. Uteri with fibroids also show higher uterine artery peak velocity and lower RI (mean: 0.74 ± 0.09).

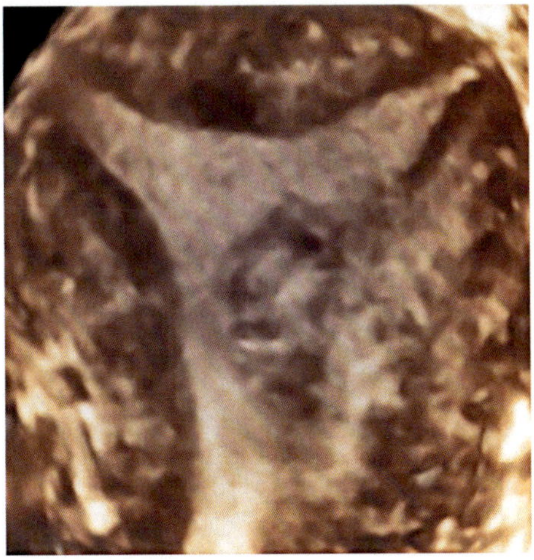

Fig. 14: Three-dimensional ultrasound showing fibroid on left wall.

Volume Ultrasound

Three-dimensional US is also useful for the exact localization of the fibroid and precisely estimates the relationship between submucous fibroid and endometrial cavity **(Fig. 14)**.

Adenomyosis

Patients present with similar signs and symptoms as fibroid. The incidence is very high, but is not correctly known as patients may not report for minor symptoms. It is common in multiparous women.

Adenomyosis is ectopic growth of endometrium in myometrium. Being an invasive lesion it has indistinct margins. It may involve whole uterus or may be localized to one wall or a part of it and may lead to symmetrical or asymmetrical thickening of the myometrial wall with heterogeneous echogenicity. The heterogeneity is due to hyperechoic dots, hyperechoic lines, hyperechoic endometrial islands or anechoic myometrial cysts **(Fig. 15A)**. Because of these echogenic differences it leads to posterior shadowing and posterior enhancement respectively leading to alternate, vertical hyperechoic, and hypoechoic bands known as fan shadows. This was earlier called vanishing blind pattern **(Fig. 15A)**. Junctional zone is irregular or interrupted **(Fig. 15B)** and echogenic flecks are seen at endometriomyometrial junction. Junctional zone is best assessed by 3D US **(Fig. 15C)** and can give results comparable to MRI. Uterus is tender on probe pressure if the disease is severe.

On color Doppler, affected myometrium shows vessels with larger diameter **(Fig. 15D)** and these are not arranged perpendicular to the endometrium like normal spiral vessels.

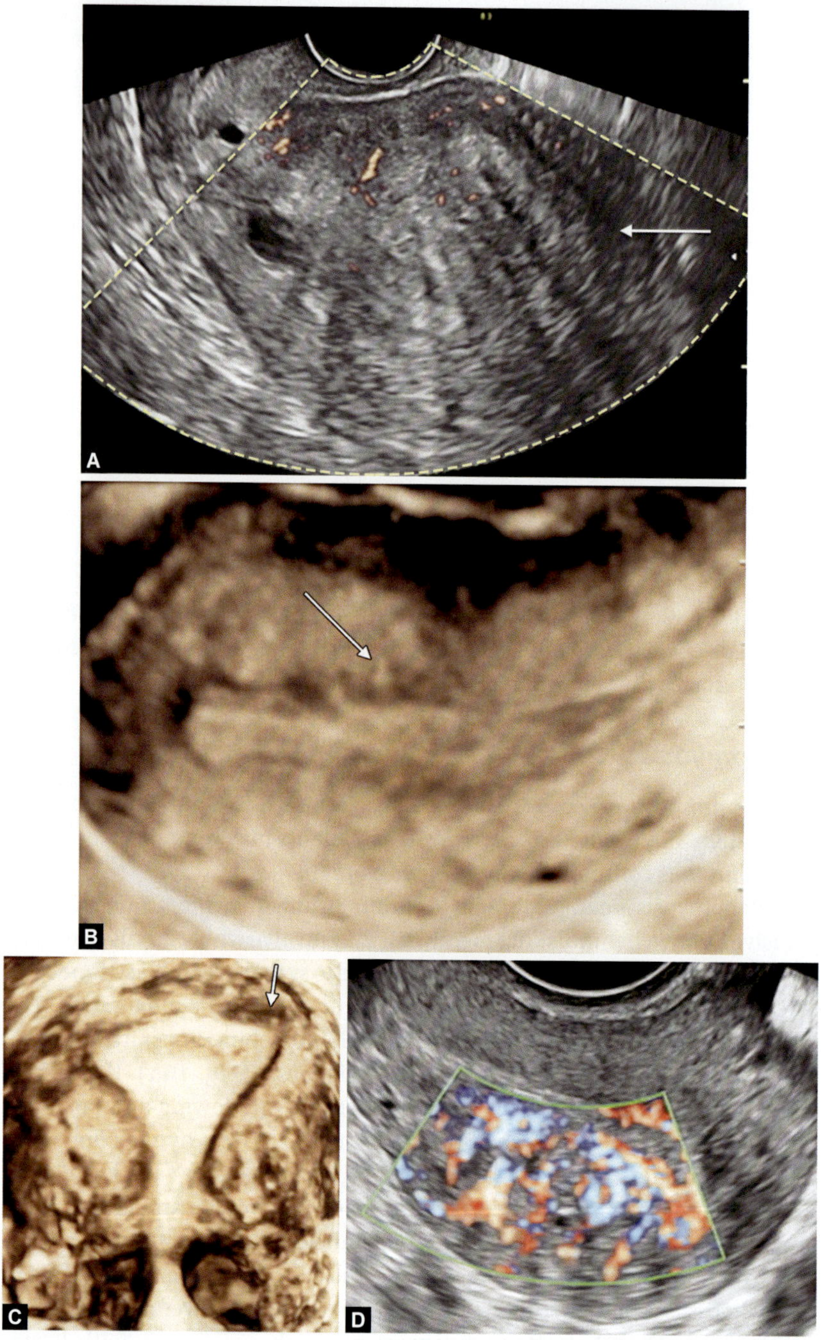

Figs. 15A to D: Adenomyosis uterus. (A) Heterogeneous myometrium and fan shadows (arrow); (B) Irregular junctional zone on two-dimensional ultrasound; (C) Three-dimensional ultrasound with irregular junctional zone; (D) Doppler in adenomyosis.

Localized adenomyosis when it is well contained in a small area is adenomyoma. When seen in the follicular phase it appears hypoechoic like a fibroid and if fibroid is degenerated it looks like adenomyoma. The main differentiating point between the adenomyoma and the fibroid is the capsular vascularity that is seen in fibroid but is never seen in adenomyoma, though both show internal vascularity, edge shadows that are present in fibroid are not seen in adenomyoma and junctional zone is interrupted in adenomyoma and not in fibroid.

ENDOMETRIAL PATHOLOGIES

Common endometrial pathologies are endometritis, polyps, endometrial hyperplasia, endometrial malignancies, synechiae, and other miscellaneous conditions with residual products of conception in endometrial cavity.

Endometritis

Acute endometritis presents as thick, isoechoic endometrium with altered junctional zone **(Fig. 16A)**, at times minimal fluid in endometrial cavity and increased vascularity in early proliferative phase. This condition often goes undiagnosed. Chronic endometritis presents as persistently thin avascular endometrium with altered junctional zone. These patients present with scanty periods or amenorrhea **(Fig. 16B)**. Tuberculosis is the common cause.

Tuberculous endometritis is a chronic endometritis with typical features. There is a large panorama of US findings that have been correlated with Koch's endometritis, though no definite features have been assigned to it, the list of possible US findings of tuberculous endometritis are as follows **(Figs. 17A to F)**.

Ultrasound features raising a doubt for Koch's endometritis:

- Persistently thin endometrium
- Echogenic spots in myometrium, endometrium, and junctional zone
- Myometrial cysts with no vascularity
- Vertically-oriented interstitial part of the tube
- Echogenic inner most layer of endometrium, with fluid in endometrial cavity in mid proliferative phase of menstrual cycle.

Endometrial Hyperplasia

This is a localized overgrowth of endometrium with normal histology. On US it is a thick echogenic endometrium with anechoic areas of varying size **(Fig. 18A)**. Endometrial thickness >15 mm in premenopausal patient and >5 mm in postmenopausal patients is hyperplasia. The endometriomyometrial junction is well maintained. On color Doppler, it shows regular distribution

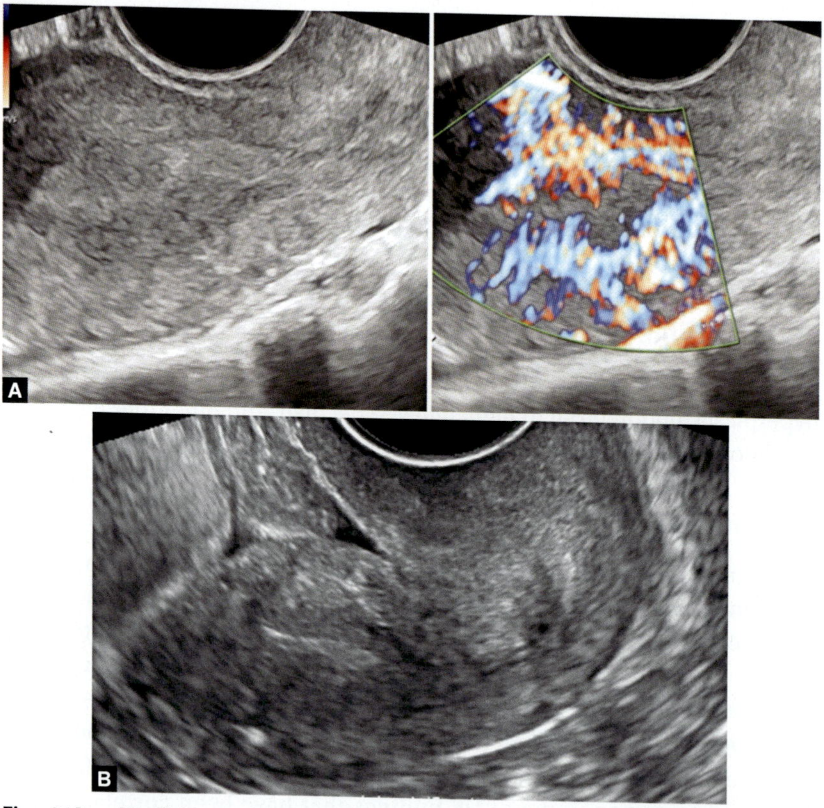

Figs. 16A and B: (A) B-mode (thick endometrium and ill-defined junctional zone) and Doppler (increased endometrial and subendometrial vascularity) image of acute endometritis, Day 3 scan; (B) Thin endometrium in secretory phase.

of vessels **(Fig. 18B)** with normal branching pattern. Patients present with intermenstrual bleeding and spotting associated with or without history of amenorrhea. Thermal balloon ablation is a popular treatment for endometrial hyperplasia.

Polyp

Endometrial polyp is a projectile lesion from the endometrial wall into the endometrial cavity. On US this appears as solid echogenic lesions in the endometrial cavity **(Fig. 19A)**. Polyps are best visible in the periovulatory phase. These are usually homogeneous but may appear heterogeneous with atypia. SIS is the best modality to demonstrate polyps and 3D adds to the information **(Fig. 19B)**. Larger lesions fill up the cavity and look like generalized endometrial thickening but color Doppler helps for differentiation. Polyp shows a single feeding vessel **(Fig. 19C)**.

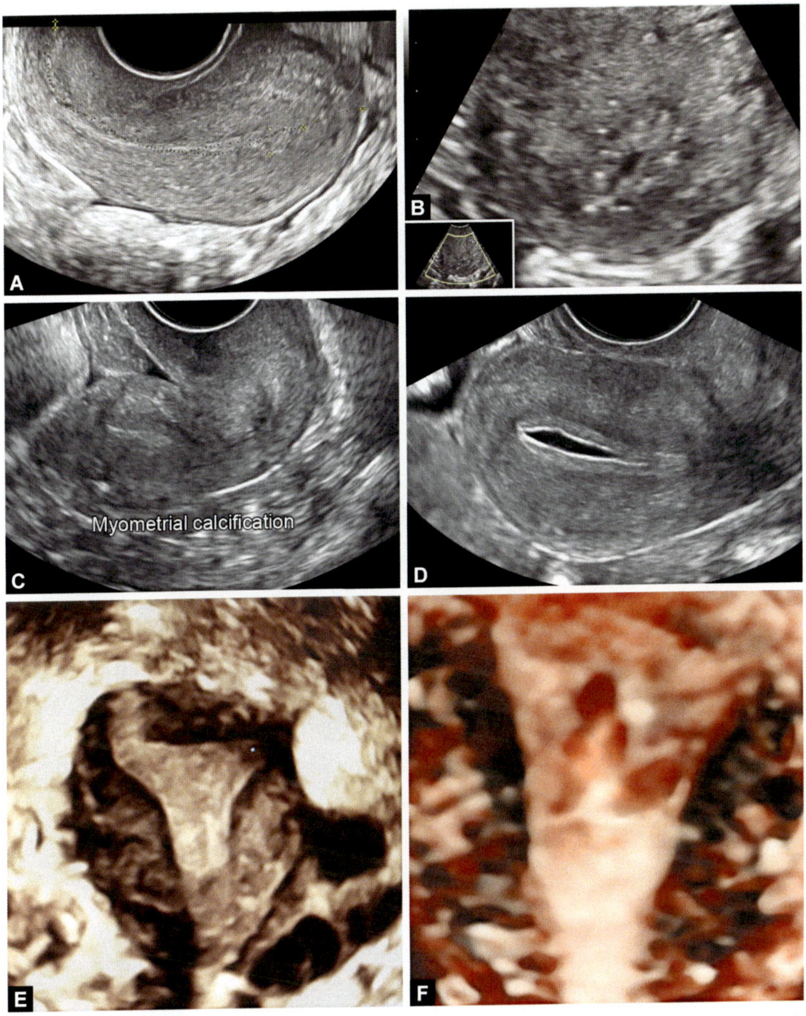

Figs. 17A to F: (A) Persistently thin endometrium with altered endometriomyometrial junction; (B) Flecks of endometrial calcification; (C) Myometrial calcification; (D) Fluid in endometrial cavity in mid proliferative stage with hyperechoic inner margin; (E) Vertical orientation of interstitial part of the tube; (F) Scarred endometrium as seen on three-dimensional ultrasound.

Vascular pattern has a high accuracy for differential diagnosis of endometrial lesions.

Single vessel pattern for polyp:[12]

- Sensitivity—81.2%
- Specificity—88.2%
- Positive predictive value—92.9%
- Negative predictive value—71.4%

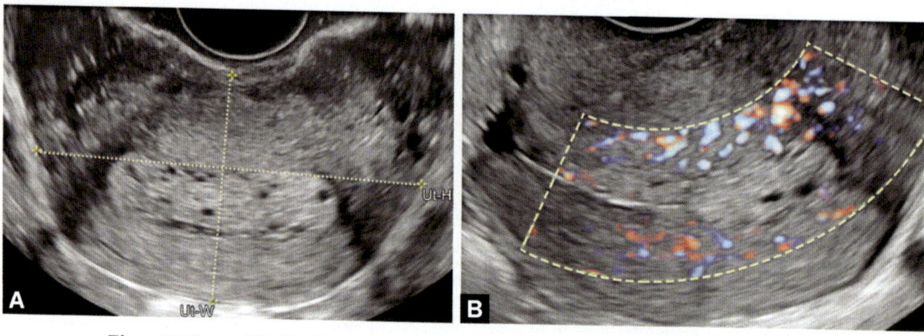

Figs. 18A and B: Endometrial hyperplasia: B-mode and power Doppler.

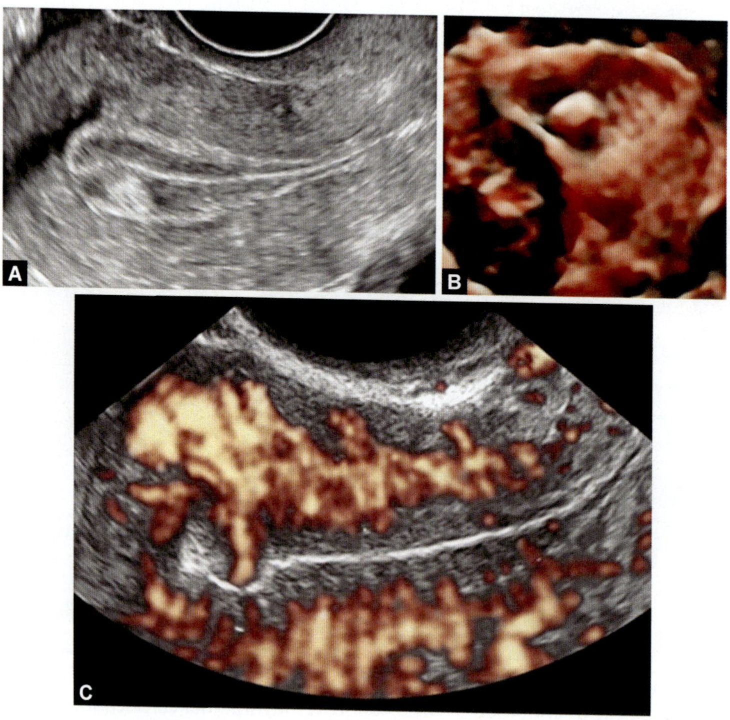

Figs. 19A to C: Endometrial polyp. (A) Two-dimensional ultrasound; (B) Saline infusion sonohysterography (SIS) with three-dimensional ultrasound coronal view; (C) Power Doppler showing vessel in pedicle of polyp.

Infection, necrosis or atypia may increase the vascularity in the polyp. Polyps may arise in the cervix or may prolapsed into cervix of they have long pedicle **(Figs. 19A to C)**.

Endometrial fibroid is hypoechoic, well demonstrated in echogenic endometrium of secretory phase and has peripheral vascularity, typical of fibroids **(Figs. 20A to C)**.

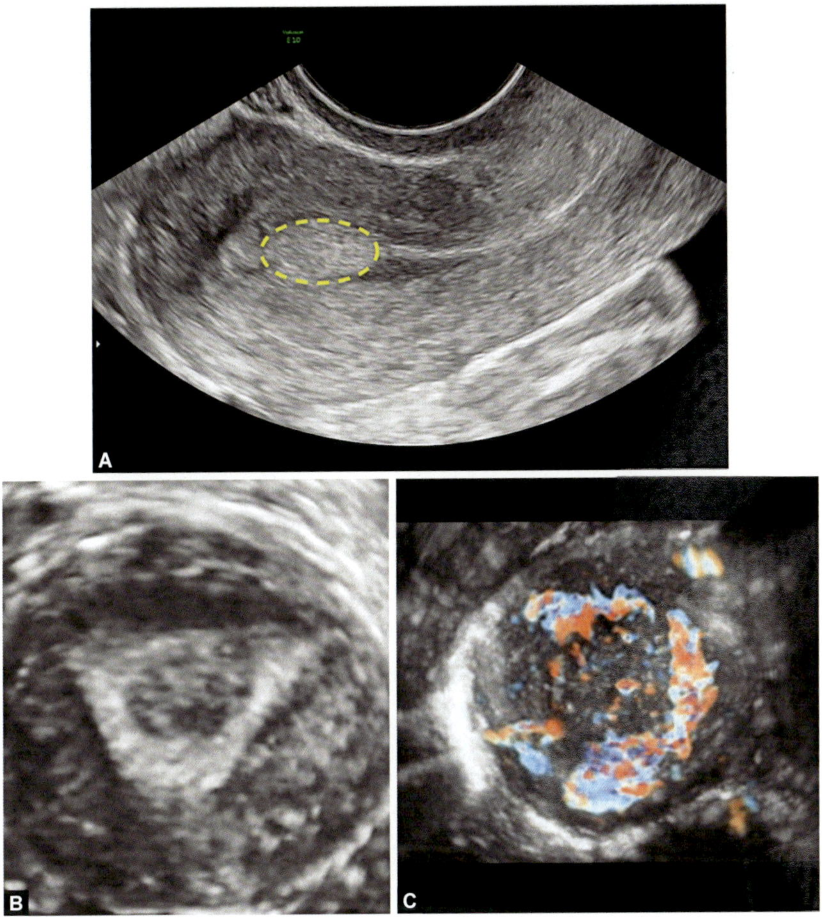

Figs. 20A to C: Endometrial fibroid. (A) Two-dimensional ultrasound; (B) Three-dimensional ultrasound coronal view; (C) Three-dimensional power Doppler showing peripheral vascularity.

Rim-like vessels for fibroid:[12]

- Sensitivity—70.6%
- Specificity—100%
- Positive predictive value—100%
- Negative predictive value—86.5%

Synechiae

Synechiae are fibrous strands between the endometrial walls, due to infection or surgical insult. When the endometrium is triple line or the cavity

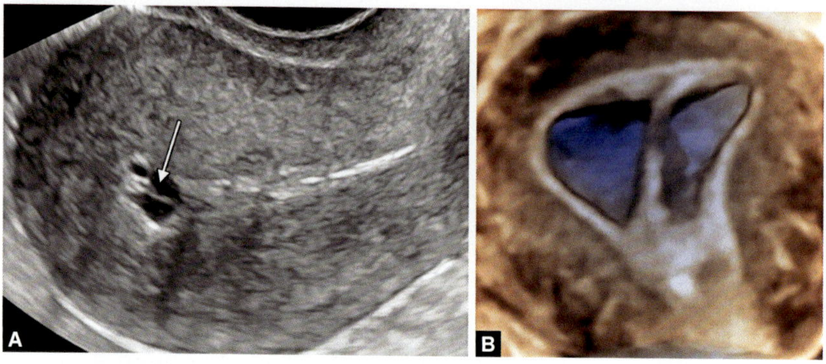

Figs. 21A and B: (A) Synechiae seen on B-mode (arrow); (B) Synechiae seen on saline infusion sonohysterography.

is distended with the fluid, synechiae are seen as lines bridging between layers of endometrium **(Fig. 21A)**. 3D US and saline infusion hysterography help in exact assessment of restriction of cavity **(Fig. 21B)** in case of bridging adhesions.

Sonohysterography has almost 100% sensitivity for the differentiation of all endometrial pathologies.

Method

- Lithotomy position of the patient.
- 6/8 Fr (external diameter 1.6 mm, internal diameter 1.1 mm) Foley catheter is placed in cervix with the help of speculum, anterior retractor and tenaculum. Catheter balloon in cervical canal.
- Distend balloon with 1.5–2 mL of fluid depending on laxity of cervix.
- Slowly inject 5 mL of normal saline with 10 mL syringe to distend the uterine cavity.
- Remove all metal instruments and introduce the probe into the vagina with catheter in situ.
- TVS shows fluid distended endometrial cavity.
- Endometrial lesions will be clearly seen.

Other endometrial lesions are postcurettage endometrial collection, vesicular mole, missed abortion, incomplete abortion, etc.

Postcurettage endometrial collection has blood in the endometrial cavity that may be partially clotted giving heterogeneous shadows filling endometrial cavity. These are avascular and have history of curettage in recent past **(Figs. 22A and B)**. Patients with missed and incomplete abortions have a history of missed period, with or without documented pregnancy earlier. Products of conception are seen in the endometrial cavity with or without fluid (blood) in the endometrial cavity. Vascularity of viable pregnancy is absent in these conditions.

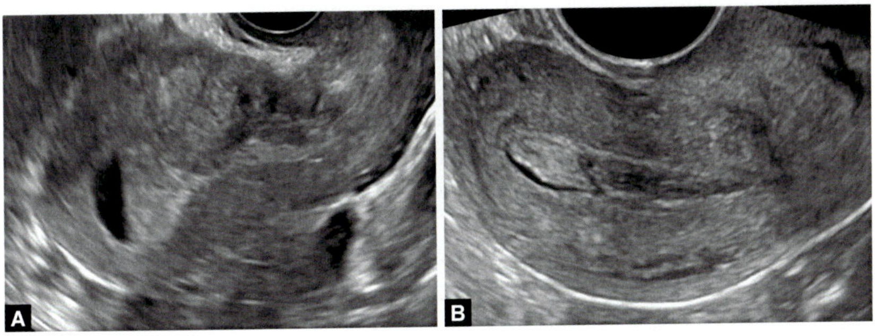

Figs. 22A and B: (A) Blood in endometrial cavity; (B) Fresh blood (hyperechoic) in endometrial cavity.

Vesicular mole shows a thick echogenic endometrium with small anechoic areas **(Fig. 23A)**—snow storm appearance. This echogenicity is higher than that of a normal secretory endometrium as it is because of decidual reaction. If it becomes invasive or malignant, it would break the endometrial-myometrial interface. On color Doppler, it shows low resistance, low velocity vessels **(Fig. 23B)**. But in early stages Doppler may not pick up the velocity because of low velocity. Extension of the same vascular pattern into the myometrium indicates myometrial invasion by the vesicular mole. Of course β-human chorionic gonadotropin (β-hCG) levels and its correlation with US findings are diagnostic. When there is a pregnancy with molar changes in the chorionic tissue, it is called partial mole. This is more difficult to diagnose. But the abnormal chorionic tissue echogenicity may be suggestive **(Fig. 23C)**.

Endometrial calcifications are common after curettage and medical termination of pregnancy **(Figs. 24A and B)**. Large calcified areas are also known as endometrial osseous metaplasia, though the cause is not known.

Intrauterine contraceptive device (IUCD) placement can also be checked by US. Even in large or very small uteri if distance from tip of IUCD to outer wall of uterine fundus ≤ (anterior wall + posterior wall)/2 ± 1.33, **(Fig. 25A)**. It indicates a proper placement. Though with 3D US these measurements are not essential. For displaced IUCD **(Fig. 25B)**, US is the investigation of choice as it determines the exact location and therefore route of removal of IUCD.

ENDOMETRIAL MALIGNANCY

Endometrial carcinoma is more common in postmenopausal age and is suspected in patients with postmenopausal bleeding.

On US it shows thickened endometrium (localized or generalized) with heterogeneous texture **(Fig. 26A)**. Fluid may or may not be seen in endometrial cavity. If the lesion is contained in the endometrium, the junctional zone is normal but if it has grown beyond the endometrium, the junctional zone is interrupted or inaccessible **(Fig. 26A)**. On color Doppler, endometrium

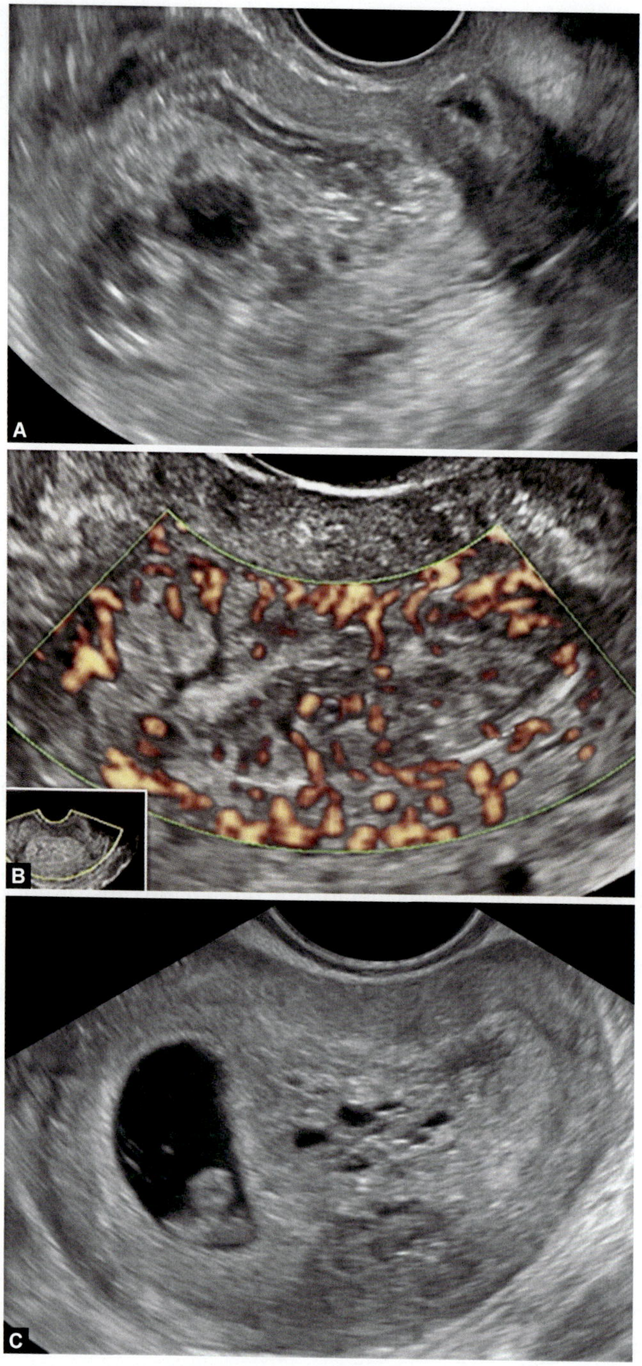

Figs. 23A to C: Vesicular mole. (A) Two-dimensional ultrasound; (B) Power Doppler; (C) Partial mole with normal gestational sac with fetal pole and yolk sac seen.

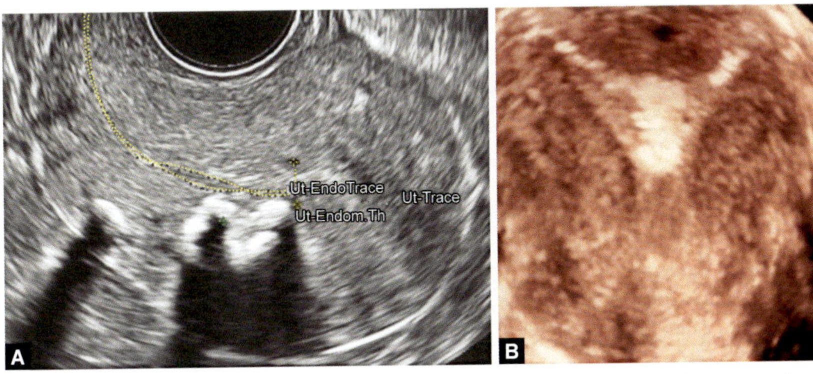

Figs. 24A and B: Endometrial calcification—two-dimensional and three-dimensional.

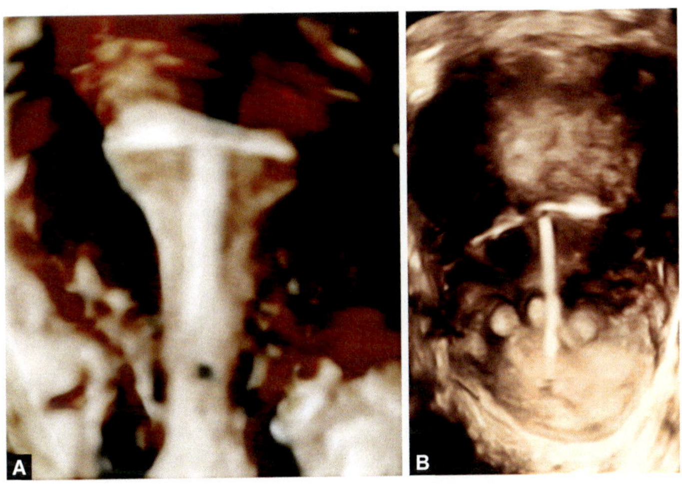

Figs. 25A and B: (A) Three-dimensional ultrasound showing intrauterine contraceptive device (IUCD) in situ; (B) Three-dimensional ultrasound showing displaced IUCD.

shows heterogeneously distributed, increased vascularity and on pulse Doppler these vessels show low RI (<0.4) **(Fig. 26B)**. With increase in size of lesion and invasion the resistance further decreases. Three-dimensional power Doppler shows dichotomous branching, intermittent narrowing and ballooning due to microaneurysms **(Fig. 26C)**. It has a sensitivity of 100%, specificity of 94.44%, and positive and negative predictive values of 83.33% and 100%, respectively.[13]

Tamoxifen has been thought to be causative of endometrial carcinoma. But this is a very late and not very common side effect of tamoxifen.

Effects of Tamoxifen on Endometrium

Tamoxifen treatment leads to endometrial metaplasia. Initially endometrium thickens but is homogeneous and junctional zone is maintained, then

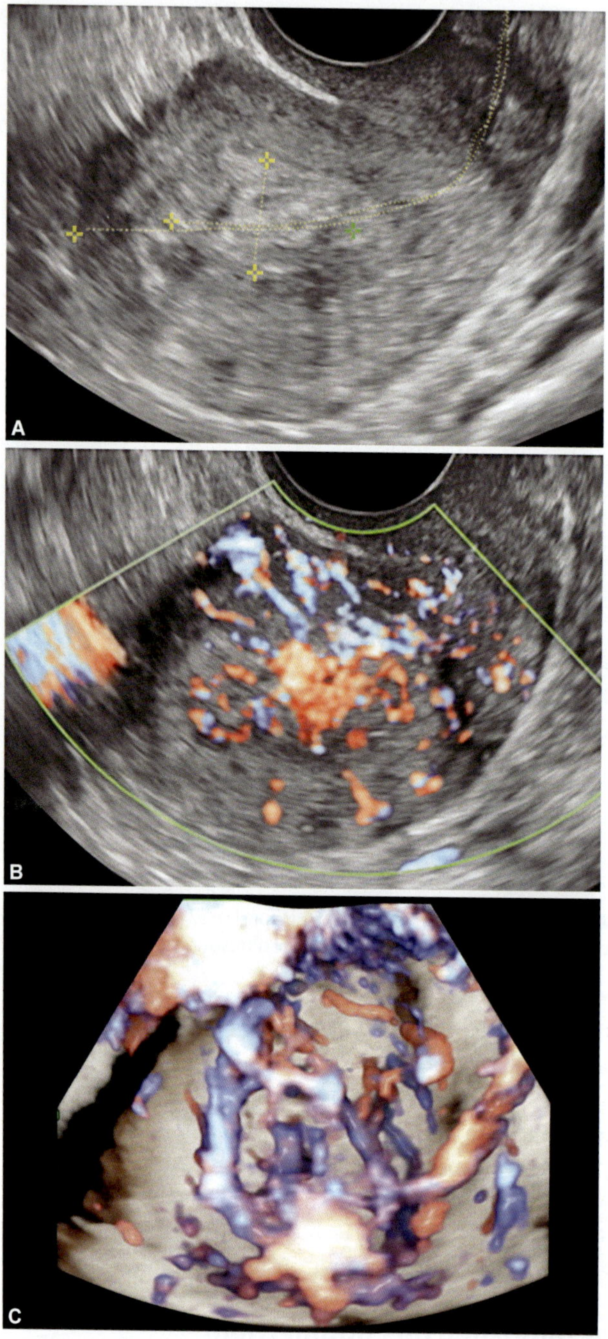

Figs. 26A to C: (A) Endometrial mass with interrupted junctional zone; (B) Doppler showing markedly increased vascularity extending beyond endometrial margins; (C) Three-dimensional power Doppler chaotic vasculature.

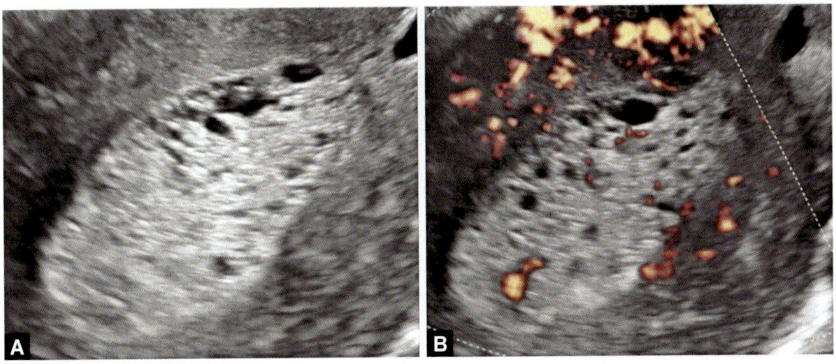

Figs. 27A and B: (A) B-mode image of cystic atrophy (tamoxifen exposed); (B) Doppler of the same patient.

small anechoic cystic areas develop in it followed by then blurring of the endometrial margins and the junctional zone. Endometrial cystic atrophy mimics hypertrophy **(Figs. 27A and B)**. Thickening of the subendometrial zone/endometrial stroma with irregular endometrial-myometrial junction are then seen. Doppler shows high resistance endometrial flow.

Interruption of the junctional zone and low resistance (RI < 0.5) endometrial blood flow suggest atypia and risk of malignancy.

UTERINE SCAR

Intact fibrous cesarean scars are seen as thick linear echogenic shadows traversing the whole myometrium at the level of internal os. When these scars show dehiscence a small anechoic triangle is seen with the base at the endometrium **(Fig. 28A)**. Scar thickness is measured as distance from the apex of the triangle to serosa. The scars sometimes are completely open and may show fluid movement into the endometrial cavity throughout the menstrual cycle **(Fig. 28B)**. 3D can be very helpful for exact assessment of the lesion. Elastography may help to assess the firmness of the scar.

Red color on elastography is an indicator of a weak scar and blue color indicates firm fibrous scar **(Fig. 28C)**.

CERVICAL LESIONS

Apart from fibroids and polyps **(Figs. 29A and B)** of cervix, the most common lesions in cervix are Nabothian cysts. These appear as well-defined anechoic rounded lesions in cervix **(Fig. 29C)**.

Cervical malignancies are solid lesions in cervix and on US present as heterogeneous lesions with irregular margins **(Fig. 30A)**. When the lesion grows beyond the cervix, US shows obliteration of tissue planes. Color Doppler

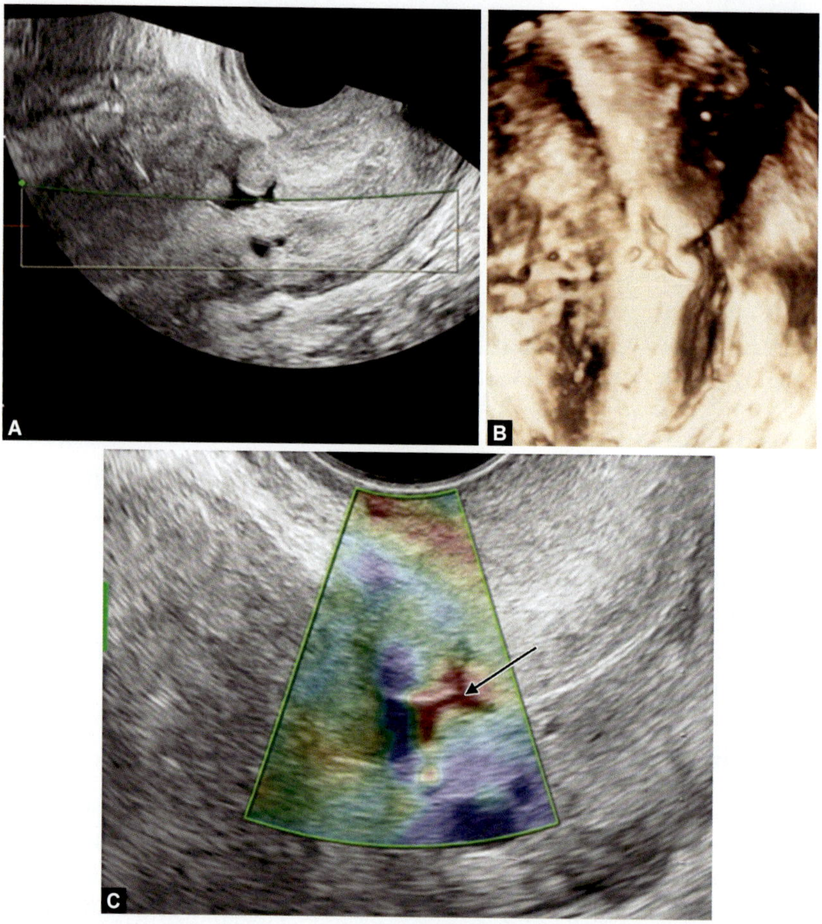

Figs. 28A to C: Weak cesarean scar. (A) On B-mode; (B) Three-dimensional ultrasound; (C) Elastography.

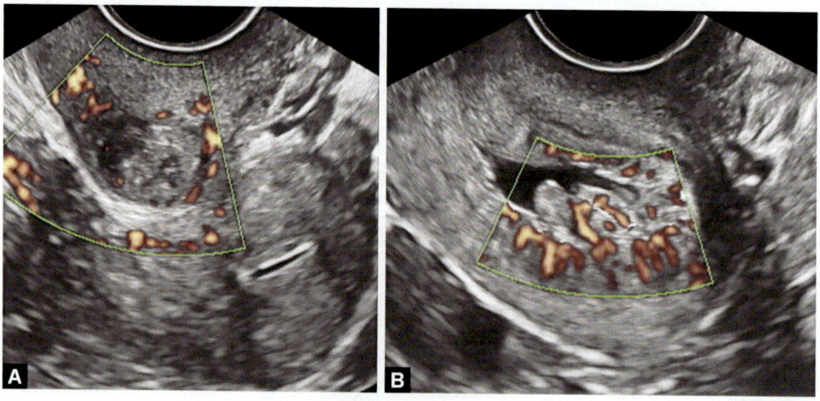

Figs. 29A and B

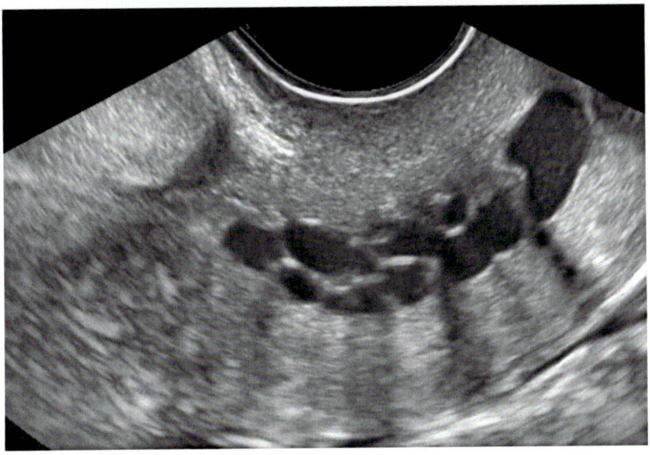

Fig. 29C

Figs. 29A to C: (A) Power Doppler image of cervical fibroid; (B) Power Doppler image of cervical polyps; (C) Nabothian cysts.

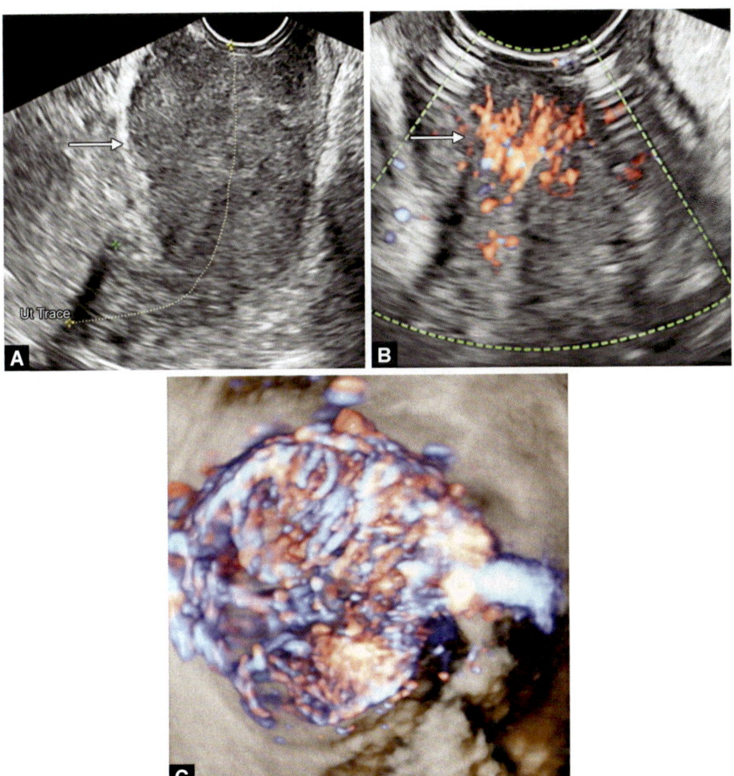

Figs. 30A to C: (A) Cervical mass on B-mode; (B) Doppler; (C) Three-dimensional power Doppler cervical malignancy.

shows significantly increased low resistance vascularity **(Fig. 30B)** and vessels with dichotomous branching and asymmetrical caliber. Three-dimensional US is an excellent tool to assess the extent of the lesion **(Fig. 30C)**.

Carry Home Message

- Müllerian duct abnormalities are diagnosed chiefly by assessment of the uterus in mid-coronal plane and observing the outer fundal contour and the endometrial cavity contour.
- For Müllerian duct abnormalities 3D US is the modality of choice.
- Fibroids are confidently diagnosed by B-mode US and Doppler showing peripheral vascularity.
- Adenomyosis can be diagnosed by interrupted or irregular junctional zone and thick heterogeneous myometrium.
- Tuberculous endometritis can be strongly suspected but not confidently diagnosed by US.
- Polyps, endometrial fibroids, and hyperplasia can be confidently differentiated by B-mode US and Doppler.
- Heterogeneity of texture, irregular margins, affection of junctional zone, and low-resistance abundant vascularity suggest malignancy.

REFERENCES

1. Raga F, Bonilla-Mosules F, Blanes J. Congenital Müllerian anomalies: diagnostic accuracy of three-dimensional ultrasound. Fertil Steril. 1996;65(3):523-8.
2. The American Fertility Society classification of adnexal adhesions, distal tubal occlusion secondary to tubal ligation, tubal pregnancies, Müllerian anomalies and intrauterine adhesions. Fertil Steril. 1998;49:944-55.
3. Rock JA, Roberts CP, Jones HW. Congenital anomalies of the uterine cervix: lessons from 30 cases managed clinically by a common protocol. Fertil Steril. 2010;94:1858-63.
4. Grimbizis GF, Tsalikis T, Mikos T, Papadopoulos N, Tarlatzis BC, Bontis JN. Successful end-to-end cervico-cervical anastomosis in a patient with congenital cervical fragmentation: case report. Hum Reprod. 2004;19:1204-10.
5. Grimbizis GF, Gordts S, Spiezio Sardo AD, Brucker S, De Angelis C, Gergolet M, et al. The ESHRE/ESGE consensus on the classification of female genital tract congenital anomalies. Human Reprod. 2013;28(8):2032-44.
6. Kupesic S, Kurjak A. Septate uterus: detection and prediction of obstetrical complications by different forms of ultrasonography. J Ultrasound Med. 1998;17:631-6.
7. Salim R, Woelfer B, Backos M, Regan L, Jurkovic D. Reproducibility of three-dimensional ultrasound diagnosis of congenital uterine anomalies. Ultrasound Obstet Gynecol. 2003;21:578-82.
8. Kupesic S. Clinical implications of sonographic detection of uterine anomalies for reproductive outcome. Ultrasound Obstet Gynecol. 2001;18:387-400.
9. Richman TS, Viscomi GN, Cherney AD, Polan A. Fallopian tubal patency assessment by ultrasound following fluid injection. Radiology. 1984;152:507-10.

10. Graupera B, Pascual MA, Hereter L, Browne JL, Ubeda B, Rodriguez I, et al. Accuracy of three-dimensional ultrasound compared with magnetic resonance imaging in diagnosis of Müllerian duct abnormalities using ESHRE-ESGE consensus on the classification of congenital anomalies of the female genital tract. Ultrasound Obstet Gynecol. 2015;46(5):616-22.
11. Munro MG, Critchley HO, Broder MS, Frase IS, FIGO working group on menstrual disorders. FIGO classification system (PALM-COEIN) for causes of abnormal uterine bleeding in nongravid women of reproductive age. Int J Gynecol Obstet. 2011;113(1):3-13.
12. Kurjak A, Kupesic-Urek S, Miric D. The assessment of benign uterine tumor vascularization by transvaginal color Doppler. Ultrasound Med Biol. 1992;18:645-9.
13. Lee CN, Cheng WF, Chen CA, Chu JS, Hsieh CY, Hsieh FJ. Angiogenesis of endometrial carcinomas assessed by measurement of intratumoral blood flow, microvessel density and vascular endothelial growth factor levels. Obstet Gynecol. 2000;96(4):615-21.

CHAPTER 15

Ultrasound in Gynecology: Adnexal Diseases

Sonal Panchal

INTRODUCTION

Ultrasound (US) is accepted as the primary imaging modality for evaluation of adnexal masses. It is a very useful tool for localizing the origin of pelvic mass and to study the morphological characteristics of the mass. Based on US morphology, these masses can be categorized as benign, possibly malignant or malignant. Doppler is an important tool for differential diagnosis of adnexal lesions. Several meta-analyses have revealed significant higher performance for combined techniques using morphologic assessment and Doppler US indices than B-mode evaluation alone.[1] It is true that in all the cases of doubtful nature of the lesion, International Ovarian Tumor Analysis (IOTA) guidelines must be used.[2] But it is also true that majority of the cystic lesions seen in the ovary are physiological. Though ovarian cancers are common, benign or lesions due to abnormal physiology are much more common. It is therefore very essential to first get acquainted to the common pathologies and then when in doubt surely use IOTA.

Adnexal lesions can be divided as:

- Ovarian lesions
- Tubal/tubo-ovarian lesions
- *Miscellaneous lesions*: Paraovarian cysts, peritoneal inclusion cyst, and broad ligament fibroids.

Ovarian lesions: Ovaries are physiologically active organs and continuous change is seen in their morphology throughout the menstrual cycle. This is in the form of follicle recruitment, maturation, rupture, and formation of corpus luteum. Therefore cystic structures appear and change in morphology from time to time in the ovaries. Apart from this, ovaries also play a host for several other pathological lesions such as endometriomas, dermoid cysts, serous and mucous cystadenomas, endometriomas, fibromas, and ovarian epithelial carcinomas.

Tubal lesions: These are mainly inflammatory lesions of the fallopian tube. They may be acute or chronic and may present as salpingitis, hydrosalpinx or complex tubo-ovarian masses. Tubal neoplasms are not common. Ectopic pregnancy, tubal or ovarian is an adnexal lesion that is very important to diagnose early but is often missed.

Adnexal lesions: Common lesions other than of tubal or ovarian origin are broad ligament fibroids or paraovarian lesions. These lesions need to be differentiated from pedunculated subserosal fibroids.

OVARIAN LESIONS

Before describing a lesion, it is important to decide the origin of the lesion.

The signs used to confirm the origin of the lesion from the ovary or otherwise are:

- Place a probe in such a way that the lesion and the ovary are seen in the same frame on the screen. Apply pressure with the probe, to separate the two. If probe pressure can displace the two away from each other, or allows these to slide over each other, the lesion is not arising from the ovary. If the two cannot be separated, the lesion is either adherent to the ovary or it is arising from the ovary.
- If the lesion is arising from the ovary, then lesion will be completely or partially covered by normal ovarian tissue and is typically described as a "rim sign" or "beak sign" respectively **(Figs. 1A and B)**.

Having confirmed the origin of the lesion from the ovary, the differential diagnosis of these lesions can be thought of. We would prefer to do this by dividing these lesions into different categories based on their US appearance.

Ultrasound-based Classification of Ovarian Lesions

- Nonseptated clear cysts
- Cysts with internal echogenicities
- Solid lesions
- Complex lesions with cystic and solid areas.

Nonseptated Clear Cysts

These cysts are thin walled, have no internal echogenicities, no septae or no solid areas in it.

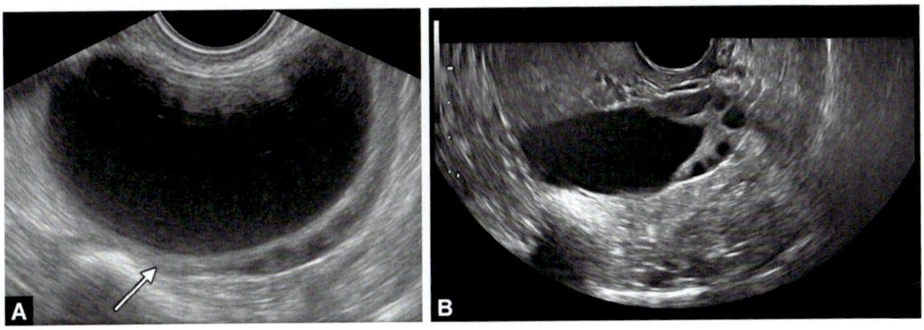

Figs. 1A and B: (A) Beak sign—intraovarian lesion; (B) Beak of ovarian tissue seen overlying the cystic lesion.

The lesions/structures in this category are:

- Follicle
- Follicular cyst
- Simple cyst

Follicle: If the scan is done in the proliferative phase of the menstrual cycle and one sees a thin-walled anechoic lesion, with no internal echogenicities or septa, the first consideration should be a follicle. For confirmation, use Doppler and if that shows vascularity around, it is a follicle.

Follicular cyst: Follicle grows till 18–24 mm in diameter before it ruptures due to the surge of luteinizing hormone to release the ovum that it contains. But if it does not rupture and keeps on increasing in size, it is termed as follicular cyst, especially when it grows to 30 mm or more. On follow-up after 2 weeks, it is replaced by a corpus luteum. It may persist in luteal phase of the cycle or even in the subsequent cycle. Contrary to the normal follicle, the follicular cyst shows scanty and high resistance flow. But it is ultimately a physiological cyst and would resolve on its own over a maximum period of 4–6 weeks **(Fig. 2A)**.

Simple cyst of the ovary: It is a thin-walled intraovarian cystic structure usually larger than 5 cm. Doppler shows no flow because it is hormonally inactive. It does not resolve on its own and may require US-guided aspiration **(Fig. 2B)**. Though if it is asymptomatic, it may be left alone.

Cysts with Internal Echogenicities and No Septae

The most common lesions in this category are:

- Corpus luteum
- Hemorrhagic cyst
- Luteinized unruptured follicle (LUF)
- Endometrioma

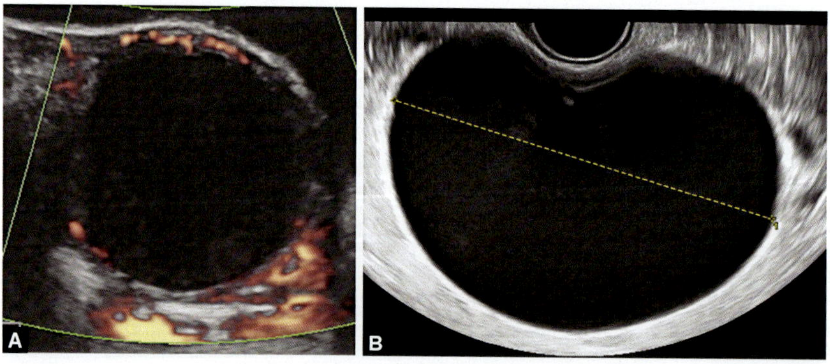

Figs. 2A and B: (A) Follicular cyst on power Doppler showing scanty pericystic flow; (B) Large anechoic cystic lesion with no internal echogenicity and thin walls—simple cyst of ovary.

All these structures have thick walls, internal echogenicities, and no septae. The appearance may vary, viz. absolutely isoechoic homogeneous, clear fluid, lace-like or cobweb pattern or ground-glass appearance.

- *Corpus luteum* is a physiologically active cyst. It appears as a result of ovulation from the follicle. Its existence usually is till the end of the luteal phase. It has thick, crenulated walls. Contents of the cyst show heterogeneous echogenicity without septae. The echogenicity and appearance of the contents may change at different times depending on the stage of degeneration of the blood that it contains. It may appear hyperechoic with fresh blood, clots may be seen and solid components with fluid content, fibrin formation may show strands or cobweb appearance. Doppler gives almost a complete ring of color with low resistance [resistance index (RI) < 0.5]. That is the most characteristic feature to differentiate it from other lesions with similar appearance on B-mode **(Figs. 3A to D)**.
- *Hemorrhagic cyst* is a cyst-containing blood in any of its forms. It is most of the times a result of nonresolved corpus luteum but is hormonally inactive and therefore shows no vascularity. If it shows minimal high resistance flow, then it is named as residual active corpus luteum and not a hemorrhagic cyst. It may persist into the proliferative phase of the next cycle, but is a physiological cyst and resolves completely over a period of 4–6 weeks. It shares the same appearance as corpus luteum on B-mode US. It changes echogenicity over time due to fibrinolysis of the clot **(Fig. 3E)**.
- *Luteinized unruptured follicle* has thick, echogenic walls, but does not contain blood or blood products. Therefore, it does show low level

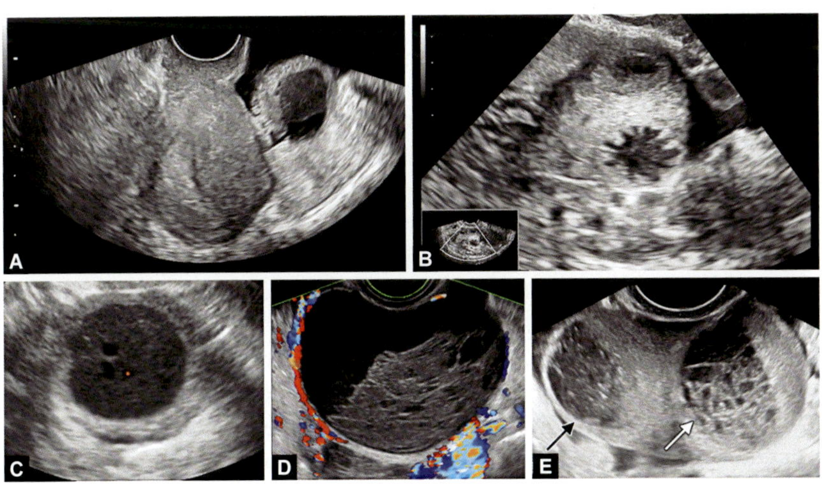

Figs. 3A to E: Different appearances of corpus luteum, also showing ring of color in the last frame. Hemorrhagic cyst (white arrow) and endometrioma (black arrow).

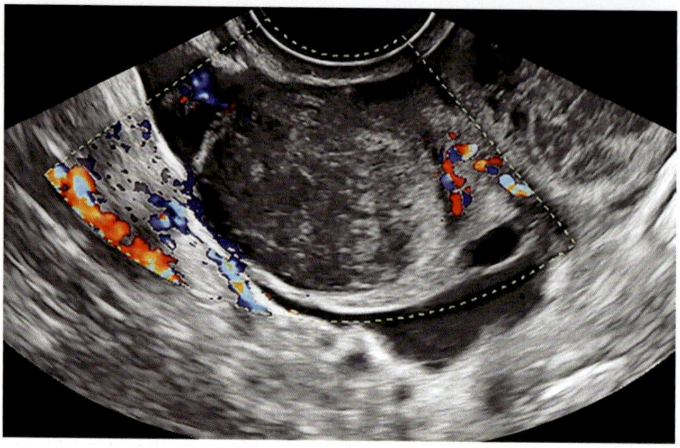

Fig. 4: Luteinized unruptured follicle (LUF)—echogenic margins and internal echogenicity.

internal echogenicity but is less heterogeneous and never shows lace-like or cobweb echogenicity **(Fig. 4)**. On Doppler, it shows variable amount of peripheral vascularity that typically has RI >0.51.

The three above-described lesions are physiological ovarian cysts and 53–89% of these show spontaneous regression on follow-up after 4–6 weeks.[3] To avoid confusing these with malignancies, scan must be done in early proliferative phase or two examinations 2–3 weeks apart should be done so that assessment can be done in two different phases of menstrual cycle, and complete or partial resolution of these lesions can be demonstrated.

- *Endometrioma*: Endometriosis is detected in 15% of infertile women. It commonly presents as dysmenorrhea, dyspareunia, irregular bleeding, and infertility. Endometriosis may be seen in various locations—ovary; uterus (adenomyosis), rectovaginal septum, bowel involvement, and bladder are the most common sites, though more distant spread and atypical presentations are also known. Endometriosis in the ovary develops as a cystic lesion and is named as endometrioma. One-third to half of the ovarian endometriotic cysts are bilateral. Ovaries with endometriomas are commonly positioned medially or retrouterine.

Features typical of endometriomas are thick shaggy walls with or without septae, ground-glass appearance, internal echogenicities similar to hemorrhagic collection, fluid levels, linear echogenic flecks in its walls **(Figs. 5A to C)** and pain on pressure with the probe. Adhesions are very common. Solid areas may be sometimes seen. Streaming sign is often seen. This is slow downward movement of small low level echogenicities seen in endometrioma (chocolate cyst). Mean gray value (MGV) is significantly higher in ovarian endometrioma compared to all other kinds of ovarian cysts. MGV cut-off >15.560 had a sensitivity of 85% and specificity of 76.5%

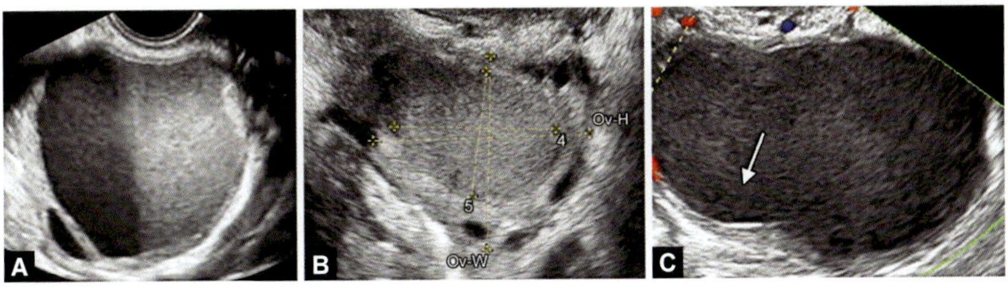

Figs. 5A to C: Endometrioma showing fluid level, ground-glass appearance, and echogenic flecks in wall.

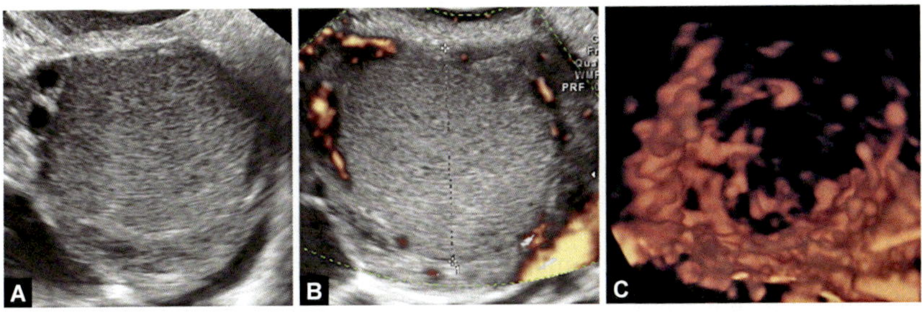

Figs. 6A to C: Endometrioma—B-mode, power Doppler showing short-coursed peripheral vessels and three-dimensional power Doppler (3D PD) showing bird's nest appearance.

for diagnosis of endometrioma.[4] But this needs to be evaluated on three-dimensional US, and is also not specific for endometriomas and therefore may be omitted.

On Doppler: Scattered vascularity at ovarian hilus with moderate vascular impedance has been described in literature. The ovarian hilar RI varies between RI 0.40 and 0.56. The lesion typically shows short-coursed vessels at its periphery. It is higher during menstruation and in symptomatic patients.[5] Vascularity can be used as a means to decide the mode of therapy for endometriomas. Avascular lesions indicate scarification and are less convenient for delivery of medication, and therefore should be considered for surgical therapy.[6]

Kurjak et al. have shown a sensitivity of 83.9%, specificity of 97.1%, positive predictive value (PPV) 82%, and negative predictive value (NPV) 97.5% of vaginal sonography for characterization of endometriomas. If CA 125 >35 IU/mL was added as a cut-off to these parameters, the sensitivity and specificity reached 99.04% and 99.64%, and PPV and NPV reached 98.10% and 99.82%.[7] Similar results were also confirmed by several other workers.

Three-dimensional US allows detection of surface of the endometrioma, visualization of preserved ovarian tissue, and assessment of the ovarian relationship with neighboring pelvic structures. 3D power Doppler (PD) typically shows multiple short-coursed regularly separated pericystic vessels giving a typical bird's nest appearance **(Figs. 6A to C)**.[8]

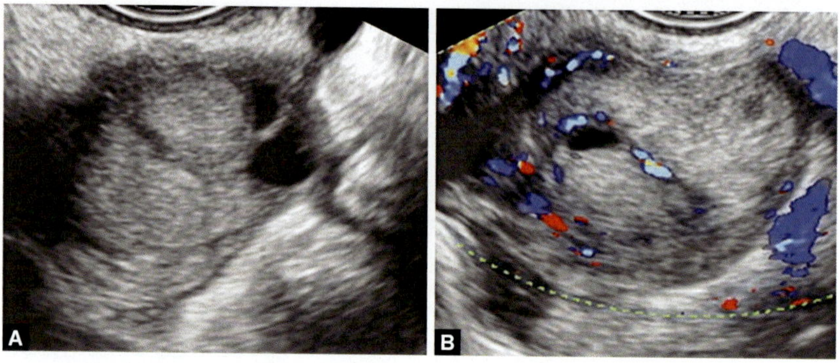

Figs. 7A and B: Ovarian fibroma with peripheral vascularity.

Solid Lesions

There is a long list of solid lesions seen in the ovary with different histopathologies but the lesions that can be included in this group are fibroma, fibrothecoma, thecoma, Brenner's tumor, etc. All except fibromas are extremely rare and also cannot be differentiated from each other by US alone. Moreover, fibroma also has a typical identifiable US appearance. Fibroma is well-defined round/oval lesion with echogenicity like that of a fibroid-hypoechoic, homogeneous, but sometimes may be heterogeneous and may also show calcifications **(Figs. 7A and B)**. Fibromas when homogeneous are isoechoic to normal ovarian stroma and may be difficult to identify on B-mode scan. The ovary may then look more solid. Therefore, Doppler study of a solid-looking ovary is a must. This will show peripheral ring of vascularity typically like fibroid.

Pedunculated fibromas need to be differentiated from pedunculated subserosal fibroids or broad-ligament fibroid and that can be done by tracing the blood supply to this lesion. Fibromas are often bilateral and may also be associated with ascites and pleural effusion. This complication is known as Meig's syndrome.

Solid-looking ovaries may also be seen in ovarian torsion. In ovary with torsion, stroma is hypoechoic with peripherally placed small follicles. Vascularity may or may not be present and that decides the viability of the ovary. It must be remembered that presence of vascularity does not exclude torsion, because when torsion occurs, first the venous flow stops and then when the torsion becomes more tight or complete, the arterial flow also stops. Definitive sign is a whirl pool sign in adnexa due to twisting of vessels but it is not always easy to locate because this is usually seen posterior to the ovary and the patient is in severe pain so examination is difficult **(Figs. 8A and B)**.[9] Follicular ring sign has been described as the earliest sign of ovarian torsion.[10] This is a complete echogenic rim surrounding small follicles **(Fig. 9)**.

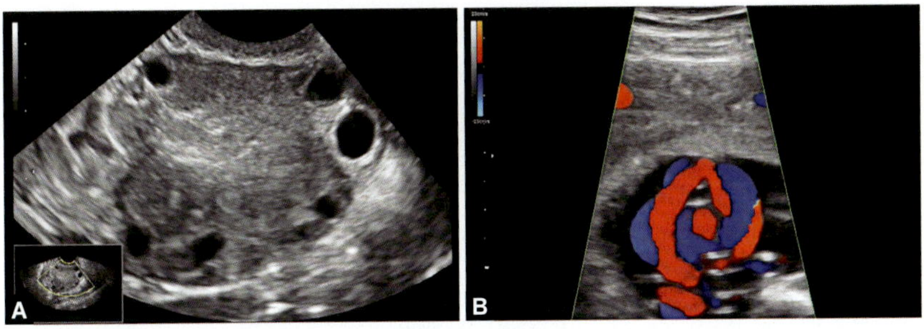

Figs. 8A and B: Solid-looking ovary with peripherally placed small follicles and whirlpool sign.

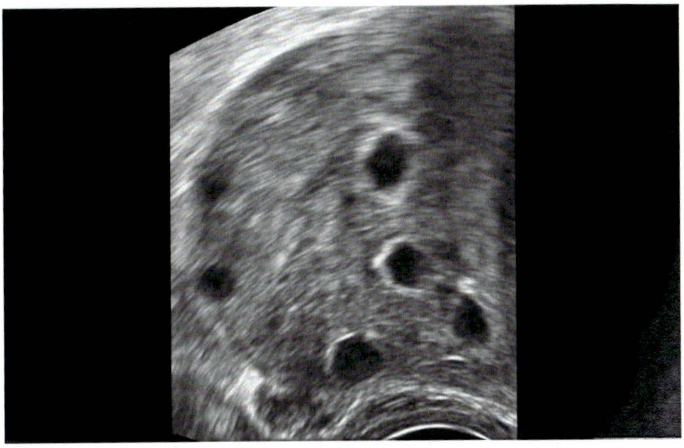

Fig. 9: Follicular ring sign in ovarian torsion.
(*Courtesy:* Dr Mala Sibbal, Bengaluru, Karnataka)

Solid-looking ovary is also seen in patients with ovarian neoplasm. In that case also ovarian vascularity helps to reach to the correct diagnosis.

Complex Lesions with Cystic and Solid Areas

Lesions in this group have thick walls with internal echogenicities, and also solid projections arising from the walls. Common lesions included in this group are:

- Dermoids
- Epithelial tumors
- Endometrioid tumors

Dermoids: Dermoids or teratomas are often an incidental finding. These are well-defined lesions with thick walls, low level echoes, fluid-fluid level, hyperechoic lines and dots due to hair, hyperechoic/calcified echoes such as teeth or bones with posterior shadowing, regional diffuse bright echoes with or without acoustic shadowing due to hair clumps or fat in Rokitansky's

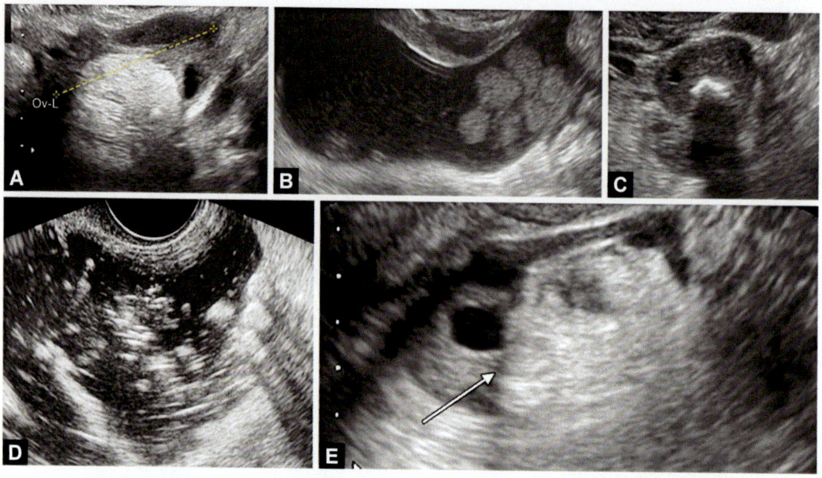

Figs. 10A to E: Dermoids—echogenic mass, hairballs in cyst, small echogenic area, teeth with posterior shadowing and echogenic lines and dots, and large Rokitansky's tubercle (arrow).

protuberance **(Figs. 10 A to E)**. Hyperechoic ball-like lesions may be seen, the posterior margin of which is not identifiable snowballs. These are very similar to bowel gas shadows but when these shadows are intraovarian this is dermoid. About 72% of cystic teratomas are avascular. Vascularity in these teratomas may be an indicator of malignant change.

These features have been assigned definite PPV.[11]

- 80% for shadowing echodensity
- 75% for regionally bright echoes
- 50% for hyperechoic lines and dots
- 20% for fluid-fluid level
- Positive predictive value for more than two features is 100%.

Morphologic scoring system for dermoids by Kurjak et al. has sensitivity of 93.1% and specificity of 99.4%. Including color Doppler, sensitivity of 99% and specificity of 99.8% can be achieved.[12]

Epithelial tumors: Surface epithelial-stromal tumors account for 60% of ovarian neoplasms and 80–90% of ovarian malignancies. Of all these 46% are serous, 36.5% are mucinous, and 7.5% are endometrioid. These tumors are chiefly cystic, have septae, internal echogenicities, and projections arising from its walls. Solid projections can be differentiated from internal echogenicities, by in and out movement of the probe with solid projection of the lesion in view. If the lesion slides against the cyst wall, then it is internal echogenicity due to debris and if it does not, it is a lesion arising from the cyst wall. Moreover solid projections more commonly have convex walls unlike internal echogenicities due to debris. Benign and malignant counterparts of these tumors have similar but overlapping US appearances. On US, therefore it is not possible to give a histopathological diagnosis. Though depending on US appearances, these lesions are divided into benign, possibly malignant, and malignant tumors.

Tumors with thin walls, clear contents, thin septae, no solid projections or papillarities, and no vascularity in septae are benign lesions. These lesions have no papillarities or solid projections.

Whereas lesions having following features have higher chance of malignancy.[13] With ovary >20 cc in premenopausal patient and >10 cc in postmenopausal patient malignancy is suspected. Though waiting till this size may be waiting too long. Other US features that suggest malignancy are:

- Cyst wall thickness >3 mm and with papillarities of >3 mm
- Septae thicker >3 mm thickness **(Fig. 11A)**
- Solid parts >1 cm
- Mixed or high level internal echoes
- RI ≤ 0.42 is suggestive of malignancy. RI < 0.41 can be used as a cut-off for the screening of ovarian malignancy and can detect ovarian cancer as early as International Federation of Gynecology and Obstetrics (FIGO) stage Ia.[14] But there are pitfalls to this generalization. Variable caliber of vessels in malignant lesion may show variable resistance and velocity. Pre-existing vessels in the lesion may not show low resistance like the newly formed once with the growth of the tumor and in postmenopausal patients, the resistance may not be as low as in premenopausal women with ovarian tumor. Therefore, a low resistance flow has a PPV for malignancy but high resistance flow does not rule out malignancy.
- *Chaotic vascular architecture*: Dichotomous branching, microaneurysms, and small arteriovenous fistulae seen on 3D PD **(Fig. 11C)**.
- Bilaterality—ascites
- Adhesions and disturbed relationship with structures around.

  Different scoring systems have been established combining all the above-mentioned features. Using 3D US and 3D PD **(Figs. 11B and D)** improves the diagnostic accuracy as it is superior in evaluating.[15]
- Papillary projections
- Characteristics of cystic walls so it is especially helpful in evaluating cystic tumors (surface mode) **(Fig. 11B and Figs. 12A and B)**
- Calcifications and bone densities (transparent mode)
- Identifying the extent of capsular infiltration of tumors
- Calculating the volume
- 3D PD has improved specificity (75% as compared to 54%) for ovarian malignancy and staging though the detection rate is 97.7%.[16]

  Typical vascular criteria seen on 3D PD in malignant tumors[17] **(Fig. 11D and Fig. 12C)**:

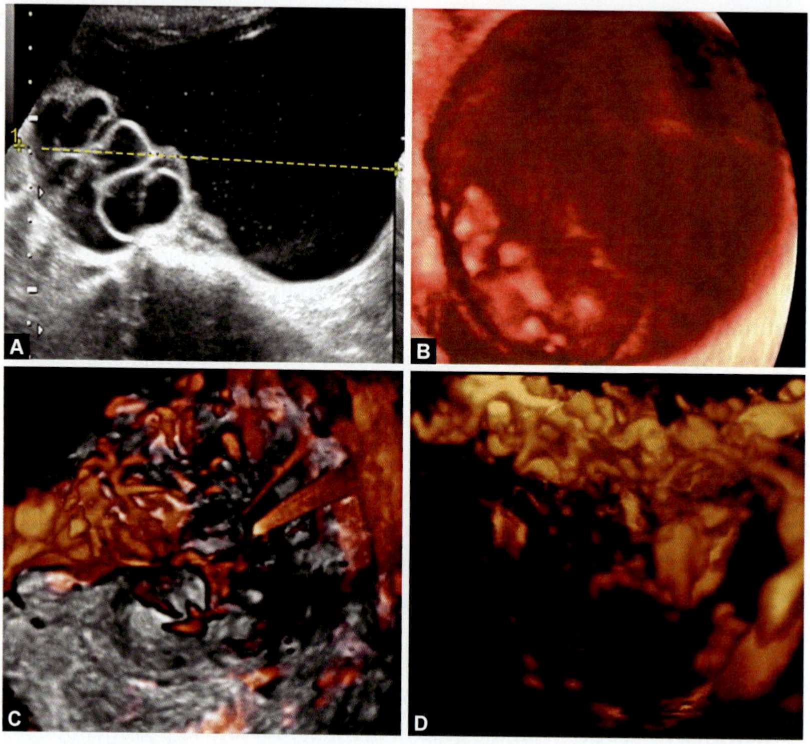

Figs. 11A to D: Multilocular mass on B-mode, on three-dimensional ultrasound (3D US) and on 3D power Doppler (PD), and Angio mode showing chaotic malignant vascular pattern.

- Loss of tree-like branching pattern of vessels
- Sacculation of arteries and veins
- Focal narrowing of arteries
- Internal shift in velocity within arterial lumen
- "Beach ball" finding of increased and disorganized blood flow
- Increased flow to center of a solid region
- Crowding of vascularity
- Abruptly stopping vessels

The advantage of being able to visualize the vascular pattern better has improved the predictability of ovarian cancer significantly as seen in several studies.[18] 3D PD allows accurate detection of the earliest appearance of ovarian malignancy at FIGO stage 1 **(Table 1)**.

But 3D PD cannot differentiate between advanced stage tumors and metastatic tumors.[18] Contrast enhancement on US further enables the visualization of very small vessels that were not otherwise seen. This improves the definition of small vessels in the tumor and their architecture. Accuracy of differentiation between benign and malignant lesions by contrast induced 3D PD are shown in **Table 2**.[19]

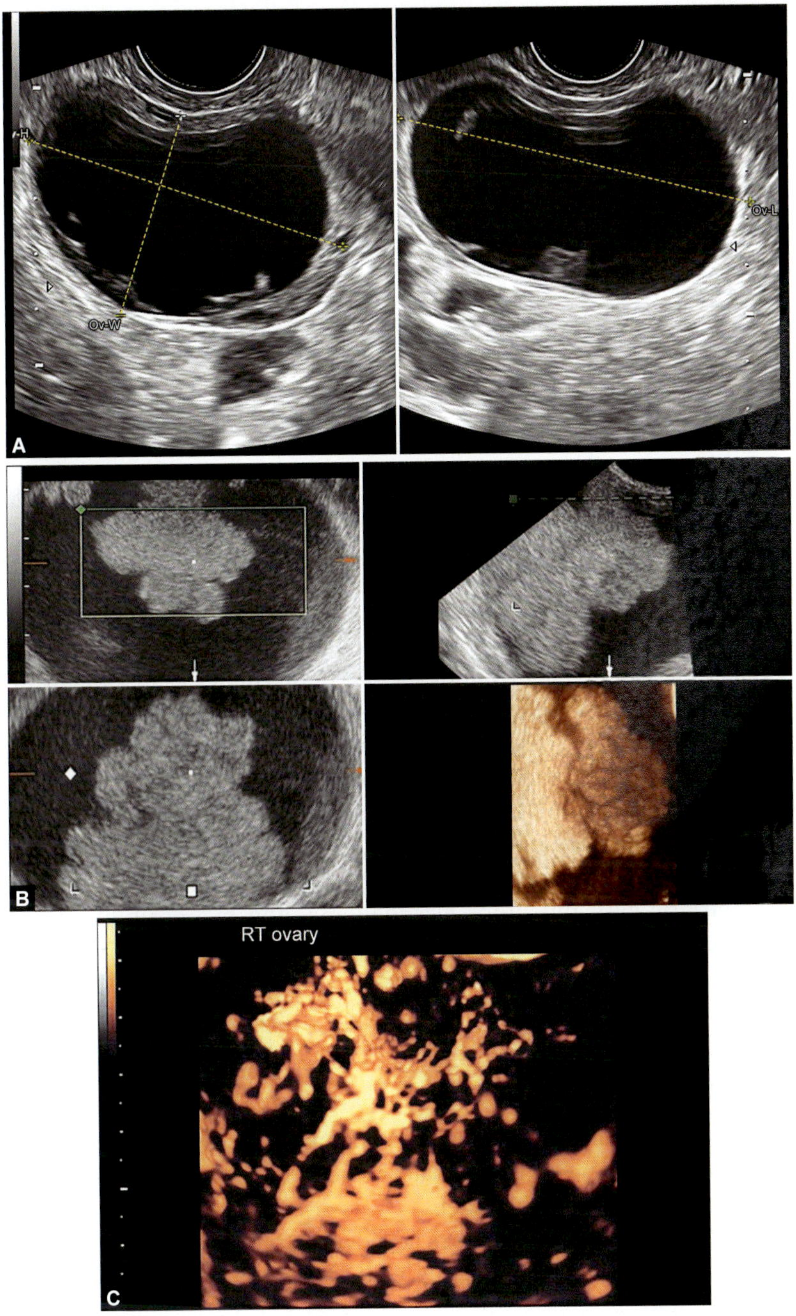

Figs. 12A to C: (A) B-mode image of an intraovarian cystic lesion with irregular internal echogenicities; (B) Three-dimensional ultrasound acquired volume of cauliflower-like solid projection from the wall seen in three orthogonal planes and rendered image; (C) Three-dimensional power Doppler showing typical malignant vascular pattern (RT: right).

Table 1: Accuracy for stage I ovarian cancer.[16]

2D US abdominal	69.8%
TVCD	86%
3D US	74.4%
3D PD	95.3%
3D PD + 3D US	97.7%

(2D: two-dimensional; 3D: three-dimensional; PD: power Doppler; TVCD: transvaginal color Doppler; US: ultrasound)

Table 2: Accuracy of differentiation between benign and malignant lesions.

Sensitivity	100%
Specificity	93.9%
PPV	85.7%
NPV	100%

Further risk factors such as postmenopausal age and family history of breast or ovarian cancer are also added to it, along with assessment of chemical markers for malignancy like CA 125. Though it is thought that ovarian malignancies are common in postmenopausal age there are a few very interesting and noteworthy facts about postmenopausal ovaries. Simple asymptomatic ovarian cyst may be found in 5–17% of menopausal population. Most likely these are inclusion cysts or neoplastic cysts and may resolve spontaneously. Amongst those which do not resolve, the most common found pathologies are serous cystadenoma, paratubal or paraovarian cysts, endometriotic cyst, mucinous cystadenoma, and hydrosalpinx. Risk of malignancy in unilocular ovarian cystic tumors <10 cm size, in women ≥50 years is very low.[20]

TUBAL LESIONS

Pelvic Inflammatory Disease

The most common of tubal lesions are inflammatory in origin. These lesions are usually a part of pelvic inflammatory disease (PID) and may also involve uterus and ovaries to variable extent.

Inflammation of fallopian tubes is known as salpingitis. Like inflammation anywhere in the body salpingitis leads to edema and hyperemia. On US, acute salpingitis is seen as thickened adnexal soft-tissue band, extending from the transverse section of the uterus to ovary >10 mm in transverse diameter. If there is fluid around the tube (free fluid), thickened tube walls may be appreciated with central hyperechoic mucosa. Normally, blood vessels seen in adnexa on color Doppler are parallel to the long axis of adnexa. But in acute salpingitis several small vessels are seen and these run across the width of this adnexal band width. On pulse Doppler, these vessels show low resistance (RI < 0.45). Acute salpingitis is almost always associated with acute oophoritis. This leads to hypoechogenicity of the ovarian stroma that is not easily identified and ovarian parenchymal blood flow also shows low to moderate RI: 0.53 + 0.09. But in chronic stage, adnexal as well as ovarian stromal vessels RI increases to 0.71 + 0.09.[21] Regression of the infection on its own or in response to antibiotics, decreases the flow in tubes and ovaries.

As this inflammation progresses towards fimbriae, it leads to adhesions of fimbriae and fluid collection in the tube, commonly described as hydrosalpinx. Patient presents with dull ache and feels ill.

On US, hydrosalpinx is seen as an extraovarian adnexal cystic lesion. On rotating the probe 90°, it changes its shape and becomes elongated **(Figs. 13A and B)**. It may typically show a retort, sausage or serpiginous shape. It can be differentiated from bowel by lack of peristalsis and from blood vessel by Doppler as it shows no flow.

It may show incomplete septae which are due to tubal haustra **(Fig. 13B, arrow)**. On transverse section, this tube gives a cog-wheel appearance, due to fibrotic remnants of endosalpingeal tissue, or beads on string appearance on long axis.[22] The fluid may show low level echoes, if the collection becomes thicker due to blood or pus. Three-dimensional US with inversion mode rendering is a very good tool to demonstrate such lesions as a whole **(Figs. 14A and B)**. Tube wall that is >5 mm thick in acute inflammation becomes thinner in chronic stage and the vascularity also decreases.

Extension of the inflammatory process further also may involve the ovary and also sometimes bowel or omentum in vicinity and forms tubo-ovarian abscess **(Fig. 15)**. It is seen as a complex lesion (with cystic and solid

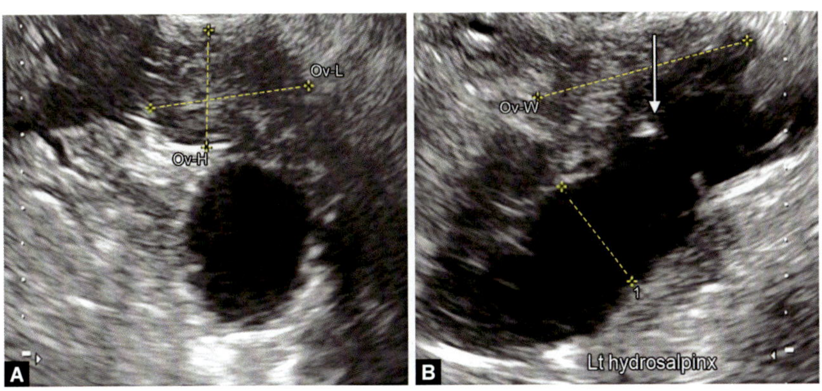

Figs. 13A and B: Hydrosalpinx—cystic roundish lesion in adnexa changes in shape on rotating the probe (Lt: left).

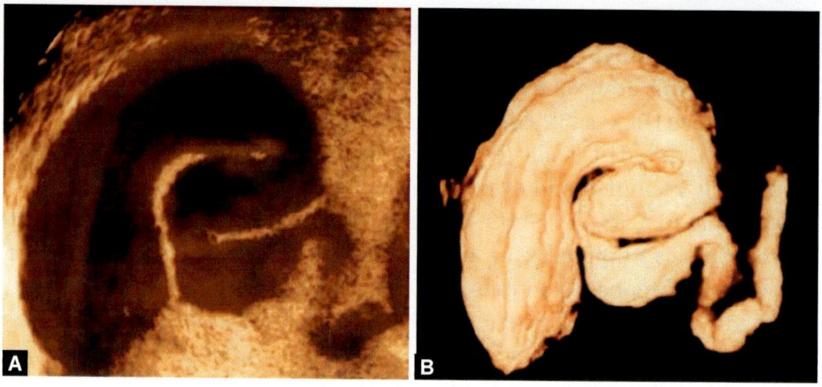

Figs. 14A and B: Hydrosalpinx—three-dimensional ultrasound (3D US); surface-rendering and inversion mode.

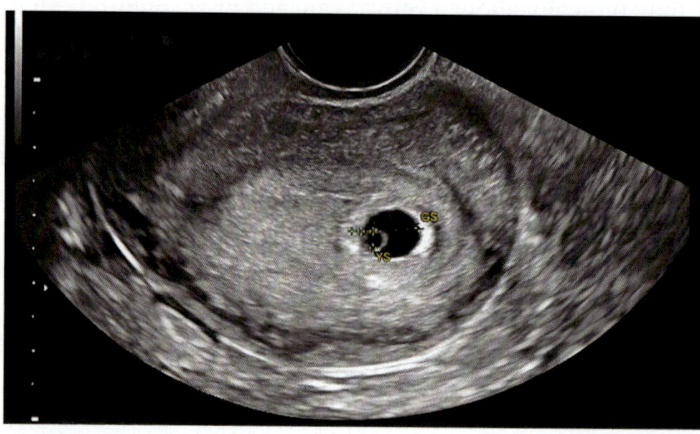

Fig. 15: Pelvic inflammatory disease (PID)—adherent ovary and distended tube, tubo-ovarian abscess where tube and ovary cannot be separately identified.

components) on US with low resistance (RI: 0.44 + 0.04)[23] vascularity in its solid areas and wall. Free fluid may be seen in pelvis.

Timor Tritsch et al. defined the sonographic markers for the tubal inflammation **(Table 3)**.[24]

On B-mode and Doppler because of the complex lesion with increased vascularity, it looks very similar to malignancy. It can be differentiated from malignancy as patient shows signs and symptoms of acute inflammation. Abscess when heals still leaves a cyst behind or it causes fibrous scarring—tubo-ovarian adhesions and then shows high resistance vascularity (RI: 0.75 + 0.04).

Clinical evaluation and correlation are very essential to differentiate inflammatory process from neoplastic process. Though US has a very high accuracy for diagnosis of adnexal malignancies as shown in **Table 4**.

Table 3: Sonographic markers for the tubal inflammation.

	Acute	*Chronic*
Thickened tube wall ≥5 mm	100%	3%
Cogwheel sign	86%	3%
Incomplete septa (92%)		
Beads on string app (flattened/fibrotic endosalpingeal folds 2–3 mm hyperechoic nodules on cross-section of fluid-filled structure)	0%	57%
Tubo-ovarian complex	36%	2%
Tubo-ovarian abscess		
Fluid in cul-de-sac	50%	10%

Table 4: Detection of adnexal malignancy.[25]

	Sensitivity	*Specificity*	*PPV*	*NPV*
TVCD	89%	98%	86%	99%
3D + 3D PD	97%	99%	97%	99%
Contrast 3D PD	100%	99%	93%	100%

(3D: three-dimensional; NPV: negative predictive value; PD: power Doppler; PPV: positive predictive value; TVCD: transvaginal color Doppler)

Ectopic Pregnancies

These are the most dreaded, often missed adnexal lesions. By definition, an ectopic pregnancy is an implantation of gestational sac in a place other than the endometrial cavity. It can be in the fallopian tube (95%), abdominal cavity, ovary, broad ligament, uterine cornu, myometrium or cervix. Though we shall here discuss only tubal and ovarian ectopic pregnancies.

Salpingitis and PID significantly increases the risk of ectopic pregnancy. Patient presents with a period of amenorrhea, positive urine pregnancy test or positive β-human chorionic gonadotropin (β-hCG) for pregnancy, with vaginal spotting and irregular vaginal bleeding abdominal pain, vasomotor shock, and fainting attacks. On examination, she will have tenderness in fornices. Patient may be stable but may show hypotension and tachycardia, if this pregnancy invades through the tube wall.

Ultrasound is considered to be the gold standard for diagnosis of ectopic pregnancy. Since it is more common in the patients on treatment for infertility.

On Ultrasound

Uterus: It shows no gestational sac in endometrial cavity and symmetrical endometrial cavity on transvaginal scan even when β-hCG > 1,000 IU. Symmetry of the endometrial cavity in frontal plane is seen in 90% of

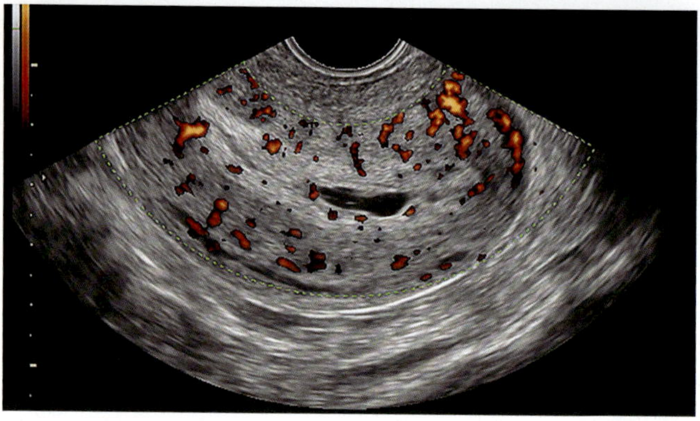

Fig. 16: True gestational sac abutting the endometrial cavity and asymmetrically placed and centrally placed pseudo sac.

extrauterine pregnancies (it is asymmetrical in 84% of normal pregnancies).[23] Uterus may or may not show increased endometrial thickness due to decidual like reaction. Pseudogestational sac may be seen. It can be differentiated from true gestational sac by its situation in the center of the uterine cavity, absence of the double decidual sign, change in shape with uterine contractions and absence of perisac vascularity **(Fig. 16)**.

Adnexa: In case of tubal pregnancy, US shows mass, separate from ovary. It may be homogeneous or heterogeneous, may or may not show gestational sac in early phase and shows a ring of vascularity with low resistance, high velocity blood flow. Ipsilateral corpus luteum is seen. Even before the gestational sac appears, tubal ectopic pregnancy can be diagnosed, if it is suspected, and clinical and biochemical factors are correlated. Adnexal mass must be differentiated from corpus luteum, hemorrhagic cyst or any other complex mass.

Volume US can especially be useful for early diagnosis of tubal pregnancy because it shows symmetry of the uterine cavity in ectopic pregnancy and distended fallopian tube, with thin hypoechoic border **(Figs. 17A and B)**.

Three-dimensional PD can also be used for follow-up of these pregnancies. Decreasing vascularity index (VI), flow index (FI), and vascularity flow index (VFI) values (3D PD indices), suggest that this pregnancy can be treated conservatively provided the patient is clinically stable, US does not show fetal pole with cardiac activity in the mass, the mass is <20 mm in diameter and β-hCG level is <2,000 IU.

Free fluid is seen in pelvis mostly only if bleeding has occurred because of invasion of tubal wall.

Ovarian ectopic pregnancy is rare, but should be differentiated from corpus luteum. Both the lesions show similar morphology and ring of

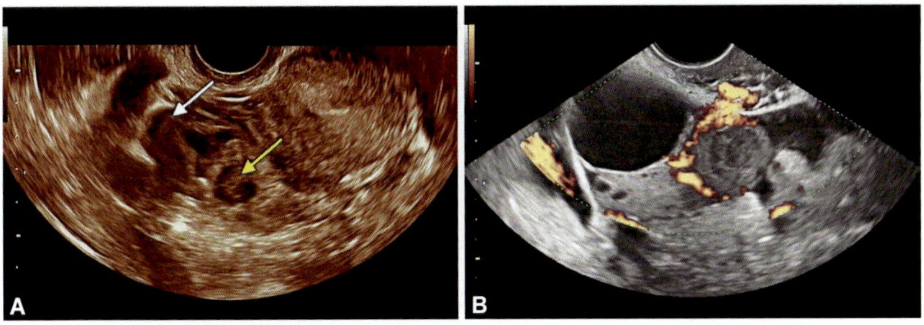

Figs. 17A and B: Tubal ectopic pregnancy in cross-section—tubal lumen (white arrow), gestational sac (yellow arrow), and ring of vascularity.

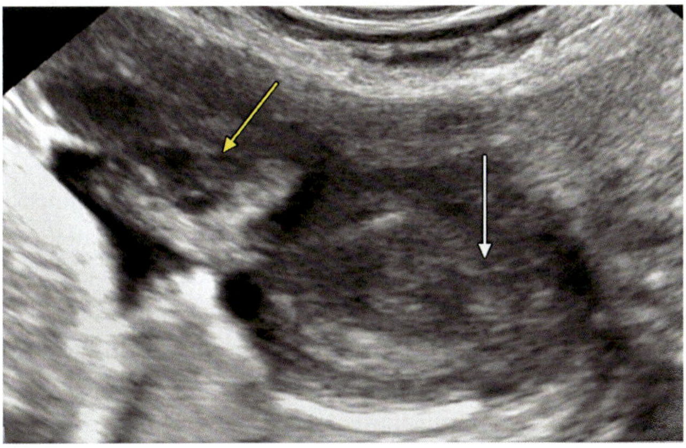

Fig. 18: Ectopic pregnancy, echogenic walls (yellow arrow), corpus luteum, and isoechoic walls (white arrow).

vascularity with low resistance flow. It is the echogenicity of its thick walls surrounding the anechoic center that gives a clue to the diagnosis. This wall is isoechoic in corpus luteum but is significantly hyperechoic (like that of decidual reaction in uterus) in an ovarian ectopic pregnancy **(Fig. 18)**.

MISCELLANEOUS LESIONS

- Broad ligament fibroid
- Peritoneal inclusion cyst
- Paraovarian cyst

Broad Ligament Fibroid

This is a fibroid arising from broad ligament. On US, it is a well-circumscribed, usually round, hypoechoic lesion. It can be separated from both uterus and ovary by probe pressure and shows peripheral vascularity.

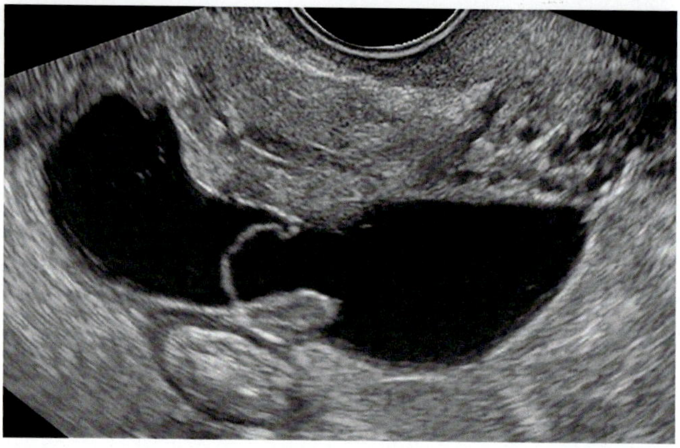

Fig. 19: Peritoneal inclusion cyst—irregular shape and lax septum.

Peritoneal Inclusion Cyst

This is a fluid collection in the pelvic peritoneum with septations. This fluid collection is not under pressure, and therefore is irregular in shape and changes shape on probe pressure. The septae inside, move with respiration, pressure or with pulsations of nearby vessel. These lesions typically do not show any vascularity **(Fig. 19)**. It may show peritoneal papillae and usually is seen close to the ovary. Since the fluid is loculated, floating bowel loops or fallopian tube is not seen in this fluid.

Paraovarian Cyst

Up to 20% of adnexal masses may be paraovarian cysts. These are extraovarian, freely mobile, benign, avascular lesions with thin walls and anechoic contents. The shape does not change with pressure but can be easily separated from ovary. Adhesions indicate infection and solid projections in it may raise a possibility of malignancy **(Fig. 20)**.

SUMMARY

Ultrasound is a very efficient tool for assessment of adnexal lesions. With advent of new US technologies, Doppler, 3D US, 3D PD, and contrast-enhanced US, this efficacy has further increased.

Pelvic US is especially important to decide the site of origin of the lesion, differentiation of pathological and physiological lesions, and for differentiation of benign from malignant masses which will help decide the line of treatment. US is also useful for management of some of these lesions, e.g., for cyst aspirations or biopsies under US guidance.

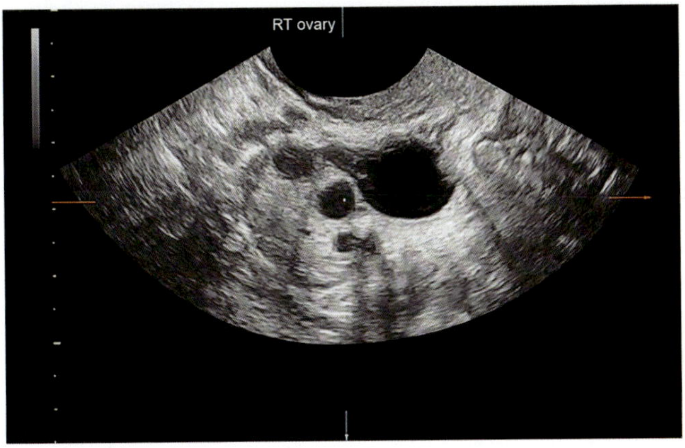

Fig. 20: Cystic lesion seen outside the ovary, with absent rim or beak sign—paraovarian cyst.

TIPS TO REACH TO CORRECT DIAGNOSIS

- Every lesion must be assessed in two orthogonal planes.
- Dynamic assessment to check for mobility of lesion or its contents is essential.
- Doppler is important to differentiate between pathologies.
- The lesions must be correlated with physiology.
- Lesions that are not proved to be malignant on the first assessment must be re-evaluated after 2–3 weeks for confirmation of diagnosis.
- Any lesion that does not appear in 4–6 weeks or is associated with other signs such as adhesions and free fluid, demands further investigation.
- In all cases of confusion, IOTA guidelines should be used and expert opinion should be sought.

REFERENCES

1. Kinkel K, Hricak H, Lu Y, Tsuda K, Filly RA. US characterization of ovarian masses: a meta-analysis. Radiology. 2000;217:803-11.
2. Timmerman D, Valentin L, Bourne TH, Collins WP, Verrelsts H, Vergote I. Terms, definitions and measurements to describe the sonographic features of adnexal tumors: a consensus opinion from the International Ovarian Tumor Analysis (IOTA) group. Ultrasound Obstet Gynecol. 2000;16:500-5.
3. Osmers R. Sonographic evaluation of ovarian masses and its therapeutic implications. Ultrasound Obstet Gynecol. 1996;8:217-22.
4. Alcazar JL, Leon M, Galvan R, Guerriero S. Assessment of cyst content using mean gray value for discriminating endometrioma from other unilocular cysts in premenopausal women. Ultrasound Obstet Gynecol. 2010;35:228-32.
5. Alcazar JL. Transvaginal colour Doppler in patients with ovarian endometriomas and pelvic pain. Hum Reprod. 2001;16(12):2672-5.
6. Kurjak A, Kupesic S. Scoring system for prediction of ovarian endometriosis based on transvaginal colour and pulsed Doppler sonography. Fertil Steril. 1994;62(1):81-8.

7. Raine-Fenning N, Jayaprakasan K, Deb S. Three-dimensional ultrasonographic characteristics of endometriomata. Ultrasound Obstet Gynecol. 2008;31:718-24.
8. Patel MD, Feldstein VA, Lipson SD, Chen DC, Filly RA. Cystic teratomas of the ovary: diagnostic value of sonography. Am J Roentgenol. 1998;171:1061-5.
9. Vijayaraghavan SB. Sonographic whirlpool sign in ovarian torsion. J Ultrasound Med. 2004;23(2):1643-9.
10. Mala S. Follicular ring sign: a simple sonographic sign for early diagnosis of ovarian torsion. J Ultrasound Med. 2012;31(11):1803-9.
11. Kurjak A, Kupesic S, Babic MM, Goldenberg M, Ilijas M, Kosuta D. Preoperative evaluation of cystic teratoma: What does colour Doppler add? J Clin Ultrasound. 1997;25:309-16.
12. Lerner JP, Timor-Tritsch IE, Federman A, Abramovich G. Transvaginal ultrasonographic characterization of ovarian masses with an improved, weighted scoring system. Am J Obstet Gynecol. 1994;51:81-5.
13. Kurjak A, Zalud I, Jurkovic D, Alfirevic Z, Miljan M. Trnsvaginal colour Doppler for the assessment of pelvic circulation. Acta Obstet Gynecol Scand. 1989;68:131-7.
14. Bonilla-Musoles F, Raga F, Osborne NG. Three-dimensional ultrasound evaluation of ovarian masses. Gynecol Oncol. 1995;59:129-35.
15. Kurjak A, Kupesic S, Sparac V, Prka M, Bekavac I. The detection of stage 1 ovarian cancer by three-dimensional sonography and power Doppler. Gynecol Oncol. 2003;90:258-64.
16. Crade M. Tissue block ultrasound and ovarian cancer: a pictorial presentation of findings. Donald School J Ultrasound Obstet Gynecol. 2009;3(1):41-7.
17. Alcazar JL. Tumor angiogenesis assessed by three-dimensional power Doppler ultrasound in early, advanced and metastatic ovarian cancer: a preliminary study. Ultrasound Obstet Gynecol. 2006;28(3):325-9.
18. Kupesic S, Kurjak A. Contrast enhanced three-dimensional power Doppler sonography for the differentiation of adnexal masses. Obstet Gynecol. 2000;96(3):452-8.
19. Bailey CL, Ueland FR, Land GL, DePriest PD, Gallion HH, Kryscio RJ, et al. Malignant potential of small cystic ovarian tumors in postmenopausal women. Gynecol Oncol. 1998;69:3-7.
20. Kupesic S, Kurjak A, Pasalic L, Benic S, Ilijas M. The value of transvaginal color Doppler in the assessment of pelvic inflammatory disease. Ultrasound Med Biol. 1995;21(6):733-8.
21. Timor-Tritsch IE, Rottem S, Lewitt N. The fallopian tube. In: Timor Tritsch IE, Rottem S (Eds). Transvaginal Sonography, 2nd edition. New York: Chapman and Hall; 1991. pp. 131-44.
22. Zalel Y, Soriano D, Lipitz S, Mashiach S, Achiron R. Contribution of color Doppler flow to the ultrasonographic diagnosis of tubal abnormalities. J Ultrasound Med. 2000;19(9):645-9.
23. Timor Tritsch IE, Lerner JP, Monteagudo A, Murphy KE, Heller DS. Transvaginal sonographic markers of tubal inflammatory disease. Ultrasound Obstet Gynecol. 1998;12:56-66.
24. Kurjak A, Kupesic S, Sparac V, Bekavac I. Preoperative evaluation of pelvic tumors by Doppler and three-dimensional sonography. J Ultrasound Med. 2001;20(8):829-40.
25. Rempen A. The shape of endometrium evaluated with three-dimensional ultrasound: an additional predictor of extrauterine pregnancy. Hum Reprod. 1998;13(2):450-4.

CHAPTER 16

Cycle Assessment for Infertility Treatment by Ultrasound

Sonal Panchal

INTRODUCTION

Fertility is a complex equation of continuous hormonal changes. Therefore, treatment of infertility needs a thorough assessment of the hormonal changes occurring during menstrual cycle in a female and therefore evaluation of the complete cycle instead of only pretrigger scan is essential. This consists of three scans: (1) baseline scan, (2) preovulatory scan, and (3) secretory scan.

Route of scan has to be transvaginal always. Using transabdominal approach for ovarian assessment may miss at least 42% of the ovarian anatomical details.[1] All scans are done using not only B-mode or two-dimensional (2D) ultrasound (US) but also color Doppler, pulse Doppler, three-dimensional (3D) US, and 3D power Doppler. Using color Doppler in this assessment is mandatory because a large number of biochemical or hormonal changes occur during the cycle, and these reflect as vascular and morphological changes in ovaries and uterus and these vascular changes can be assessed by Doppler. 3D US is especially useful for volume measurements. 3D power Doppler has also been proved to be highly promising in several studies, as it gives idea about the global vascularity of the structure examined.

BASELINE SCAN

This scan is done on second or third day of the cycle. It is known as a baseline scan because at this time of the cycle, the ovaries have no active follicles and estrogen and progesterone are both at lowest levels, endometrium is thin like a single line as it has shed off during menstruation and this is a baseline status of the ovaries **(Fig. 1)**.

This scan consists of transvaginal sonography (TVS), transvaginal color Doppler (TVCD) and volume US of ovaries and uterus. It is done to classify the ovaries in one of the four categories: Polycystic ovaries (PCO), normal ovaries, low reserve ovaries, and poorly responding ovaries. Or in other words to predict the ovarian reserve and response which can guide to decide the stimulation protocols for assisted reproductive technology (ART). Ovarian reserve assesses the number of follicles likely to develop or mature by ovarian stimulation and assessing response is to calculate the dosage of

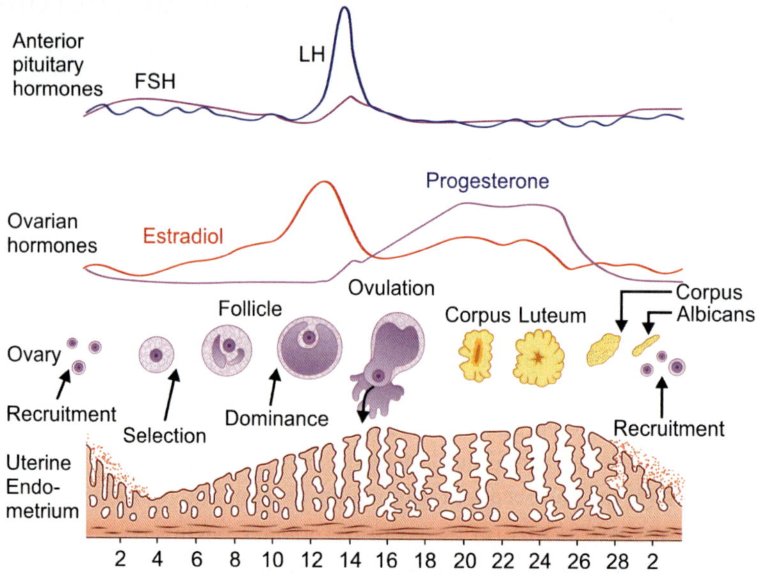

Fig. 1: Diagrammatic representation of hormonal and morphological changes during menstrual cycle (FSH: follicle-stimulating hormone; LH: luteinizing hormone).

drugs required for these follicles to grow. Uterus is assessed for the procedure: intrauterine insemination (IUI) or embryo transfer (ET), and for receptivity.

BASELINE SCAN OF OVARIES

Two-dimensional US assessment of the ovaries consists of assessment of ovarian diameters and volume and counting of antral follicles as quantitative assessment and qualitative assessment of stromal density. Color or power Doppler is used to see the presence of vessels in the stroma and pulse Doppler is used for quantitative assessment of the flows—intraovarian stromal resistance index (RI) and peak systolic velocity (PSV). Then 3D and 3D power Doppler volume of the ovary is acquired for ovarian volume and stromal volume calculation and counting number of antral follicles. Global vascular indices, vascularity index (VI), flow index (FI), and vascularity flow index (VFI) may be calculated by volume histogram. VI indicates abundance of flow in the calculated volume, FI indicates average intensity of flow, and VFI indicates perfusion of this volume.

Normal ovaries have (ovaries with normal reserve and response):

- Diameter (longest): 2–3.5 cm
- Volume: 3–6.6 cc
- Stromal RI: 0.6–0.7
- Stromal PSV: 5–10 cm/sec
- Follicle number per ovary (FNPO): 19

ULTRASOUND AND DOPPLER FEATURES FOR POLYCYSTIC OVARIES

Enlarged ovaries, multiple antral follicles, stromal abundance, and atypical endometrium are features of PCO as described in literature. But each feature needs to be evaluated independently. According to Rotterdam criteria [European Society of Human Reproduction and Embryology/American Society for Reproductive Medicine (ESHRE/ASRM) 2003 consensus and updated 2018 ESHRE recommendations] polycystic ovarian syndrome (PCOS) is defined as.[2]

Two of the following three criteria and exclusion of other endocrinological etiologies:

1. Oligo and/or anovulation
2. Hyperandrogenism: Clinical or biochemical
3. PCO on US

According to this definition PCO on US are ovaries that are >10 cc in volume and/or has >20 antral follicles.

Enlarged Ovaries

On 2D US an ovary which has a longest diameter of >3.5 cm is considered enlarged. When scanning the ovary, the probe is rotated and spanned at various angles to find out the most longitudinal section of the ovary. To calculate the volume of the ovary on 2D US a second section is taken by rotating the probe 90° from this most longitudinal section. Longest diameter is taken on the longest section. Anteroposterior (AP) diameter is measured as the longest diameter perpendicular to the longest diameter. Transverse diameter is measured as longest side to side measurement **(Fig. 2)**. Volume is calculated by applying the formula $(x \times y \times z) \times 0.523$. Calculation of ovarian volume by virtual organ computer-aided analysis (VOCAL) (volume calculation by computer) on 3D US is much more accurate **(Fig. 3)**. For VOCAL usually rotating angle of 30° is used, but in case of an ovary is not perfectly oval, angle of 15° may be preferred.

"For an ovarian size of 10 cc a good correlation has been found between US diagnosis of polycystic morphology and histopathological criteria for PCO".[3]

The interpretation here would be, according to the above quoted reference, that if a patient has an ovarian volume of 10 cc or more, she has to have clinical features of PCOS also. But reports have also shown that an ovarian size of 6.6 cc has 91% sensitivity and 91% specificity for PCOS.[4] And yet another report says "however, ovaries which are normal in volume can be polycystic as demonstrated by histological and biochemical studies (in 20%)".[4]

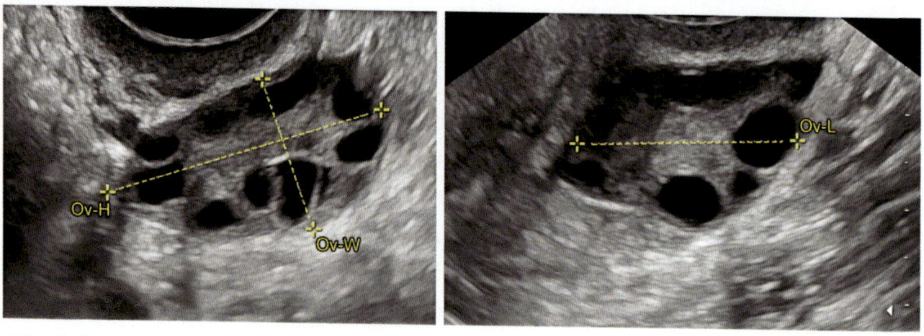

Fig. 2: B-mode image of longitudinal and transverse sections of ovary. Length, height, and width of the ovary are measured to assess the volume.

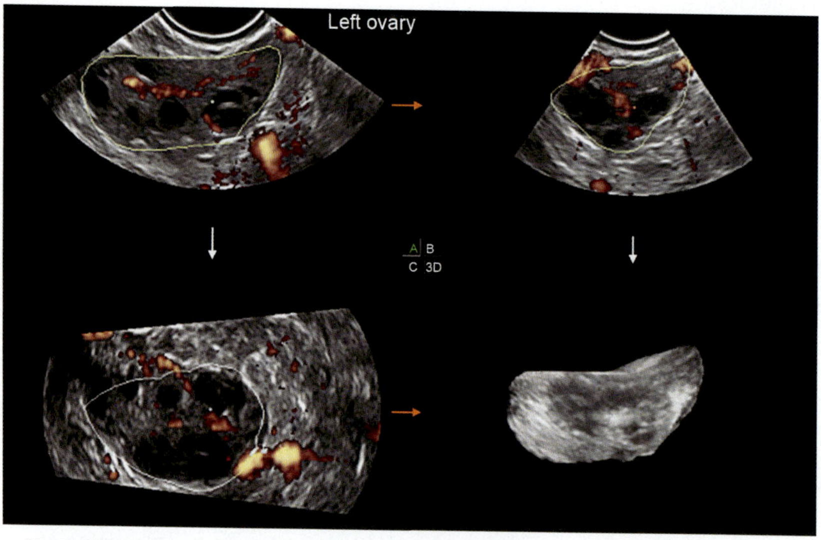

Fig. 3: Three-dimensional ultrasound with volume calculation of ovary by virtual organ computer-aided analysis.

This means ovarian volume alone cannot be used as the criteria for diagnosis of PCO.

Polycystic ovarian morphology has been found to be a better discriminator than ovarian volume between PCOS and control women.[5]

These morphological features are:

- Number of antral follicles
- Arrangement of antral follicles
- Stromal predominance.

Multiple Antral Follicles (2–9 mm)

Counting antral follicles especially in PCO patients is difficult on 2D US. There is a high chance of over or undercounting because of multiple follicles and therefore it has low interobserver and even intraobserver reliability. If 3D volume of the ovary is acquired and then is rendered in inversion mode **(Fig. 4)** or Sono AVC (automatic volume calculation) **(Fig. 5)** is used the antral follicle count (AFC) can be reliably calculated. Sono AVC color codes each follicle and on report sheet presents diameter and volume of each follicle **(Fig. 6)**. Using Sono AVC for counting antral follicles requires postprocessing (PP).

It takes longer to perform, because of the need for post processing (PP), and obtains values that are lower than those obtained by the 2D and 3D-multiplanar view (MPV) techniques. However, the AFC obtained by Sono AVC-PP is likely to be lower because this method measures and color

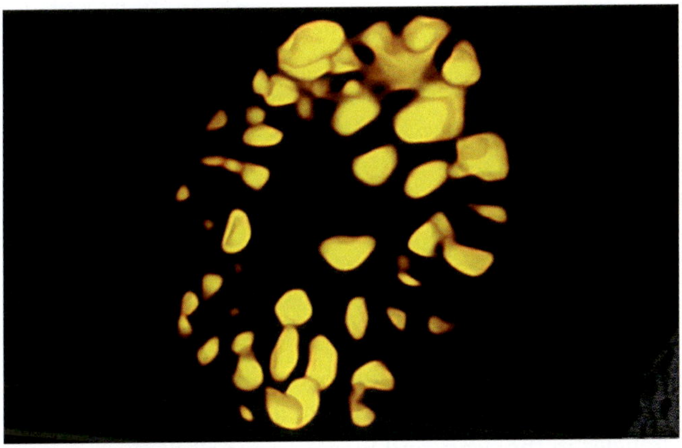

Fig. 4: Three-dimensional volume of polycystic ovary rendered in inversion mode.

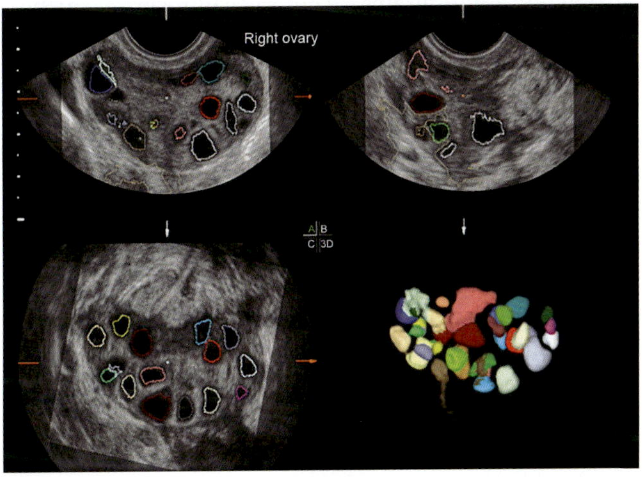

Fig. 5: Three-dimensional volume of polycystic ovary with sonoautomatic volume calculation.

DR NAGORI INSTITUTE — Date of Exam: 19.07.2014 — Page 2/4 — Exam Type:

Name: Hetal — Pat. ID: D15359-14-07-19-6

Ovary: Left — Total#: 21

Nr.	d(V) mm	dx mm	dy mm	dz mm	mn. d mm	V cm³
5	14.2	18.9	15.4	11.2	15.2	1.50
6	14.0	19.5	16.5	9.2	15.0	1.45
7	13.9	18.1	14.8	10.9	14.6	1.42
8	13.0	21.0	11.7	10.4	14.4	1.16
9	12.1	14.1	12.3	11.3	12.6	0.92
10	11.1	19.2	10.0	8.1	12.4	0.72
11	10.9	15.4	10.8	8.9	11.7	0.68
12	10.6	16.8	11.3	7.5	11.9	0.62
13	9.9	14.2	9.3	7.9	10.4	0.51
14	9.6	11.2	9.3	8.7	9.7	0.46
15	9.5	12.0	10.0	7.9	10.0	0.45
16	8.9	12.1	8.6	7.3	9.3	0.37
17	5.8	8.1	5.4	4.6	6.0	0.10
18	4.9	7.9	5.8	4.2	6.0	0.06
19	4.1	6.8	4.8	3.4	5.0	0.04
20	3.6	5.5	3.8	2.3	3.8	0.02
21	2.9	4.6	3.0	1.9	3.2	0.01

Ovary: Right — Total#: 27

Nr.	d(V) mm	dx mm	dy mm	dz mm	mn. d mm	V cm³
5	14.3	24.2	13.7	11.8	16.6	1.54
6	13.9	19.5	13.9	11.2	14.9	1.40
7	12.8	19.1	12.1	10.0	13.7	1.10
8	11.5	15.7	11.1	10.0	12.3	0.79
9	11.4	16.5	13.8	7.8	12.7	0.78
10	9.1	11.1	10.1	7.2	9.5	0.40
11	8.9	11.0	9.0	7.5	9.2	0.37
12	8.7	11.6	9.4	7.2	9.4	0.35
13	8.7	13.0	10.0	5.7	9.6	0.34
14	8.4	11.7	9.9	5.9	9.2	0.31
15	7.6	8.9	8.1	6.1	7.7	0.23
16	7.5	16.8	7.0	4.3	9.4	0.22
17	7.0	12.2	8.9	3.9	8.3	0.18
18	6.5	12.1	7.9	3.4	7.8	0.15
19	6.0	9.8	5.7	4.3	6.6	0.11
20	5.9	10.5	6.3	3.7	6.8	0.11
21	5.4	6.9	5.9	4.1	5.6	0.08

Fig. 6: Report sheet of sonoautomatic volume calculation.

codes each follicle preventing recounting. Intraobserver and interobserver reliability of automated AFCs made using 3D US and Sono AVC a preferred method.[6]

Setting the threshold at 12 for 2–9 mm FNPO offered the best compromise between specificity (99%) and sensitivity (75%).[7] The more recent studies have mentioned the follicular number per ovary of 19 and even 26.[8,9] And the new threshold for AFC for PCO is 20.[2] But females in adolescence also have multiple follicles in the ovary and these are not all PCOS patients. It is now strongly suggested that different cut-offs for AFC is required for different age groups and different ethnic groups.[10] These all controversies can be explained if we go through the evolution of PCOS.

Evolution of Polycystic Ovarian Syndrome

Polycystic ovarian syndrome is a genetic condition and insulin resistance leading to hyperinsulinemia is thought to be the root cause. This leads to androgen excess. Androgen leads to recruitment of multiple follicles in the ovaries. But under the effect of androgen these follicles cannot grow beyond 6–7 mm in size. The follicles then become follicle-stimulating hormone (FSH) sensitive. But still these small follicles do produce some estrogen. The excess androgen also is converted to estrogen. This leads to rise in estrogen levels in absence of mature follicle. This gives negative feedback to FSH, which dampens the rise in FSH levels and slows down the follicular growth. Follicles when grow to a size of 9–10 mm, then become FSH dependent. At this stage, the estrogen level further rises and gives a negative feedback to FSH and a positive feedback to luteinizing hormone (LH). In FSH lack, these follicles do

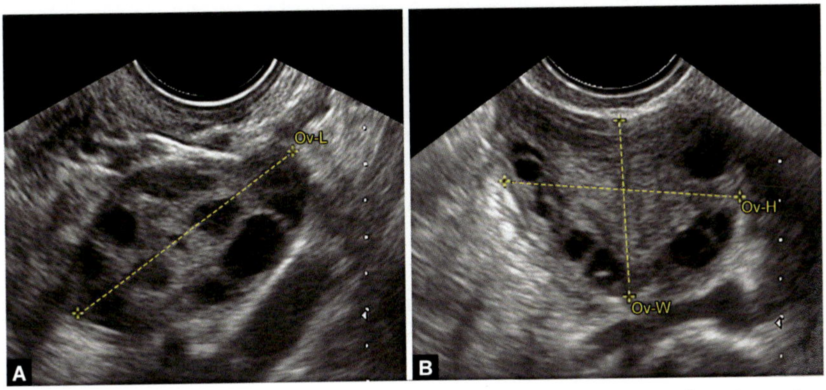

Figs. 7A and B: Generalized cystic pattern and peripheral cystic pattern in polycystic ovaries.

not grow further, instead they are exposed to LH which causes luteinization of these immature follicles and follicular atresia, with conversion of granulosa cells to theca cells and contribute to stroma.[11] This leads to stromal abundance as a result of anovulation. In the early phase of the disease the stroma becomes denser in parts and when anovulation continues, whole stroma becomes echogenic, leading to a generalized cystic pattern (GCP) of PCO. As the disease progresses, follicles are pushed to the periphery and then not only the stromal density but the stromal volume also increases, leading to enlargement of the ovary and then leading to peripheral cystic pattern (PCP) of PCO. This means that from multicystic cystic ovaries—ovaries normal in size having multiple follicles of various sizes and normal stroma—which is a normal appearance in adolescence to GCP PCO and PCP PCO is a process of evolution as a result of high basal androgen levels and chronic anovulation in these females **(Figs. 7A and B)**.[12] This explains not only the variability in the size of the ovaries but also the variability in the number of antral follicles in patients having oligoovulation and hyperandrogenism in patients with PCOS.

Predominant Hyperechoic Stroma

Stromal abundance therefore is the most consistent character and key factor for the diagnosis of PCOS.[13,14] This abundance can be known by increased stromal echogenicity. The PCO show a hyperechoic stroma but assessment of this hyperechogenicity is subjective not only to the operator but also to equipment settings.[15,16] Therefore, a more objective or reproducible criteria is required for assessment of stromal density and this is done by measuring ovarian area and stromal area on 2D US and ovarian volume and stromal volume on 3D US. Ovarian area of 5.3 cm^2 on strict longitudinal ovarian section and stromal area of 4.6 cm^2 has high sensitivity and specificity for PCOS.[17] But stromal area/ovarian area ratio has been found to be even more efficient for diagnosis of PCOS.

Sensitivity for Diagnosis of Polycystic Ovarian Syndrome[13]

▪ Ovarian volume	13.21 cc	21%
▪ Ovarian area	7 cm^2	4%
▪ Stromal area	1.95 cm^2	62%
▪ Stromal/total area	0.34	100%

Stromal volume can be calculated by acquiring a 3D volume of the ovary and calculating the volume by VOCAL, and then using threshold volume, adjusting the threshold to exclude the follicles from total ovarian volume. This helps to separately calculate the volume of the structures below threshold (follicular volume) and above threshold (stromal volume) **(Fig. 8)**.

Stromal volume to ovarian volume ratio of >75% in an ovary which has a volume of at least 6.6 cc or has >12 antral follicles was found to be diagnostic of PCOS in a study of 1,000 PCOS patients assessed at our center (unpublished data).

Apart from these major features, PCOS patients show atypical endometrium or out of phase endometrium due to the hormonal derangements like high LH and early rise of estrogen due to multiple follicle recruitment and conversion of androgen to estrogen. For these reasons, endometrium in early follicular phase appears multilayered in PCOS patients and becomes echogenic just before ovulation due to early LH surge and progesterone exposure.

There are certain Doppler characteristics of the PCO. These ovaries show low resistance stromal flow on the baseline scan. When color box is placed on the ovary the blood vessels in the stroma only are to be picked up for quantitative assessment **(Fig. 9A)**. Vessels close to the developing follicles

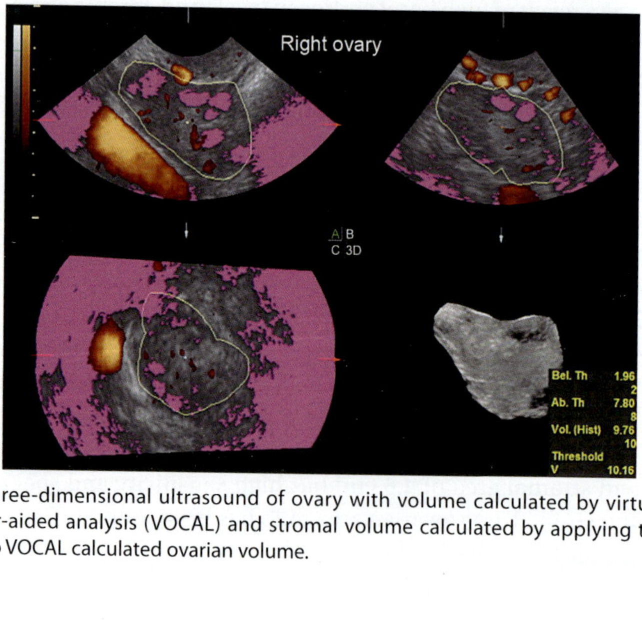

Fig. 8: Three-dimensional ultrasound of ovary with volume calculated by virtual organ computer-aided analysis (VOCAL) and stromal volume calculated by applying threshold volume to VOCAL calculated ovarian volume.

are not stromal vessels. On pulse Doppler these vessels show RI: 0.50–0.58.[18] This is because of high LH levels. If these blood vessels also show a PSV of >10 cm/sec, they are prone to hyperstimulation. High androgen levels in these patients also lead to high uterine artery pulsatility index (PI) **(Fig. 9B)**.

It is interesting to note here that higher uterine artery PI and lower ovarian stromal vessel resistance is seen in PCP ovaries than GCP ovaries, higher age, amenorrohic, rather than oligomenorrhic patients and in obese, hyperinsulinemic and hirsute patients.

Increased ovarian stromal blood flow in PCOS may be because of overexpression of vascular endothelial growth factor (VEGF), which modulates the permeability of theca cells and increase insulin-like growth factor 1 (IGF-1),[19,20] which in turn enhances gonadotropin-stimulated steroid production in granulosa cells and theca cells resulting in increased ovarian androgen production and subsequently increased anti-Müllerian hormone (AMH) production.[11]

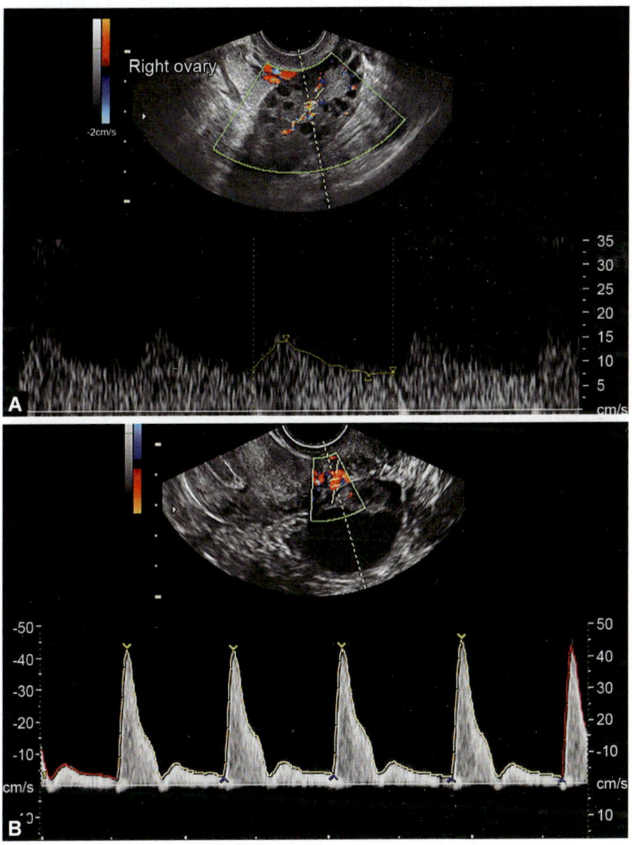

Figs. 9A and B: (A) Low resistance ovarian stromal flow; (B) High resistance uterine artery flow.

Follicle number perovary in the range of 6–9 mm is significantly and negatively related to body mass index and fasting serum insulin level.[21]

Ultrasound features of PCO:
- Longest diameter > 3.5 cm (old criteria)
- Ovarian volume at least >6.6 cc
- More than 20 antral follicles per ovary
- Hyperechoic and predominant stroma
- Intraovarian stromal flow present
- Intraovarian stromal RI 0.50–0.58
- Intraovarian stromal PSV 10 cm/sec or more
- High uterine artery PI
- Atypical endometrium
- *Stromal area:* Ovarian area ratio >0.34
- *Stromal volume:* Ovarian volume ratio >75%

Remember all features cannot be seen in all the patients.

Third type of ovaries is poorly responding ovaries. They may be of any size but have intraovarian stromal RI > 0.7, and PSV < 5 cm/sec. These ovaries have low vascularity and therefore respond only to higher doses of stimulation.

Fourth type is low reserve ovaries which are small sized ovaries with <2 cm in longest diameter or <3 cc in volume and have <3 antral follicles. They will produce very few follicles with any stimulation.

Actually any ovary has one feature from each of these two following groups:

1. Low reserve, normal reserve, and polycystic ovary.
2. Low response, normal response, and hyperresponse.

Based on this, predictors of ovarian response are:[22]

- Number of antral follicles
- Ovarian stromal FI
- Total ovarian stromal area
- Total ovarian volume

In that order of importance.

Antral follicle count is a better marker than basal FSH for selection of older patients with acceptable pregnancy offer.[23] AFC and ovarian volume showed significant correlation with AMH, total testosterone, and free androgen index.[24]

Precise calculation of AFC therefore can help in predicting the ovarian response. This can be done on 2D US by scanning across the whole ovary while counting the follicles by eyeballing. But this has high chances of error when follicles are multiple as in PCO. In these cases counting, the antral follicles by 3D US is much more precise as mentioned earlier. Antral follicle when counted by inversion mode: likely to get 60% of follicles of the counted antral follicles in vitro fertility (IVF) cycles.[25]

Sono AVC with PP is a reliable method to calculate total AFC.

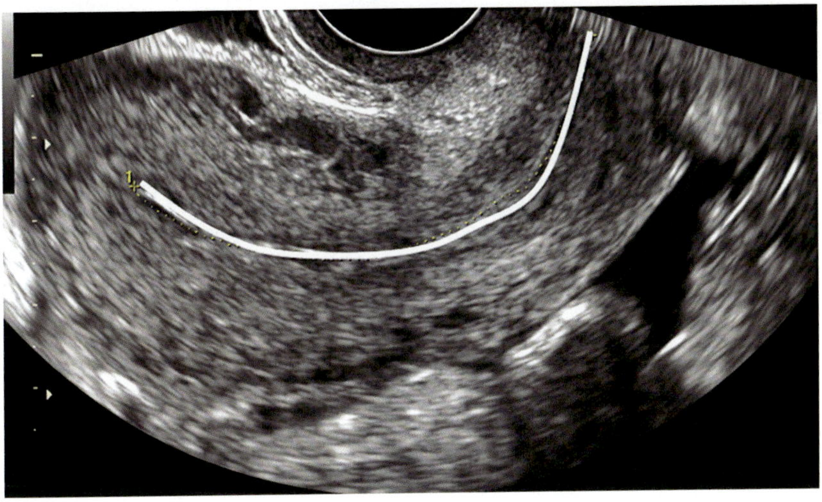

Fig. 10: Measuring functional uterocervical length.

Measurement of ovarian stromal flow in early follicular phase is related to subsequent ovarian response in IVF treatment.[26]

Blood flow is less in stromal vessels in aged patients and it is known that these patients require higher doses for stimulation.[27]

UTERUS

Baseline scan of the uterus is done to assess the uterocervical length by US. Longitudinal section of the uterus is imaged on the screen where whole of the uterus is seen with endometrial cavity starting from fundus to the internal os and external os. For all ART procedures may it be IUI or ET, the uterocervical length is measured from the fundal end of the endometrium to the external os and is known as functional or physiological uterocervical length **(Fig. 10)**. Doppler of the uterine artery is done. Uterine artery RI > 0.79 indicates that high doses of stimulation will be required for endometrial maturation.[28] Subendometrial flow on Day 2 if is present indicates a low receptive endometrium for implantation. This is so because on Day 2 ovaries are silent, estrogen levels are very low, and therefore no endometrial vascularity is expected normally. If it is present it is either high basal estrogen or inflammation of the endometrium leading to increased vascularity.

PREOVULATORY SCAN

It is known that not all antral follicles grow to become dominant and mature follicle. A follicle that grows to >10 mm is a dominant follicle, it grows at a rate of 2–3 mm/day and ovulation occurs at 18–24 mm in size usually. Follicular flow can be first detected when follicular size is 10 mm[29] and its resistance starts falling 2 days prior to ovulation.

FEATURES OF A MATURE FOLLICLE

A rounded 16–18 mm sized follicle with thin walls and no internal echogenicity is seen. A sonolucent halo appears surrounding the follicle 24 hours prior to ovulation. Cumulus oophorus a small projection from wall in the follicular lumen may be seen 24–36 hours before ovulation **(Fig. 11A)**. But since this is a very tiny structure, unless the image is optimized, it is difficult to see.

On color Doppler vascularity is seen surrounding three-fourths of the follicular circumference **(Fig. 11B)**. On pulse Doppler these vessels show RI 0.4–0.48,[30] PSV >10 cm/sec **(Fig. 11C)**. These flow indices are of perifollicular vessels and perifollicular vessels are the ones that obscure the follicular wall.

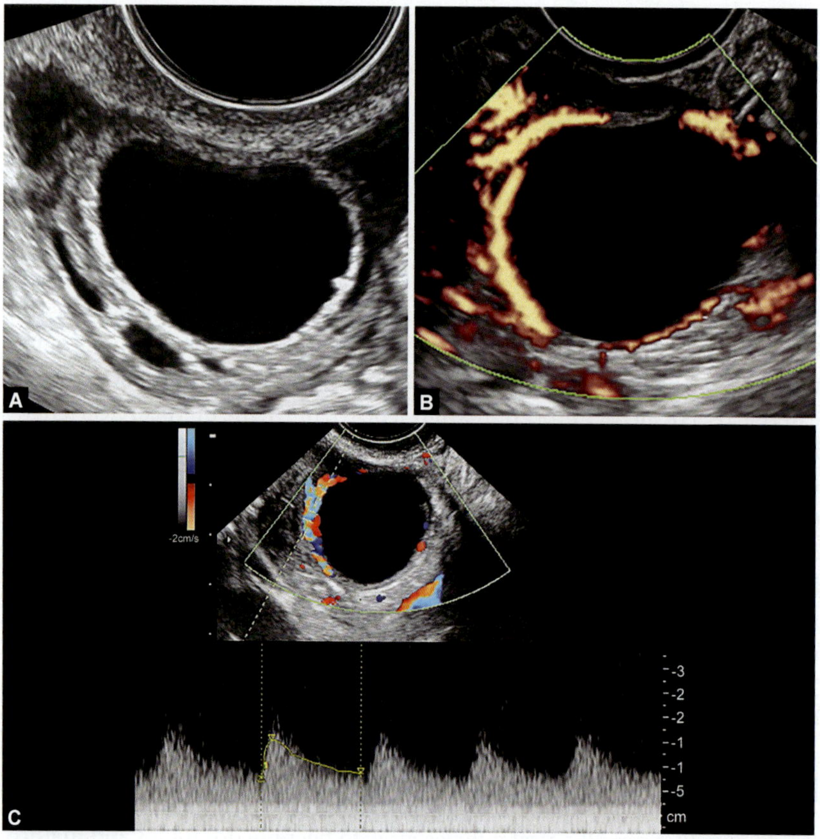

Figs. 11A to C: Mature follicle. (A) B-mode image of a round follicle with peripheral halo and cumulus-like projection; (B) Blood vessels surrounding the follicle; (C) Spectral representation of blood flow in this follicle.

If the follicular vascular indices are not in the defined range, it means that the follicle is not yet physiologically mature and therefore stimulation still needs to be continued. Size of the follicle till 24 mm is the size till which one can wait for the optimum flows to be achieved.

This means that if the follicle is said to be functionally mature when PSV is 10 cm/sec, i.e., the time when the LH surge starts and under the effect of that LH, the perifollicular PSV keeps on rising constantly.[29] Follicular blood flow velocity starts increasing approximately 26–29 hours before rupture and continues till 72 hours after rupture. The perifollicular PSV may rise as high as 35–45 cm/sec before an hour of ovulation. This means that in a follicle of >16–18 mm diameter, if the RI of the perifollicular vessels is <0.5 and the PSV is >10–15, LH surge has already started.

We have done a study of 350 IUI cycles based on these facts to find out appropriate time of IUI based on pre-perifollicular vascularity. Patients were divided into two groups randomly, in group A patients single IUI was done and in group B patients double IUI was done. Single IUI was done between 36 and 38 hours and double IUI were done one at 12–14 hours and other at 36–38 hours in all patients in whom perifollicular PSV > 15 cm/sec. When perifollicular PSV on the day of trigger was more than 20 cm/sec, and perifollicular RI was within normal range, double IUI gave significantly higher pregnancy rates.[30] This indicates that in patients with higher perifollicular pre-trigger PSV, IUI done at 12–14 hours has been fruitful **(Fig. 12)**. When this study was further extended, it derived that in patients with perifollicular PSV of 10–15 cm/sec, only one IUI is to be done at 36–38 hours, in patients with perifollicular PSV of 15–25 cm/sec, two IUIs should be done at 12–14 hours

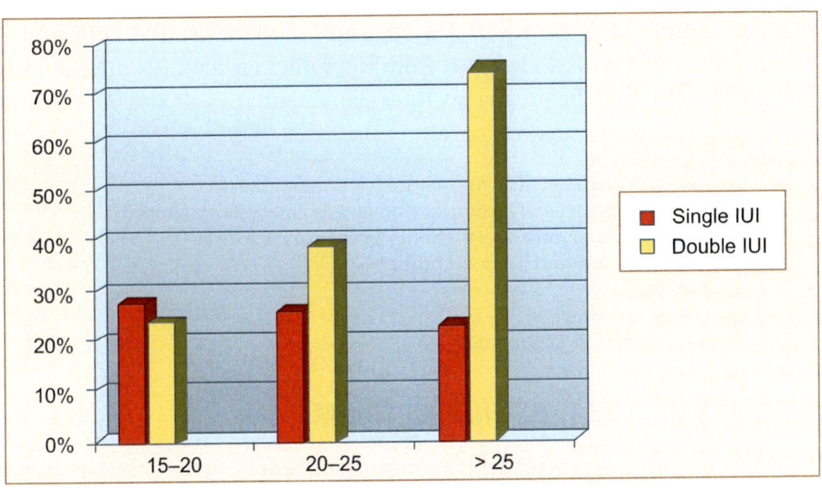

Fig. 12: Graphic representation showing increased pregnancy rates with double intrauterine insemination (IUI) in patients with perifollicular peak systolic velocity >20 cm/sec.

and at 36–38 hours after human chorionic gonadotropin (hCG) and if the perifollicular PSV is more than 25 cm/sec, only one IUI is to be done at 12–14 hours after trigger.

Fertilization of a follicle with a PSV of less than 10 cm/sec, has high chances of fertilizing into an embryo with chromosomal abnormality due to hypoxic ovum.[32]

Rising PSV with steady low RI suggests that the follicle is close to rupture. Steady or decreasing PSV with rising RI suggests that the follicle is proceeding toward luteinized unruptured follicle (LUF).

APPLICATION OF 3D US FOR FOLLICULAR ASSESSMENT

When there is multifollicular development as in PCO the follicular shapes become polygonal and therefore follicular diameter may not be a reliable parameter. Follicular volume by 3D is a more reliable parameter. Follicular volumes of between 3 and 7 cc are optimum for oocyte retrieval **(Fig. 13B)**. The limits of agreement between the volume of the follicular aspirate and 3D volume of the follicle were +0.96 to –0.43 with 3D and +3.47 to –2.42 by 2D volume estimation.[33]

Cumulus can be seen in more than almost 90% of follicles using 3D US rendering. This is possible only in up to 40–45% of mature follicles by 2D US. On the day of trigger, if cumulus like echo is not seen in all three planes in the follicle, it is less likely to be mature fertilizable oocyte **(Fig. 13A)**.[34]

Three-dimensional power Doppler gives idea about the global vascularity of the follicle **(Fig. 13C)**. The 3D power Doppler indices, VI, FI, and VFI give quantitative global assessment of vascularity **(Fig. 13D)**. We have done a large study taking this into consideration. Based on study of >1,000 cycles,[35,36] follicular volume of 3–7.5 cc, VI > 6–20, and FI > 35 if used as additional features for a mature follicle apart from the follicular features mentioned previously, increased the pregnancy rates significantly.

Features of mature follicle:
- Minimum follicular diameter of 16 mm for gonadotropin stimulation
- Minimum follicular diameter of 18 mm for clomiphene citrate (CC) stimulation
- Perifollicular flow around three-fourths circumference of the follicle
- Perifollicular RI 0.40–0.48 and PSV >10 cm/sec
- Cumulus oophorus
- Follicular volume 3–7.5 cc
- Follicular VI 6–20 and FI >27 (preferably >35).

FEATURES OF A MATURE ENDOMETRIUM

On 2D US an endometrium of 6 mm or more in thickness, preferably 8–10 mm, and multilayered is thought to be good enough. But its morphological assessment is essential. Because of orderly organization of glandular

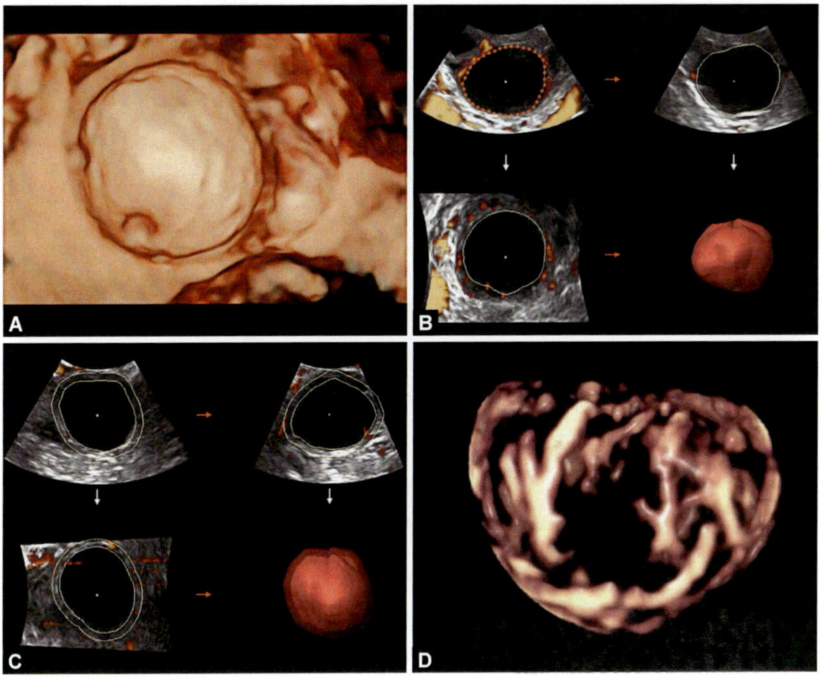

Figs. 13A to D: (A) Cumulus oophorus in follicle on three-dimensional ultrasound of follicle-rendered view; (B) 3D power Doppler volume of follicle with virtual organ computer-aided analysis (VOCAL) and shell volume calculation; (C) 3D power angiography of perifollicular flow; (D) Calculation of 3D power Doppler vascular indices (volume histogram) after VOCAL and shell volume for perifollicular flow.

elements in proliferative phase, endometrium is generally hypoechoic in this phase, though the morphology can be graded as follows.

ENDOMETRIAL GRADING (FIGS. 14A TO C)[37]

- *Grade A endometrium*: Multilayered with intervening area as echogenic as myometrium.
- *Grade B endometrium*: Multilayered with intervening area hypoechoic to myometrium or almost anechoic.
- *Grade C endometrium*: Homogeneous isoechoic endometrium.

It was earlier thought that grade A endometrium may be the best for implantation and grade may the worst. But this does not appear to prevail still. Actually the endometrium as it grows from single line, as estrogen level increases and it becomes multilayered, the intervening area is moderately hypoechoic and this is grade B endometrium. As the estrogen levels rise to more than that from one mature follicle, the intervening area starts becoming more echogenic and till it becomes as echogenic as the surrounding myometrium,

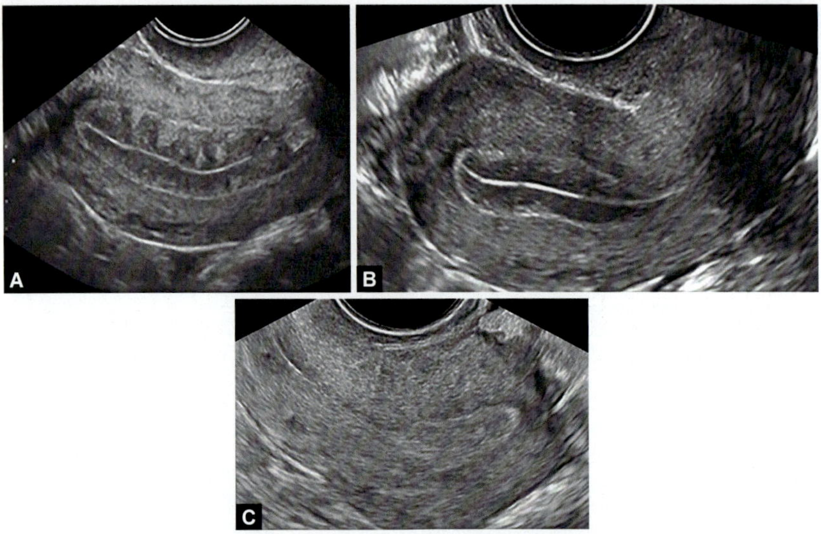

Figs. 14A to C: Grade A, B, and C endometrium.

but still maintains the multilayer look. This is grade A endometrium, seen with high estrogen levels, usually with three to six mature follicles. When the estrogen level rises beyond this, the endometrium loses its multilayered look and becomes isoechoic, and this endometrial morphology is often seen in PCO patients **(Figs. 14A to C)**.

Spiral arteries supply the endometrium and these are the vessels that undergo substantial changes during menstrual cycle. Estrogen causes vasodilatation and progesterone antagonizes the effect. Therefore, higher estradiol/progesterone (E2/P) ratio is responsible for higher blood flow through uterine vascular bed. Thus, endometrial color Doppler gives direct information about estrogen and progesterone levels and in turn also about functional maturity of the follicle and endometrium. Several studies have related better endometrial vascularity with better receptivity.[38]

On color Doppler, the vascularity of the endometrium is classified by Applebaum as follows **(Figs. 15A to D)**:[39]

- *Zone 1:* Blood vessels reaching endomyometrial junction surrounding the endometrium.
- *Zone 2*: Blood vessels reaching hyperechoic endometrial edge.
- *Zone 3:* Blood vessels reaching intervening endometrial hypoechoic zone.
- *Zone 4*: Blood vessels reaching endometrial cavity—the central line.

On pulse Doppler, these blood vessels should show RI 0.49–0.59 < 0.6. These blood vessels should cover 5 mm^2 area of a particular (3–4) zone of endometrium.[40]

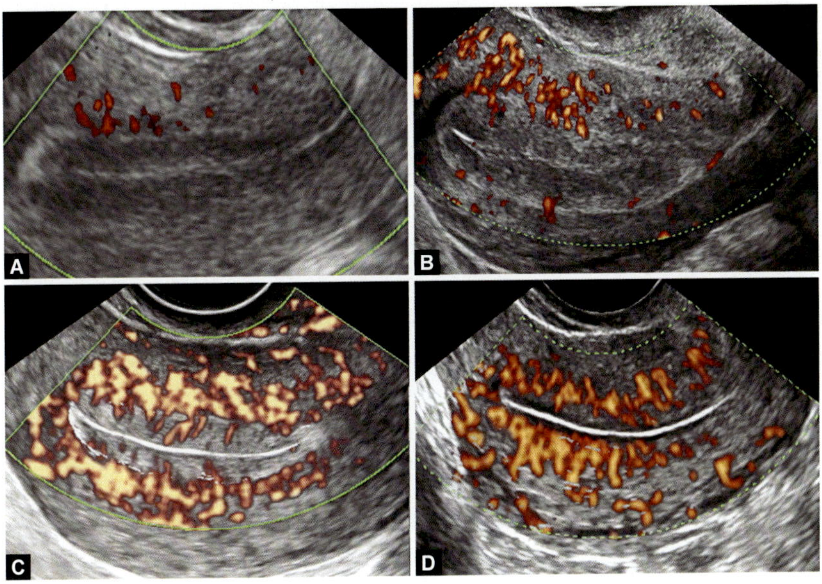

Figs. 15A to D: Zone 1, 2, 3, and 4 vascularity seen in endometrium on color and power Doppler.

Even if TVCD of follicle is normal, endometrial and the uterine artery indices should be within normal limits for implantation. Therefore, even with mature follicle if endometrial vascular parameters are not achieved, stimulation should be continued for 1 or 2 days. This will increase the estrogen produced from follicle and in turn improve the endometrial thickness and vascularity. Absent subendometrial and intraendometrial vascularization on the day of hCG appears to be a useful predictor of failure of implantation in IVF, irrespective of morphological appearance. Conception rates according to zones of vascularity in two different studies are quoted as:[41]

- Zone 1 3.5%–7.5% 5.2%
- Zone 2 15.8%–29.7% 28.7%
- Zone 3 24.2%–47.8% 52%
- Zone 4 67.3% 74%

It has also been observed that when pregnancy is achieved in absence of endometrial and subendometrial flow on the day of ET, more than half of these pregnancies will finish as spontaneous miscarriage.[41]

Though it has been observed that spiral arteries have higher PSV and lower resistance in natural cycles as compared to stimulated cycles, may it be CC or gonadotropins.

Apart from endometrium and follicle it is also essential to evaluate the uterine artery flow on the dominant side before trigger. Estrogen receptors are also present in uterine arteries and cause vasodilatation in these vessels also.

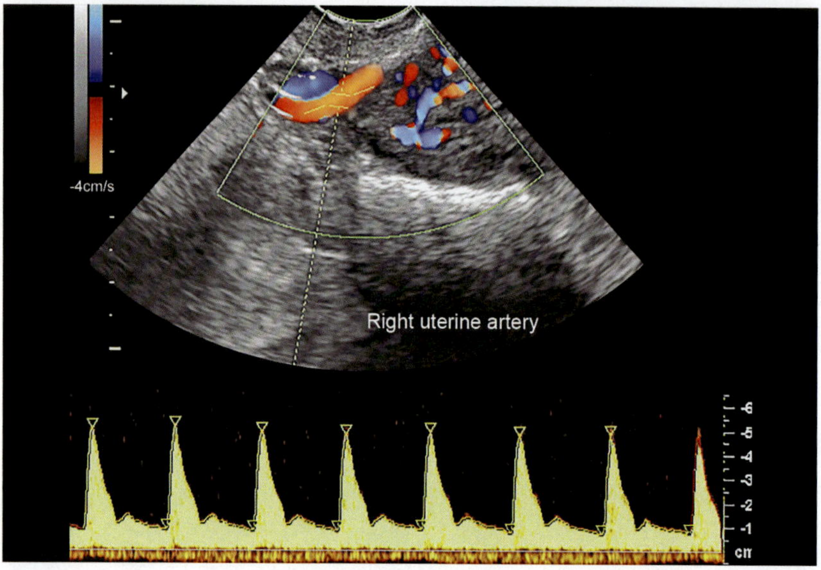

Fig. 16: Uterine artery flow.

The normal values of uterine artery should be PI < –3.16 **(Fig. 16)**.[42] Even if TVCD of follicle is normal, endometrial and the uterine artery indices should be within normal limits for implantation. ETs in IVF cycles are also cancelled if the uterine artery PI > 3.2.[43] Doppler study for uterine receptivity should be done on the day of trigger. Trigger administration induces significant increase in LH and in turn increase in the resistance of uterine artery for 48 hours which can affect its evaluation on the day of follicular aspiration/rupture, therefore Doppler study for uterine receptivity should be done on the day of hCG.[28] Moreover, the Doppler studies are better done at the same time every day as circadian rhythm is seen in uterine artery flow in periovulatory phase.

As for the follicle, the endometrium also if evaluated by 3D and 3D power Doppler for maturity before trigger, gives better implantation rates. It calculates endometrial volume instead of endometrial thickness. When we measure endometrial thickness, we measure it at the thickest part and only in midsagittal plane, and this thickness might not be uniform in the whole endometrium. Moreover, sometimes in spite of normal thickness the length of the endometrial cavity may be so short that the total endometrial volume is not enough for implantation. Therefore, volume is considered to be a better parameter than endometrial thickness. Moreover 3D power Doppler gives idea about the global vascularity of the endometrium not only in terms of quality but also in terms of quantity, which should be a more useful parameter than 2D Doppler where we can see vessels only in one plane at a time and also interrogate a few vessels not all, by pulse Doppler. In our study,[36]

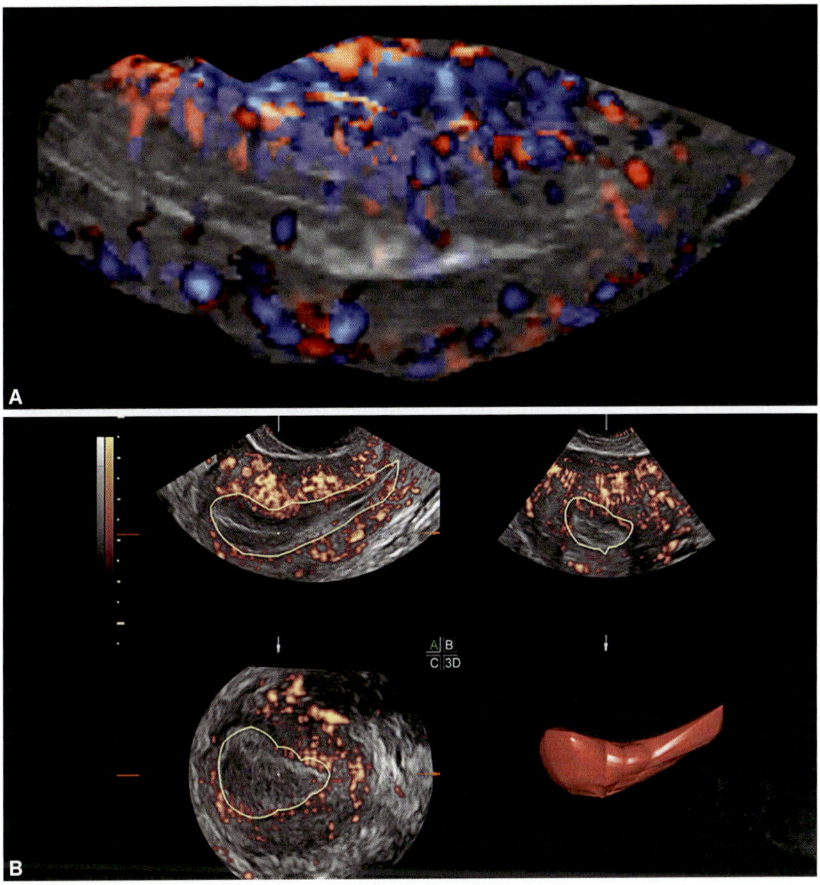

Figs. 17A and B: Three-dimensional power angiography and volume histogram of endometrium.

3D power Doppler indices that we have found good for endometrial receptivity are endometrial volume 3 cc, FI > 20, and VFI > 5 **(Figs. 17A and B)**. There are several other people who have also worked on endometrial receptivity assessment by 3D and 3D power Doppler. A study by Luis T Merce et al. of 40 IVF cycles has shown endometrial volume of 3–7 mL as most favorable for conception. Median values for a favorable endometrium according to this study is 4.28 ± 1.9 mL.[44]

According to another study, endometrial volume of >2.0 mL has a significantly higher pregnancy rates and no pregnancies were recorded with endometrial volume of <1 mL.[45]

According to one another study, no pregnancy occurred when endometrial volume < 3 mL and VI < 10. Exceptionally better pregnancy rates are achieved with endometrial volume 7 mL and subendometrial VI between 10 and 35%.[44] A study by Kupesic et al. shows lower RI of 0.49–0.57 in subendometrial vessels and FI of 11.0–15.4 in conception cycles as compared to 9.5–13.3 otherwise.[46]

Though one another study shows that VFI on the day of trigger is more sensitive than volume, VI, and FI for prediction of pregnancy. VFI > 0.24 has:

- Sensitivity of 83.3%
- Specificity of 88.9%
- Positive predictive value (PPV) 93.8%
- Negative predictive value (NPV) 72.3%

For prediction of pregnancy with 33% pregnancy rate.[47]

Scoring system has also been developed for endometrial receptivity, which apart from the endometrial thickness, morphology, vascularity, and uterine artery Doppler also includes uterine contraction count. Calculating contractions/min > 52/min is considered unfavorable for implantation and, 3 contractions 2/min is considered good for implantation.[48] This is purely based on the fact that uterus that is highly contractile and irritable, will not allow implantation, and the one that is pacified by progesterone may have better chances of implantation. This may also be one of the causes for better implantation rates for blastocyst transfer. Though this scoring system is not practically applicable as even with full scores of the often used uterine scoring systems, pregnancy might not occur.

Features of endometrium with good receptivity:
- Minimal thickness of 6 mm, preferably 8 mm
- Grade A endometrium
- Vascularity reaching zone 3–4
- Endometrial RI < 0.6
- Endometrial volume 3–7 cc
- Endometrial FI > 20 and VFI > 5
- Uterine artery PI < 3.2.

SECRETORY SCAN

With the rupture of the follicle corpus luteum is formed. Corpus luteum is a cystic structure with thick shaggy walls and echogenicity in the lumen. But it is known to have variable appearances like ground glass echogenicity in lumen or lacelike echogenicities **(Fig. 18A)**. Secretory changes are seen in the endometrium in the form of hyper echogenicity of the endometrium which starts from outside, proceeding to the central line making a ring sign of the endometrium **(Fig. 18B)**.[49] Posterior wall of the uterus also appears more echogenic in this phase due to acoustic enhancement due to fluid accumulation in the endometrium.

Assessment of the corpus luteum, endometrium and uterine artery by Doppler gives information about the luteal phase normalcy and progesterone

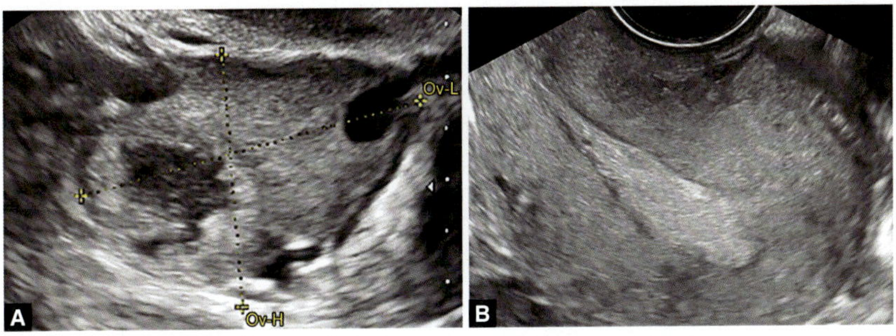

Figs. 18A and B: Corpus luteum and secretory endometrium.

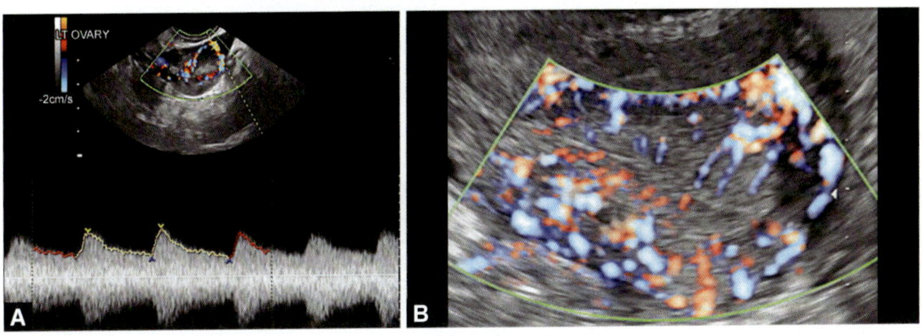

Figs. 19A and B: Corpus luteum and endometrial Doppler in secretory phase.

levels. A clear correlation between RI of corpus luteum and plasma progesterone levels has been seen in natural cycle.[50]

Resistance index of the corpus luteum can therefore be used as an adjunct to plasma progesterone assay as an index of luteal function.[50]

A healthy corpus luteum will show a vascular ring surrounding itself on color Doppler and on power Doppler these vessels show RI 0.35–0.50 and PSV 10–15 cm/sec **(Fig. 19A)**.[51,52] This resistance starts increasing on Day 23 of the cycle in a nonconception cycle.

Endometrial Doppler shows branches of spiral arteries piercing the outer echogenic margins of the endometrium and better if it reaches the central line with RI 0.48–0.52[52,53] **(Fig. 19B)**. Uterine artery at this time of the cycle has PI of 2.0–2.5. Based on these values abnormal parameters indicate luteal phase problems like LUF or luteal phase defect.

LUTEINIZED UNRUPTURED FOLLICLE

Persistent follicle with thick walls and low level echogenicities are seen on 2D US. These echogenicities are not fish net or lacelike that are seen due to blood collection. Endometrium is thick and echogenic and no fluid is seen in pouch of Douglas (POD). On Doppler perifollicular RI is 0.51–0.59, which is higher than normal and remains almost constant till the end of the cycle.

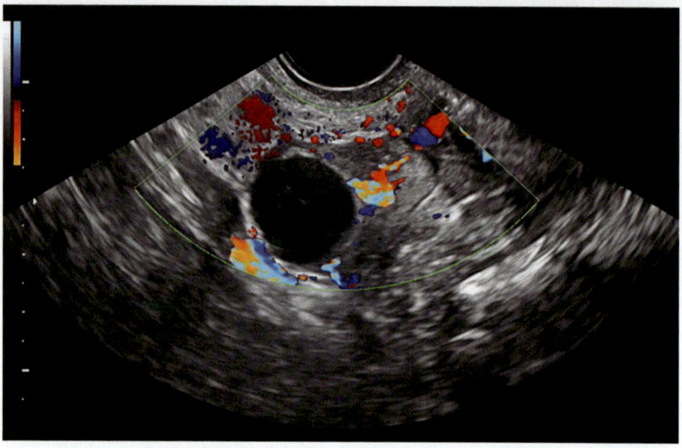

Fig. 20: *Luteinized unruptured follicle:* High resistance flow in luteinized unruptured follicle.

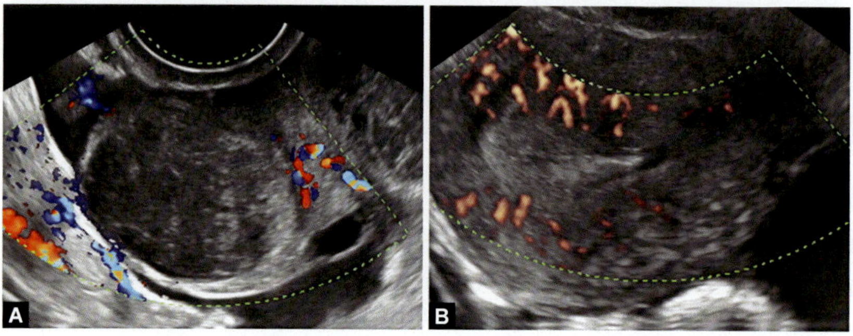

Figs. 21A and B: *Luteal phase defect:* Inadequate corpus luteal function.

Nondominant ovary also shows similar Doppler indices. Endometrium shows scanty and high resistance flow **(Fig. 20)**.[31]

LUTEAL PHASE DEFECT

In this case there is normal follicular development and ovulation with early secretory transformation of endometrium. On Doppler corpus luteum shows high resistance flow with RI: 0.58 + 0.04. Bilateral ovarian RI shows no difference, that means there is no difference in vascular resistance in dominant and nondominant ovary. Increased resistance is also seen in spiral arteries RI: 0.72 ± 0.06.[52] This is the case when luteal phase defect is due to insufficient corpus luteum **(Figs. 21A and B)**. But when luteal phase defect is due to insufficient progesterone receptors in the endometrium, the corpus luteal flow is normal but endometrium is thin, nonhyperechogenic, and shows scanty vascularity **(Figs. 22A and B)**.

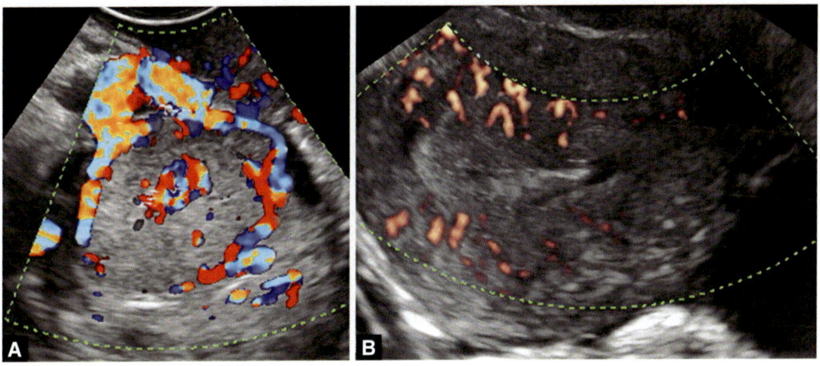

Figs. 22A and B: Luteal phase defect due to bad endometrial receptivity.

Increased resistance of uterine blood flow in the midluteal phase may be an important contributing factor to some causes of infertility and the cause of some previously "unexplained" infertility.[53]

Segmental uterine and ovarian artery perfusion demonstrates a significant correlation with histological and hormonal markers of uterine receptivity and may aid assessment of luteal phase defect.

SUMMARY

Monitoring of follicular growth with 2D and Doppler is the crux of treatment success. Doppler adds to the information available. Because the hormonal changes reflect as vascular changes, which can be studied by Doppler, it gives better understanding and closer monitoring of the treatment cycle. 3D and 3D power Doppler can help improve the results better.

As quoted by *Golan et al., Shoham et al., and Tan SL et al.* "In the hands of experienced operators, ultrasound alone suffices for cycle monitoring, with no necessity for additional hormonal estimations".

REFERENCES

1. Hull MGR. Polycystic ovarian disease: clinical aspects and prevalence. Res Clin Forums. 1989;11:21-34.
2. Rotterdam ESHRE/ASRM-Sponsored PCOS Consensus Workshop group. Revised 2003 consensus on diagnostic criteria and long-term health risks related to polycystic ovary syndrome. Fertil Steril. 2004;81(1):19-25.
3. Takahashi K, Eda Y, Abu Musa A, Okada S, K Yoshino, M Kitao. Transvaginal ultrasound imaging, histopathology and endocrinopathy in patients with polycystic ovarian syndrome. Hum Reprod. 1994;9:1231-6.
4. Kupesic S. Sonographic imaging in infertility. Donald School Textbook of Transvaginal Ultrasound. New Delhi: Jaypee Brothers Medical Publishers; 2005. pp. 357-83.
5. Legros RS, Chiu P, Kunselman AR, Bentley CM, Dodson WC, Dunaif A. Polycystic ovaries are common in women with hyperandrogenic chronic anovulation but

do not predict metabolic or reproductive phenotype. J Clin Endocrinol Metab. 2005;9:2571-9.

6. Deb S, Campbell BK, Clewes JS, Rainne-Fenning NJ. Quantitative analysis of AFC and size: a comparison of 2D and automated three-dimensional ultrasound techniques. Ultrasound Obstet Gynecol. 2010;35:354-360
7. Jonard S, Robert Y, Cortet-Rudelli C, Decanter C, Dewailly D. Ultrasound examination of polycystic ovaries: is it worth counting the follicles. Hum Reprod. 2003;18:598-603.
8. Dewailly D, Gronier H, Poncelet E, Robin G, Leroy M, Pigny P, et al. Diagnosis of polycystic ovarian syndrome (PCOS): revisiting the threshold values of follicle count on ultrasound and of the serum AMH level for the definition of polycystic ovaries. Hum Reprod. 2011;26(11):3123-9.
9. Lujan ME, Jarrett BY, Brooks ED, Reines JK, Peppin AK, Muhn N, et al. Updated ultrasound criteria for polycystic ovary syndrome: reliable thresholds for elevated follicle population and ovarian volume. Hum Reprod. 2013;28(5):1361-8.
10. Kim HJ, Adams JM, Gudmundsson JA, Arason G, Pau CT, Welt CK. Polycystic ovary morphology: age-based ultrasound criteria. Fertil Steril. 2017;108(3):548-53.
11. Kyei-Mensah AA, Lin Tan S, Zai, Jacobs HS, et al. Relationship of ovarian stromal volume to serum androgne concentrations in patients with polycystic ovary syndrome. Hum Reprod. 1998;13:1437-41.
12. Brown MA, Chang RJ. Polycystic ovary syndrome: clinical and imaging feature. Ultrasound Q. 2007;23:233-8.
13. Fulghesu Am, Ciampelli M, Belosi C, Apa R, Pavone V, Lanzone A. A new ultrasound criterion for the diagnosis of polycystic ovarian syndrome: the ovarian stroma/total area ratio. Fertil Steril. 2001;76:326-31.
14. Buckett MM, Bouzayen Rm Watkin KL, Tulandi T, Tan SL. Ovarian stroma echogenicity in women with normal and polycystic ovaries. Hum Reprod. 1999;14(3):618-21.
15. Ardaens Y, Robert Y, Lemaitre L, Dewailly D. Polycystic ovarian disease: contribution of vaginal endosonography and reassessment of ultrasonic diagnosis. Fertil Steril. 1991;55:1062-8.
16. Robert Y, Dubrulle F, Gaillandre L, Ardaens Y, Thomas-Desrousseaux P, Lemaitre L, et al. Ultrasound assessment of ovarian stroma hypertrophy in hyperandrogenism and ovulation disorders: visual analysis versus computerized quantification. Fertil Steril. 1995;64:307-12.
17. Dewailly D, Robert Y, Helin I et al. Ovarian stromal hyperandrogenic women. Clin Endocrinol (oxf). 1994;41:557-62.
18. Zaidi J, Campbell S, Pittrof R, Kyei-Mensah A, Shaker A, Jacobs HS, et al. Ovarian stromal blood flow in women with polycystic ovaries: a possible new marker for diagnosis? Hum Repro Ovsriad. 1995;10:1992-5.
19. El Behery MM, Diab AE, Mowafy H, Ebrahiem MA, Shehata AE. Effect of laparoscopic ovarian drilling on vascular endothelial growth factor and ovarian stromal blood flow using three dimensional power Doppler. Intern J Gynecol Obstet. 2011;112:119-21.
20. Abd El Aal DE, Mohamed SA, Amine AF, Meki AR. Vascular endothelial growth factor and insulin-like growth factor-1 in polycystic ovary syndrome and their relation to ovarian blood flow. Eur J Obstet Gynecol Reprod Biol. 2005;118:219-24.
21. Jonard S, Robert Y, COrtet-Rudelli C, et al. Ultrasound examination of polycystic ovaries: is it worth counting it. Hum Reprod. 2003;18(3):598-603.
22. Kupesic S, Kurjak A. Predictors of in vitro fertilization outcome by three-dimensional ultrasound. Hum Reprod. 2002;17(4):950-5.
23. Klinkert ER, Broekmans FJ, Looman CW, Habbema JD, te Velde ER. The antral follicle count is a better marker than basal follicle-stimulating hormone for the selection of older patients with acceptable pregnancy prospects after in vitro fertilization. Fertil Steril. 2005;83,811-4.

24. Chen MJ, Yang WS, Chen CL, Wu MY, Yang YS, Ho HN. The relationship between anti-Mullerian hormone, androgen and insulin resistance on the number of antral follicles in women with polycystic ovarian syndrome. Hum Reprod. 2008;23(4):952-7
25. Raine-Fenning NJ, Lam EP. Assessment of ovarian reserve using the inversion mode. Ultrasound Obstet Gynecol. 2006;27(1):104-6.
26. Zaidi J, Barber J, Kyei-Mensah A, et al. Relationship of ovarian stromal blood flow at baseline ultrasound to subsequent follicular response in an in vitro fertilization program. Obstet Gynecol. 1996;88:779-84.
27. Ng EH, Chan CC, Yeung WS, et al. Effect of age on ovarian stromal flow measured by three-dimensional ultrasound with power Doppler in Chinese women with proven fertility. Hum Reprod. 2004;19:2132-7.
28. Bassil S, Magritte JP, Roth J, Nisolle M, Donnez J, Gordts S. Uterine vascularity during stimulation and its correlation with implantation in in vitro fertilization. Hum Reprod. 1995;10:1497-501.
29. Bourne T, Jurkovic D, Waterstone J, Campbell S, Collins WP. Intrafollicular blood flow during human ovulation. Ultrasound Obstet Gynecol. 1991;1:53-9.
30. Kupesic S, Kurjak A. Uterine and ovarian perfusion during the periovulatory period assessed by transvaginal color Doppler. Fertil Steril. 1993;603:439-43.
31. Nagori CB, Panchal SY. Double IUI in cases with high pre-hCG perifollicular PSV for better pregnancy rates: a randomized study of 350 IUI cycles. Presented at 16th World Congress on Ultrasound in Obstetrics and Gynecology, 2006, London. J Ultrasound Obstet Gynecol. 2006;28(4):612.
32. Van Blerkom I, Antzak M, Schrader R. The developmental potential of the human oocyte is related to the dissolved oxygen content of follicular fluid: association with vascular endothelial growth factor levels and perifollicular blood flow characteristics Hum Reprod. 2003;18(11):2429-40
33. Kyei-Mensah A, Zaidi J, Pittrof R, Shaker A, Campbell S, Tan SL. Transvaginal three dimensional ultrasound: accuracy of follicular volume measurements. Fertil Steril. 1996;65:371-6.
34. Feichtinger W. Transvaginal three dimensional imaging for evaluation and treatment of infertility. In: Merz E (Ed). 3D Ultrasound in Obstetrics and Gynecology. Philadelphia: Lippincott Williams & Wilkins; 1998. pp. 37-43.
35. Panchal SY, Nagori CB. Can 3D PD be a better tool for assessing the pre-hCG follicle and endometrium? A randomized study of 500 cases. Presented at 16th World Congress on Ultrasound in Obstetrics and Gynecology, 2006, London. J Ultrasound Obstet Gynecol. 2006;28(4):504.
36. Panchal SY, Nagori CB. Pre-hCG 3D and 3D power Doppler assessment of the follicle for improving pregnancy rates in intrauterine insemination cycles. Journal of Human Reproductive Sciences. 2009;2(2):62-7.
37. Smith B, Porter R, Ahuja K, et al. Ultrasonic assessment of endometrial changes in stimulated cycles in an in vitro fertilization and embryo transfer program. J In Vitro Fert Embryo Transf. 1984;1:233-8.
38. Zaidi J, Campbell S, Pittrof R, Tan SL. Endometrial thickness, morphology, vascular penetration and velocimetry in predicting implantation in in vitro fertilization program. Ultrasound Obstet Gynecol. 1995;6:191-8.
39. Applebaum M. The 'steel' and 'teflon' endometrium-ultrasound visualization of endometrial vascularity in IVF patients and outcome. Presented at The Third World Congress of Ultrasound in Obstetrics and Gynecology. Ultrasound Obstet Gynecol. 1993;3(Suppl 2):10.
40. Jehn-Hsiahn Yang, Ming-Yih Wu, Chin-Der Chen, Mau-Chaio Jiang, Hong-Nerng Ho, Yu-Shih Yang. Association of endometrial blood flow as determined by a modified colour Doppler technique with subsequent outcome of in-vitro fertilization. Human Reproduction. 1999;14(6):1606-10.

41. Chein LW, Au HK, Chen PL, Xiao J, Tzeng CR. Assessment of uterine receptivity by the endometrial-subendometrial blood flow distribution pattern in women undergoing IVF-ET. Fertil Steril. 2002;78:245-51.
42. Coulam CB, Stern JJ, Soenksen DM, Britten S, Bustillo M. Comparison of Pulsatility indexes on the day of oocyte retrieval and embryo transfer. Hum Reprod. 1995;10:82-4.
43. Salle B, Bied Damon V, Benchaib M, Desperes S, Gaucherand B,Rudigoz RC. Preliminary report of an ultrasonography and colour Doppler uterine score to predict uterine receptivity as in in-vitro fertilization. Hum Reprod. 1998;13:1669-73.
44. Merce LT, Barco MJ, Bau S, Arenas JB. 2D and 3D power Doppler ultrasound study of endometrium as implantation marker. Textbook of Transvaginal Sonography. New Delhi: Jaypee Brothers Medical Publishers; 2005. pp. 241-2.
45. Raga F, Bonilla-Musoles F, Casa. EM, Klein O, Bonilla F. Assessment of endometrial volume by three-dimensional ultrasound prior to embryo transfer: clues to endometrial receptivity. Hum Reprod. 1999;14:2851-4.
46. Kupesic S, Bekavac I, Bjelos D, Kurjak A. Assessment of endometrial receptivity by transvaginal color Doppler and three dimensional power Doppler ultrasonography in patients undergoing in vitro fertilization procedures. J Ultrasound Med. 2001;20:125-34.
47. Wu HM, Chiang CH, Huang HY, Chao AS, Wang HS, Soong YK, et al. Detection of subendometrial vascularization blood flow by three-dimensional ultrasound may be useful for predicting pregnancy rate for patients undergoing in vitro fertilization-embryo transfer. Fertil Steril. 2003;79:507-11.
48. Applebaum M. The uterine biophysical profile. Ultrasound Obstet Gynecol. 1995;5(1):67-8.
49. Bald R, Hackeloer BJ. Ultraschall-darstellung verschiendener. Endometrium foramen. In: Otto R, Jan FX (Eds). Ultraschalldiagnostik 1982. Stuttgart: Thieme; 1983. pp. 187.
50. Glock JL, Brumsted JR. Color flow pulsed Doppler ultrasound in diagnosing luteal phase defect. Fertil Steril. 1995;64:500-4.
51. Salim A, Kurjak A, Zalud I. Ovarian luteal flow in normal and abnormal early pregnancies. J Matern Fetal Invest. 1992;2:119.
52. Kupesic S, Kurjak A, Vujisic S, Petrovic Z. Luteal phase defect: comparison between Doppler velocimetry, histological and hormonal markers. Ultrasound Obstet Gynecol. 1997;9:105-12.
53. Steer CV, Tan SL, Mason BA, Campbell S. Midluteal-phase vaginal color Doppler assessment of uterine artery impedance in a subfertile population. Fertil Steril. 1994;61(1):53-8.

CHAPTER 17

Normal and Abnormal First-trimester Pregnancy

Sonal Panchal

INTRODUCTION

First trimester of pregnancy is the most eventful time of human life. Study of the first trimester of pregnancy by ultrasound (US) is sonoembryology. Embryology has always been a study of specimens. It was very difficult to understand the development of human embryo until the advent of volume US. Volume US with transvaginal probe has brought a revolution in the study of embryology.

Transvaginal sonography (TVS) is so far the method of choice for earliest visual documentation of pregnancy and volume US has added value to that by various rendering modes and the multiplanar mode to understand the anatomy better.

Using transvaginal US, study of pregnancy can be started even before the sac appears. It is known that the blastocyst implants in the endometrium, 5 days after the fertilization of the ovum in the fallopian tube, i.e., approximately 18th to 20th day of the 28 days cycle. With implantation the progesterone secretion is enhanced from corpus luteum and this is reflected as increased blood flow to the corpus luteum. The receptive organ to this progesterone and proteolytic and other factors is the endometrium. It thickens due to the decidual reaction. New blood vessels develop to provide nutritional support to the embryo.

On US, these changes are represented as:

- *Two-dimensional (2D) US:*
  - Asymmetrical endometrial thickening. One of the endometrial lips is thickened as compared to other because of implanting embryo **(Fig. 1B)**.
  - Corpus luteum **(Fig. 1A)**.
- *Color Doppler:*
  - High velocity, low resistance trophoblastic flow [peak systolic velocity (PSV) >6] in the thickened endometrial lip. This is typically described as a color comet sign by Honemeyer et al. **(Fig. 2B)**.[1]
  - Corpus luteum vascularity with low RI <0.5 **(Fig. 2A)**.
- *Three-dimensional (3D) US:*
  - Asymmetrical endometrial thickening is more evident on 3D US, with thickened part showing increased echogenicity due to decidual reaction and increased vascularity **(Fig. 3)**.

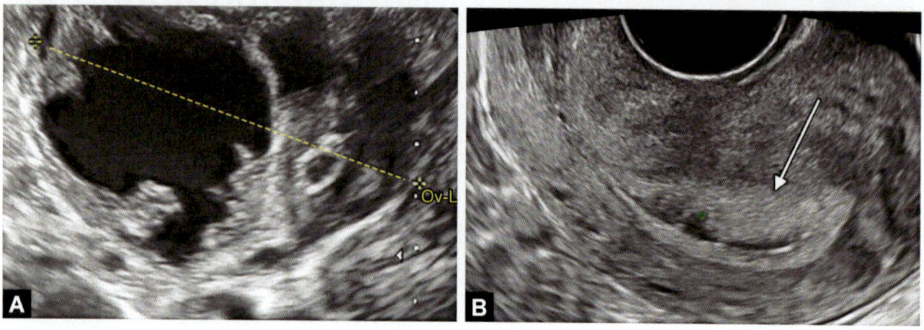

Figs. 1A and B: Corpus luteum and secretory endometrium with asymmetrical thickening on B-mode (arrow).

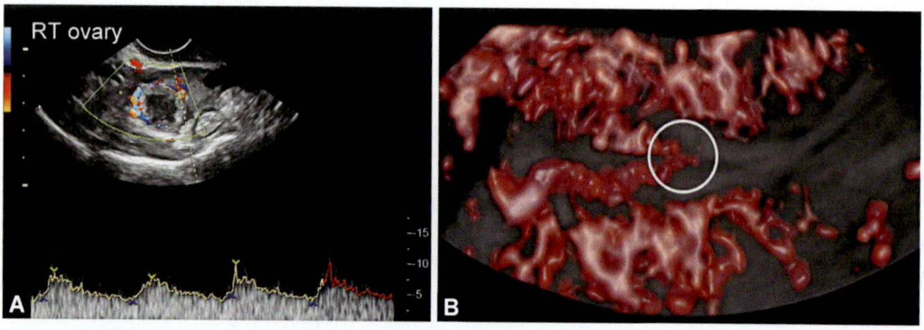

Figs. 2A and B: Corpus luteal and endometrial color comet sign on power Doppler (circle). (RT: right)

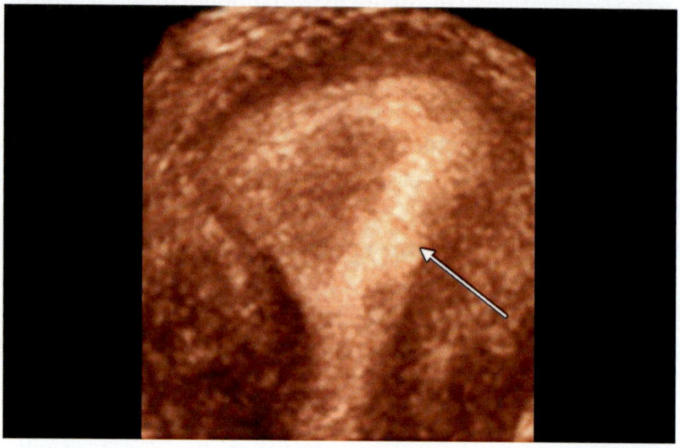

Fig. 3: Three-dimensional ultrasound—possibly conception cycle, midluteal phase (arrow).

Endometrial thickness of <6 mm and nonhyperechogenic endometrium with scanty vascularity in midluteal phase are negative predictors of conception.

Embryo is a very fast growing structure and therefore its anatomy changes every-day or may be even faster. It is very difficult to keep a day-to-day track of these changes. Therefore changes in the embryo are described week-to-week.

Scans are done during early pregnancy for:

- Confirmation of pregnancy
- Location of pregnancy
- Early detection of multiple gestation
- Assessment of progress of pregnancy
- Evaluation of abnormal early pregnancy.

CONFIRMATION OF PREGNANCY

Since the use of transvaginal US has become popular, documentation of pregnancy has become earlier. Presence of gestational sac can be confirmed in the endometrial cavity as early as four weeks and 3–4 days and is diagnostic of pregnancy. Gestational sac is a rounded anechoic structure with thick hyperechoic margins. This echogenic margin is because of decidual reaction and is known as double decidual ring sign. The true gestational sac must be differentiated from pseudo-sac that may often be seen in patients with ectopic pregnancies and the differentiating points are shown in **Table 1**.

β-human chorionic gonadotropin (β-hCG) is the earliest and the first marker for confirmation of pregnancy and gestational sac must be detected

Table 1: Difference between true sac and pseudo sac.

Features	*True sac (Fig. 4)*	*Pseudo sac (Fig. 5)*
Situation	Eccentric in endocavity	Central in endocavity
Margins	Double decidual ring	No hyperechoic ring
With uterine peristalsis	No change in shape	Changes shape
On Doppler	Peripheral vascular ring	No peripheral vascularity

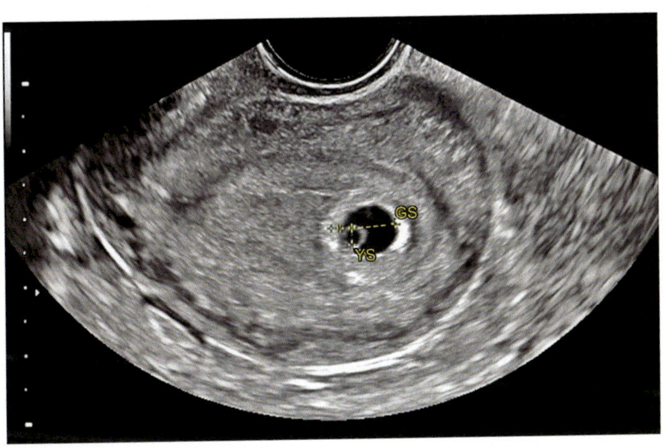

Fig. 4: True gestational sac.

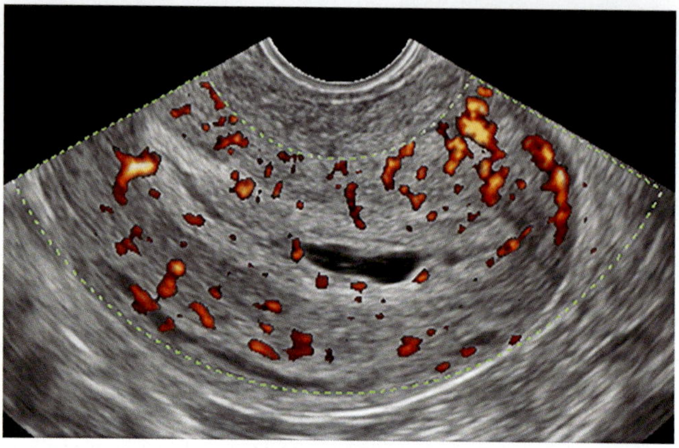

Fig. 5: Pseudo sac.

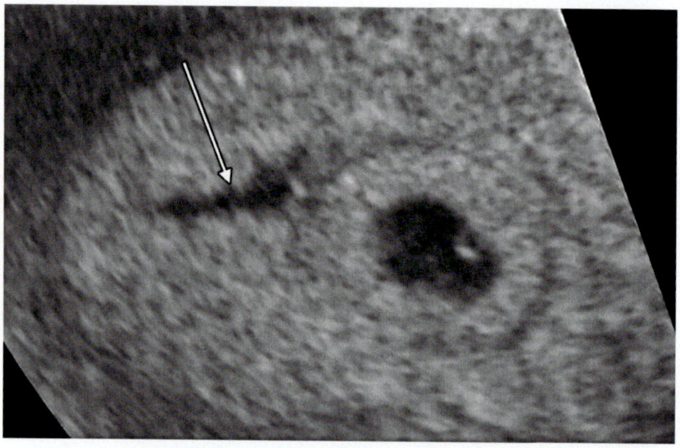

Fig. 6: Residual endometrial cavity (arrow).

in the endometrial cavity on transvaginal scan when β-hCG levels are >1,000 IU/mL.

In absence of which the possibilities are: (1) ectopic pregnancy, (2) early multiple pregnancy, and (3) early missed abortion. At appearance gestational sac it is 2–3 mm in diameter. It grows at a rate of 1 mm/day and at 7 weeks it occupies one-third of endometrial cavity. As it is implanted in one of the endometrial leaves, the endometrial cavity still persists till the sac grows large enough to abut the cavity. This residual cavity may be seen till 7 weeks and fluid seen surrounding the sac till this time should be first considered as a residual cavity, rather than perisac bleeding **(Fig. 6)**. Its continuity with the endometrial central line towards fundus or with cervical canal towards cervix confirms it is residual endometrial cavity.

A gestational sac that is not circular, does not have thick echogenic margins, appears late, is too large or too small for dates, has internal echogenicities and does not show peripheral vascularity is considered abnormal **(Figs. 7A to C)**. A gestational sac that grows <0.7 mm/day is also considered to have a bad prognosis.

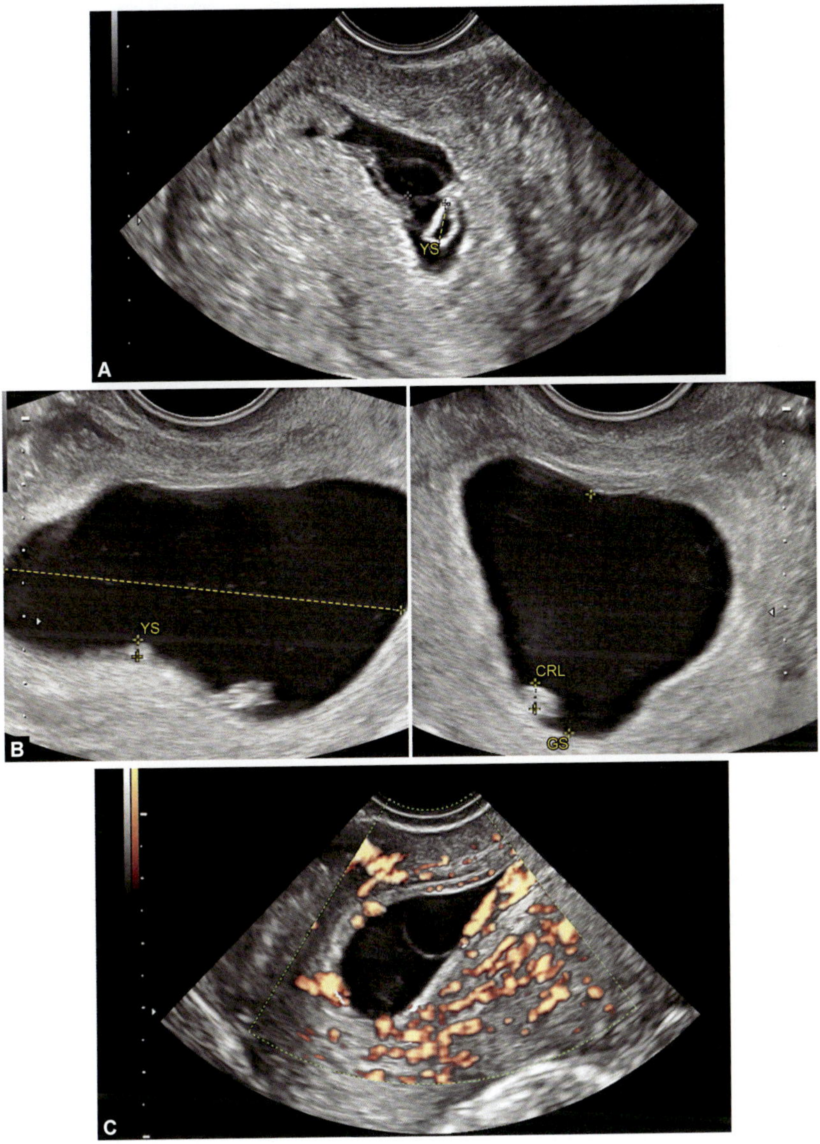

Figs. 7A to C: (A) Irregular sac with internal echogenicities; (B) Large gestational sac; (C) Gestational sac with yolk sac and minimal vascularity.

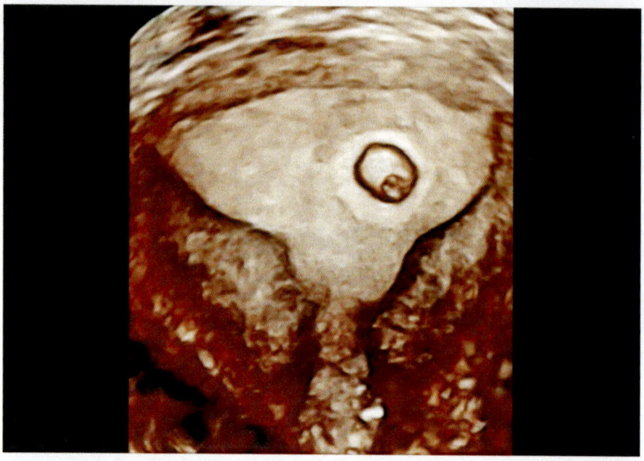

Fig. 8: Normally implanted gestational sac.

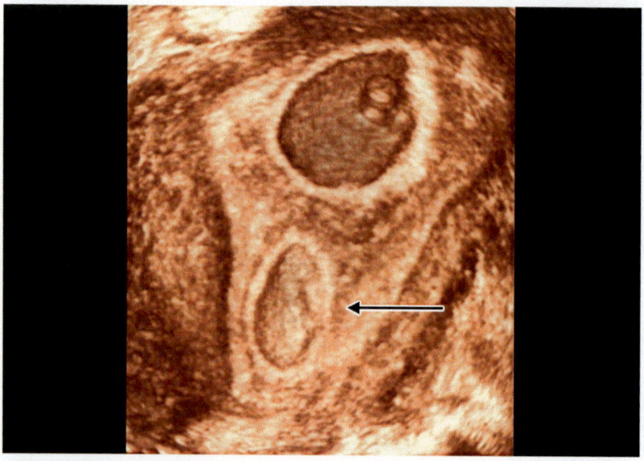

Fig. 9: Three-dimensional ultrasound image of the uterus with twin gestational sacs, one is normal in fundus and the other is low implanted (arrow).

Location of Gestational Sac

Usually, the gestational sac is implanted in the fundal area **(Fig. 8)**. Gestational sac that is implanted at any other location than this is considered abnormal or ectopic. Gestational sac that is implanted low **(Fig. 9)** in the endometrial cavity, though may not be called ectopic but has increased chance of abortion.

Other locations of gestational sac in uterine cavity that are not considered normal are angular and interstitial pregnancy. Pregnancy in the lateral angle of the endometrial cavity is called angular pregnancy and the one in the interstitial part of the fallopian tube is interstitial pregnancy. Gestational sac in angle of the endometrial cavity usually grows inside the endometrial cavity

(Fig. 10A). Pregnancy in this location is usually observed closely. The risk is only possibility of adherent placenta. Interstitial part of the tube is covered by myometrium and gestational sac in this location cannot distend beyond 6–7 weeks. Differentiation between two is also important **(Fig. 10B)**. Cornual pregnancy was the term earlier used for angular pregnancy. But now that term is reserved for the pregnancies in abnormal uterine cornu.

In interstitial pregnancy, myometrial interface is seen between the endometrium and gestational sac on transverse section of uterus that is cut at the level of the gestational sac. Where as a cornual pregnancy, transverse section of the uterus at the level of gestational sac shows endometrial shadow covering the gestational sac medially but no endometrium is seen lateral to gestational sac **(Figs. 10C and D)**.

Gestational sac may also implant in the cervix and is known as cervical pregnancy and is typically seen as ballooning of the cervix and hour glass shape of the uterus **(Fig. 11A)**.

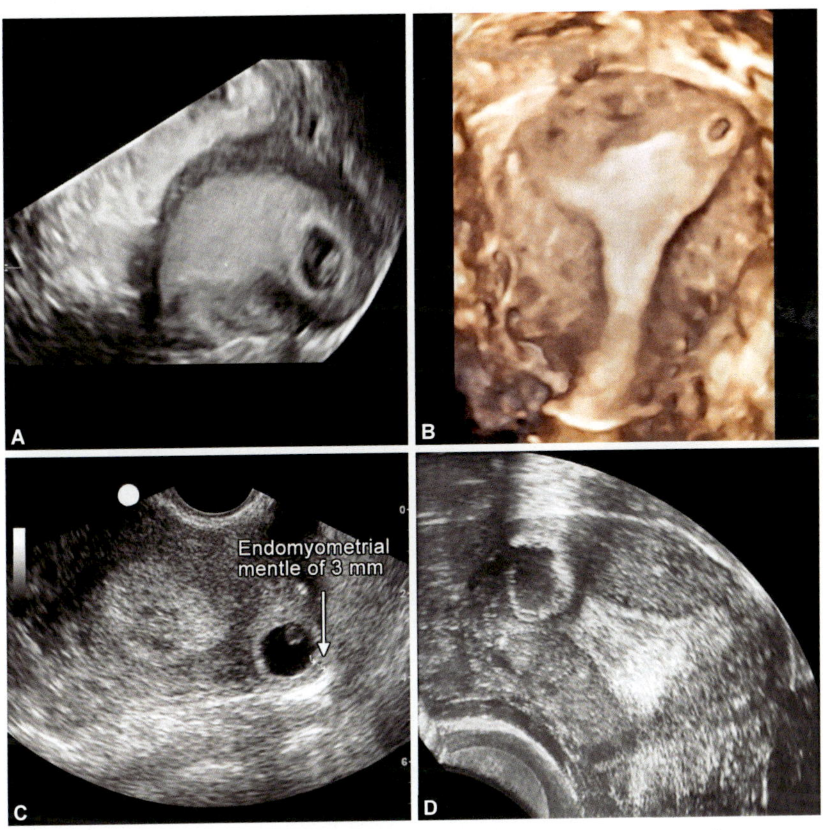

Figs. 10A to D: (A and B) Angular pregnancy on 2D and 3D ultrasounds; (C and D) Interstitial pregnancy on 2D and 3D ultrasounds.

Cervical pregnancy can be differentiated from gestational sac in process of abortion by its eccentric location and the surrounding vascularity **(Fig. 11B)**. Rarely, one may also see a gestational sac in the scar. It is called scar pregnancy and the incidence is increasing because of increased rate of cesarean sections. Scar pregnancy may be implanted in the scar or over the scar **(Fig. 11C)**. Gestational sac which implants in the scar is more dangerous as it can tear off the scar. But the gestational sac that is implanted over the scar can grow in the endometrial cavity, though there is a risk of adherent placenta.

Abnormal location of pregnancy, that are extrauterine are in the tube, ovary or free in the peritoneal cavity. Tubal ectopics are the most common of all ectopic situations.

Patients with ectopic pregnancy typically present with a history of missed period with either fainting attacks, dizziness or acute lower abdominal pain with raised β-hCG levels. The US diagnostic signs are discussed below.

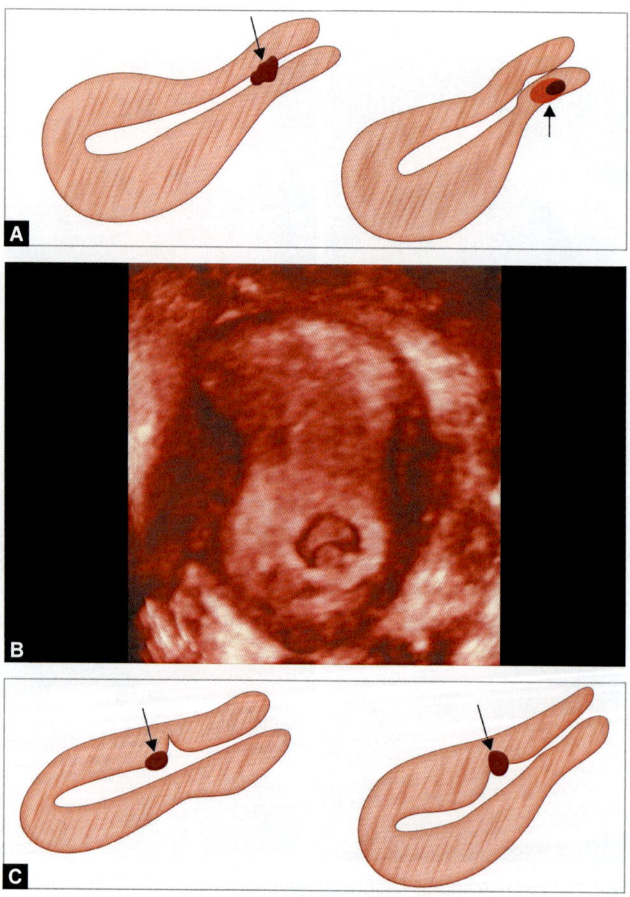

Figs. 11A to C

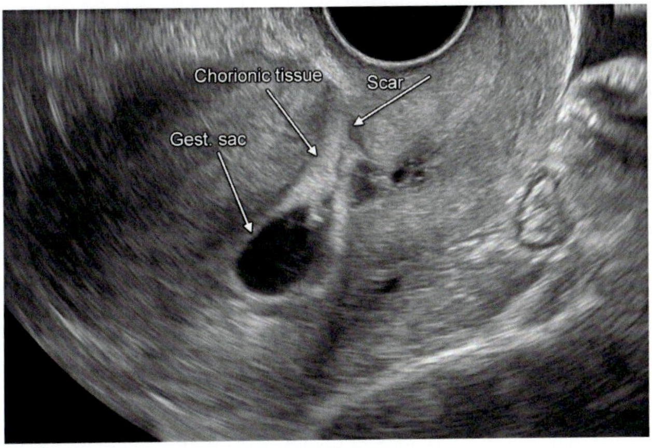

Fig. 11D

Figs. 11A to D: (A) Diagrammatic presentation of gestational sac in the cervical canal in case of abortion in process in the left side image, diagrammatic presentation of gestational sac in the cervical wall indicating cervical pregnancy in the right image; (B) 3D ultrasound of cervical pregnancy; (C) Diagrammatic presentation of scar pregnancy, over the scar in image on left and in the scar in image on right; (D) B-mode ultrasound of pregnancy over the scar pregnancy.

Tubal Ectopic Pregnancy

- No intrauterine gestational sac with symmetrical endometrial cavity **(Fig. 12A)**.
- Adnexal mass with peripheral low resistance vascularity with or without gestational sac which is tender on probe pressure **(Fig. 12B)**. In earlier stages of ectopic pregnancy, the adnexal mass only appears as an isoechoic mass, in extraovarian location with peripheral vascularity. A central hyperechoic shadow then becomes visible, followed by central anechoic are (gestational sac). It is important to diagnose ectopic pregnancy early. This can minimize the risk to the patient. It is also true that this ectopic pregnancy can be followed up closely without any intervention. If the mass size increases, gestational sac appears with cardiac activity or patient becomes unstable, intervention is justified.
- Ipsilateral active corpus luteum.
- Free fluid in pelvis. This sign is seen only when the pregnancy completely invade the tubal wall and bleeding starts from the tube.

Ovarian Ectopic Pregnancy (Fig. 12C)

- No intrauterine gestational sac with symmetrical endometrial cavity.
- Anechoic circular gestational sac in ovary with typical hyperechoic decidual reaction like rim, with peripheral vascularity.
- This can be differentiated from a corpus luteum only by its hyperechoic rim.

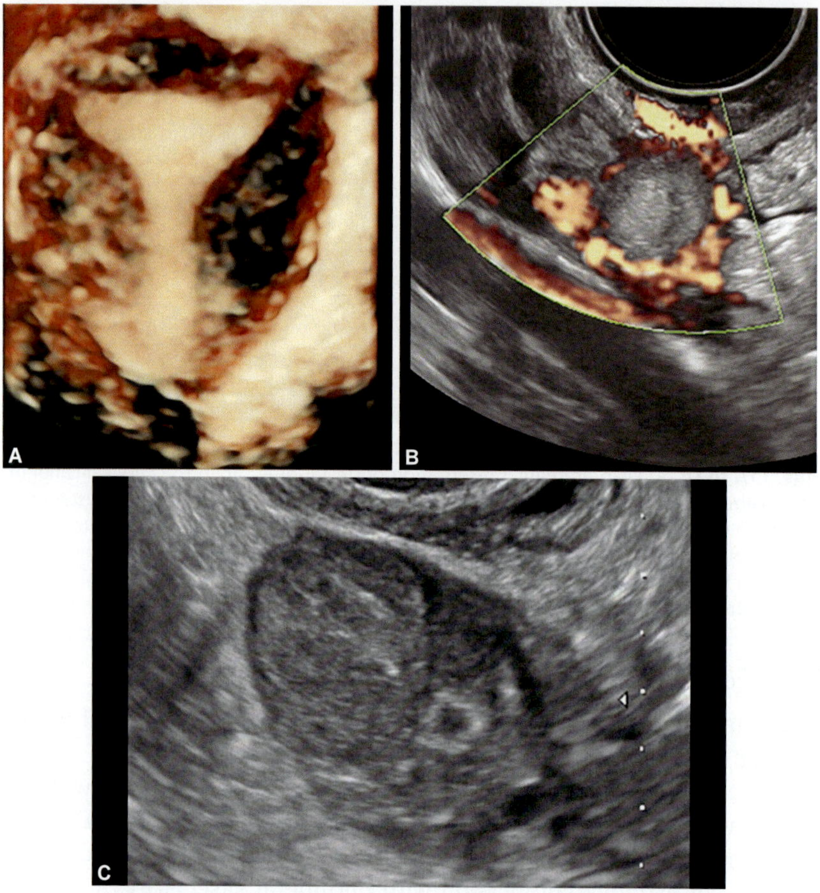

Figs. 12A to C: (A and B) Tubal ectopic pregnancy; (C) Ovarian ectopic pregnancy.

Abdominal/Peritoneal Ectopic Pregnancy (Fig. 13)

- No intrauterine gestational sac with symmetrical endometrial cavity.
- Gestational sac is seen lying free outside uterus, tubes or ovaries.
- It is usually surrounded by fluid.
- Is very difficult to locate as it can be placed anywhere in the peritoneal cavity?

It must be remembered that ectopic pregnancy may coexist with intrauterine pregnancy and is known as heterotopic pregnancy.

Early Detection of Multiple Gestation

Multiple gestations have much higher complication rate than singleton pregnancy. The complication rate and management are different for monochorionic and dichorionic and monoamniotic and diamniotic pregnancies.

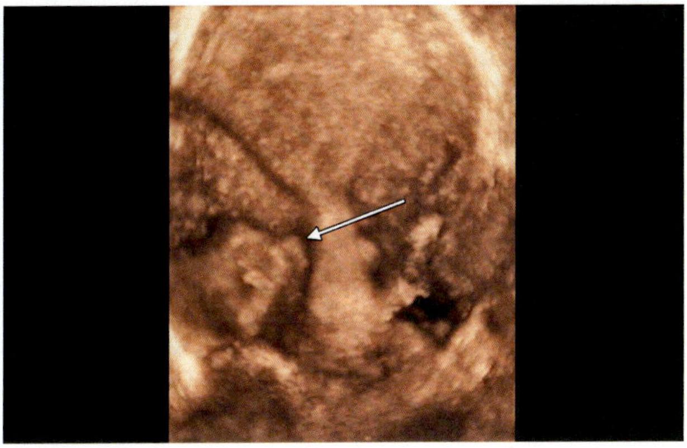

Fig. 13: Abdominal ectopic pregnancy (arrow).

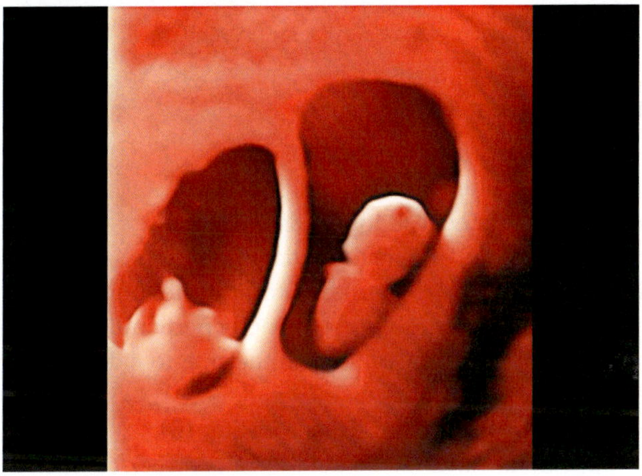

Fig. 14: Multiple gestations (dichorionic diamniotic twins).

It is therefore essential to confirm the chorionicity and amnionicity of any multiple gestation. This can be best done at 8 weeks of pregnancy. This is the time when gestational sacs are small and therefore individual sac margins can be confidently identified **(Fig. 14)**. Without mentioning the chorionicity and amnionicity, no report of multiple gestation is to be considered complete.

Growth and Progress of Pregnancy

Growth of pregnancy is assessed by increase in the size of gestational sac or fetal pole and appearance of new structures in the fetus. Gestational sac, yolk sac, amniotic sac, and fetal pole, all have a definite time of appearance and pace of growth. These growth rates are very precise in first trimester and do not have genetic or individual variation. The technique for these measurements therefore should be standardized.

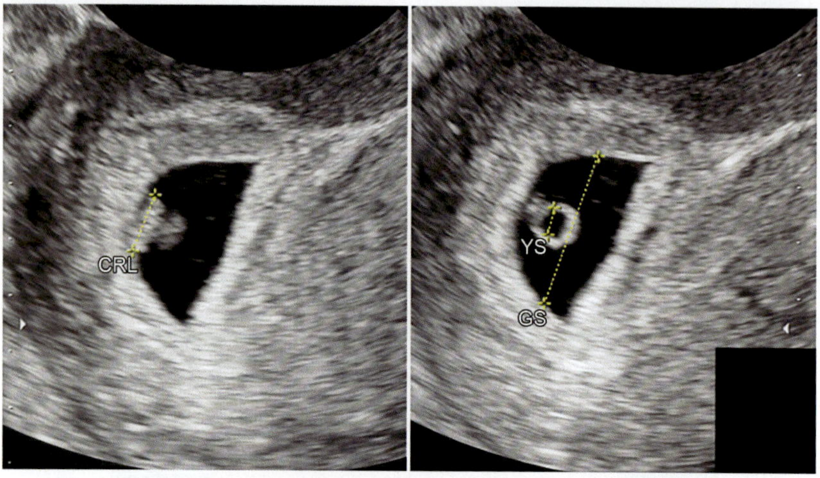

Fig. 15: Measuring gestational sac (GS), yolk sac (YS), and crown-rump length (CRL).

Gestational Sac (Fig. 15)

- Gestational sac appears at 4 weeks 5/6 days.
- It should grow at a rate of 1 mm/day.
- Measured from inner edge to inner edge.
- Always take a mean of 3 orthogonal diameters. After locating the gestational sac, the probe is rotated to find the longest diameter. The second measurement is the longest diameter perpendicular to the longest diameter. The probe is rotated 90° and the side-to-side longest diameter parallel to X-axis is transverse diameter.
- Volume is now considered more reliable **(Fig. 16)**.

Yolk sac appears towards the end of the fourth week or when gestational sac is 10 mm in diameter. Fetal pole must be seen when gestational sac is 15 mm in diameter.

Yolk Sac

Yolk sac has nutritive, metabolic, endocrine, immunological, and hematopoietic functions. It must be seen after 7–8 days of visualization of the gestational sac. It is a confirmatory sign of true gestational sac:

- Measured inner wall to inner wall
- Increases 0.1 mm/day till 10 weeks—maximum 5-6 mm.

Yolk sac is an indicator of poor outcome if it is **(Figs. 17A to D)**:

- Too small yolk sac <2 mm
- Too large yolk sac >6 mm
- Thick walled yolk sac
- Irregular yolk sac
- Solid yolk sac.

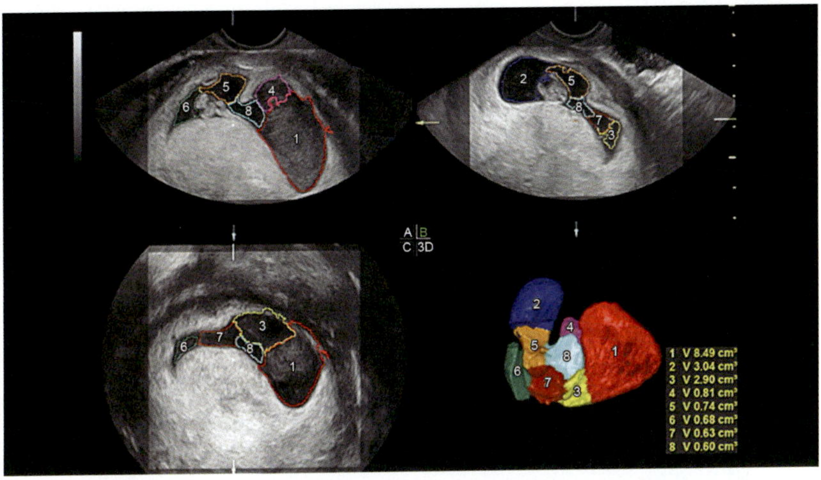

Fig. 16: Gestational sac volume measured by three-dimensional ultrasound.

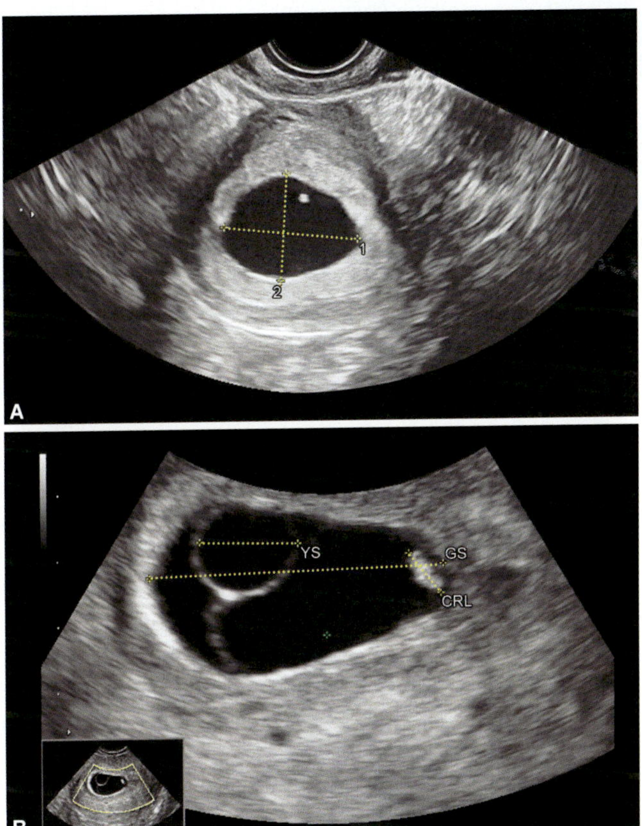

Figs. 17A and B

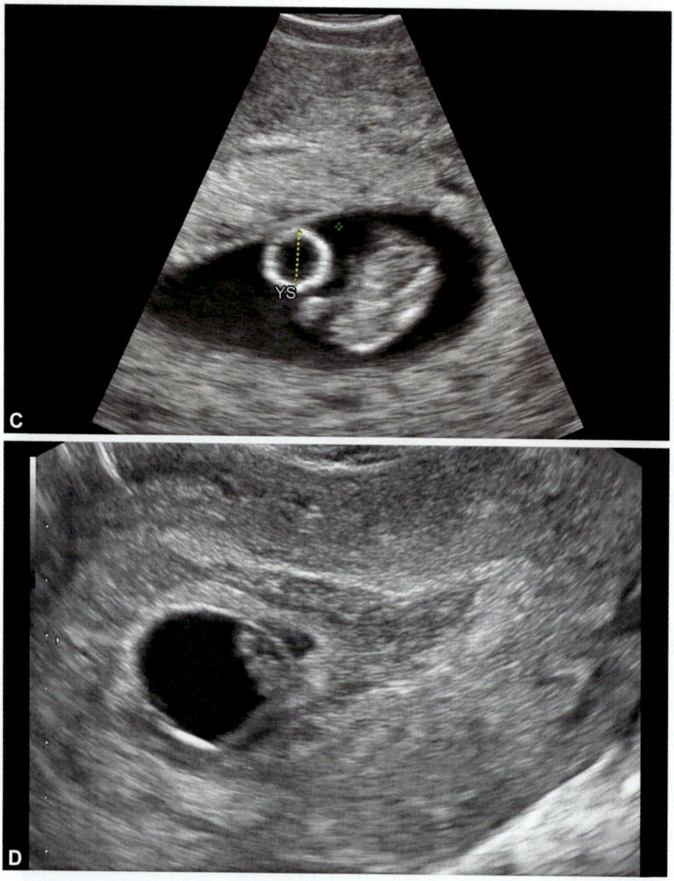

Figs. 17C and D

Figs. 17A to D: (A) Tiny yolk sac; (B) Large yolk sac; (C) Thick-walled yolk sac; (D) Solid yolk sac.

Fetal Pole

Fetal pole is the structure to follow the yolk sac. Detection of the fetal pole is actually by visualization of the cardiac activity. By transvaginal US fetal cardiac activity can be detected at 5.6 weeks approximately, when the fetal pole appears like a linear structure by the side of the yolk sac approximately 1–2 mm in length. Its length is measured from end to end. Fetal pole grows at a rate of 1 mm/day. Size to date discrepancy of up to 5 days can be considered to be within normal limits. Difference in crown rump length (CRL) of >7 mm of normal indicates three times higher risk of aneuploidy.

Cardiac activity must always be seen at all times after 6 weeks of pregnancy. Appearance of a fetal pole, without cardiac activity is a sign of abnormal pregnancy.

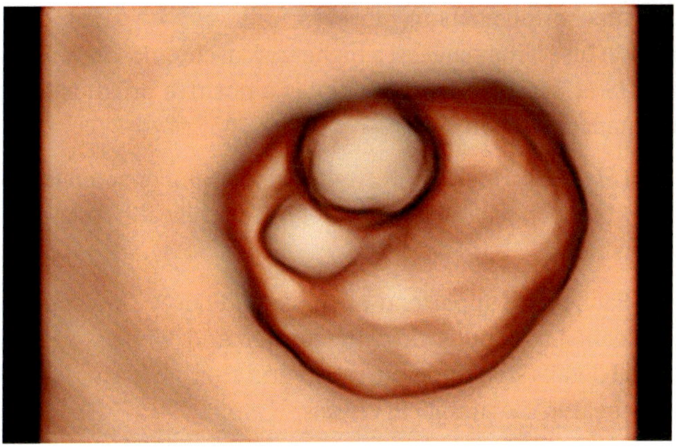

Fig. 18: Six weeks pregnancy.

Cardiac Activity (Rate at Different Gestational Age)

- 5th week—slow-like peristalsis—60–80/min
- End of 5th week—100/min
- End of 6th week—105–130/min
- 9 weeks—160–170/mt, then 120–160/min
- Heart rate of >200/min is termed as tachycardia and <100/min is termed as bradycardia in the first trimester.

Persistently, abnormal heart rate and late appearance of cardiac activity also indicates pregnancy with bad prognosis.

Structures then to appear by completion of each following week after 5 weeks are as follows:

*Six weeks **(Fig. 18)**:*
- Fetal pole it is seen and cephalic and caudal poles are identified
- Omphalomesenteric duct is seen.

Seven weeks:
- Cephalic pole shows the first brain vesicle—rhombencephalon
- Amnion is seen around the fetal pole
- Chorionic tissue around the gestational sac starts differentiating into chorion frondosum and chorion leave.

Amniotic Membrane

- It is seen when CRL is 5–7 mm.
- When it starts appearing with tiny fetal pole, it appears to be the same size as the yolk sac and is mistaken by some as double yolk sac. But presence of fetal pole in this cyst like structure, confirms it is amniotic sac.
- It grows at a rate of 1 mm/day.

- It fuses with chorion at about 14 weeks.
- If it does not fuse it may suggest a higher risk of chromosomal abnormality.

Normal US at 8 weeks of pregnancy is a positive prognostic sign for a normal pregnancy outcome.

Eight weeks **(*Fig. 19*)***:* Fetal trunk straightens, rhombencephalon becomes evident, limb buds appear, and physiological umbilical hernia develops by the end of this week.

Nine weeks: Fetal neck, upper end of spine, and coccyx lower end of spine are clearly seen. Limb buds develop further and elbows and knees are formed. Facial details start appearing. Falx and choroid plexus start showing. Pulsations appear in the umbilical vessels.

Ten weeks **(*Fig. 20*)***:* Brain further develops and now three brain vesicles; prosencephalon, mesencephalon, and rhombencephalon are seen. The limb

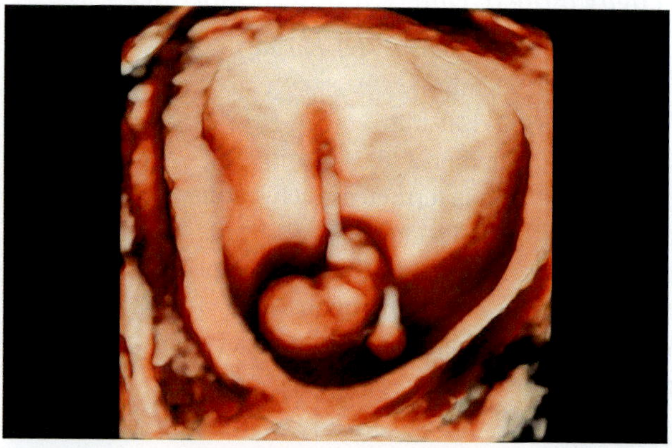

Fig. 19: Eight weeks pregnancy.

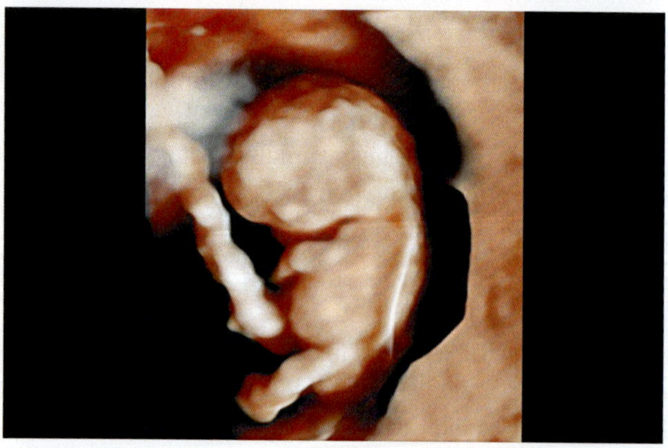

Fig. 20: Ten weeks pregnancy.

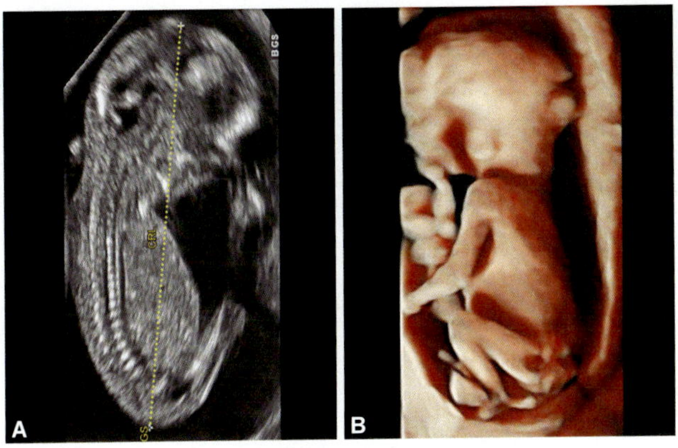

Figs. 21A and B: Twelve weeks pregnancy.

buds start showing fingers and toes. With that the knees bend and the two feet approach each other in midline. There is further development of the circulatory system and ossification of the spine starts.

Eleven weeks: Spinal column is well seen. Facial details are well developed, abdominal organs, liver, and stomach is seen. Umbilical hernia starts getting smaller and disappears almost completely at 11 weeks and 5 days.

Twelve weeks ***(Figs. 21A and B)****:* Kidneys and urinary bladder are developed. Ears, nose, orbits, lens, lips, and jaws can be seen. Heart is well seen but still does not clearly show four chambers.

Thirteen weeks: Facial features and individual vertebrae in the spine are seen. Diaphragm can be appreciated; heart clearly shows four chambers and umbilical hernia is no more seen.

Beyond 12 weeks fetus is fully formed and therefore that is the time for nuchal scan. This shall be discussed in Chapter 19 of this book. But there are abnormalities that can be suspected or even at times diagnosed earlier in the first trimester.

These include:

- *Acrania* ***(Fig. 22)***: Acrania is lack of skull bone development. This leads to abnormal head shape as the developing brain tissue is directly exposed to amniotic fluid. This can be diagnosed as early as 10 weeks of gestation.
- *Holoprosencephaly* ***(Fig. 23)***: This is absence of development of falx. It has been discussed earlier that falx can be seen at all times after completion of ninth week. If it is not seen beyond tenth week, holoprosencephaly must be suspected.
- *Major limb abnormalities*: All limb buds appear at 8 weeks and by the end of 10 weeks, all the segments of all four limbs are formed. Complete or partial absence of any of the limbs can be detected at all times after 10 weeks.

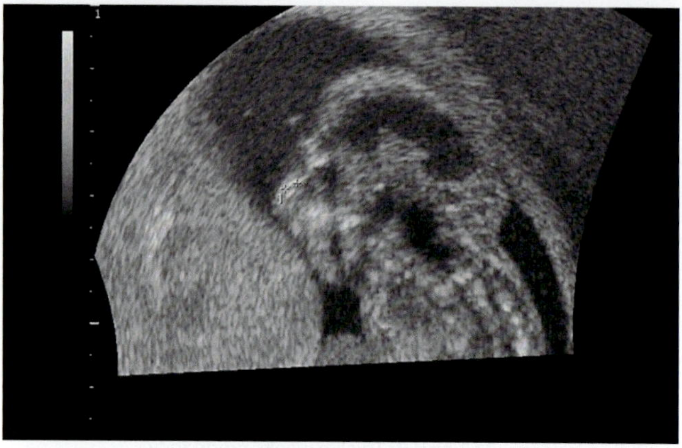

Fig. 22: Acrania.

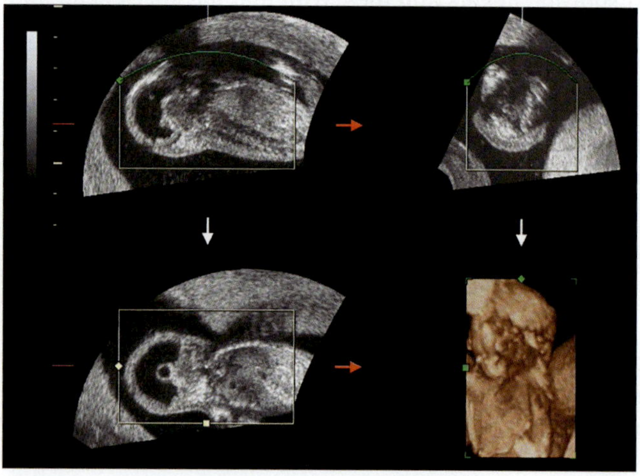

Fig. 23: Holoprosencephaly.

- *Situs inversus*: Situs inversus is complete reverse position of all fetal organs: a mirror image, where heart, aorta, and stomach are on right side and liver, gallbladder and inferior vena cava (IVC) are on left side. As heart and stomach are developed and are evident at 10 weeks, their position can be checked and situs inversus can be diagnosed in first trimester. All situs abnormalities can be diagnosed.
- *Dextrocardia*: Solitary dextrocardia is heart in the right hemithorax. This can be diagnosed in first trimester of pregnancy.
- *Major cardiac abnormalities* ***(Figs. 24A and B)***: By 11 weeks, four-chambered heart is formed and can be seen clearly on transvaginal scan. Major cardiac abnormalities like single ventricle, truncus arteriosus, etc., can be diagnosed on first trimester scans.

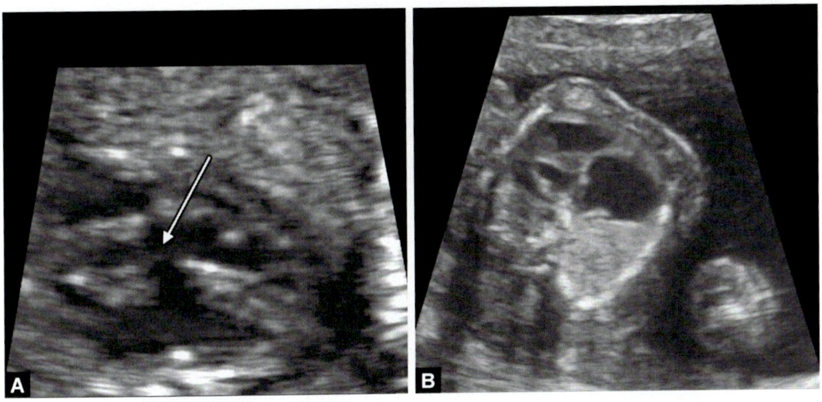

Figs. 24A and B: (A) Major septal defect; (B) Ebstein's anomaly.

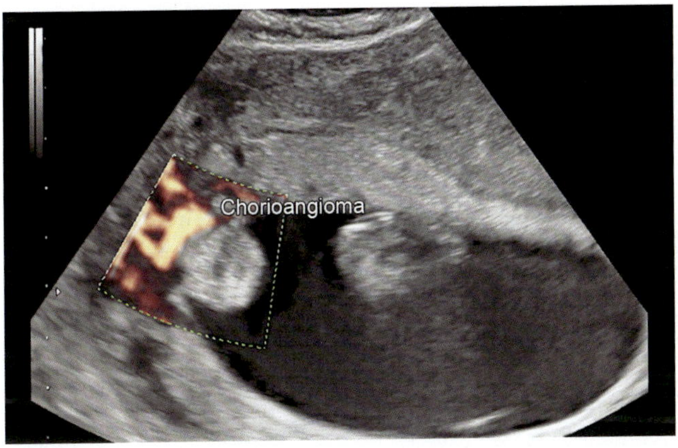

Fig. 25: Chorioangioma.

- *Major spinal defects*: Ossification centers of the spine are formed at the end of 10 weeks. Major spinal defects, multiple vertebral abnormalities, hemivertebrae, etc., can be diagnosed on first-trimester scans.
- *Chorioangioma **(Fig. 25)***: Chorioangioma is an overgrowth, tumor of the chorionic tissue. Chorioangiomas can be seen very early in pregnancy, 7–8 weeks of pregnancy. Small chorioangiomas do not affect the pregnancy, but larger ones may lead to circulatory failures in fetus.
- *Vesicular mole **(Fig. 26)***: This is another chorionic lesion. High β-hCG levels with absent gestational sac with thick echogenic endometrium, that has small anechoic areas is diagnostic of vesicular mole. In early phases, vascularity may not be picked up on Doppler studies due to low velocity flow. Only when it becomes invasive it disrupts the endometrio-myometrial junction and then is usually large enough to show abundant low resistance vascularity.

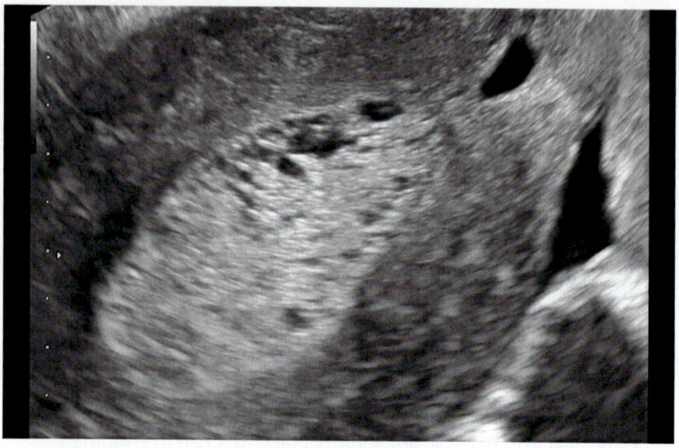

Fig. 26: Vesicular mole.

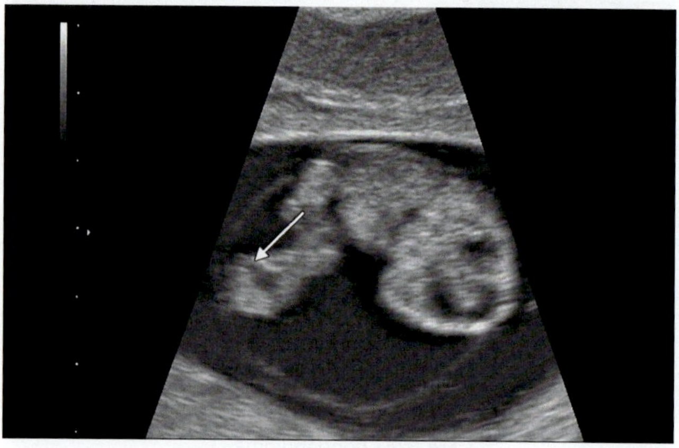

Fig. 27: Umbilical cord cyst (arrow).

Umbilical cord cyst is another not so uncommon lesion that can be picked up in first trimester, but is not clinically significant **(Fig. 27)**. Amniotic bands also can be picked up by the end of the first trimester.

Detailed and careful systematic scanning technique can therefore help in early diagnosis of several fetal abnormalities. Volume US is very informative for first-trimester scanning.

REFERENCE

1. Honemeyer U, Kurjak A, Monni G. Normal and abnormal early pregnancy. In: Kurjak A, Chervenak FA (Eds). Donald School Textbook of Ultrasound in Obstetrics and Gynecology, 2nd edition. New Delhi: Jaypee Brothers Medical Publishers. 2008. pp. 106-29.

CHAPTER 18

Normal Fetal Anatomy in Second Trimester

Sonal Panchal

INTRODUCTION

Second trimester scan is done for detailed structural assessment of the fetus. It carries the importance almost equal to the 11 – 13 + 6 weeks scan. This scan is usually done between 18 and 20 weeks and maximum up to 22 weeks. The optimum time period of doing this scan may vary a little in different parts of the world depending on the local rules for permission of legal abortions.

At this gestational age, most fetal structures are already functional, and therefore a detailed scan at this time is planned. Moreover, the bones are also not too dense at this stage to obstruct the view of the soft tissues of the fetus. Though usually this scan is not done before 18 weeks, it may be planned at 16–18 weeks, especially for fetuses at a higher risk of abnormalities. This group may include those with abnormal ultrasound findings or abnormal biochemical markers in the first trimester, fetuses of mothers with previous abnormal babies, old age mothers, etc.

As mentioned earlier, this scan is done to assess the complete fetal anatomy and a systematic approach is required. It is ideal to move from crown to feet or feet to crown in any fetus, so that no part of the body would be left out. But it is known that fetus is moving and sometimes may be very active to allow assessing the intended part of its body. Therefore when doing fetal assessment one has to be opportunistic and start with imaging the part of the fetal body that is readily seen. In this case it might be possible to skip or forget to image and assess certain parts of the fetal body, therefore it is best to make a checklist of the sections and measurements of the fetal body required and confirm that all the items on the checklist are assessed before the scan is declared complete.

A list of sections suggested by Fetal Medicine Foundation (FMF), UK and most authentic workers in the field for this scan is as follows:

- *Head and face:*
  - *Axial sections:*
    - Transventricular plane
    - Transthalamic plane
    - Transcerebellar plane
    - Transorbital plane
    - Maxillary plane

- *Coronal plane:*
  - Lips
  - Lenses
- *Midsagittal plane:* Nasal bone and frontomaxillary facial angle

- *Trunk:*
  - Axial sections
  - *Thorax:*
    - Four chamber heart
    - Right ventricular outflow tract (RVOT)
    - Left ventricular outflow tract (LVOT)
    - Three-vessel trachea view
  - *Abdomen:*
    - Stomach section for abdominal circumference (AC)
    - Kidneys
    - Umbilical cord insertion
    - Sacrum transverse
  - *Sagittal plane:*
    - Spine
    - Bladder
    - Aortic arch—optional
    - Ductus arch—optional
  - *Coronal plane:* Spine
  - *Limbs:*
    - All four limbs and all three segments
    - Sagittal leg and foot
    - Forearm with hand

It is very essential that all these sections are imaged in a standardized manner to be reliable and comparable, with least interobserver and intraobserver variations. It is also important for optimal anatomical analysis and also for the measurements (biometry) that are to be used for assessment of fetal growth or prediction of any abnormalities of the fetus. To minimize the errors in anatomical details and measurements, it is also essential that the image is optimized and area of interest must be in the center of the screen and sufficient zoom should be used so that the image covers at least two-thirds of the screen.

So let us discuss the details of each of these sections and the fetal anatomy that these demonstrate.

HEAD

Axial Sections

These sections are usually easiest to achieve, especially in a singleton fetus.

Transventricular Plane

This plane cuts through the ventricles as shown in figure as line (a) **(Fig. 1)**. The optimum section must show posterior horns of lateral ventricles, choroid plexus, lateral sulcus, falx, cavum septum, and anterior horns of lateral ventricles **(Fig. 2)**. The oval shape of the skull vault is seen in this section and the calvarial thickness should be symmetrical all around, and not more than 3 mm in second trimester. Thicker calvarial thickness and especially asymmetrical may suggest an oblique section.

Thalami must not be seen in this section, as this section cuts higher up in the head. This is an ideal plane for assessment of the ventricles and choroid plexus. The abnormalities that can be picked up on this section are

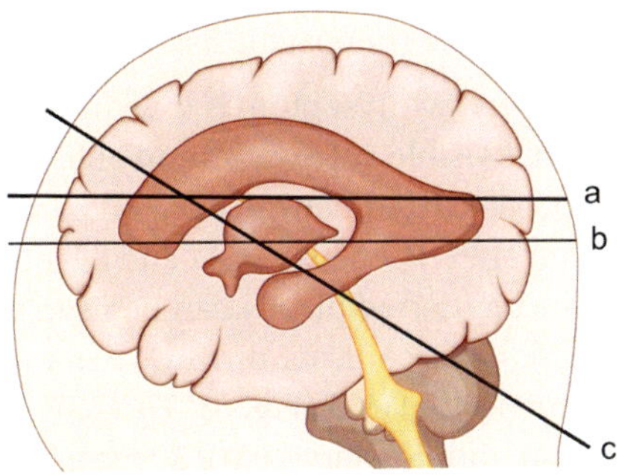

Fig. 1: The three basic axial sections of the head: (a) Transventricular section, (b) Transthalamic section, and (c) Transcerebellar section.

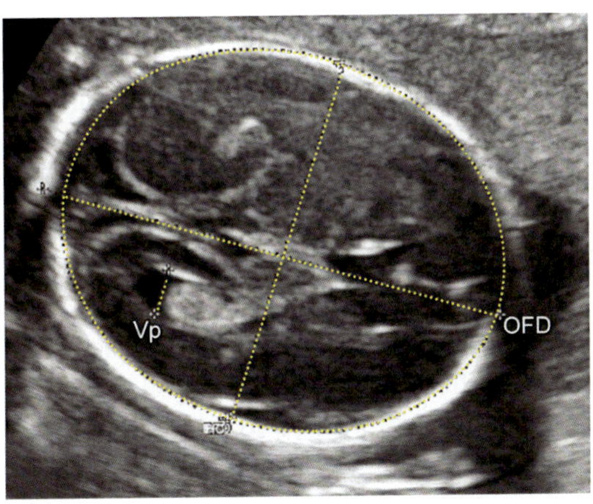

Fig. 2: Transventricular section of the fetal head showing falx, cavum septum pellucidum, and choroid plexuses in posterior horns of lateral ventricles.

ventriculomegaly, hydrocephalus, choroid plexus cysts, holoprosencephaly, corpus callosal defects, skull vault defects, and abnormal skull shape-like brachycephaly or dolichocephaly **(Figs. 3A to H)**.

Transthalamic Plane (Line B in the Fig. 4)

This plane cuts through the thalamus. The optimum section must show the thalami, cavum septum pellucidum, anterior horns of lateral ventricle, falx cerebri, and lateral sulcus. It also shows hippocampal gyrus, posterolateral to the thalami **(Fig. 5)**. The complete oval skull vault should be seen, with symmetrical skull thickness all around and it should not be more than 3 mm. This plane must not show cerebellum or orbits. This plane shows abnormalities of cavum septum pellucidum and corpus callosum, midline shift if present, is evident on this plane. Absence of lateral sulcus is an earliest indicator of lissencephaly. Coronal sutures can be identified in this plane and therefore abnormalities such as craniostenosis can be diagnosed.

Cavum septum pellucidum: Cavum septum is a cavity in the midline inferior to the corpus callosum. It is visible at 16 weeks and obliterates near term. This means it must always be visualized between 18 and 37 weeks, which means when biparietal diameter (BPD) of between 44 and 88 mm.

Both of these above-mentioned planes can be used for the quantitative assessment of the head. This consists of BPD, occipitofrontal diameter (OFD), and head circumference (HC) **(Fig. 6)**. Though conventionally these were measured in transthalamic plane, FMF suggests to measure these in transventricular plane. Transventricular plane is also used to assess the ventricular diameter.

There also is a suggestion that transthalamic plane may be omitted from the routine protocol of second trimester targeted scan. But another consideration is that in the late trimester as the brain matter develops, there is compression on the ventricles and ventricular size decreases. This might at times make identification of ventricles difficult and therefore transventricular plane may be difficult to obtain. In this case, if head parameters were measured in transventricular plane during second trimester scan, its comparison for growth assessment might become difficult or less accurate in third trimester.

Biparietal diameter: This measurement is taken perpendicular to falx cerebri, at the broadest part of the oval skull vault; this is usually at the midpoint between the frontal and the occipital end of the oval skull vault as seen in this axial section. The measurement is taken from outer margin of the proximal parietal bone to the inner margin of the distal parietal bone.

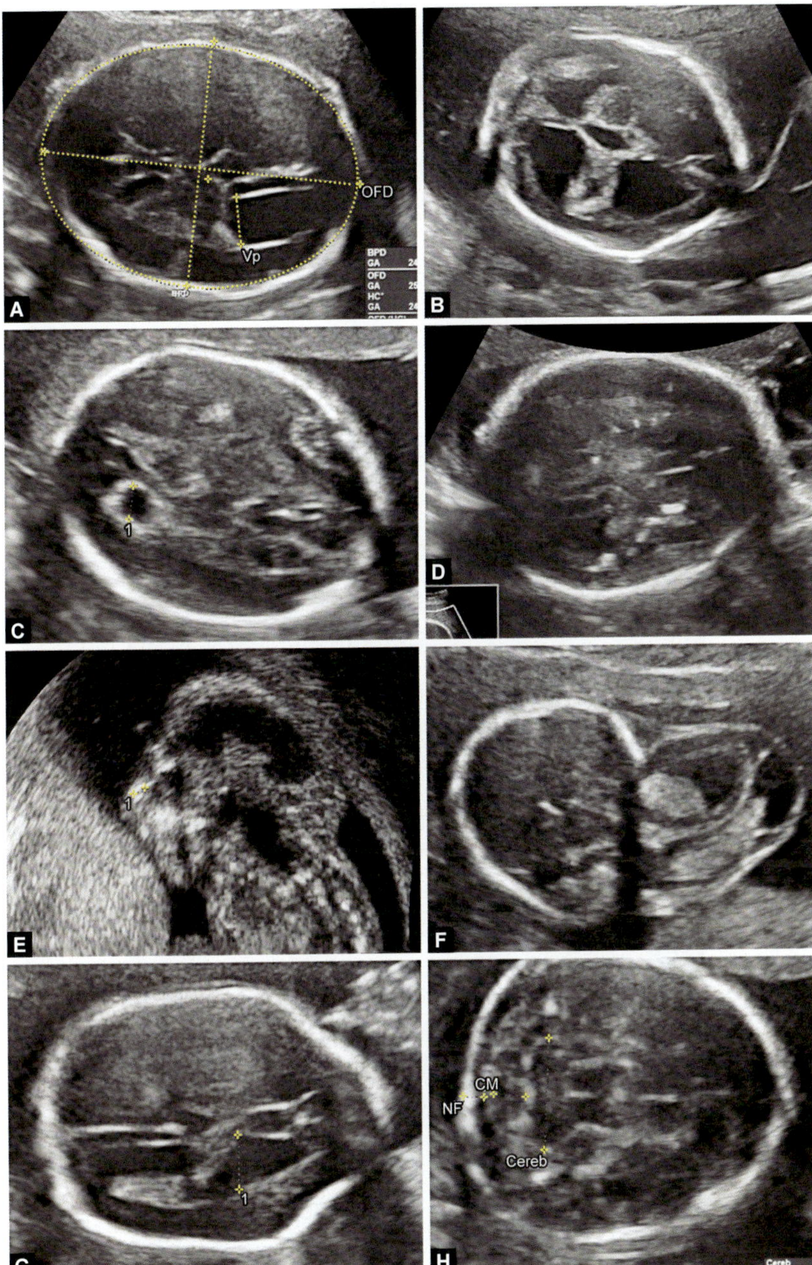

Figs. 3A to H: (A) Ventriculomegaly; (B) Hydrocephalus; (C) Choroid plexus cyst; (D) Ventricular calcifications; (E) Anencephaly; (F) Exencephaly; (G) Lemon skull; (H) Braphycephaly.

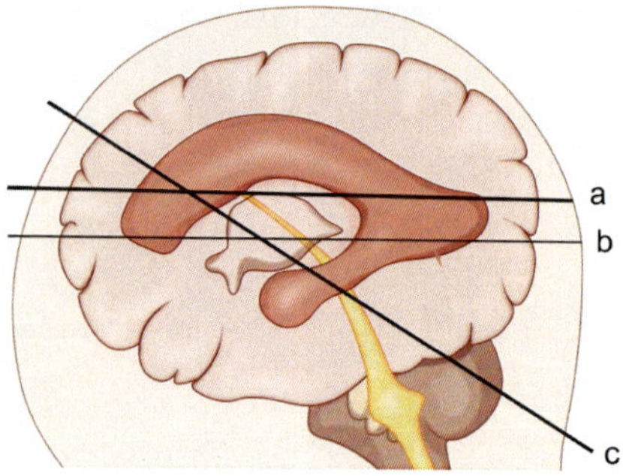

Fig. 4: The three basic axial sections of the head: (a) Transventricular section, (b) Transthalamic section, and (c) Transcerebellar section.

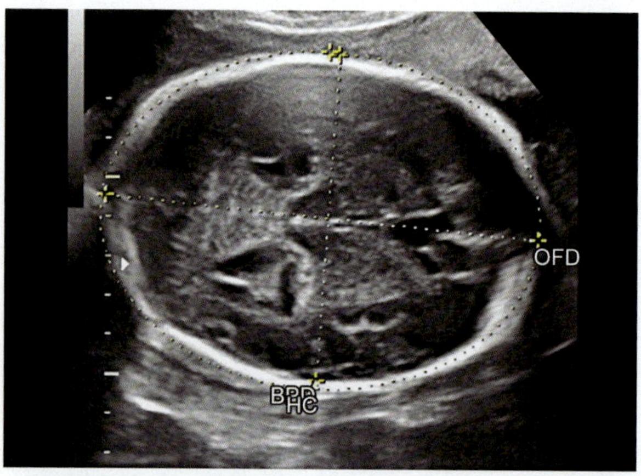

Fig. 5: Transthalamic section showing falx, cavum septum pellucidum, and thalami.

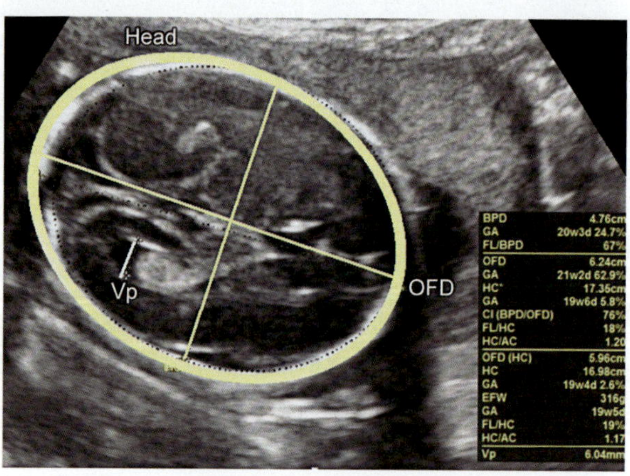

Fig. 6: Transventricular section of the head showing the assessment of biparietal diameter (BPD), occipitofrontal diameter (OFD), head circumference (HC), and ventricular width.

Biparietal diameter increases by:

- 3 mm/week till 30 weeks
- 1.5 mm/week between 30 and 38 weeks
- 1 mm/week after 38 weeks
- Nil at 42 weeks

Intrauterine growth restriction (IUGR) is suspected if growth rate is decreased by <5th percentile. There is a high chance of error when the measurements are between 5th and 10th percentile.

Sensitivity of BPD is considered as only 45% at 34–36 weeks for prediction of gestational age. Though its sensitivity for growth assessment is much higher in earlier pregnancy. As such as the pregnancy advances the genetic factors play a role in controlling the growth pattern and so with advancing pregnancy the accuracy of growth assessment with all biometric parameters decrease. This measurement is not much affected by placental insufficiency or nutritional deprivation and so is more reliable than AC, though it is variable with change in skull shape, like brachycephaly or dolichocephaly. In such cases, it is considered reliable only when confidence interval (CI) is 70–85% (CI: BPD/OFD × 100). As long as the CI is within normal limits, the head shape is considered normal. But when CI is <70 or >85, these are indicators of pathologically abnormal head shape.

Head circumference: It is measured on the outer edges of calvarium, not the scalp on the same plane as BPD. It is the better predictor of gestational age as compared to other commonly used predictors.

This parameter is not affected by change in head shape as long as CI is within limits (70–85). Its sensitivity is 52% and specificity is 80% for prediction of age in the third trimester.

It is altered in trisomy 18, where the head is strawberry shaped or in craniosynostosis.

Depending on the head parameters the IUGR can be classified as:

- *Type I (symmetrical)*: Below –2 standard deviation (SD) in early pregnancy and remains parallel to the normal growth curves.
- *Type II (asymmetrical)*: Falls below line after 30 weeks and therefore it cuts across the normal growth curves.
- *Type III*: Intermediate pattern when there is early deviation of the growth curves, usually in the second trimester.

Ventricular atrium: It is the measurement of the size of the lateral ventricles. It is measured at the level of parieto-occipital sulcus, perpendicular to the medial ventricular wall and not perpendicular to the midline. Calipers are placed inside the ventricular walls **(Figs. 7A and B)**.

The lateral ventricle to hemisphere ratio decreases from 70% at 18–20 weeks to 30% at 28–29 weeks and remains steady thereafter.

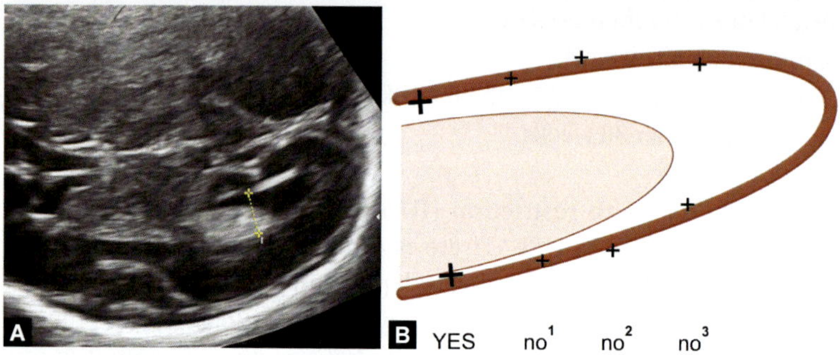

Figs. 7A and B: Ultrasound and schematic diagrams showing assessement of ventricular width.

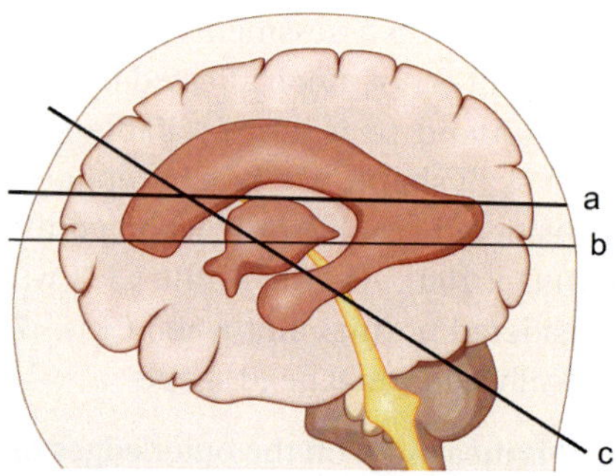

Fig. 8: The three basic axial sections of the head: (a) Transventricular section, (b) Transthalamic section, and (c) Transcerebellar section.

In second and third trimesters, it measures 6–8 mm, 8–10 mm is borderline ventriculomegaly and >10 mm is ventriculomegaly. Ventricular diameter of up to 10 mm is treated expectantly, if it is a solitary finding. Larger ventricular diameters may be considered as a soft marker for chromosomal abnormality. Ventricular diameter of 10–12 mm is ventriculomegaly and >15 mm with increased pressure is called hydrocephalus and may be associated thinning of skull vault and widening of sutures. It is also a marker of abnormal cerebral development. This may require *in utero* or immediate postnatal treatment of the fetus.

Transcerebellar Plane (Line C on the Fig. 8)

This section passes through the cerebellar hemispheres. It is obtained by angulating the probe towards fetal back from the transthalamic plane. Optimum transcerebellar section will show the cerebellar hemispheres, cisterna magna, falx cerebri, septum pellucidum, and also cuts through the thalamus **(Fig. 9)**. Lateral sulcus also extends to this level. As for the previous two sections, the skull vault should be seen as a complete oval outline and should be symmetrical. Orbits should not be seen on this section. Cerebellar

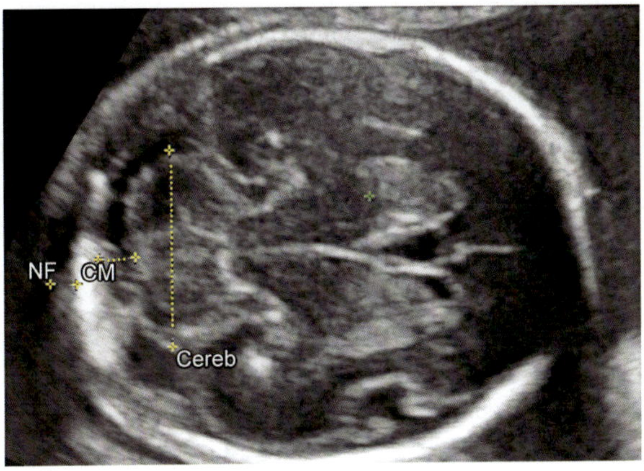

Fig. 9: Transcerebellar section of fetal head showing falx, cavum septum pellucidum, thalamus, cerebellum (Cereb), cistern magna (CM), and nuchal fold (NF).

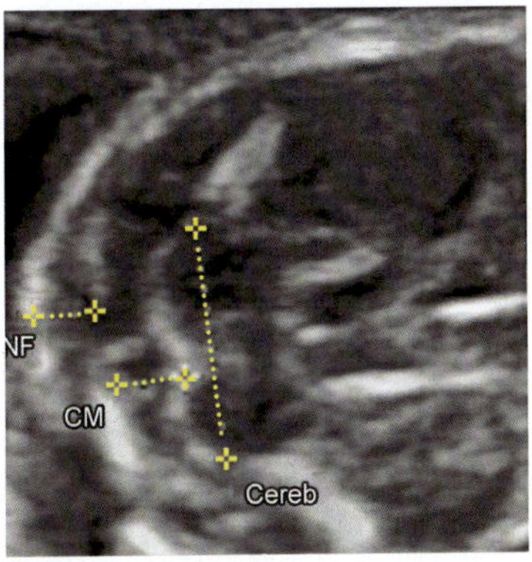

Fig. 10: Transcerebellar section of the head (magnified view) showing measurements of cerebellum (Cereb), cistern magna (CM), and nuchal fold (NF) thickness.

hypoplasia, mega cisterna magna, Dandy-Walker syndrome and variant, and Blake's pouch cyst are the lesions diagnosed on this section.

Cerebellum: It is measured from outer-to-outer margin of the cerebellum on transcerebellar section. Transverse cerebellar diameter increases by 1 mm every week from 14 to 21 weeks. Diameter corresponds to the weeks of gestation in second trimester and is not affected by IUGR. Therefore in cases of severe IUGR, it can be used as a parameter for estimation of correct gestational age **(Fig. 10)**.

Cisterna magna: It is measured from posterior margin of cerebellar vermis to the anterior margin of overlying occipital bone **(Fig. 10)**. Cisterna magna is traversed by thin septa and this is a normal appearance. These represent remnants of the walls of Blake's pouch. These are markers of development of roof of rhombencephalon.

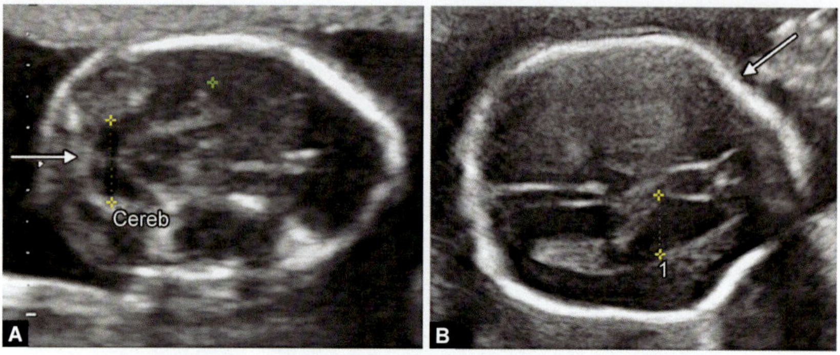

Figs. 11A and B: (A) Obliteration of the posterior concavity of the cerebellum (Cereb) due to open spinal canal defect making cerebellum look-like a banana; (B) Collapsing of the frontal bones due to open spinal canal defect make the calvarial shape look like a lemon-lemon skull.

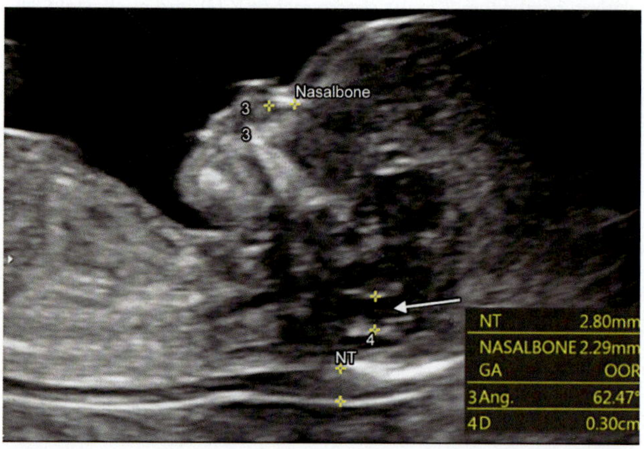

Fig. 12: Midsagittal section of 11–14 weeks fetus showing intracranial translucency.

It measures 2–10 mm but is slightly more in dolichocephaly. It is enlarged in cerebellar pathologies, especially in vermian pathologies, like vermian hypoplasia, Dandy–Walker malformations or variants, but in neural canal defects when cerebellum is pulled caudally and cistern magna is obliterated. This is known as "banana sign" of cerebellum. This is also associated with collapsed frontal bones and makes the skull shape-like a lemon and is called "lemon sign" **(Figs. 11A and B)**.

Though major open spinal canal defects can be suspected as early as the 11 – 13 + 6 weeks scan. Cisterna magna is seen as intracranial translucency in the midsagittal section of 11–14 weeks fetus **(Fig. 12)**.

Transorbital Plane

This plane cuts through the middle of the orbits. It is obtained by slight angulation of the probe towards fetal anterior aspect. It shows both bony

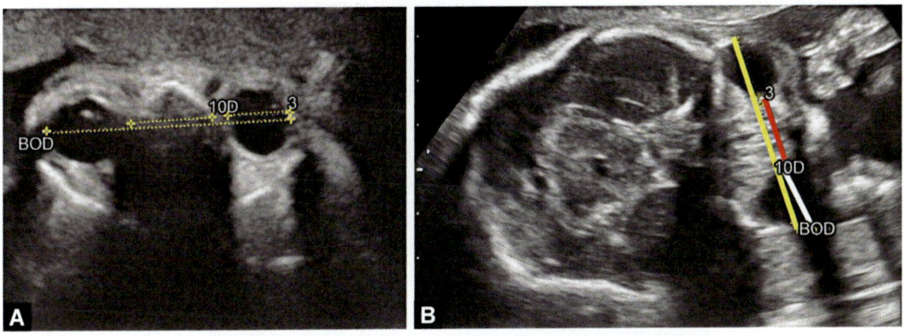

Figs. 13A and B: (A) Transorbital section showing both orbits with lenses; (B) Transorbital section showing the binocular (yellow), interocular (red), and ocular (white) diameters.

orbits in transverse section with nasal bones in between. It might cut through the upper part of the thalamus, but should not show the cerebellum. Bony orbits on this plane show lens—one in each orbit and may also show the artery posterior to it **(Fig. 13A)**.

The quantitative assessment on this plane includes the binocular diameter, interocular diameter, and ocular diameter **(Fig. 13B)**.

Binocular diameter is measured as the largest distance between from lateral inner wall of one orbit to the lateral inner wall of another orbit. Interocular diameter is measured broadest diameter from medial inner bony wall of one orbit to medial inner bony wall of another orbit. Ocular diameter is measured as broadest diameter of orbit from medial inner bony wall to lateral inner bony wall. Interocular distance and ocular diameter are almost equal always. This plane is used to diagnose abnormalities of the orbits such as hypotelorism, hypertelorism, single orbit, and anophthalmia.

Increased interocular diameter is hypertelorism and decreased interocular diameter is hypotelorism. It is best to take the measurements when the fetus is facing the probe. Though lenses are best seen when the fetal face is not towards the probe but on one of the sides.

Plane of Maxilla

This plane is just slightly caudal to the transorbital plane. This plane shows the tooth line of maxilla. This plane is best achieved in a fetal position where the fetus faces the probe. It is used to exclude maxillary abnormalities like cleft palate. The soft tissues seen anterior to the maxilla is the upper lip and so it is one of the views suggested for diagnosis of cleft lip and palate **(Fig. 14)**.

Head: Coronal Section

Lips (Figs. 15A and B)

From the previous plane, 90° rotation of the probe shows coronal or sagittal plane. If sagittal plane is seen on this rotation, lift up the probe to place it on

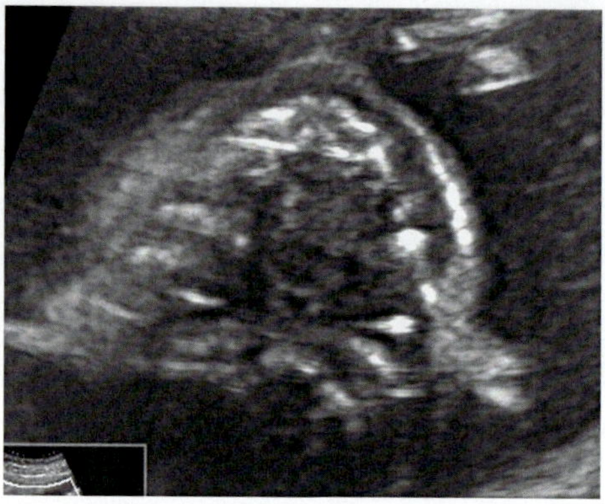

Fig. 14: Maxilla in transverse section.

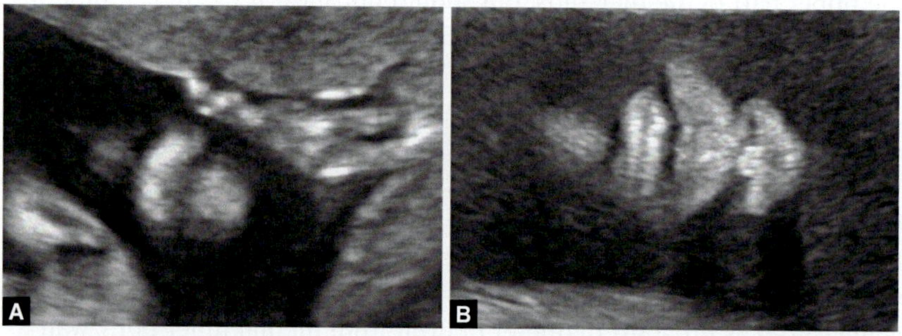

Figs. 15A and B: Nostrils, upper lip, lower lip, and chin seen in coronal section.

one of the sides of the abdomen to see the coronal plane. Move the probe then towards anterior aspect of the fetus and this will show the tip of the nose/nostrils, upper lip, and the lower lip. This plane is used for diagnosis of cleft lip. Fetuses with cleft lip may also show asymmetry of the nostrils which may be seen on this section as well.

Midsagittal Plane

This plane is same as the midsagittal plane taken for nuchal translucency on nuchal scan. A true plane will show the tip of the nose, maxilla in sagittal section as a bold line and not as a triangle, nasal bone, mandible is seen as a dot, no zygoma between nasal bone and maxilla. Because of the ossification of the frontal bone, brain anatomy is not much seen on this section at this stage of pregnancy. This plane is obtained in a fetal position when the fetus is preferably facing the probe. Nasal bone length and frontomaxillary facial angle are the two measurements taken on this plane **(Figs. 16A and B)**. Nasal bone length is measured end-to-end. Frontomaxillary facial angle is measured by drawing one line on the superior surface of the maxilla and the other line is a line joining anterior-superior end of maxilla to the nasion.

Nasion is the point where the nasal bone is attached to the frontal bone. Frontomaxillary facial angle is 66.6–89.5° in normal fetus with a mean of 78.5°. In trisomy 21 fetuses because of the flat face or a flat nasal bridge, this angle is increased to 75.4–104°, with a mean of 88.7°. Even a rotation of the fetal face of 2–3° can lead to a measurement error of 5–15°. Therefore a correct fetal position is very essential. Prenasal thickness (thickness of the skin anterior to the nasion) is also assessed now as one of the markers for trisomy 21.

It is this section which will also demonstrate micrognathia **(Fig. 17)**. This can also quantitatively assessed. Cephalometric analysis by prenatal sonography can be performed to study the anteroposterior jaw relationship. We think that this procedure could be useful to improve prenatal diagnosis of retrognathism in high-risk pregnancies.[1] Inferior facial angle (IFA) and the frontal nasomental angle has been used on stored gray scale images

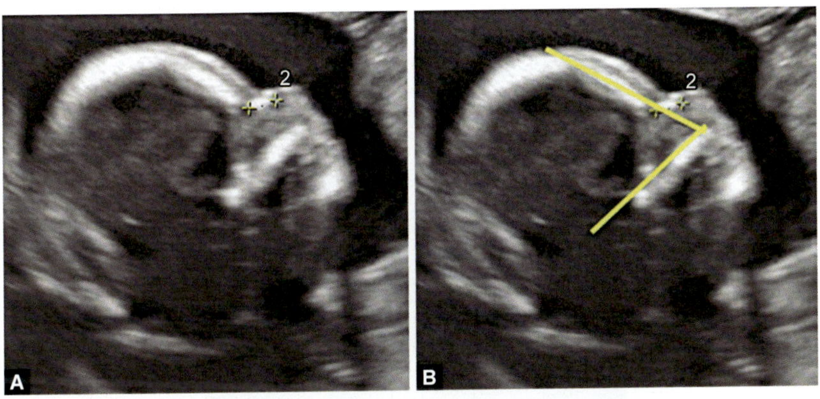

Figs. 16A and B: (A) Midsagittal section of the head showing nasal bone assessment; (B) Frontomaxillary facial angle assessment.

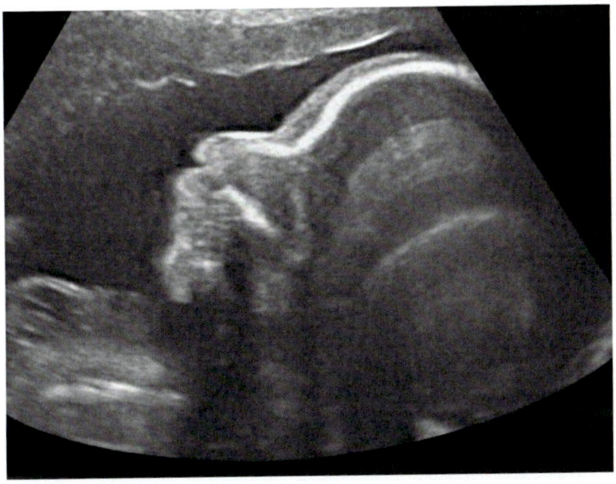

Fig. 17: Midsagittal section of the head showing a small receding chin—micrognathia.

to objectively establish the diagnosis. The mean values for IFA and frontal nasomental angle were 44.8° and 123.3°, respectively.[2]

TRUNK

Axial Sections: Chest

- Four chamber view of heart **(Fig. 18)**
- Left ventricular outflow tract **(Fig. 19)**
- Right ventricular outflow tract **(Fig. 20)**
- Three vessel view **(Fig. 21)**

In above-mentioned four planes will be discussed in detail in the chapter 21 of the book.

Axial Sections: Abdomen

- Section through stomach
- Section through renal pelvis

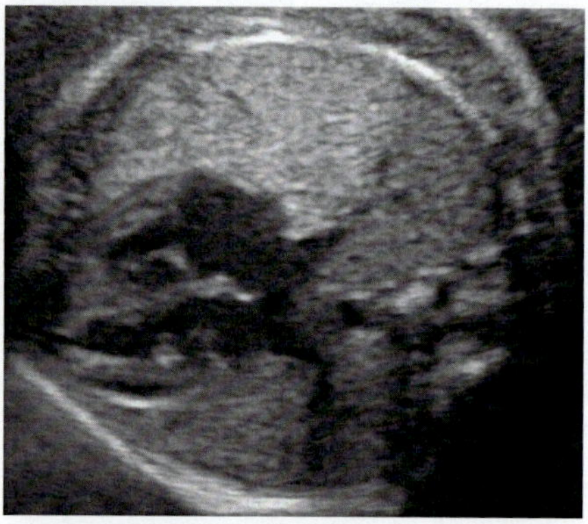

Fig. 18: Four chamber view of the heart.

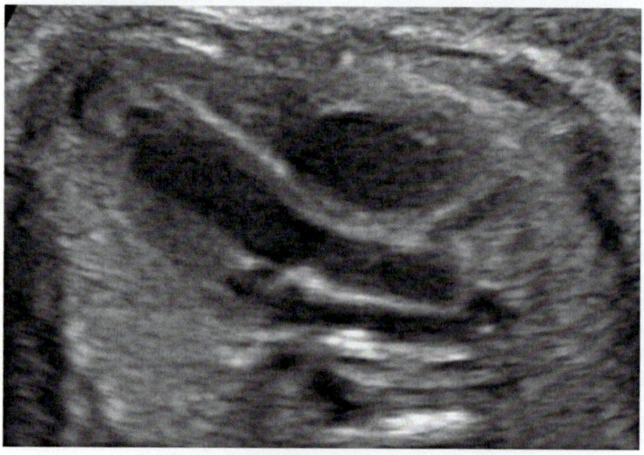

Fig. 19: Left ventricular outflow tract.

- Section through umbilical cord attachment
- Section through sacrum (transverse sacrum section)

Section through the Stomach for Abdominal Circumference

As mentioned, this section passes through the stomach and entry of umbilical vein to hepatic vein seen as a J with curve of the J concave towards fetal right **(Figs. 22A and B)**. The ribs cover the contour symmetrically on both sides. This ensures it is a true transverse section and the section is achieved during fetal apnea. Kidneys must not be seen on this plane.

Abdominal circumference is measured on the outer margin of this section. Most accurate is the smallest measurement. It shows linear rise till 36 weeks of 11–12 mm per week and fall thereafter. It is the first measurement to show alteration in IUGR. This is the single most sensitive measure of fetal growth and so it is better to measure accurately, than to add other parameters.

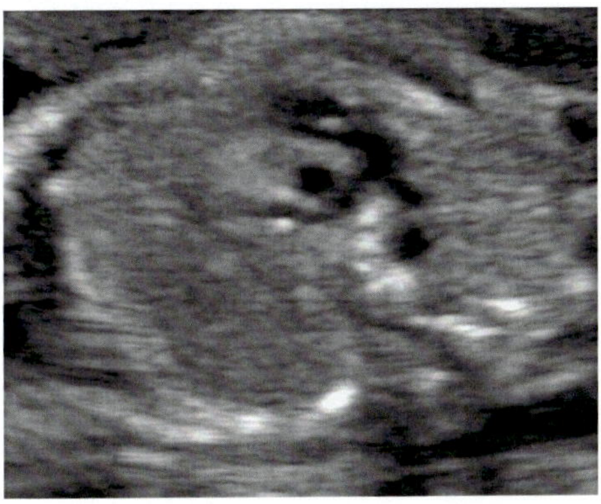

Fig. 20: Right ventricular outflow tract.

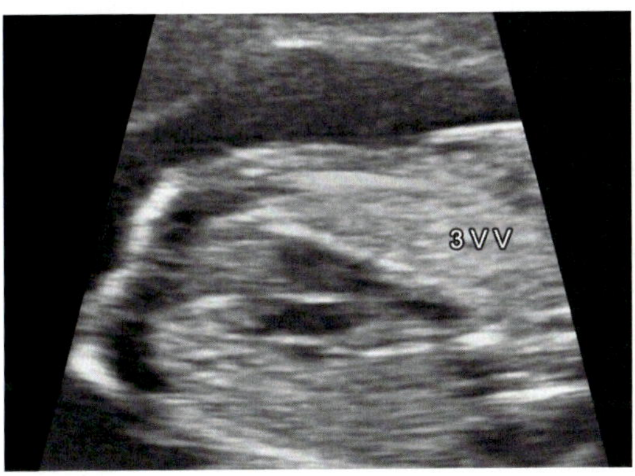

Fig. 21: Three vessel view.

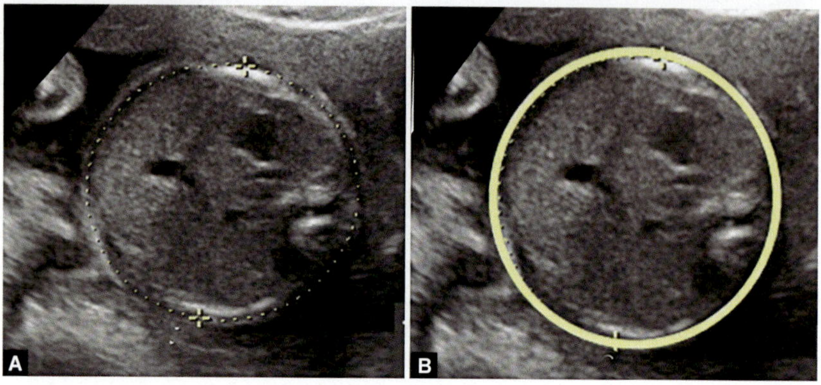

Figs. 22A and B: Axial section of the abdomen showing stomach and mid-third of the vein above-mentioned in the text. Figure B shows the same plane with the measurement of abdominal circumference (AC).

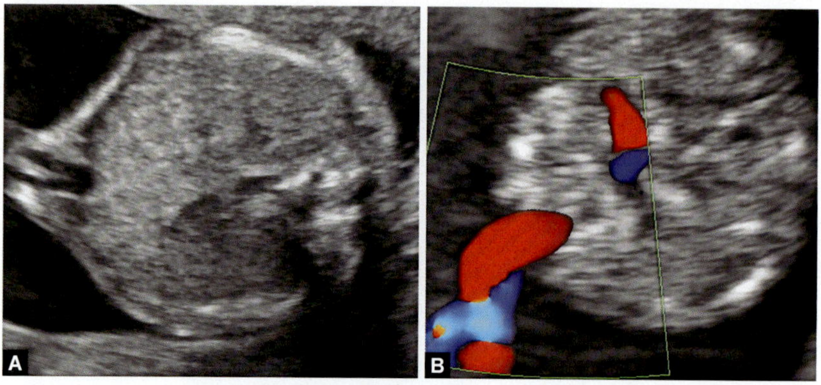

Figs. 23A and B: Axial section of the abdomen showing insertion of the umbilical cord. (A) B-mode; (B) Color Doppler.

Umbilical Cord Insertion Plane

This plane is a true transverse plane again and is caudal to the AC plane. It is at the level where the umbilical cord enters the fetal abdomen.

This plane may be imaged on B-mode or with Doppler **(Figs. 23A and B)**. Doppler has an advantage of showing the entry of cord vessels into fetal abdomen more clearly. This plane helps to exclude abnormalities such as omphalocele and gastroschisis **(Figs. 24A and B)**.

Alternatively, some workers would prefer to demonstrate the cord vessels with the urinary bladder to confirm the presence of two umbilical arteries.

Renal Pelvis Plane

This plane is caudal to the plane of cord insertion and it cuts the abdomen through both renal pelvises. This plane should not include the stomach

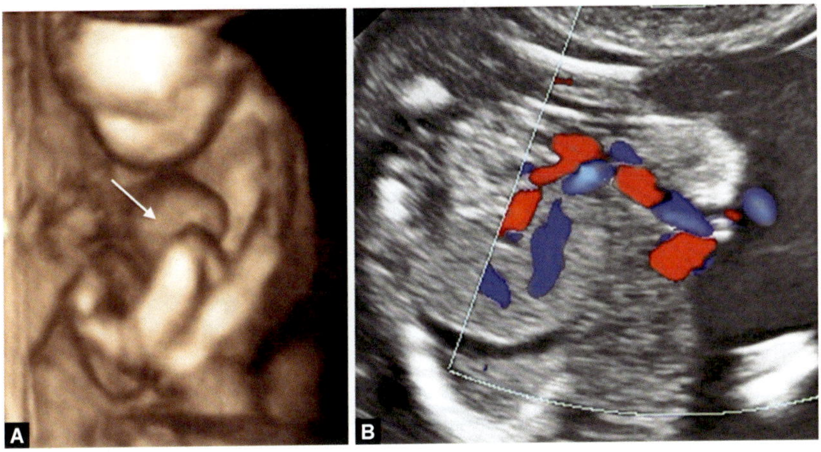

Figs. 24A and B: (A) Omphalocele with the umbilical cord arising from the dome of the herniation; (B) Gastroschisis where the cord is seen arising from the side of the herniation in color Doppler.

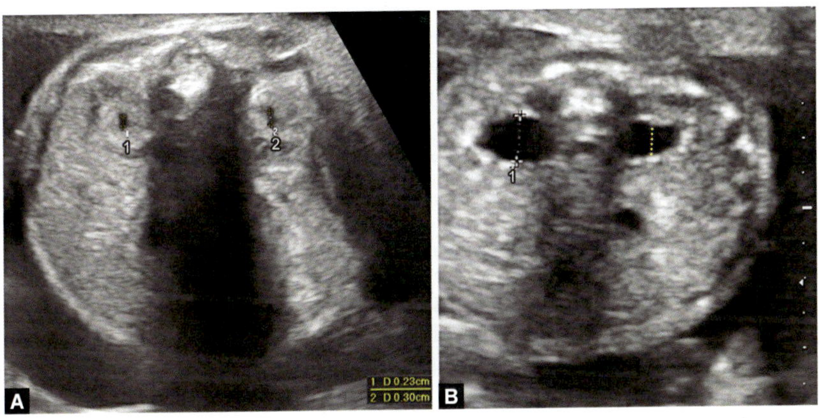

Figs. 25A and B: (A) Transverse section of the abdomen at the level of renal pelvis; (B) Assessment of renal pelvic diameter.

shadow and should be symmetrical and circular. This plane is used to measure the diameter of the renal pelvis. It is best to obtain this section with the fetus in a position, spine anterior or spine posterior. The renal pelvis diameter is measured anteroposteriorly, inner margin to inner margin **(Figs. 25A and B)**.

Normal measurements:

- 16–20 weeks, 4 mm
- 20–30 weeks, 5 mm
- 30–40 weeks, 7 mm

Dilated renal pelvis may be indicative of chromosomal abnormality. There may also be an obstructive lesion in the ureter or bladder leading to dilatation of renal pelvis and may be unilateral or bilateral.

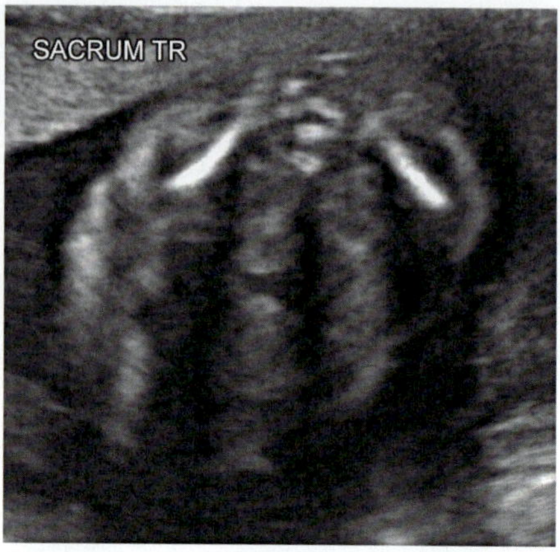

Fig. 26: Transverse section of sacrum.

Transverse Sacral Plane (Fig. 26)

This is the lowest transverse section through the fetal trunk. Two iliac bones are seen with three ossification centers of the sacrum seen in the centre. This helps to confirm absence of spina bifida or open sacral defects at the level of the sacrum.

Abdomen

Midsagittal Section (Figs. 27A and B)

This section is taken to assess the spine in sagittal section. It is seen as two parallel lines of echogenic dots (ossification centers). It is essential to establish the continuity of the overlying skin. It is also important to observe the whole spine, establish the continuity and also to confirm tapering of ossification centers of the sacrum. Though chiefly aimed to assess the spine this plane also shows the bladder.

Coronal Plane

A posterior coronal plane section is essential to observe the whole spine in coronal section **(Figs. 28A and B)**. At the level of vertebral bodies, it is seen as a single line of ossification centers and at the transverse process level, it appears like two parallel lines. Widening of the distance between two lines may be indicative of spina bifida or open spinal canal. Both lines if do not make pairs of ossification centers; it may be indicative of hemivertebrae. On this plane also, it is essential to establish the tapering of ossification in the sacral spine. The vertebral body plane which is a slightly anterior to this plane may also show kidneys in coronal plane.

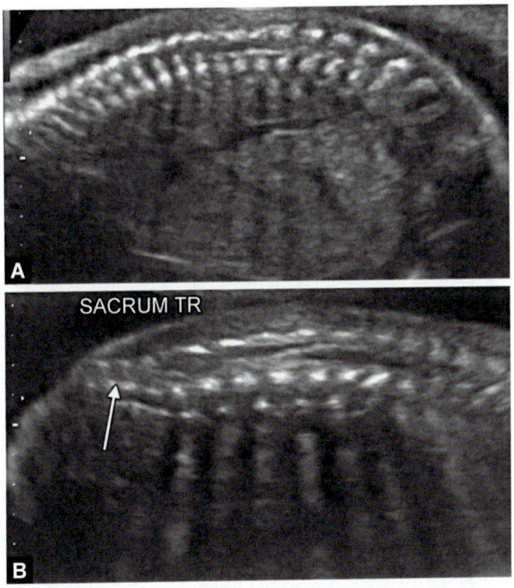

Figs. 27A and B: Midsagittal section of the trunk showing the spine in sagittal plane. (A) Cervicothoracic and upper lumbar spine; (B) Lumbosacral spine (arrow shows the sacral tapering).

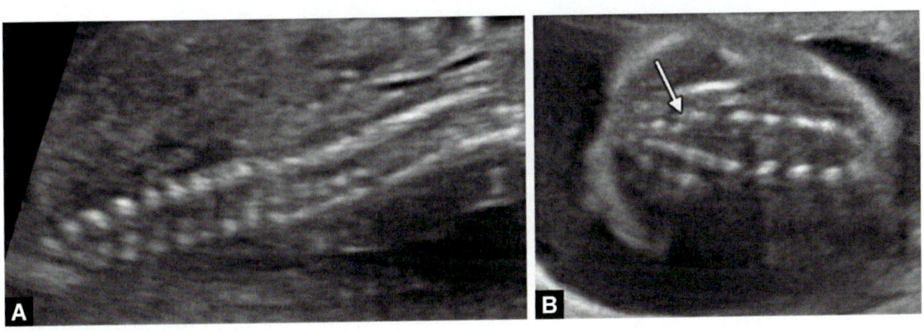

Figs. 28A and B: Coronal section of the spine showing transverse processes of vertebral bodies. (A) Thoracolumbar spine; (B) Lumbosacral spine with sacral tapering (arrow).

Seeing kidneys in this plane is especially important for diagnosis of renal parenchymal disorders and renal dysplasias **(Fig. 29)**.

Limbs

It is essential to document the presence of all four limbs and all three segments of all the limbs. It is best to demonstrate both forearms and hands in a single image and both legs and feet in a single image to establish both limbs have been assessed.

In leg and forearm, presence of two long bones must be documented. Relation of foot to leg and forearm to hand must be established

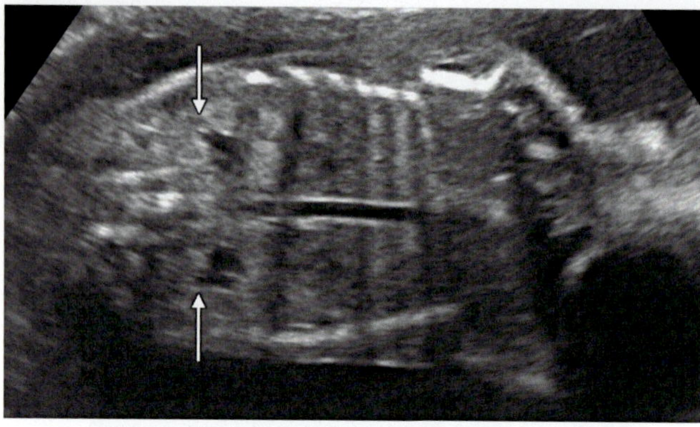

Fig. 29: Coronal section of the abdomen showing renal pelvis on both the sides (arrow).

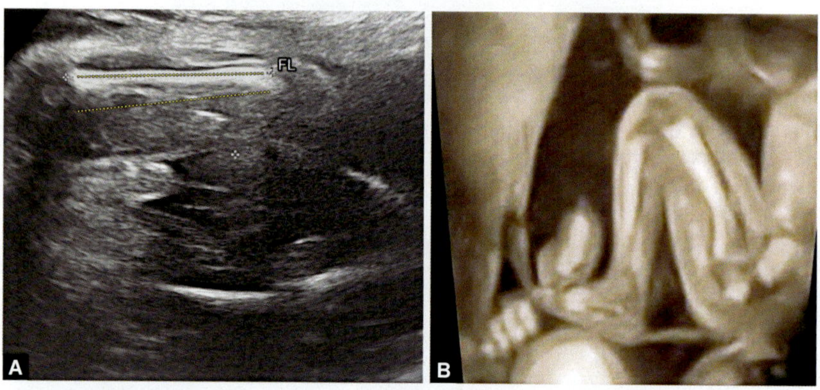

Figs. 30A and B: (A) Femur and its longitudinal measurement; (B) Full lower limb. The special attention is towards the normal relationship of leg to foot.

(Figs. 30A and B). Long bones must be measured end to end **(Figs. 30A and B)**, excluding the epiphysis. Though counting fingers and toes may be done, it is not mandatory for the detailed second trimester scan. If an open hand can be demonstrated with the thumb outside it would be of significance **(Fig. 31)**.

When measuring the femur length (FL), long axis of femur should be aligned with the transducer and only osseous part of diaphysis and metaphysis is measured. Femur grows 3 mm/week from 14 to 27 weeks and 1 mm/week in third trimester.

It shows moderate curvature from 18 weeks onwards giving a typical "golf-club" like appearance. It is not affected in asymmetrical IUGR, but is affected in symmetrical IUGR. But as compared to FL only, FL/AC has been considered to be more reliable. This is so because independent of gestational age the ratio remains constant after 22 weeks. Its sensitivity is

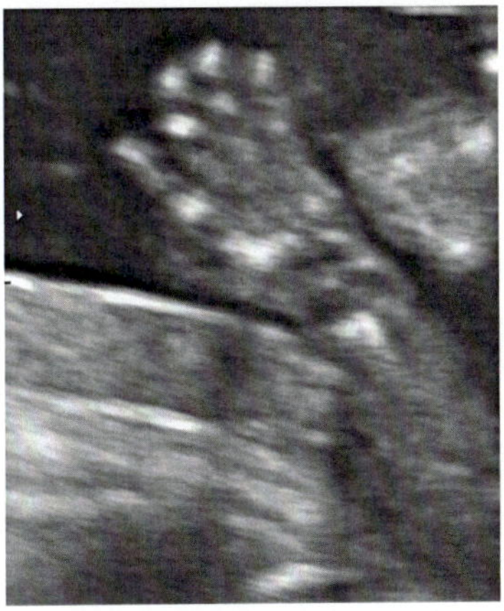

Fig. 31: Open hand with fingers and thumb seen individually.

63% and positive predictive value is 30% for IUGR. We prefer to measure femur, humerus, and tibia in all fetuses.

Apart from assessment of the fetus, it is preferable to assess the placenta and the umbilical cord insertion in the placenta.

It is essential to document the placental location, anterior, posterior or lateral wall and upper or lower part of the uterus. If it is not implanted in the fundal part, it is important to mention the distance of the lower end placenta to internal os. If placental lower end is less than 4 cm from the internal os, it needs a special mention and of it all placenta preavia is present, its grade needs to be mentioned.

- *Grade 0:* Lower segmental-distance from internal os <10 mm
- *Grade 1:* Marginal
- *Grade 2:* Incomplete
- *Grade 3:* Complete

Moreover, it is also essential to conform the interface between the placenta and the myometrium to confirm that the placenta is not adherent to uterus or is not invading into the myometrium or beyond **(Figs. 32A and B)**. If it is a morbidly adherent or invading placenta, the placental vessels will be seen till the depth of the placenta **(Figs. 32C and D)**. Accessory placental lobe is also reported. Placental calcification may be mentioned but according to the latest studies, this calcification that is used for placental grading is now not considered to be of clinical importance as placental grading cannot be correlated to pregnancy-induced hypertension or fetal growth retardation.

Placental attachment of the umbilical cord is also to be documented. Abnormalities of the cord insertion of the placenta are important for management **(Fig. 32E)**.

Amniotic fluid index is assessed as vertical fluid pouch in all four quadrants. The probe must be always kept vertical during assessment of the

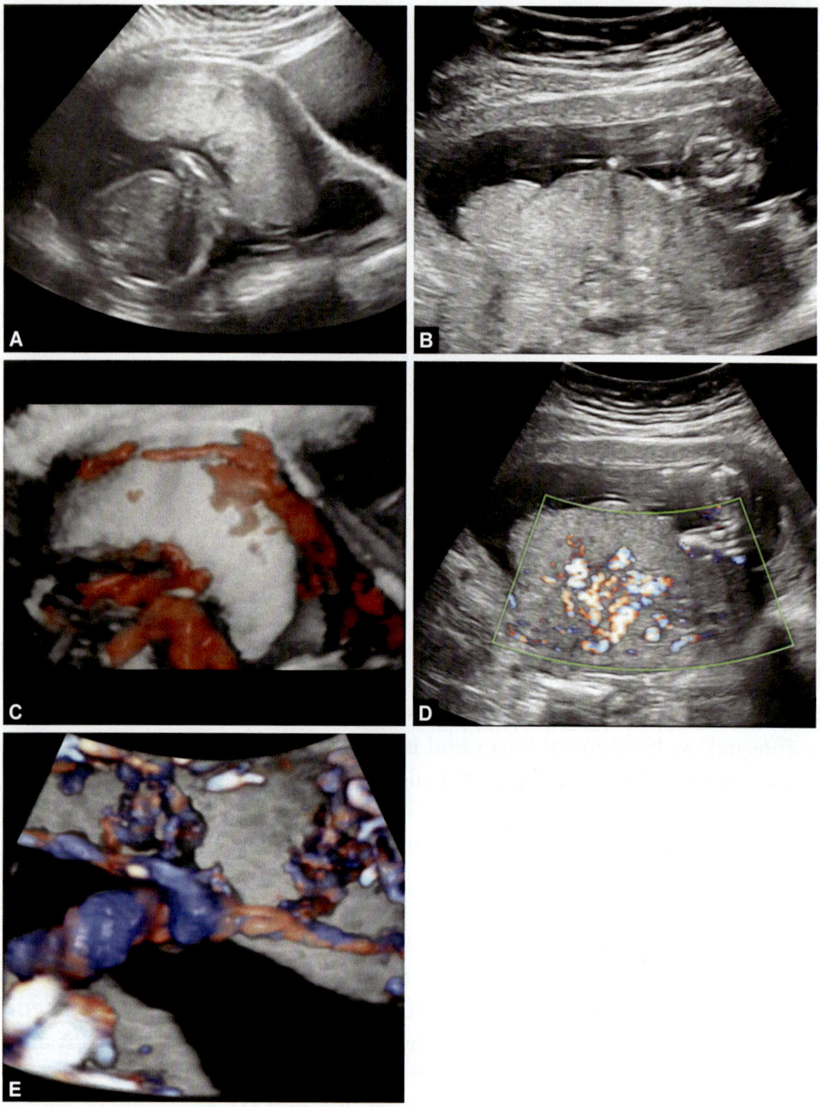

Figs. 32A to E: (A) Anterior placenta with normal placenta-myometrial interface on B-mode ultrasound; (B) Posterior placenta with obliterated placenta-myometrial interface on B-mode ultrasound-morbidly adherent placenta; (C) Normal placental vasculature in the same case as in Figure A, seen on 3D power Doppler; (D) Placental vasculature in the same case as in Figure B, seen on HD flow; (E) Normal cord insertion in placenta seen on 3D HD flow.

amniotic fluid index and the deepest pouch clear of umbilical cord loops or fetal limbs is selected **(Fig. 33)**. Though many workers would prefer to assess only the depth of one largest pocket of amniotic fluid. And a single pocket of 5–8 cm may be considered adequate.

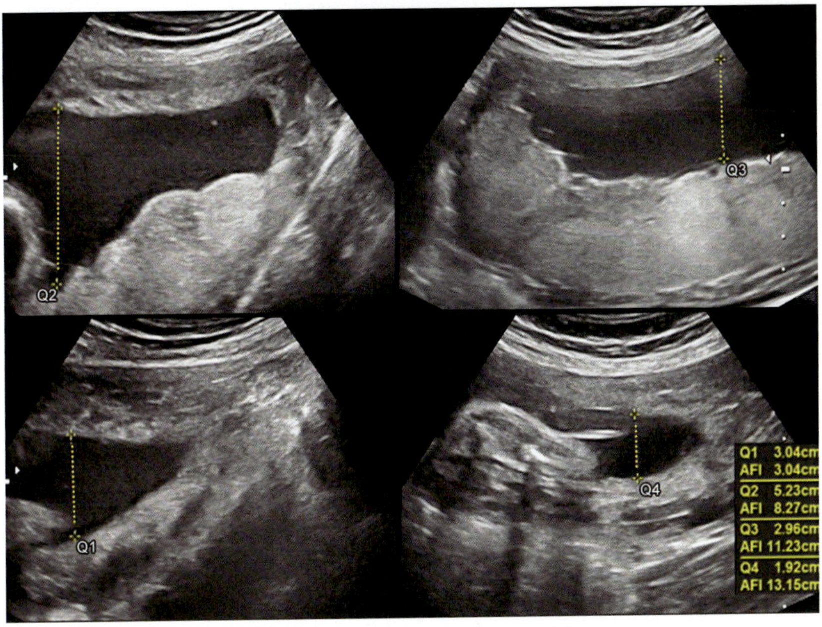

Fig. 33: Assessment of the amniotic fluid index in four quadrants.

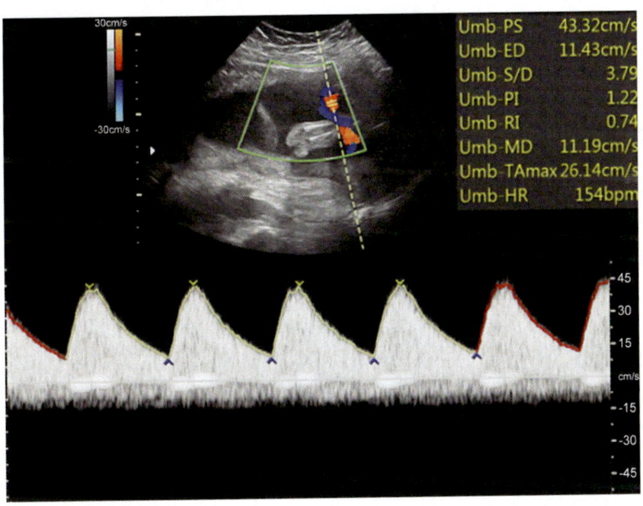

Fig. 34: Spectral Doppler of umbilical artery showing its normal waveform.

Apart from this, the second trimester scan must include assessment of the uterine artery and umbilical artery Doppler. Umbilical artery flow can be assessed in any free loop of umbilical cord but in very mobile fetus, the cord insertion at the placenta may be selected as a site of preference for Doppler assessment of the umbilical artery. Though is thought that the resistance is a

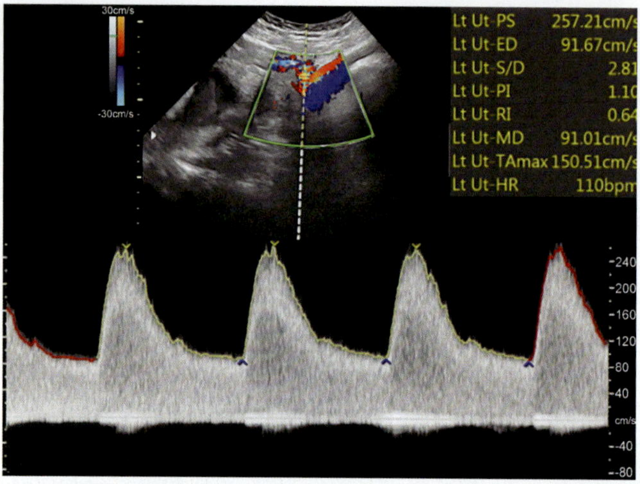

Fig. 35: Spectral Doppler of uterine artery normal waveform in second and third trimesters.

little different at the fetal end and the placental end, this difference is not of much clinical significance.

Umbilical artery flow is usually a moderate resistance flow **(Fig. 34)** and normally the resistance keeps on decreasing as age advances.

The uterine artery is localized by moving the probe from the symphysis pubis laterally without angulating it. Where the iliac vessels are seen in long axis, a slight medial angulation of the probe shows uterine artery crossing iliac vessels perpendicular to the iliac vessels. Uterine arteries are usually high-resistance flow in the early pregnancy but are fairly low resistance vessels in later pregnancy **(Fig. 35)**, especially on the side of the placenta, if the placenta is not central.

A systematic scan thus done in the second trimester is capable to excluding almost all major and especially nonprogressive abnormalities of the fetus.

REFERENCES

1. Captier G, Faure JM, Bäumler M, Canovas F, Demattei C, Daures JP. Prenatal assessment of the anteroposterior jaw relationship in human fetuses: from anatomical to ultrasound cephalometric analysis. Cleft Palate Craniofac J. 2011;48(4):465-72.
2. Rotten D, Levaillant JM, Martinez H, Ducou le Pointe H, Vlcaut E. The fetal mandible: a 2D and 3D sonographic approach to the diagnosis of retrognathia and micrognathia. Ultrasound Obstet Gynecol. 2002;19(2):122-30.

CHAPTER 19

Fetal Screening for Chromosomal Anomalies

Sonal Panchal

INTRODUCTION

As seen in sonoembryology, at 12–13 weeks, the fetus is a fully developed human being and naturally therefore, if only one scan is to be done in the first trimester to detect abnormalities, it should be done after 10 weeks, preferably 11–12 weeks. The purpose of this scan is to look for structural abnormalities, but more importantly for chromosomal abnormalities and the most feared of the chromosomal abnormalities is trisomy 21 (T21) or Down's syndrome. Though trisomy 13 (T13) and trisomy 18 (T18) are though not uncommon, fetuses with these abnormalities either die intrauterine or soon after birth. T21 babies wherein have a nearly normal life-span, and because of the marked mental retardation that they have as a result of their aneuploidy, they are not capable most of times of independent existence and so they suffer a lot and also are burden on the society. For this reason when we discuss about fetal screening for chromosomal abnormalities, it is chiefly about Down's syndrome, though we shall also discuss the markers for the other two aneuploidies.

It is important here to understand that screening means segregating the high-risk patients from the low-risk patients. Screening does not diagnose an aneuploidy; it only tells as to how much is the risk of a particular fetus being chromosomally abnormal. There are different tests offered for screening. The most primary is the age of the patient.

It has been studied that the risk of chromosomal abnormalities increases as the maternal age advances and is very high when maternal age is more than 35 years. These women are considered, high-risk mothers. But that does not mean that only the fetuses of the mothers of 35 years of age or more are at risk, because as seen on the graph **(Fig. 1)**, only 30% of the babies having Down's syndrome have been born to the mothers of more than 35 years of age. This clearly means that 70% of the Down's babies are born in the low-risk group mothers.

The risk of chromosomal abnormalities is higher in those fetuses whose siblings have chromosomal abnormalities, or mother has a family history of chromosomal abnormalities, or is the fetus has any structural abnormalities, etc. Apart from the history, other screening tests include hematological investigations such as dual marker, triple marker, and quadruple marker.

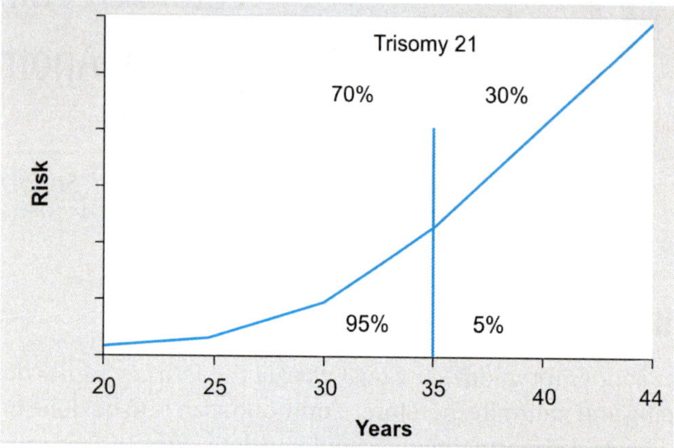

Fig. 1: From Fetal Medicine Foundation, 11–13+6 weeks scan.

Though triple marker is not commonly used now. A dual marker test consisting of free β-human chorionic gonadotropin (β-hCG) and pregnancy-associated plasma protein-A (PAPP-A) can be done from 10 to 14 weeks. Free β-hCG and PAPP-A increases and decreases with the gestational age, respectively. In order to standardize and eliminate the variation associated with gestational age, they are converted to multiples of median (MoM). In euploid pregnancies the average free β-hCG is 1.0 MoM and PAPP-A is 1.0 MoM. In T21 at 12 weeks, the maternal serum concentration of free β-hCG is about twice as high (2 MoMs) and PAPP-A is reduced to about half (0.5 MoM) compared to chromosomally normal pregnancies. In T18 and T13, both the serum markers are reduced. The individual risk is derived by the laboratories using software and this risk is compared to the cut-off risk for final interpretation, follow-up, and management. But the testing and risk assessment should be done by the laboratories that are conscious for their quality of work.

Quadruple marker includes alpha-fetoprotein, unconjugated estriol (uE3), free β-hCG, and inhibin A and is done between 15 and 19 weeks. The detection rate (DR) for quadruple tests is 65–75% respectively, for a false positive rate (FPR) of 5%.

Ultrasound (US) is also used as an important modality for screening these fetuses. If by screening a particular fetus proves to be at high risk then diagnostic test is done. These include chorion villous biopsy, amniocentesis, etc.

Down's or any other chromosomal abnormalities can be most confidently diagnosed by invasive testing like amniocentesis and chorion villous biopsy followed by chromosomal study. But these invasive tests have 1% risk of abortion. Moreover being invasive can be offered only to the high-risk mothers, which means detecting only 30% of Down's babies, and if this method was preferred 70% of the Down's babies will be missed on antenatal screening.[1]

ULTRASOUND AS A SCREENING MODALITY

In early 90s, some subtle anatomical variations were detected in the fetuses with chromosomal abnormalities. Though these subtle variations could be detected in about 2% of normal fetuses, their frequency was very high in fetuses with aneuploidies. These subtle anatomical variations are called markers for aneuploidies. It is important to remember here that markers are subtle variations in the usual features and these are not abnormalities.

Based on this knowledge of markers, a detailed scan was designed that could be best done between 11 and 13+6 for detection of aneuploid fetuses and was called a *genetic scan*.

By definition, a genetic sonogram is defined as an US scan that can modify the *a priori* risk of fetal aneuploidy, typically based on a panel of US markers. The background risk which depends upon the maternal age and gestational age is referred to as the "a priori risk". To this the risk (0.75%) of previous chromosomally abnormal fetus is added if the patient has such a history. Screening is started after that. Depending on the positive or negative likelihood ratio (LR) of present or absent abnormal marker.[2,3]

This scan is done for detection of:

- *Major structural anomalies in aneuploidies:*
  - Compatible with life
  - Incompatible for independent existence
- *Chromosomal markers:*
  - Most indicative or major markers
  - Soft markers

Structural abnormalities that must be looked for and are detectable on early 11–13+6 weeks scan can be listed as follows:

- *Neural tube abnormalities:*
  - Holoprosencephaly
  - Anencephaly and/or acrania
  - Iniencephaly
  - Spina bifida
- *Facial abnormalities:*
  - Cleft palate
  - Ocular abnormalities
  - Micrognathia
  - Short/low placed ears
- Cardiovascular abnormalities
- *Abdominal abnormalities:*
  - Diaphragmatic hernia
  - Duodenal atresia

- Omphalocele
- Mega cystitis

- Limb reduction abnormalities
- Hydrothorax-ascites.

NEURAL TUBE ANOMALIES

Holoprosencephaly (Fig. 2)

This abnormality is complete or partial deficiency of falx leading to alobar, semilobar or lobar type of holoprosencephaly. Lobar is the mildest form with defect of the falx only in mid hemispheric region and often not diagnosed till late pregnancy and also has least neurological implications. Whereas alobar is the most extensive defect leading to severe neurological deficits and can be diagnosed as early as 12–14 weeks of gestational age. This shows single spherical cerebral structure, with single common ventricle, posterior large cyst of third ventricle known as dorsal sac, absent olfactory bulbs and tracts and single optic nerve. Septum pellucidum is always absent with midline fusion of cingulated gyrus and frontal horns of lateral ventricles. These have flat roof and freely communicate with third ventricle.

About 40–60% of the holoprosencephalic fetuses have chromosomal abnormalities, of which 50% are T13. Of those which are euploids, 90% have facial abnormalities. The commonly seen abnormalities include cyclopia, hypotelorism, proboscis, and median cleft lip.[4,5] About 70% have other structural abnormalities.[6] Alobar and semilobar holoprosencephaly are more likely to be associated with aneuploidies, rather than the lobar ones.

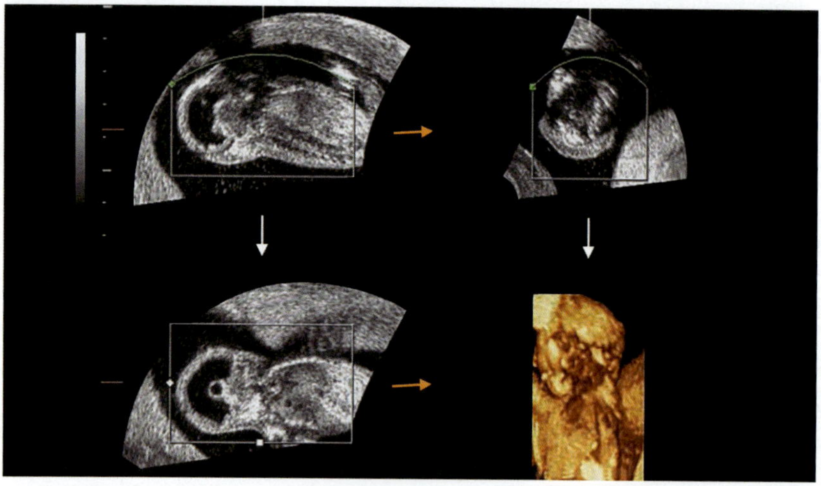

Fig. 2: Holoprosencephaly.

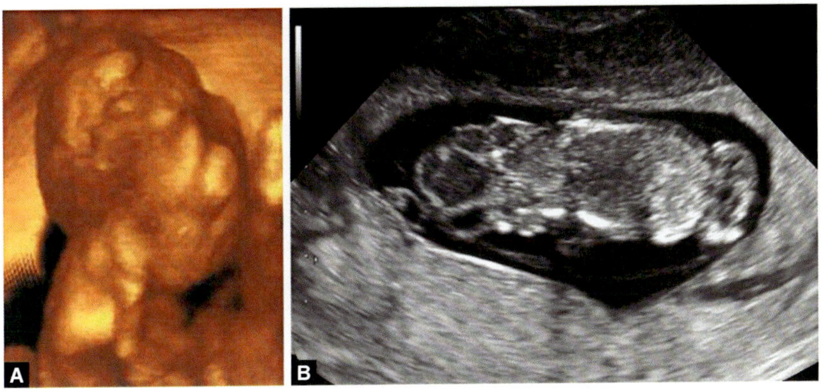

Figs. 3A and B: Exencephaly and acrania.

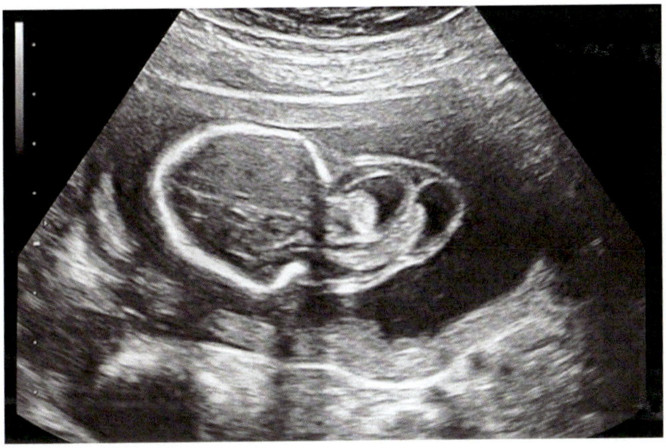

Fig. 4: Encephalocele.

Acrania/Exencephaly and Anencephaly (Figs. 3A and B)

Acrania is total nonossification of skull vault bones and exencephaly is partial (above the orbits) nonossification of skull vault bones. It may evolve from exencephaly. Ossification of the skull bones starts and accelerates at 9 weeks of gestation. Acrania can, therefore, be diagnosed after 11 weeks. In acrania, brain matter lies free in the amniotic cavity and shows abnormal shape of the head due to disintegration of brain matter. Typical shape of the head is described as Mickey Mouse head when majority of the brain matter is disintegrated.

Smaller defects in skull vault with herniation of the meninges or brain matter is described as cephaloceles **(Fig. 4)**.

Anencephaly is a neural tube defect. Total disintegration of brain matter and appearance is described as frog face as the orbits become the most protruding structures. There is no forehead or calvarium **(Fig. 5)**.

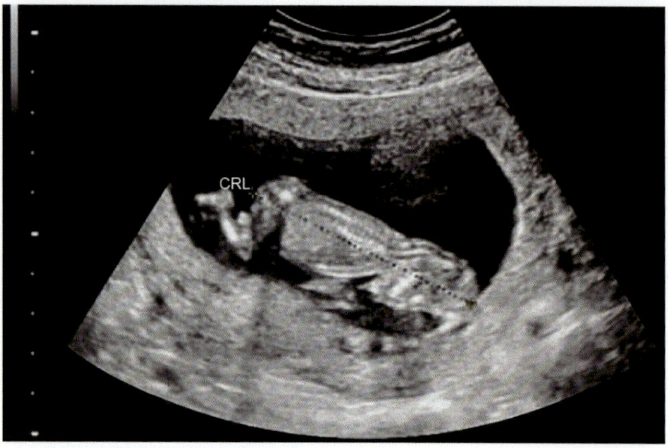

Fig. 5: Acrania.

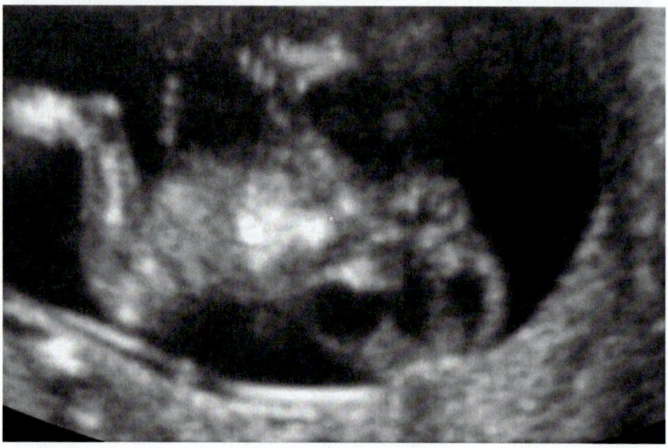

Fig. 6: Iniencephaly.

Iniencephaly (Fig. 6)

This is a lethal anomaly with defect in occiput involving foramen magnum, a complete spinal bifida, retroflexion of entire spine—star gazing fetus and open spinal canal defects of variable degrees. Associated abnormalities such as hydrocephaly, microcephaly, ventricular atresia, and holoprosencephaly are also known. It may also be associated with diaphragmatic hernia, urinary tract abnormalities, cleft lip and palate, omphalocele, and thoracic cage abnormalities with polyhydramnios; though these associated abnormalities may be more evident only in second trimester.

Spina Bifida and Hydrocephalus (Figs. 7A and B)

The most common abnormality of spine, detectable in first trimester is open spinal canal defects or spine bifida. About 14% fetuses with spina bifida have

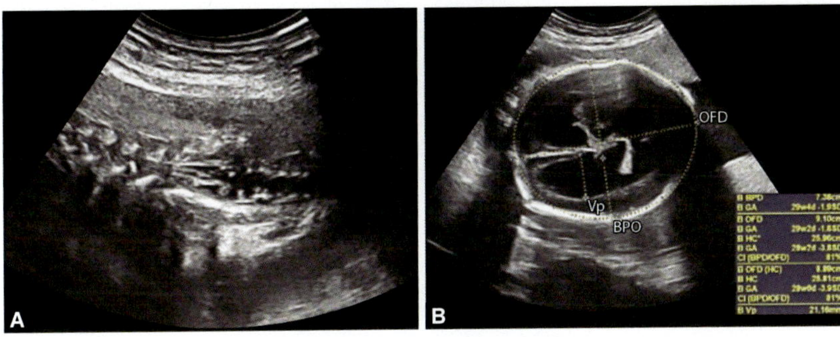

Figs. 7A and B: Spina bifida with hydrocephalus.

aneuploidy, most commonly trisomies 18, 13, triploidy, and translocation.[7] Hydrocephalus is a common association and consequence. About 22% of the fetuses with chromosomal anomalies may present only with spina bifida and hydrocephalus in first trimester.

The earliest sign for open spinal canal defects is measuring intracranial translucency (IT). This requires the same section as that for nuchal translucency (NT) and, therefore, we shall discuss it later in this chapter.

FACIAL ANOMALIES

The midline facial anomalies especially with holoprosencephaly are commonly associated with trisomies 18 and 13 and so, whenever found detailed study for chromosomal abnormalities is mandatory. Facial abnormalities are best diagnosed by volume US, rendered imaging as coronal view of the face is required which is more easily obtainable on three-dimensional (3D).

Cleft Lip and Palate

Lip becomes continuous at 8 weeks and, therefore, a cleft can be diagnosed at 11–14 weeks scan. On nuchal scan, on the coronal plane of the face, prenasal triangle is seen, on a plane just anterior to the coronal section of orbits. This triangle is formed of two tiny nasal bones (NBs) at the apex, sides formed by frontal process of maxillary bone and base formed by maxillary plate. Incomplete bas on this plane indicates cleft palate. The imaging plane for this is considered correct when the two echogenic dots of ossification centers of maxillary bone are placed within the width of the base of this triangle This has been discussed in Chapters 17 and 18.

The chances of aneuploidy with cleft palate are:

- 20–30%, if unilateral cleft palate (more common on left side and in females)
- 30–50%, if bilateral cleft palate
- 50–80%, if median cleft palate

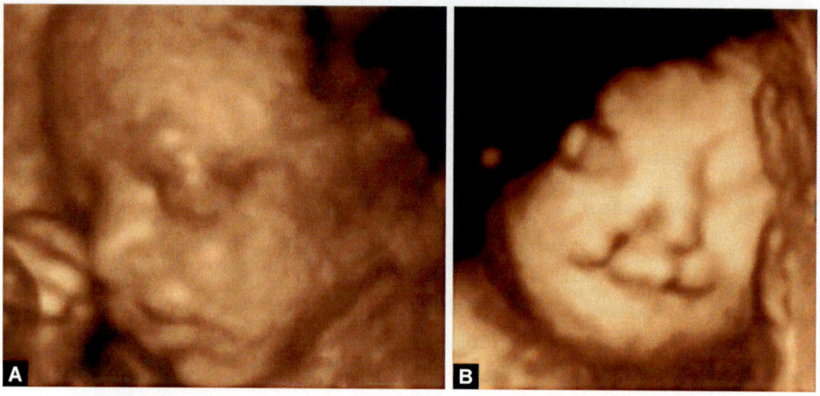

Figs. 8A and B: Cleft lip and cleft palate on three-dimensional ultrasound.

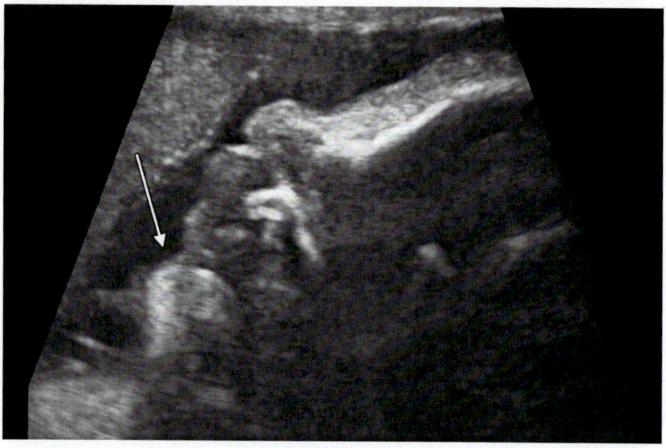

Fig. 9: Micrognathia.

Isolated cleft lip without a cleft palate is not commonly associated with aneuploidies.[8] Three-dimensional ultrasound is an impressive modality to demonstrate this abnormality **(Figs. 8A and B)**.

OCULAR ABNORMALITIES

Cyclopia (single orbit in the center), hypotelorism (closely placed orbits) or hypertelorism (widely placed orbits) are associated with trisomies 13, 18, and nonchromosomal syndromes. These are best demonstrated on coronal or transverse plane of the face.

Micrognathia (receding small chin) may be an indicator of T18 or triploidy **(Fig. 9)**. This is best seen on the midsagittal plane, which is same as the plane for NT.

Short low placed ears **(Fig. 10)** are typically associated with trisomies 21, 18, and 13 and have similar value as increased NT in detection of fetal

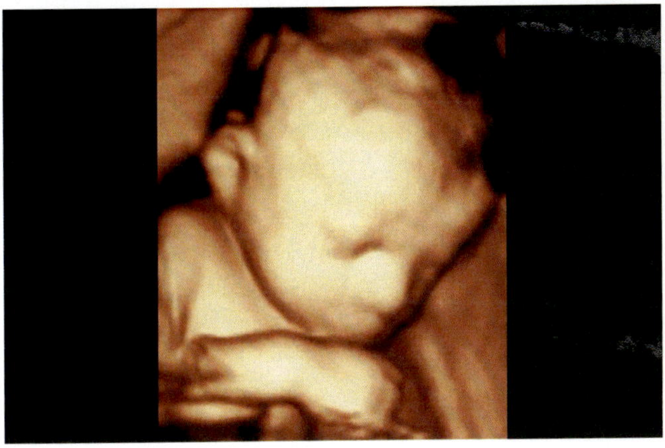

Fig. 10: Low placed ear.

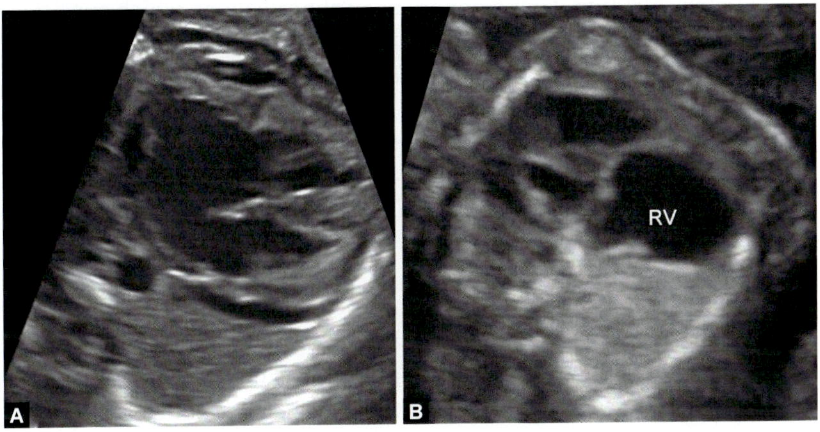

Figs. 11A and B: (A) Complete atrioventricular septal defect; (B) Ebstein's anomaly.

aneuploidies. But these are not easy to diagnose on B-mode US and so are not included in major markers. Though volume US can be diagnostic.

Prominent occiput may be seen in T18 fetuses.

CARDIAC ABNORMALITIES

About 22–32% of fetuses with cardiac anomalies have chromosomal anomalies.[9] Only 0.1% of euploid neonates have cardiac abnormalities but 13% of the aneuploid neonates have cardiac abnormalities.

Atrioventricular septal defects (AVSDs) **(Fig. 11A)**, ventricular septal defect (VSD), Ebstein's anomaly **(Fig. 11B)**, Fallot's tetralogy **(Fig. 12)**, and hypoplastic left heart are often associated with aneuploidies.[10] Ectopia cordis, only when associated with pentalogy of Cantrell, is associated with trisomies.

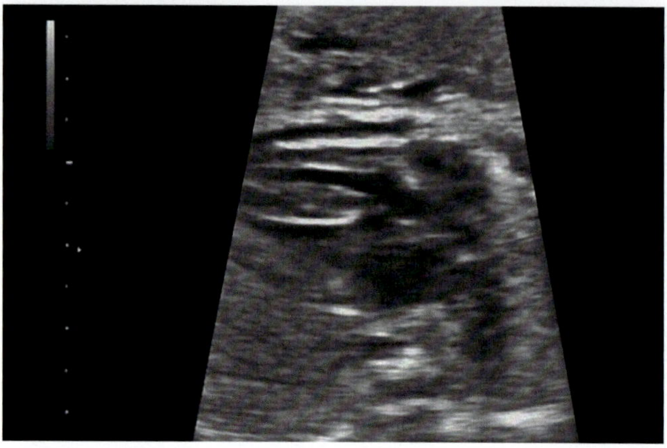

Fig. 12: Fallot's tetralogy.

(Pentalogy of Cantrell has a panorama of abnormalities, which consist of median supraumbilical abdominal defect, defect in lower sternum, defect of diaphragmatic pericardium, defect of anterior diaphragm, and intracardiac abnormality).

Isomerism, transposition of great arteries, pulmonary atresia, and stenosis are never associated with aneuploidies.

The incidence of cardiac abnormalities in fetuses with chromosomal abnormalities is:

- 90% in T13
- 40–50% in T21
- 15–20% in Turner's syndrome

Detailed echocardiography is out of the scope of this chapter. But it is still essential to emphasize at this point that with advancing technology of US, it is now possible to study fetal heart transvaginally in late first trimester in detail.

ABDOMINAL ABNORMALITIES

Diaphragmatic Hernia (Fig. 13A)

About 10–20% of fetuses with diaphragmatic hernias have chromosomal anomalies, the most common being T18, but are more significant when associated with other abnormalities, especially increased NT. Diaphragmatic hernia is diagnosed on US by assessing the transverse section of the thorax at the level of four chamber heart. Heart is displaced to right side and stomach shadow or bowel shadows are seen at the same level as the four chamber heart. Stomach shadow may not be seen in the abdomen. Though, liver herniation in the thorax is rare, if present displaces the heart to extreme left side. In cases of diaphragmatic hernia, prognosis depends on the resultant pulmonary hypoplasia.

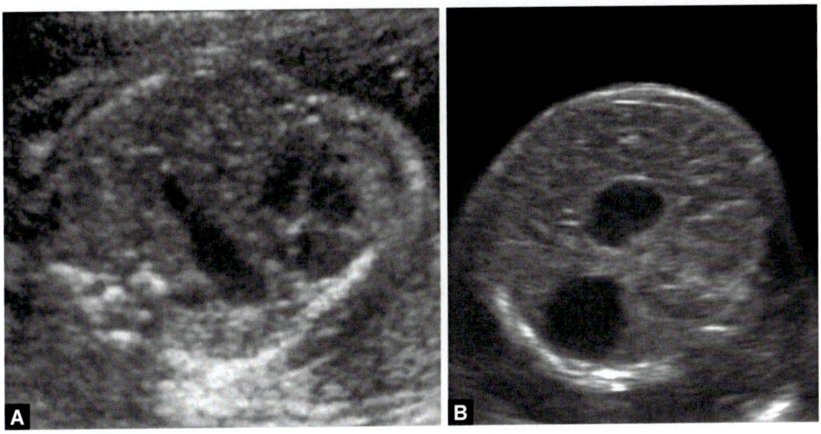

Figs. 13A and B: (A) Diaphragmatic hernia; (B) Double bubble sign—duodenal atresia.

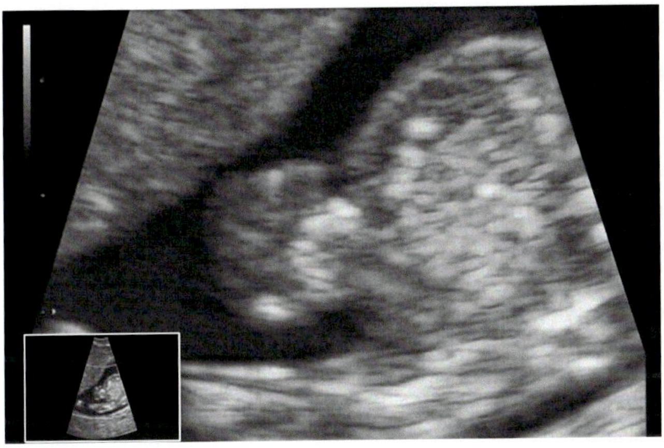

Fig. 14: Omphalocele—three-dimensional ultrasound and two-dimensional ultrasound.

Duodenal Atresia (Fig. 13B)

One-third of the fetuses with duodenal atresia have T21.[11] Typical sign described to diagnose duodenal atresia is "double bubble sign", where one bubble is the distended stomach and the other one is the distended duodenal cap. But duodenal atresia is very difficult to diagnose before 20–24 weeks. Karyotyping is a must when duodenal atresia is diagnosed.

Omphalocele (Fig. 14)

It is physiologically present from 8th to 12th weeks of gestation but is considered abnormal if it persists after 12th week of gestation. It increases the risk of T18. Even before 12th week, an omphalocele may be considered abnormal if:

- Has a neck of more than 7 mm
- It is larger than or of the size of the abdomen or
- There is herniation of the liver.

An omphalocele may contain bowel or liver, but those containing liver are usually not associated with aneuploidies.[12] The bowel containing omphalocele is commonly associated with syndromes and 50% of bowel containing omphaloceles are associated with cardiac anomalies also.

When it contains bowel, it appears more echogenic than abdomen which contains liver, and when it contains liver, abdomen is more echogenic, which contains bowel.

About 40–60% of the fetuses with omphalocele have chromosomal anomalies and is 10 times more common in fetuses with increased NT. Others are likely to have nonchromosomal syndromes like Turner's syndrome or uniparental disomies.

Gastroschisis (Fig. 15)

This is another anterior abdominal wall defect. This defect is usually to the right of the umbilicus with evisceration of abdominal organs. Gastroschisis can be diagnosed as early as 12 weeks of gestation. This condition is not often associated with chromosomal abnormalities, but is associated with other structural abnormalities such as exstrophy of bladder, intrauterine growth restriction (IUGR), and malrotation of gut.

Genitourinary Anomalies

The most common ones associated with chromosomal abnormalities are bladder outlet obstruction and megacystis **(Fig. 16)** and are most commonly

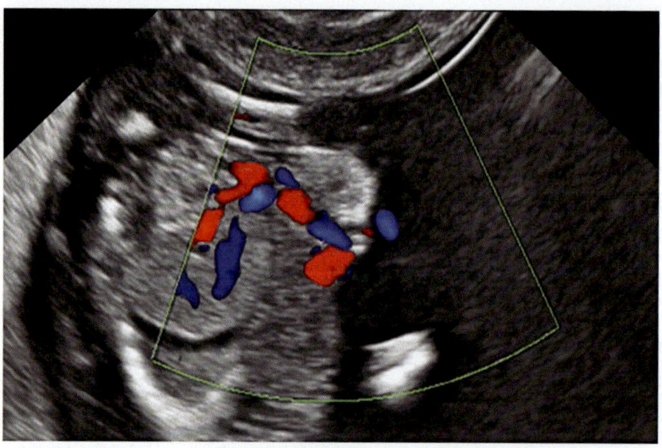

Fig. 15: Gastroschisis—cord insertion is seen by the side of the anterior abdominal wall defect.

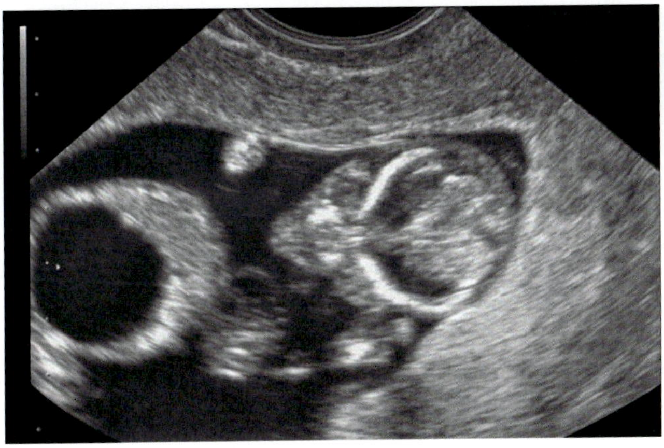

Fig. 16: Megacystis.

associated with trisomies 18 and 13.[13] More proximal genitourinary tract malformations are less associated with chromosomal abnormalities, and the risk is still lower with unilateral affections. More over these are less likely to be diagnosed in the first trimester.

Fetal kidneys are consistently seen after 11 weeks of gestation normally. Their absence may indicate agenesis which may be confirmed by absence of renal vessels also (unilateral or bilateral) on Doppler examination. Kidneys are hyperechoic oval structures at 12 weeks. Dysplastic kidneys though may appear large with cystic lesions. Renal pyelectasis has been discussed with chromosomal markers.

SKELETAL ABNORMALITIES

Limb reduction deformities and radial aplasia indicate a risk of T18. Isolated club foot is not commonly associated with chromosomal abnormality, especially in an otherwise low-risk patient. But there is a consensus that whenever a club foot **(Figs. 17A to C)** is seen, a fetal karyotyping must be done because there is a possibility of presence of many other subtle abnormalities, which are very likely to be missed on first trimester scan, if a very careful detailed search is not done.

Hand makes an important landmark for chromosomal abnormalities. Clinodactyly is seen in T21, clenched hands in T18, polydactyly in T13, and syndactyly in triploidy.

Generalized skeletal dysplasias such as achondroplasia **(Fig. 17C)** and achondrogenesis can be diagnosed on late first trimester scan by disproportionately short long bones. It is easy to note this disproportion in the first trimester as the whole fetus can be seen in a single frame. Osteogenesis imperfecta is diagnosed by nonossified bones. This may be seen as less echogenic bones of skull and limbs.

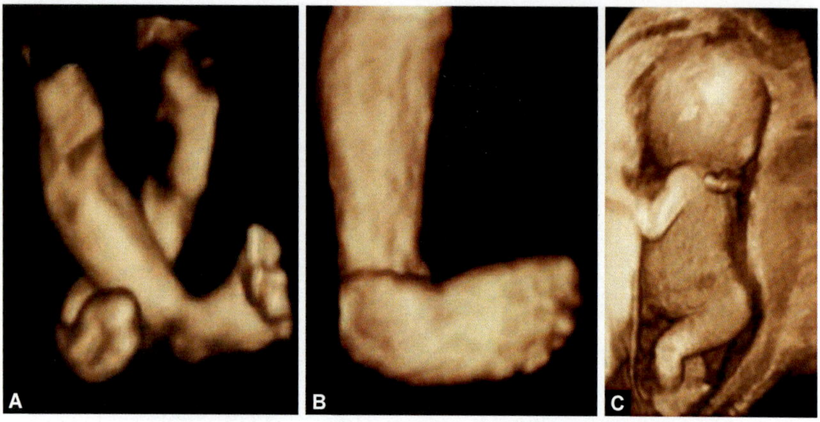

Figs. 17A to C: (A and B) Club feet; (C) Achondroplasia.

Sirenomelia (fusion of lower limbs) if present can be diagnosed as early as 10–11 weeks and is commonly associated with other abdominal structural abnormalities and single large umbilical artery.

MISCELLANEOUS ABNORMALITIES

Ascites and hydrothorax suggest possibility of aneuploidy or infection, especially when present without hydrops.

As such any abnormalities in the fetus should lead the sonographer towards the search for the chromosomal anomalies, except the acquired disorders which are a result of tissue or vascular disruption, e.g., tumors, hydranencephaly, amniotic band syndrome, limb body wall complex, jejunal atresia due to vascular insufficiency, and gastroschisis and complex anomalies like cardiosplenic syndrome. The identification of a major anomaly obviates the need for further screening tests and calls for diagnostic invasive test because:

- If the abnormalities are lethal or associated with severe handicap, invasive testing and fetal karyotyping may determine the possible cause and predict the risk of recurrence in future pregnancy.
- If pregnancy is to be continued in case of a potentially correctable defect it is essential to exclude chromosomal defect.

CHROMOSOMAL MARKERS

Markers, as already been discussed, are not structural abnormalities but are subtle variations in the normal anatomy, that indicate the presence of chromosomal abnormalities. If sonographic markers for fetal anomalies are taken into consideration with other sonographic findings, 50–70% of T21, 80% of T18, and 90% of T13, fetuses will show positive genetic sonogram.

These markers are divided into major and soft markers depending on their sensitivity for the diagnosis of aneuploidies.

Major or most indicative markers:

- Nuchal translucency—cystic hygroma
- Ductus venosus flow
- Nasal bone length

Nuchal Translucency

Nuchal translucency (NT) refers to the sonographic appearance of subcutaneous accumulation of fluid behind the fetal neck in the first trimester. Normally, NT is 1.5–2.5 cm between 10 and 12 weeks and 2–3 mm between 12 weeks and 14 weeks. NT increases by 17% every week. It must be remembered that there is no cut-off value for NT. It has definite values for definite gestational age so ideally the calculated values must be placed on the nomograms for correct risk assessments. Though any value above 3 mm surely requires counseling. These nomograms are based on the NT values in relation to crown-rump length (CRL). Therefore, correct assessment of CRL is essential. CRL is measured in midsagittal plane of the fetus, when the fetal trunk and neck are neither extended nor flexed. In the correct plane the proximal long bones (femur and humerus) are never seen. Both crown and the rump must be clearly seen and the straight distance from crown to rump is measured **(Fig. 18)** The prevalence of defects increase from 0.8 to 65.8 per thousand as the NT increases from below 95th percentile to above 99th percentile **(Fig. 19)**.

Measuring Nuchal Translucency (The Fetal Medicine Foundation) (Fig. 20A)[14]

Nuchal translucency can be measured accurately by transabdominal route in 95% of cases, while in others transvaginal ultrasonography would be required.

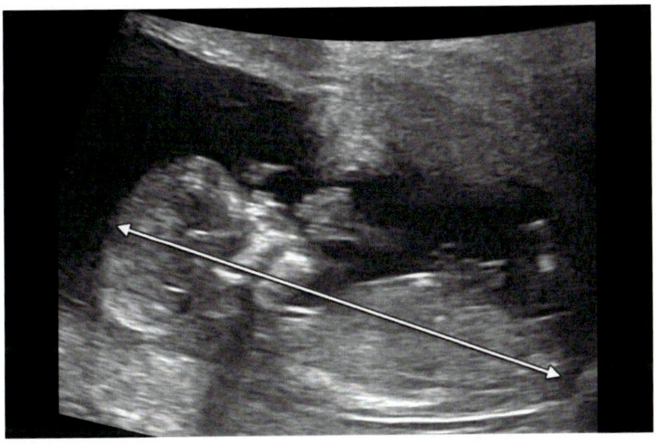

Fig. 18: Measurement of crown-rump length.

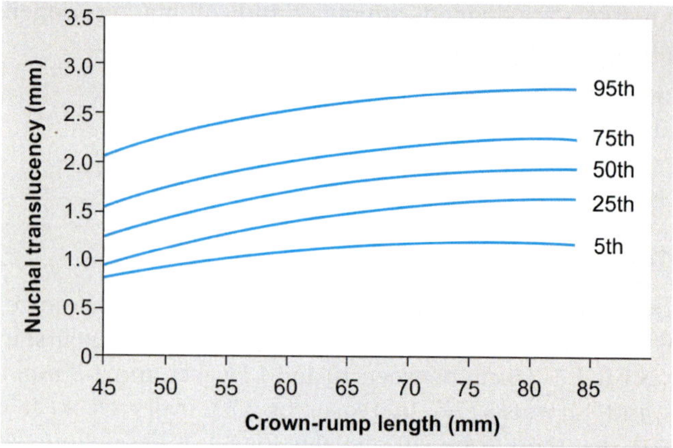

Fig. 19: Chart of 95th, 75th, 50th, 25th and 5th centile values of nuchal translucency varying with CRL.

- When CRL is between 45 and 84 mm, preferably 45–84 cm.
- In true sagittal section, in which:
  - Echogenic tip of the nose
  - Nasal bone
  - Rectangular shape of palate anteriorly
  - No bone is seen between NB and palate (zygoma)
  - Fluid in third ventricle between thalami
  - Diencephalon is seen
  - Aqueduct of Sylvius in between cerebral peduncles
  - Mandible is seen as a point.
- With maximum magnification—75% should cover the screen (caliper 0.1 mm).
- Neutral position—neither extension, nor flexion of the head, because NT increases by 0.6 mm on extension and reduces up to 0.4 mm on flexion of the fetal neck. Cord round neck leads to false increase in NT up to 0.8 mm measurements above and below the cord depending on how tight is the loop tied.
- Maximum width of the translucency between the skin and soft tissues posterior to the cervical spine.
  - The calipers should be placed on the interface between the tissue (white line) and nuchal fluid that describes the NT—the horizontal line of the crossbar of the caliper should merge with the white line of the margin and not seen in the nuchal fluid.
  - It is important to take more than one measurement and record the maximum one **(Fig. 20B)**.
  - Care must be taken to distinguish between fetal skin and amnion.

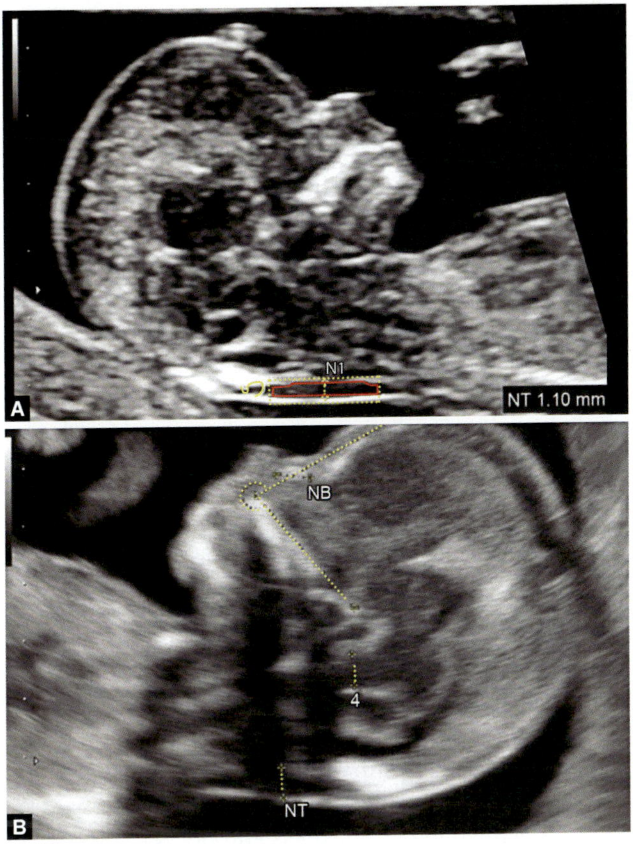

Figs. 20A and B: Measuring nuchal translucency (NT)(NB: nasal bone).

When NT is measured in this way, the interobserver and intraobserver error is only of <0.5%. Accurate measurement of NT requires adequate training, expertise, and adherence to the standard protocols laid by the Fetal Medicine Foundation (FMF), UK. The individual measuring NT should be ideally certified by FMF and his/her performance should be regularly audited.

About 75–80% of the fetuses with trisomies 21 and 5–10% of euploid fetuses may show increased NT. But even in euploid fetuses with increased NT prevalence of major defects was 7.3%. NT may be increased due to several causes apart from aneuploidies.

Causes of Increased Nuchal Translucency

- *Chromosomal anomalies*: Altered extracellular matrix composition is seen in chromosomal abnormalities as the component proteins of extracellular matrix is encoded on chromosomes 21, 18, and 13. The diagnosis can be guided by a few associated features and dual marker tests.

- *Trisomy 18:* Early IUGR, relative bradycardia, and omphalocele (both free β-hCG and PAPP-A are low)
- *Trisomy 13:* IUGR, relative tachycardia, omphalocele, and holoprosencephaly
- *Turner's syndrome:* Early IUGR and tachycardia
- *Triploidy:* Asymmetrical IUGR, bradycardia, holoprosencephaly, omphalocele, posterior fossa cyst, and molar changes in placenta.

It has also been found in other genetic syndromes like achondrogenesis type II due to altered collagen metabolism in achondroplasia and thanatophoric dysplasia due to abnormal fibroblast growth factor receptors and in Zellweger's syndrome due to disturbed metabolism of peroxisome biogenesis factor.

- *Cardiac abnormalities and overload in T-T transfusion*: The prevalence of the cardiac defects increased from <3% at NT of <3 mm at 14 weeks, to 15% if it was >5.4 mm.[15]
- *Venous congestion* due to fetal constriction due to amniotic rupture or superior mediastinal compression due to diaphragmatic hernia or narrow chest due to skeletal dysplasias.
- *Delayed development of lymphatic drainage*: Neuromuscular defects such as fetal akinesia sequence leading to impaired lymphatic drainage.
- *Congenital infection* causing fetal anemia and cardiac dysfunction.
- *Anemia and hypoproteinemia*: Increased NT may resolve at and after 16 weeks. Moreover the subcutaneous fat deposition starts after 16 weeks and then the significance of NT decreases. What we measure after 16 weeks is nuchal fold thickness and not NT. It is very important to remember here that spontaneous resolution of increased NT does not exclude chromosomal defects. A normal karyotype in the fetuses with increased NT also does not exclude structural abnormalities, especially cardiac abnormalities and abnormalities of abdomen.

Significance

- Nuchal translucency only picks up Down's syndrome in 85% of high-risk patients and in 75% of low-risk patients.
- Maternal age + NT + NB + serum parameters 97% sensitivity with 5% false negative (FMF, London 2004).

The Fetal Medicine Foundation Multicenter Project Report

Assessment of risk by combination of maternal age and NT followed by invasive diagnostic testing for 5% of pregnancies with screen positive result and selective termination of affected fetuses, would reduce the live birth incidence of T21 by 75%.[16]

Nuchal translucency scan with dual marker test for risk assessment can be done according to following two schedules depending on the convenience of the doctor and the patient:

1. Both the NT measurement and the biochemical markers can be analyzed at the same time at 12 weeks. This option is employed in United Kingdom at OSCAR (One-Stop Clinic for Assessment of Risk) clinics, where the results of the combined screen are available in 30 minutes. The DR is 85–90% for a FPR of 5%.
2. Serum biochemical analytes are measured at 10 weeks and NT is done at 12 weeks in two separate visits. It has been estimated that this approach would improve the DR to 93–94%. But, the disadvantage will be an increase in the noncompliance rate that is associated with this method.

In twin babies with twin-to-twin transfusion, NT is frequently increased. In recipient fetus, it is a manifestation of heart failure due to hypervolemic congestion. As the gestation advances, there would be diuresis, which will correct the hypervolemia, decrease the heart strain and resolve the NT.

Limitations

- If normal NT is considered as THE sign for a normal embryo, chances are there to miss a significant percentage of abnormal babies, so detailed structural scan is always a must.
- Increased NT, as a single sign may be rarely seen in a normal baby also.

Nuchal Fold Thickness (Fig. 21)

Nuchal fold thickness is measured as the total soft tissue thickness behind the cervical spine. It is measured in axial plane on transcerebellar section.

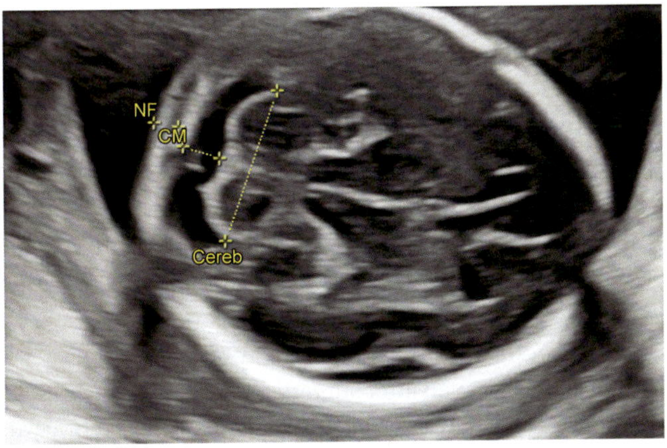

Fig. 21: Nuchal thickness (BPD: biparietal diameter; HC: head circumference; OFD: occipitofrontal diameter).

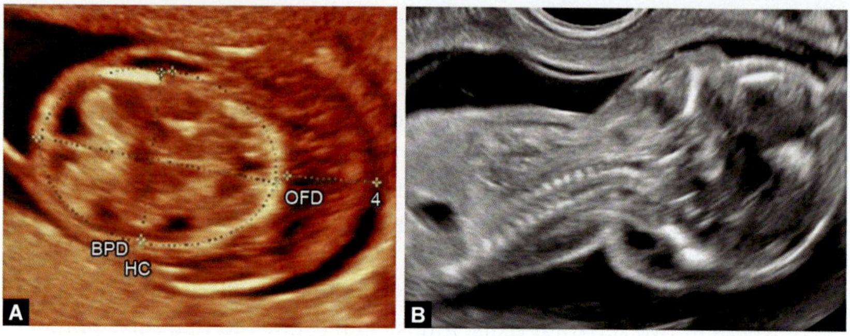

Figs. 22A and B: Cystic hygroma (BPD: biparietal diameter; HC: head circumference; OFD: occipitofrontal diameter).

It is to be measured only between 15 and 20 weeks when the skin thickness is constant. It is normally ≤5 mm, though if plotted on graphs as MoM, it has specific LRs at a particular thickness and particular gestational age. It is found to be increased in 0.1% of normal but 80% of Down's fetuses, and is also seen in fetuses with Noonan's syndrome and cardiac abnormalities. Like NT, this also may be a transient sign or may be present after resolution of cystic hygroma, but that does not decrease the risk of aneuploidy and must be considered as important as NT for the suspicion of aneuploidy or cardiac defect.

Cystic Hygroma (Figs. 22A and B)

It is grossly increased nuchal edema which extends beyond neck to involve the back and the head also. Cystic hygroma may or may not be septated. Nonseptated nuchal edema increases the risk of cardiac defects or trisomies, whereas septated cystic hygroma is almost invariably associated with Turner's syndrome.

Cystic hygroma is the one isolated abnormality, where invasive testing is must because 47–73% of fetuses with cystic hygroma have cytogenetic anomalies and one-third fetuses have nonimmune hydrops. But isolated cystic hygromas in atypical location are not notably associated with chromosomal abnormality.

In 37% of fetuses, cystic hygroma will resolve in second trimester. If it progresses to lymphangiectasis or persists in second trimester, chances of Turner's syndrome are more and it may be fatal.

Milder cases of cystic hygroma have better prognosis. Surgical correction after birth is possible. But even after surgery for correction of cystic hygroma, bony abnormalities of mandible, occipital bone and vertebrae and facial palsy may persist. Counseling for cystic hygroma therefore should be done very carefully.

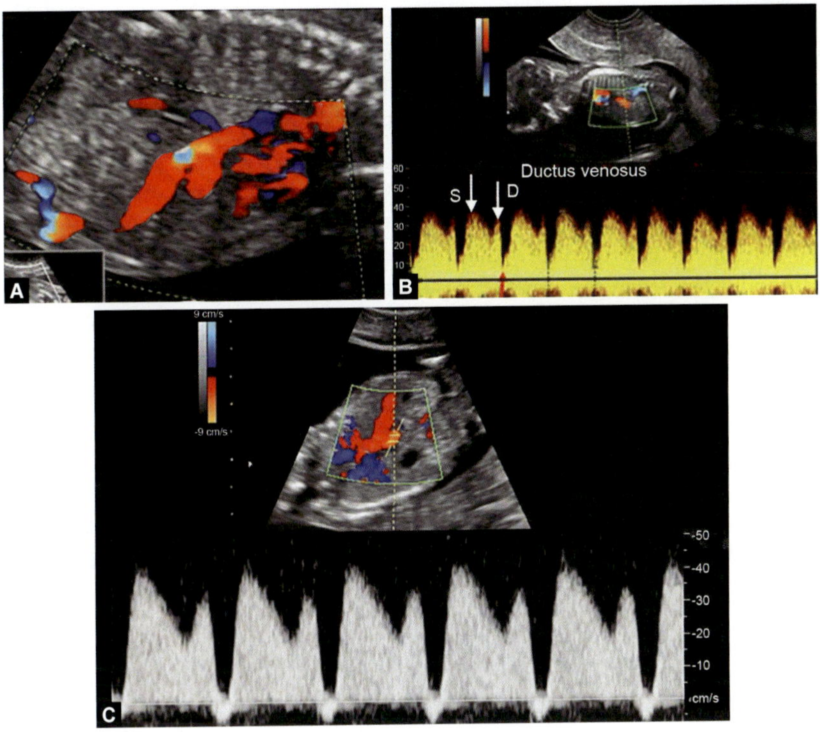

Figs. 23A to C: (A and B) Ductus venosus flow; (C) Abnormal ductus venosus flow.

Ductus Venosus Flow

Ductus venosus is a vessel that connects the umbilical vein to the right atrium of the fetal heart. It has no anatomical continuity with the umbilical vein but connects portal sinus to the umbilical sinus. It is only 2 mm in diameter at its inlet into the umbilical sinus but carries 56% of the total fetal oxygenated blood. Ductus venosus flow velocity is approximately three times higher than the flow velocity in the umbilical vein or inferior vena cava. This vessel can be visualized in midsagittal longitudinal section or oblique transverse section through upper abdomen as a most bright spot on color Doppler. It shows a continuous forward triphasic flow **(Figs. 23A and B)** normally, where the first peak indicates the ventricular systole, the second peak corresponds to ventricular diastole, and the deepest point after the second peak corresponds to the atrial systole and is known as the A wave. Reversed diastolic flow that means an absent flow or flow reversal at A wave, indicates chromosomal or cardiac anomalies **(Fig. 23C)**. Though early in first trimester an immature sphincter of ductus venosus would give a reversal if the A wave due to back flow of blood into the ductus with atrial systole. Absent/inverted A wave has been seen in about 70–90% with chromosomal anomalies.[17] About 40%

fetuses having an abnormal ductus venosus waveform show increased NT. Evaluating it inversely, fetuses with increased NT showed abnormal ductus flow in 90% of chromosomally abnormal fetuses or with cardiac defects. With the addition of new sonographic markers to the combined test, the DR would be 93–96% for a FPR of 2.5%.[18]

An abnormal ductus flow in T21 can be explained by increased levels of atrial and brain natriuretic peptide messenger ribonucleic acid in fetal heart suggesting heart strain. This abnormal waveform may be in the form of reversal of the A wave or increased pulsatility index.

But this alteration in the waveform must be very carefully evaluated as it is very common to make a mistake of examining the hepatic vein instead of ductus venosus, which would show a reversal of A wave normally. Ductus venosus is best picked up in midsagittal plane as the brightest color spot below the diaphragm on color Doppler. Doppler sample should be small (0.5–1.0 mm) to avoid contamination from the adjacent veins. The insonation angle should be less than 30°. The filter should be set at a low frequency (50–70 Hz) to allow visualization of the whole waveform. The sweep speed should be high (2–3 cm/s) so that the waveforms are assessed better.

Nasal Bone (Figs. 24A and B)

As is often observed that Down's syndrome babies have a flat nasal bridge and a flat nose. This observation was applied into the fetal evaluation for diagnosis of Down's syndrome. It was observed that 40% of Down's syndrome fetuses have absent NB but no euploid fetuses showed this finding.[19] LR of absent NB for Down's syndrome is as high as 83.

So that makes NB a very important marker, independent of NT for diagnosis of aneuploidies. The NB is nonossified in 60% of fetuses with T21. In the normal population, the frequency of nonossified NB is related to the ethnicity of the mother. It is 2.2% in Caucasians, 5% in Asians, and 9% in the Afro-Caribbeans. This needs to be taken into account while evaluating the individual patient risk.

Earlier NB length was considered important but since the huge variation according to ethnicity has been recognized, it is now believed that it is presence or absence (ossification or nonossification of the NB that is important rather than the length of the NB). Its presence is confirmed in the same plane as for NT. Looking at the profile of the face, the top line represents the skin, the underlying line, which is thicker and more echogenic than the overlying skin, represents the NB. These two parallel lines of echogenicity have the shape of an "equal sign". A third line in front of the bone and at a higher level than the skin represents the tip of the nose. But the recent school of thoughts now is that the NB can be short in certain ethnic groups and it is only the presence of the NB that is important at nuchal scan. Of course further in second and third

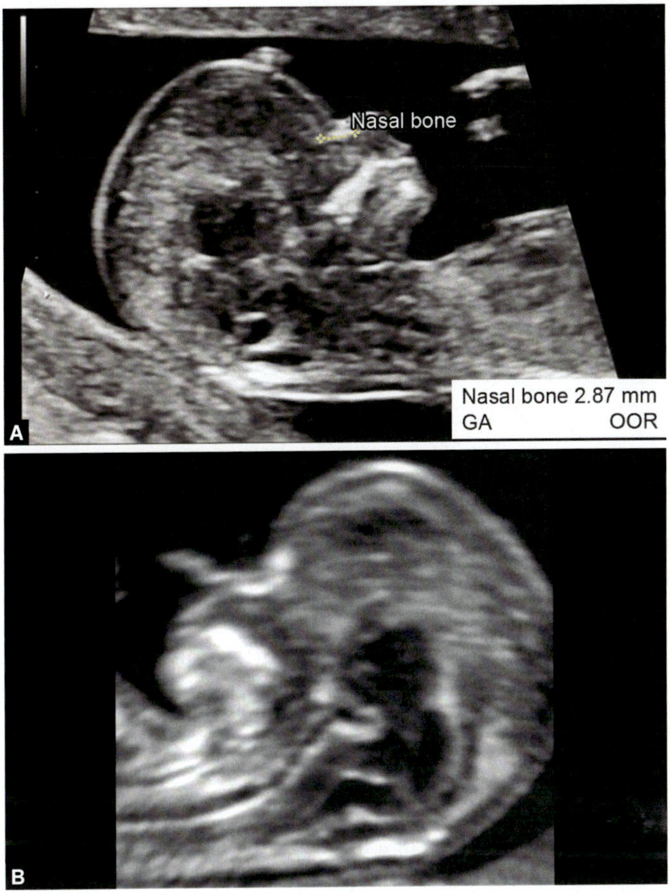

Figs. 24A and B: Nasal bone.

trimester then, the values of NB length are to be plotted on the nomogram. It must be remembered that 0.5% of normal patients have absent NB and if a detailed US and a marker test does not show any indication of T21, follow-up scans should be done and any structural abnormalities must be looked for.

It must be remembered that incidence of absent NB decreased with fetal CRL, increased with NT thickness, and was substantially high in Afro-Caribbeans than in Caucasians.[20]

Though the sensitivity for Down's syndrome as individual marker is as follows:

- Nuchal translucency—80.4%
- Nasal bone—58.7%
- Ductus venosus flow—93.5%.

All three together have a sensitivity for Down's syndrome of 94% with LR for negative test only 0.08%.

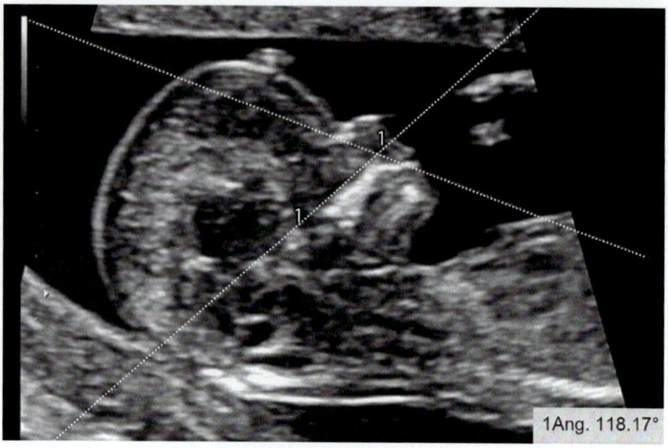

Fig. 25: Frontomaxillary facial angle.

Apart from these, there are some new markers for aneuploidies that are gaining a lot of importance and significance lately. These are:

- Facial angle or frontomaxillary facial (FMF) angle
- Tricuspid regurgitation
- Though not a marker for chromosomal abnormalities, it is also an important measurement to exclude open spinal defects that may be a part of chromosomal abnormality.

Frontomaxillary Facial Angle (Fig. 25)

In midsagittal plane of the face, a line is drawn on the superior surface of the maxilla that is rectangular in shape and a second line is drawn from the anterior point of maxilla to the nasion. But it needs to be a true midsagittal plane. Rotation of even 5–15° will lead to error of 2–3°. In normal fetuses this angle is 66.6–89.5°, mean 78.1° but it decreases with increase in CRL. It is 84° at CRL 45 mm and 76.5° at CRL 84 mm.

Incorporating FMF angle in first trimester combined screening *increased the estimated DR of T21 from 90% to 94% at FPR 5%* and from 85% to 92% at FPR of 3%.[21]

Tricuspid Regurgitation (Fig. 26)

Four chamber heart view is the section required for assessing the tricuspid valve flow. With the new advances in US technology, now this view can be achieved at the nuchal scan. The sample volume of pulse Doppler is placed across the tricuspid valve with a sample volume of 2–3 mm and the spectrum of flow is documented. The insonation angle to the direction of flow should be less than 30° from the direction of the interventricular septum. The sweep

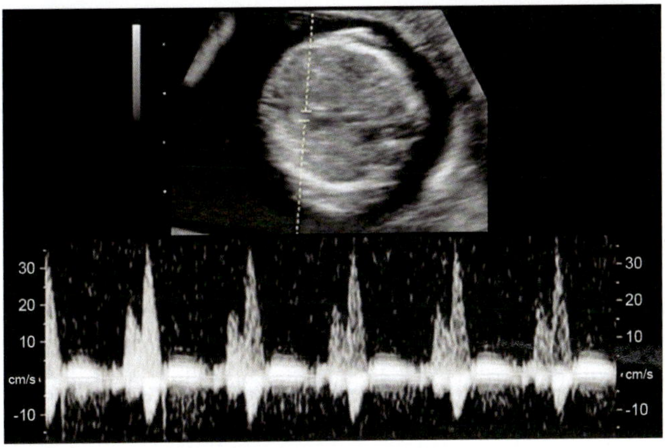

Fig. 26: Normal tricuspid flow.

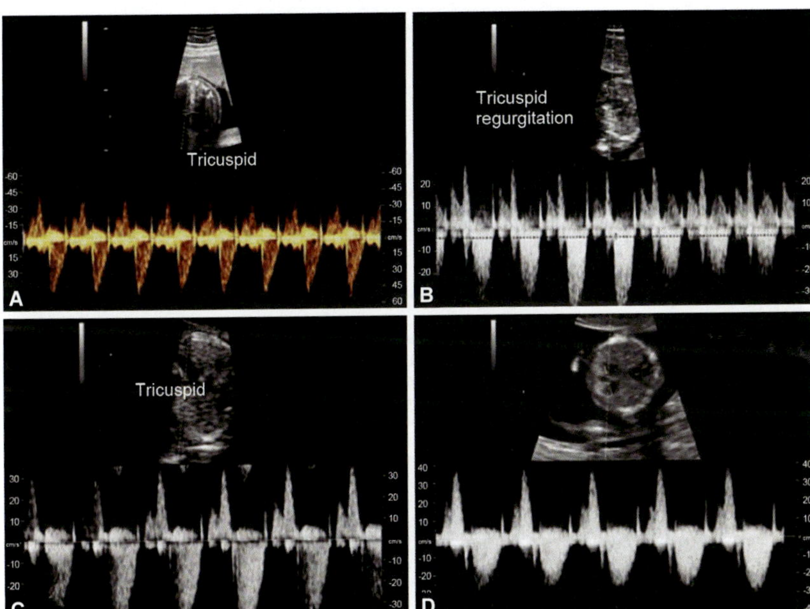

Figs. 27A to D: (A to C) Tricuspid regurgitation, but (D) is not true tricuspid regurgitation.

speed should be high (2–3 cm/s) so that the waveforms are widely spread for better assessment. Tricuspid flow is a positive flow during ventricular diastole and is absent during ventricular systole. Reverse flow during ventricular systole that involves more than half of the systolic phase and has a velocity of 60 cm/s or more is defined as tricuspid regurgitation. This is a marker for chromosomal and/or cardiac abnormality in the fetus **(Figs. 27A to D)**.

Tricuspid regurgitation is seen in:[22]

- Euploid: 0.9%
- T21: 55.7%
- T18: 33.3%
- T13: 30.0%
- Turner's: 37.5%.

Intracranial Translucency (Fig. 28)

Midsagittal plane (same as the plane for NT) is absolutely essential. This is the space between the posterior margin of the brainstem and anterior margin of choroid plexus of fourth ventricle. It is measured in the same plane as that for NT and parallel to NT. It is a curved translucency, widest in the middle of the fourth ventricle. IT is normally 2–3 mm, anything less than 2 mm, open spinal canal defect is suspected.

Apart from these markers, there are some other markers, which though have a lower sensitivity for aneuploidies than the major markers, are seen much more often in the aneuploidies rather than normal fetuses. It should be noted that in the absence of major congenital anomalies and normal karyotype of the fetus, they do not carry any significance and do not affect the fetal prognosis as they are not pathological except for ventriculomegaly.

These markers are picked up in second trimester except echogenic cardiac focus, megacystis, echogenic bowel, clinodactyly/syndactyly/polydactyly and aberrant right subclavian artery (ARSA).

In women found to be at low risk through first trimester combined test or second trimester quadruple test, should not be referred for further assessment. Such low-risk women would require further assessment only if the following markers are identified:

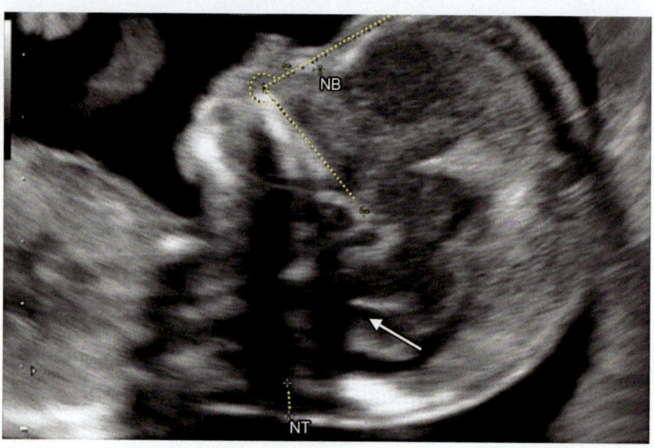

Fig. 28: Intracranial translucency (arrow)(NT: nuchal translucency; NB: nasal bone).

- Nuchal fold >6 mm
- Ventriculomegaly (atrium >10 mm)
- Echogenic bowel
- Renal pelvic dilatation >7 mm
- Small measurements <5th centile

These are soft markers and can be listed as follows:

- Ventriculomegaly
- Choroid plexus cyst (CPC)
- Strawberry-shaped head
- Echogenic cardiac focus
- Renal pyelectasis
- Megacystis
- Hyperechoic bowel
- Clinodactyly/syndactyly/polydactyly
- Short long bones
- Aberrant right subclavian artery
- Umbilical cord abnormalities
- Extrafetal abnormalities

Ventriculomegaly ***(Fig. 29)****:* The ventricular size remains relatively constant throughout gestation at 6.1 ± 1.3 mm, though is slightly larger in males and smaller in females.[23] As a rule ventricular width less than 8 mm is considered as normal. 8–10 mm is borderline and 10–12 mm is mild ventriculomegaly. The ventricular size larger than that is called a hydrocephalus and not a ventriculomegaly. Visually, when the choroid plexus of the dependent ventricle is seen hanging away from the medial ventricular wall (separation of >3 mm), is considered as ventriculomegaly. Ventriculomegaly as an isolated

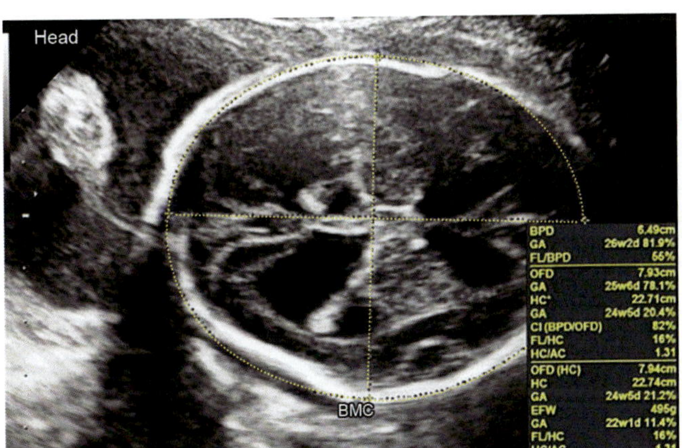

Fig. 29: Ventriculomegaly.

sign is not a very significant marker and demands only a close follow-up, but may be one of the markers of trisomies 18, 13, and 21 and triploidy. The odds ratio of mild ventriculomegaly for chromosomal abnormality is 4.4%.[24]

Strawberry-shaped skull **(Fig. 30)** is anteroposteriorly flattened head which on transthalamic section looks like a strawberry in shape. It is seen in T18, but associated findings must be looked for. Its combination with CPC increases the risk of T18.

*Choroid plexus cyst **(Fig. 31)**:* Choroid plexus cyst (CPC) is seen in 0.3–3.6% of the population between 16 and 24 weeks. These are transient in 80–94% and disappear at 24 weeks in euploid or aneuploid fetuses. CPCs have no adverse fetal outcome, if the karyotype is normal.

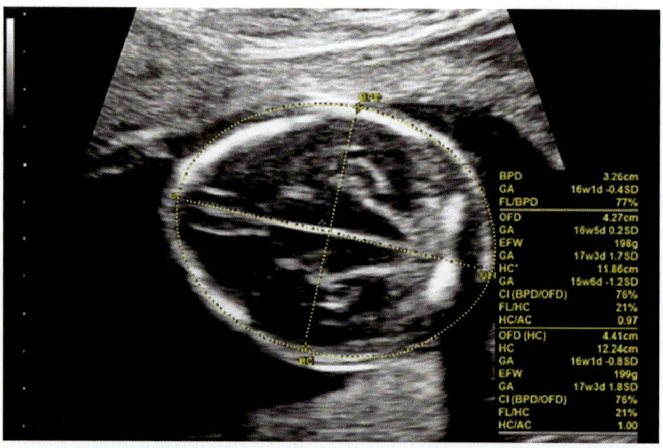

Fig. 30: Strawberry-shaped skull.

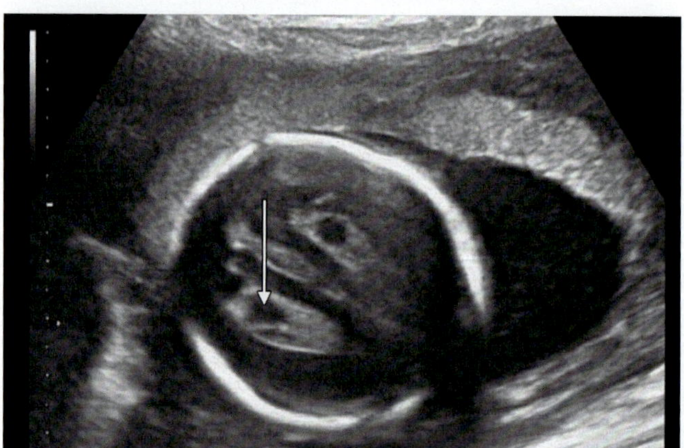

Fig. 31: Choroid plexus cyst.

Table 1: Approximate risk of trisomy 18 in fetuses with choroid plexus cyst.[25]

Gestation weeks	*Baseline*	*Isolated cyst*	*Other abnormalities*
20–24	1:4,500	1:2,950	1:225
25–29	1:3,600	1:2,300	1:175
30–34	1:2,000	1:1,300	1:100
35–39	1:750	1:470	1:35
40–44	1:400	1:100	1:10

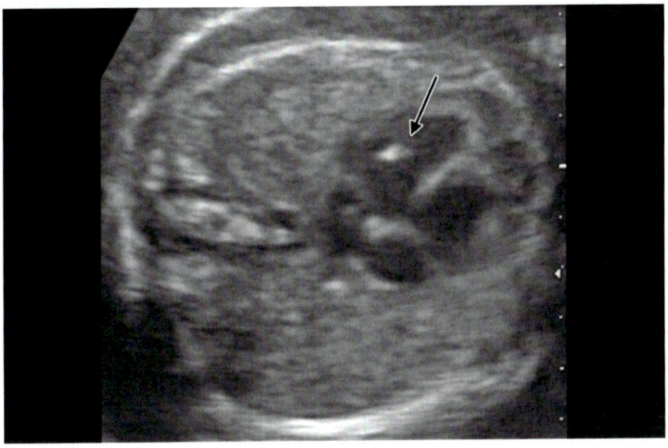

Fig. 32: Echogenic focus in left ventricle.

Though CPCs are seen in 1% of normal fetuses but are seen in 50% of T18 fetuses **(Table 1)**. Single CPC that are <3 mm in size and that are transient are less likely to be associated with aneuploidies. Multiple or bilateral CPCs and especially which persist for a longer time or disappear late have higher risk for aneuploidies, but any associated abnormality with CPC increases the LR by as much as 20 times.[25] The LR of CPC is 13.8 for T18 and for T21.[26]

A quadruple marker must be done for fetuses with isolated CPC, to select the ones which need amniocentesis. If karyotyping is not done, there is no point in doing a follow-up scan for CPC as they are almost always transient. A follow-up scan only helps to detect other abnormalities which may be missed.

Echogenic cardiac focus ***(Fig. 32)****:* An echogenic dense spot of 1–6 mm is sometimes seen in the cardiac ventricles which moves in the heart like a golf ball with each ventricular contraction, as it is attached to the papillary muscle or chordae tendineae. A single such focus may be seen in the left ventricle in 3–10% of the population and is more often seen in fetuses of Asian mothers than in fetuses with Down's syndrome. The sensitivity and the specificity

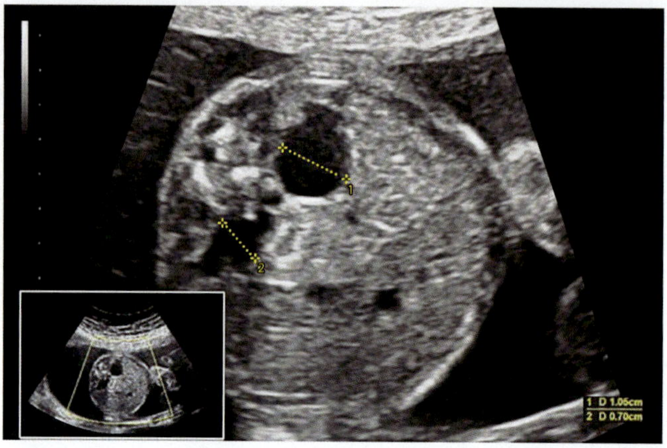

Fig. 33: Renal pyelectasis.

of this marker are low. It has a LR for Down's syndrome of 1.8–4.2%.[27] But when such foci are multiple or are in the right ventricle or bilateral, the risk increases to double. Less than 20% of aneuploid fetuses have echogenic cardiac focus. It is seen in 16% of fetuses with T21, 39% of fetuses with T13, and in 2% of normal fetuses.[28]

Its significance as a marker for aneuploidies is very low especially when isolated.

Renal pyelectasis ***(Fig. 33)****:* Renal pelvis diameter is 3–4 mm at 14–15 weeks in anteroposterior (AP) plane when fetal abdomen is seen in transverse section. It must be a true transverse section when renal pelvis are seen but stomach or bladder is not seen. The measurement is taken from inner margin to inner margin of renal pelvis. When this diameter increases to >4 mm it is called pyelectasis and it increases the risk for T21 by 1.6 folds.[29] Though 2–3% of normal fetuses have pyelectasis, it is seen in 17–25% of Down's syndrome fetuses. Though often a transient sign, renal pelvic diameter of:

- >4 mm between 16 and 20 weeks,
- >5 mm between 20 and 30 weeks, and
- >7 mm between 30 and 40 weeks is considered abnormal.

Megacystis: Normally in all fetuses beyond 67 mm CRL, the bladder is visible. Normal emptying time cycle is 30–155 minutes CRL. Megacystis is defined when the bladder vertically measures >8 mm or bladder diameter/CRL >13%. About 20% of the fetuses with megacystis have aneuploidies. It resolves in second trimester, but that does not exclude the risk of aneuploidy. Risk is significant when due to megacystis is due to obstructive uropathy and associated with other abnormalities.

Hyperechoic bowel ***(Fig. 34)****:* The bowel is normally a little hyperechoic to the liver due to multiple tissue interfaces, but when it is as dense as bone it

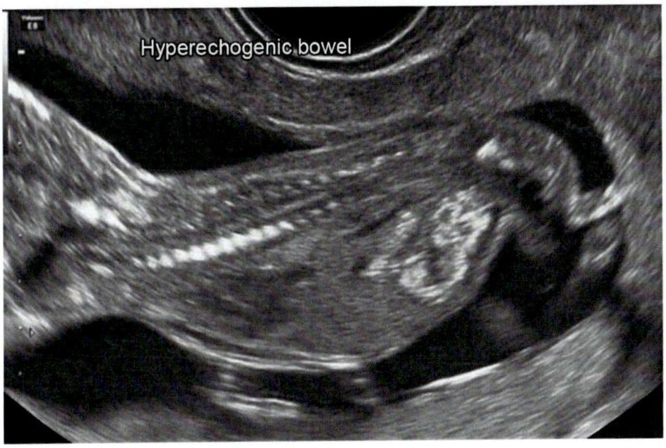

Fig. 34: Hyperechoic bowel.

is termed hyperechoic bowel and is a marker for aneuploidies. Hyperechoic bowel increases the risk for T21 by 6–7 folds.[30] It is found in 12% of fetuses with T21.

It is seen in late trimester in presence of fetal growth restriction or intrauterine death in second trimester.

According to the density and the uniformity it can be graded as:[31]

- *Grade I*: Homogeneously mildly hyperechoic
- *Grade II*: Focal hyperechogenicities
- *Grade III*: As echogenic as bone

Hyperechoic bowel may be seen in fetuses with:

- Aneuploidies
- Meconium ileus—due to cystic fibrosis
- Bowel atresia
- Congenital infections like cytomegalovirus (CMV)

Phalangeal abnormalities:

- *Clinodactyly*: T21 [ratio of middle phalanx of fifth digit to middle phalanx of fourth digit in Down's is 0.59 (median), normal 0.85]
- *Polydactyly*: T13
- *Syndactyly*: Triploidy

Short long bones: When femoral length shows a difference of 2 weeks or more than the other biometric parameters, it has a significant risk of aneuploidies, especially T21 and T18. But short humerus is considered to be more sensitive for T21 than short femur.

Umbilical cord abnormalities: Umbilical cord diameter, though is not normally measured routinely, has its own nomographic values. When it is above 95th percentile, it is considered as abnormal and may increase the risk

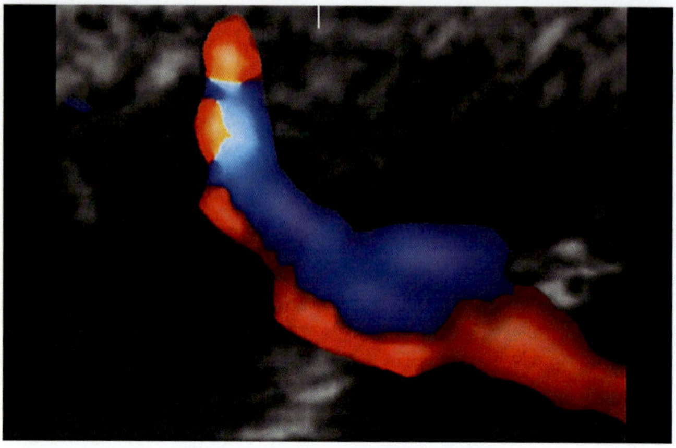

Fig. 35: Single umbilical artery.

of aneuploidy.[32] Single umbilical artery **(Fig. 35)** was though once considered a very significant marker, is often seen in normal fetuses also. Single umbilical artery should definitely lead to a detailed search for chromosomal or cardiac abnormalities, but has a significant value only when associated with other abnormalities.

Reversed end-diastolic flow in umbilical artery at 10–14 weeks is thought to be associated with chromosomal anomalies.

Extrafetal markers: Placental thickening or cystic areas are associated with aneuploidies. Cystic areas in the placenta suggest a possibility of trisomies 18 and 13, especially when associated with oligohydramnios or IUGR.

The risk for aneuploidies increases when:

- Multiple markers are present.
- Markers are seen at the higher age of gestation.
- Fetus shows delayed development—the risk of aneuploidy increases by 9.04 odds ratio if the CRL was 14 mm or more decreased than the expected. Early onset IUGR is usually associated with T18 or T13. About 96% of the fetuses with IUGR have multisystem abnormalities, characteristic of type of aneuploidy. Though usually symmetric IUGR is seen in most chromosomal abnormalities, triploidy shows asymmetric IUGR. IUGR with polyhydramnios/oligohydramnios has higher risk for aneuploidies.
- Gestational sac is large for dates.
- Cardiac anomaly or duodenal atresia is present.

  But when we say that the risk is increased, does not suffice. It is important to exactly calculate the risk in order to allow the patient take a balanced, informed decision regarding the continuation or termination of pregnancy.

Calculating the Risk

- Background risk × LRs of the risk factors or markers
- *Likelihood ratio of positive scan*: Sensitivity/FPR, LR for a normal scan:false negative rate/specificity. Positive LR of a marker is derived by dividing the percentage of confirmed Down's syndrome having the marker by the percentage of normal fetus with the same marker. Negative LR results from dividing the number of T21 fetuses that do not exhibit the marker by the number of normal fetuses that do not exhibit the marker.
- *Background risk*: Maternal age + gestational age + previous pregnancy with aneuploidy.

Background Risk Factors

- Maternal age > 35.
- Paternal age > 39—three times increased risk.
- *Previous chromosomal anomaly*: Previous aneuploid child increases an additional risk of 0.75% to the risk otherwise calculated as background risk.
- Biochemical screening positive.
- *Increasing gestational age*: About 30% of T21 fetuses die between 12 weeks of gestation and full-term and 20% between 16 weeks and full-term. That means that with increasing age of gestation the number of aneuploid fetuses decreases due to nature's law of existence of the strongest. So, if the markers for chromosomal abnormality are detected at the higher gestational age means that the likelihood of this fetus being abnormal increases.
- The actual sensitivity of a genetic sonogram depends on various factors, including the markers sought, gestational age, reasons for referral, and quality of US. The increasing DR of cardiac abnormalities has increased the DR of aneuploidies by sonography from 60 to 90%.

Chart of Likelihood Ratios

Likelihood ratio = Cases%/Controls%.

Likelihood ratio is calculated for a particular finding by dividing the percentage of abnormal fetuses/percentage normal fetuses with that particular finding/measurement. Each marker has independent LR and increases the risk of aneuploidy accordingly **(Table 2)**.

Moreover, more the markers, more is the risk **(Table 3)**. A single marker increases the risk two-fold, two markers increase the risk nearly ten-fold, and three or more markers increase the risk to more than 100 folds. Though the actual risk depends on the type and number of markers that are present.

Table 2: Likelihood ratios of different markers for trisomy 21.

Marker	*Isolated*	*In combination*
Increased NT	15	60–95
Short humerus	05	15–23
Short femur	04	06–10
Echogenic cardiac focus	04	06–08
Hyperechoic bowel	03	15–33
Choroid plexus cyst	1.5	Same
Mild hydronephrosis	1.5	05–09
Normal scan	0.2	–

(NT: nuchal translucency)

Table 3: Number of markers and likelihood ratio for trisomy 21.

Number of markers	*Likelihood ratio*
1	0.2
2	1.9
3	6.2
4	80

A normal US has a LR for aneuploidy of only 0.2–0.4 and decreases the risk by 60–80%.[33] About 45% of risk of chromosomal anomalies is decreased if US is normal, though the biochemical markers are positive.[33]

The pooled estimates of DR, FPR, positive and negative LR for T21 for each marker are summarized in **Table 4**.

Ventriculomegaly, nuchal fold thickness, and ARSA each one of them increase the risk by three to four times. All the other markers in isolation do not have significant effect on the risk, while the presence of two or more markers will produce significant modification of the risk.

Another method of risk assessment based on US is age-adjusted US risk assessment. Here a priori risk of the maternal age is multiplied by the LRs of the individual sonographic marker. This in low-risk group gives a sensitivity of 61.5% with a FPR of only 4%.

NONINVASIVE PRENATAL TESTS

Since the discovery of cell-free fetal deoxyribonucleic acid (cffDNA) in the maternal plasma, there has been major progress in the field of prenatal diagnosis. cffDNA is employed in noninvasive prenatal testing (NIPT). NIPT has been endorsed by the American College of Obstetricians and

Table 4: Screening performance of second-trimester soft markers.

Marker	*DR%*	*FPR%*	*LR+*	*LR–*	*LR isolated marker*
Intracardiac echogenic focus	24.4	3.9	5.83	0.80	0.95
Ventriculomegaly	7.5	0.2	27.52	0.94	3.81
Increased nuchal fold	26.0	1.0	23.30	0.80	3.79
Echogenic bowel	16.7	1.1	11.44	0.90	1.65
Mild hydronephrosis	13.9	1.7	7.63	0.92	1.08
Short humerus	30.3	4.6	4.81	0.74	0.78
Short femur	27.7	6.4	3.72	0.80	0.61
ARSA	30.7	1.5	21.48	0.71	3.94
Absent or hypoplastic nasal bone	59.8	2.8	23.27	0.46	6.58

(ARSA: aberrant right subclavian artery; DR: detection rate; FPR: false positive rate; LR: likelihood ratio: LR+: positive likelihood ratio; LR–: negative likelihood ratio)
(*Source*: Data from Agathokleous M, Chaveeva P, Poon LCY, Kosinski P, Nicolaides KH. Meta-analysis of second-trimester markers for trisomy 21. Ultrasound Obstet Gynecol. 2103;42:247-61.)

Gynecologists and the Society for Maternal-Fetal Medicine as screening option for aneuploidy in 2011.

The majority of cell-free DNA is maternal in origin, with the fetal origin constituting about 3–13% after 10 weeks of gestation. The fetal DNA is derived from the placental trophoblasts. Testing can be performed at any period of gestation after 10 weeks. Results are generally available within 7–10 days of maternal sampling. NIPT has a sensitivity of 99.3% and a specificity of 99.8% for the detection of T21.

The reported FPR is 1% and is due to vanishing twin, confined placental mosaicism, and maternal malignancy.

Prerequisites

- Baseline US is mandatory to determine the viability, number of fetus, and gestational age.
- The couple should be counseled about the benefits and limitations of NIPT. A negative test does not assure a chromosomally normal fetus in a very small percentage of patients.

Limitations

- NIPT is expensive and is not applicable for screening general obstetric population. It is not universally available.

Table 5: Sensitivity and specificity of NIPT.

Condition	*Sensitivity*	*Specificity*
Trisomy 18	97.4%	99.8%
Trisomy 13	91.6%	99.9%
Sex chromosome aneuploidy	91%	99.6%

- Only T21, T18, and T13 can be detected. Information about sex chromosomal aneuploidies and other trisomies (T16 and T22) would be available only if requested for.
- It cannot determine if the trisomy is due to translocation. This information would be important for predicting the risk of recurrence.
- NIPT cannot routinely be offered for the detection of microdeletions. Hence, for the above reasons, NIPT cannot replace conventional karyotype.
- Laboratories require a minimum of 4% fetal fraction for a reportable result, irrespective of the methodology used. Maternal obesity is associated with lesser fetal fraction, leading to 1–8% screen failure.

Recommendations

- *NIPT can be offered **(Table 5)***:
  - As a follow-up test for pregnant women with a high or intermediate risk from a conventional screening test before proceeding for invasive tests. But a normal NIPT result does carry a residual risk of 2% of a chromosomal abnormality in such a situation.
  - To any pregnant woman, provided she understands the benefits and drawbacks of this screening strategy in the context of alternative screening tests. But the use of NIPT to the general obstetric population may produce higher screen false-positives because the positive predictive value is lower in this population due to the lower prevalence of aneuploidy in the general obstetric population.
- *NIPT cannot be offered in the following situations*:
  - In the event of identification of a structural anomaly by US which needs a diagnostic test
  - Multiple pregnancy as it provides only a single composite result for the entire gestation
  - Couple is unaffordable
  - Nonavailability of NIPT
- Women with a positive test should undergo invasive diagnostic test since NIPT does not replace the accuracy of invasive tests. Knowing the type of trisomy from the karyotype becomes essential for purposes of prediction

of recurrence. Management decisions should not be based solely on NIPT results.

- For women, whose NIPT results are not reported or indeterminate should be offered comprehensive US evaluation, genetic counseling, and invasive diagnostic test for confirmation.
- In addition to NIPT, parallel or simultaneous testing with multiple screening methodologies for aneuploidy is not necessary and should not be performed. But comprehensive anomaly scan should be offered as NIPT does not diagnose structural malformations.

Over and above this, every screening procedure for aneuploidy should commence with a counseling session. The aim of pretest counseling is to facilitate the couple to make informed choices concerning the pregnancy outcome. It is the prime responsibility of the clinician and his/her team to explain to the couple about the condition to be screened (Down's syndrome) and the disabilities and morbidities which the child would face. Information about the screening options relevant to their gestational age and the screening process should be provided. Patient should be explained the difference between screening and diagnosis and should also be explained the consequences in case the fetus turns out to be at high risk, or aneuploid at the end of invasive testing.

The scanner's aim should be to minimize the false positive results in low-risk group and maximize the sensitivity in the high-risk group. With this aim a scoring index system has been devised by Benacerraf et al. She decided a score of 2 for structural abnormalities and nuchal thickening and 1 point for other markers. All those having a score of more than 2 were offered amniocentesis. Some prefer to modify this system by adding 1 point for maternal age of 35 or more and 2 points for the age of 40 and more.

Though being so significantly helpful for the diagnosis of aneuploidies, sonography is not useful for diagnosis of single gene disorders such as thalassemia or muscular dystrophy, which show no structural variations or abnormalities.

A detailed, well-performed anomaly scan can reduce the rate of invasive testing and less number of abnormal births.[34]

The combined first and second trimester screening strategies that have been developed in our country are as follows **(Table 6)**:

- *Integrated screening*: It incorporates the results of the combined test and quadruple test into a single risk. The integrated test has the highest DR and least FPR, thereby reducing unwanted amniocentesis in normal pregnancies. The disadvantage associated with integrated screening strategy lies in ethical issue of not conveying the first trimester result and denying them the option of chorionic villus sampling (CVS).

Table 6: Performance of different screening protocols for Down's syndrome.

Screening test	*Detection rate*	*False +ve rate*
First-trimester tests		
MA + NT	75–80%	5%
MA + first trimester serum markers	60–70%	5%
Combined test (MA + NT + serum markers)	85–90%	5%
Contingent I trimester test (Combined test + NB/TR/DV flow)	93–96%	2.5%
Second-trimester tests		
Triple test	60–70%	5%
Quadruple test	65–75%	5%
Genetic sonogram	56%	NA
Quadruple test + genetic sonogram	80%	NA
Combined first- and second-trimester tests		
Integrated test	90–94%	5%
Stepwise sequential test	90–94%	5%
Contingent sequential test	90–94%	5%
Combined test + genetic sonogram	88%	NA
Noninvasive prenatal test (NIPT)	99%	NA

(DV: ductus venosus; MA: maternal age; NA: not available; NB: nasal bone; NT: nuchal translucency; TR: tricuspid regurgitation)

Source:

1. Benn P, Borrell A, Chiu RW, Cuckle H, Dugofff L, Faas B, et al. Position statement from the Chromosome Abnormality Screening Committee on behalf of the Board of the International Society for Prenatal Diagnosis. Prenat Diagn. 2015;35(8):725-34.
2. Nicolaides KH. Screening for fetal aneuploidies at 11–13 weeks. Prenat Diagn. 2011;31: 7-15.

- *Sequential screening*: First trimester combined test is the primary screening modality. The results of the combined test are stratified into low (risk <1:1,000), intermediate (risk ≥1:1,000 and ≤1:51), and high (risk >1:50) risk groups. The results are informed only to women at high risk, thus allowing them to choose the option of CVS. There are two testing strategies in this category:
  - *Stepwise sequential screening*: Both the low- and intermediate-risk group would be offered the quadruple test in the second trimester.
  - *Contingent sequential screening*: No further testing would be required for low-risk group. For those in the intermediate-risk group, quadruple test will be offered. This approach is the most effective for population screening as it obviates the need for second trimester screening in low-risk group, who constitute about 85%.

Following the quadruple test, the final risk is calculated after incorporating both the first and second trimester results. When the risk is below the established cut-off, no further screening would be required. When the risk is above the established cut-off, amniocentesis should be offered.

One must also confirm patient's wish in case the abnormality detected turns out to be incompatible with life, will she be ready for termination. The information should be in simple language, balanced, and nondirective. The couple should be given every opportunity to discuss with the clinician before they make a final decision. This counseling is as important as post-test counseling where the results their meanings are explained to the patient, the directive is suggested but the final proceedings should be a joint decision of the couple and the doctor.

REFERENCES

1. Evans MI, Galen RS, Drugan A. Biochemical screening. In: Evans MI, Johnson MP, Yaron Y (Eds). Prenatal Diagnosis: Genetics, Reproductive Risks, Testing and Management. New York: McGraw-Hill; 2006. pp. 277-88.
2. Snijders RJ, Sundberg K, Holzgreve W, Henry G, Nicolaides KH. Maternal age- and gestation-specific risk for trisomy 21. Ultrasound Obstet Gynecol. 1999;13:167-70.
3. Snijders RJ, Nicolaides KH. Sequential screening. Ultrasound Markers for Fetal Chromosomal Defects. Carnforth, UK: Parthenon Publishing; 1996. pp. 109-13.
4. Blaas HG, Eriksson AG, Salvesen KA, Isaksen CV, Christensen B, Mollerlokken G, et al. Brains and faces in holoprosencephaly: pre- and postnatal description of 30 cases. Ultrasound Obset Gynecol. 2002;19(1):24-38.
5. Blass HG, Eik-Nes SH, Vainio T, Isakesen CV. Alobar holoprosencephaly at 9 weeks gestational age visualized by two- and three-dimensional ultrasound. Ultrasound Obset Gynecol. 2000;15(1):62-5.
6. Bullen PJ, Rankin JM, Robson SC. Investigation of the epidemiology and prenatal diagnosis of holoprosencephaly in the North of England. Am J Obstet Gynecol. 2001;184:1256-62.
7. Babcook CJ, Goldstein RB, Filly RA. Prenatally detected fetal myelomeningocoele: is karyotype analysis warranted? Radiology. 1995;1949(2):491-4.
8. Nyberg DA, Sickler GK, Hegge FN, Kramer DJ, Kropp RJ. Fetal cleft lip with and without cleft palate: US classification and correlation with outcome. Radiology. 1995;195(3):677-84.
9. Benacerraf BR, Pober BR, Sanders SP. Accuracy of fetal echocardiography. Radiology. 1987;165:847-9.
10. Chaoui R, Körner H, Bommer C, Göldner B, Bierlich A, Bollmann R. Prenatal diagnosis of heart defects and associated chromosomal aberrations. Ultraschall Med. 1999;20(5):177-84.
11. Fonalsrud EW, DeLorimier AA, Hays DM. Congenital atresia and stenosis of the duodenum. A review complied from the members of surgical section of the American Academy of Pediatrics. Pediatrics. 1969;43:79-83.
12. Nyberg DA, Fitzsimmons J, Mack LA, Hughes M, Pretorius DH, Hickok D, et al. Chromosomal anomalies in fetuses with omphalocele. Significance of omphalocele contents. J Ultrasound Med. 1989;8:299-308.

13. Nicholaides KH, Snijders RJ, Gosden CM, Berry C, Campbell S. Ultrasonographically detectable markers of fetal chromosomal abnormalities. Lancet. 1992;340(8821): 704-7.
14. Nicolaides KH (2004). The 11–13+6 weeks scan. London: Fetal Medicine Foundation; 2004.
15. Zosmer N, Souter VL, Chan CS, Huggon IC, Nicolaides KH. Early diagnosis of major defects in chromosomally normal fetuses with increased nuchal translucency. Br J Obstet Gyneacol. 1999;106:829-33.
16. Snijders RJ, Noble P, Sebire N, Souka A, Nicolaides KH. UK multicentre project on assessment of risk of trisomy 21 by maternal age and fetal nuchal-translucency thickness at 10–14 weeks of gestation. Fetal Medicine Foundation First Trimester Screening Group. Lancet. 1998;352:343-6.
17. Zoppi MA, Putzolu M, Ibba RM, Floris M, Monni G. First-trimester ductus venosus velocimetry in relation to nuchal translucency thickness and fetal karyotype. Fetal Diagn Ther. 2002;17:52-7.
18. Nicolaides KH. Nuchal translucency and other first-trimester sonographic markers of chromosomal abnormalities. Am J Obstet Gynecol. 2004;191:45-7.
19. Bromley B, Lieberman E, Shipp TD, Benacerraf BR. Fetal nose bone length: a marker for Down's syndrome in second trimester. J Ultrasound Med. 2002;21:1387-94.
20. Cicero S, Longo D, Rembouskos G, Sacchini C, Nicolaides KH. Absent nasal bone at 11–14 weeks of gestation and chromosomal defects. Ultrasound Obstet Gynecol. 2003;22:31-5.
21. Borenstein M, Persico N, Kagan KO. Frontomaxillary facial angle in screening for trisomy 21 at 11+0 to 13+6 weeks. Ultrasound Obstet Gynecol. 2008;32:5-11.
22. Kagan KO, Valencia C, Livanos P, Wright D, Nicolaides KH. Tricuspid regurgitation in screening for trisomies 21, 18 and 13 and Turner's syndrome at 11+0 to 13+6 weeks of gestation. Ultrasound Obstet Gynecol. 2009;33:18-22.
23. Patel MD, Goldstein RB, Tung S, Filly RA. Fetal cerebral ventricular atrium: difference in size according to sex. Radiology. 1995;194(3):713-5.
24. Sohl BD, Scioscia AL, Budorick NE, Moore TR. Utility of minor ultrasonographic markers in prediction of abnormal fetal karyotype at prenatal diagnostic center. Am J Obstet Gynecol. 1999;181(4):898-903.
25. Snijders RJ, Shawa L, Nicolaides KH. Fetal choroids plexus cysts and trisomy 18: assessment of risk based on ultrasound findings and maternal age. Prenat Diagn. 1994;14(12):1119-27.
26. Yoder PR, Sabbagha RE, Gross SJ, Zelop CM. The second-trimester fetus with isolated choroids plexus cysts: a meta-analysis of risk of trisomies 18 and 21. Obstet Gynecol. 1999;93(5 Pt 2):869-72.
27. Achiron R, Lipitz S, Gabbay U, Yagel S. Prenatal ultrasonographic diagnosis of fetal heart echogenic foci: no correlation with Down's syndrome. Obstet Gynecol. 1997;89(6):945-8.
28. Roberts DJ, Genest D. Cardiac histologic pathology characteristic of trisomies 13 and 21. Hum Path. 1992;23:1130-40.
29. Snijders RJ, Sebire NJ, Faria M, Patel F, Nicolaides KH. Fetal mild hydronephrosis and chromosomal defects: relation to maternal age and gestation. Fetal Diagn Ther. 1995;10(6):349-55.
30. Nyberg DA, Souter VL, El-Bastawissi A, Young S, Luthhardt F, Luthy DA. Isolated sonographic markers for detection of fetal Down's syndrome in second trimester of pregnancy. J Ultrasound Med. 2001;20(10):1053-63.

31. Nyberg DA, Resta RG, Mahony BS, Dubinsky T, Luthy DA, Hickok DE, et al. Fetal hyperechogenic bowel and Down's syndrome. Ultrasound Obstet Gynecol. 1993;3:330-3.
32. Ghezzi F, Raio L, Di Naro E, Franchi M, Buttarelli M, Schneider H. First-trimester umbilical cord diameter: a novel marker of fetal aneuploidy. Ultrasound Obstet Gynecol. 2002;19:235-3.
33. Nyberg DA, Souter VL, El-Bastawissi A, Young S, Luthhardt F, Luthy DA. Isolated sonographic markers for detection of fetal Down's syndrome in second trimester of pregnancy. J Ultrasound Med. 2001;20:1053-63.
34. Nicholaides KH, Bindra R, Heath V, Cicero S. One-stop clinic for assessment of risk of chromosomal defects at 12 weeks of gestation. J Matern Fetal Neonatal Med. 2002;12:9-18.

CHAPTER 20

Systematic Examination of Fetal Central Nervous System: How Much Should an Obstetrician Know?

Sonal Panchal

INTRODUCTION

Abnormalities of central nervous system (CNS) are the most common of all congenital anomalies. Neural tube defects are most frequent of these and the incidence is 1–2 per 1,000 births. Intracranial anomalies with intact neural tube are often missed antenatally so exact incidence of CNS abnormalities is not known but is estimated to be approximately 1 in 10.

Ultrasound (US) has been used for nearly 30 years now for diagnosis of fetal CNS abnormalities. With increasing efficacy of technology, the anatomy of CNS can now be studied much more in detail than ever before and as early as late first trimester.

To study and diagnose CNS abnormalities precisely, it is important to know the development of the brain, as brain has the most dynamic anatomy amongst all the body organs during embryonic life. The developmental maturation of the normal brain follows a predictable sequence and this maturation can be followed by ultrasonography (USG).[1]

Though in selected cases, fetal magnetic resonance imaging (MRI) after 20–22 weeks has given promising results, its advantage over US remains debated.[2]

To make the examination standardized, of this quick changing anatomy, International Society of Ultrasound in Obstetrics and Gynecology (ISUOG) has established guidelines of CNS examination. According to these guidelines the examination has been staged as:

- *Optimized approach to the evaluation of fetal CNS:* Basic examination
- *Detailed evaluation of fetal CNS:* Fetal neurosonogram; indicated for pregnancies at high-risk for CNS abnormalities and may need three-dimensional ultrasonography (3D USG).

TIME OF EXAMINATION

For basic studies in low-risk population, around midgestation—20 weeks—is a good time for the study of fetal CNS. Studies later in gestation hampers visualization of intracranial structures because of calvarial ossification. First or early second trimester scans at 14–16 weeks has an advantage that bones are thin and brain evaluation at all angles is possible. Though with high-end scanners it is now possible to assess the fetal neural development from as early as 8–9 weeks, especially by transvaginal scans.

EQUIPMENT AND APPROACH (ACCORDING TO ISUOG GUIDELINES)

Transabdominal Approach

Transabdominal scan is done with transducer frequency of 3–5 MHz. This is the most commonly used approach and is used for basic examination. It is adequate for any fetal presentation. The sections most easily obtained by this approach are axial and sometimes coronal. But transabdominal approach is considered adequate for axial sections only. Sagittal sections are very difficult by this approach except in odd fetal lies, which are common in multiple pregnancies. The quality of image is deteriorated by factors like maternal obesity, adverse fetal position inadequate liquor, and advanced pregnancy leading to calcification of fetal calvarium.

Transvaginal Approach

Transvaginal scans are done with 5–9 MHz or 6–12 MHz intracavitary probes. Transvaginal probe being a high frequency probe gives much more details and is a more preferred approach for sagittal and coronal planes detailed fetal neurosonogram. Whenever fetus is in cephalic presentation and fetal head is not too high, this route of examination is chosen. Gentle manipulation of the fetus may be required for correct sections and planes.

METHOD OF TRANSVAGINAL SCAN

This scan is done through anterior fontanelle of the fetus. All sections are fanning from front to back or side to side respectively parallel to coronal and sagittal sutures. Transvaginal probe sound beam is aligned with sutures and fontanelle. Transverse or axial sections cannot be obtained by this approach.

The coronal sections obtained are divided as frontal 1, 2, midcoronal 1, 2, 3 and occipital 1, 2 and the side to side sections obtained are median, paramedian 1, 2 **(Figs. 1 and 2)**. These sections are similar to the neonatal scans and so easier to understand for pediatricians.

Three-dimensional may be used with both the approaches, whenever indicated.

IMAGING SPECIFICATIONS

Primary assessment of the fetal head-brain is done with B-mode scan. Scanning on B-mode can be made better with the technology advances such as

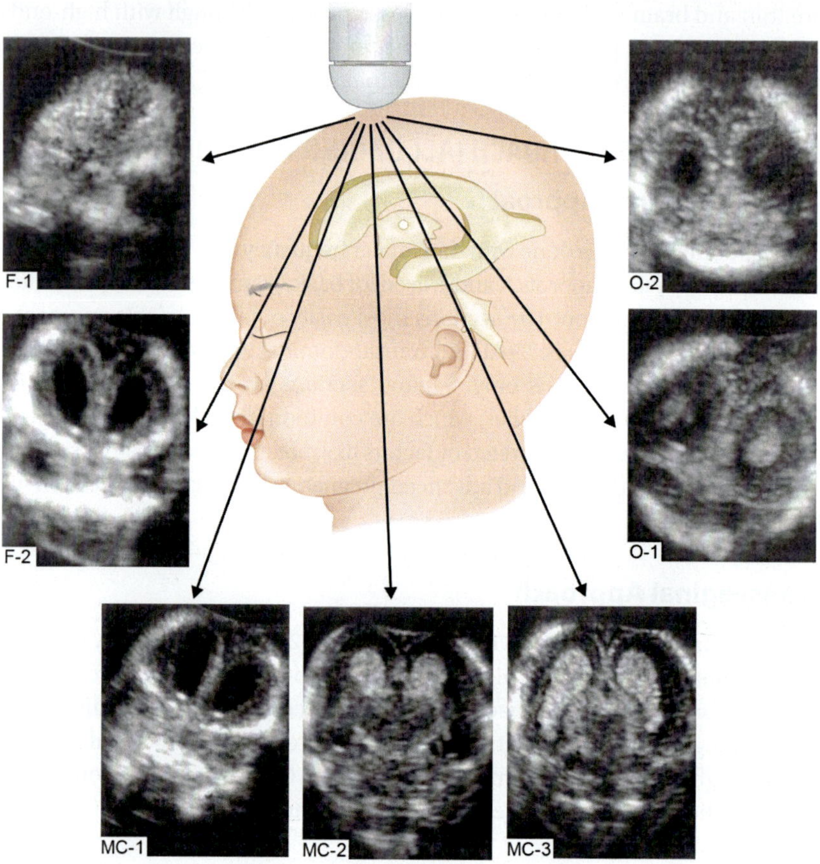

Fig. 1: Diagrammatic definition of various coronal planes of the fetal head and their ultrasound images. Figure from prenatal diagnosis, Marks I Evans et al. 203.

speckle reduction imaging, compound resolution imaging, and harmonics, all these enhance subtle anatomical details. Color and power Doppler are used for vascular studies. Increased persistence on color Doppler settings is required to pick-up small vessels.

The basic fetal CNS evaluation is divided into qualitative and quantitative evaluation (according to ISUOG guidelines):

- *Qualitative evaluation of head* consists of three axial planes **(Fig. 3)**:
  - Transventricular plane
  - Transthalamic plane
  - Transcerebellar plane
- *Qualitative evaluation of the spine* requires at least two of the three planes:
  - Longitudinal/sagittal
  - Transverse/axial
  - Coronal

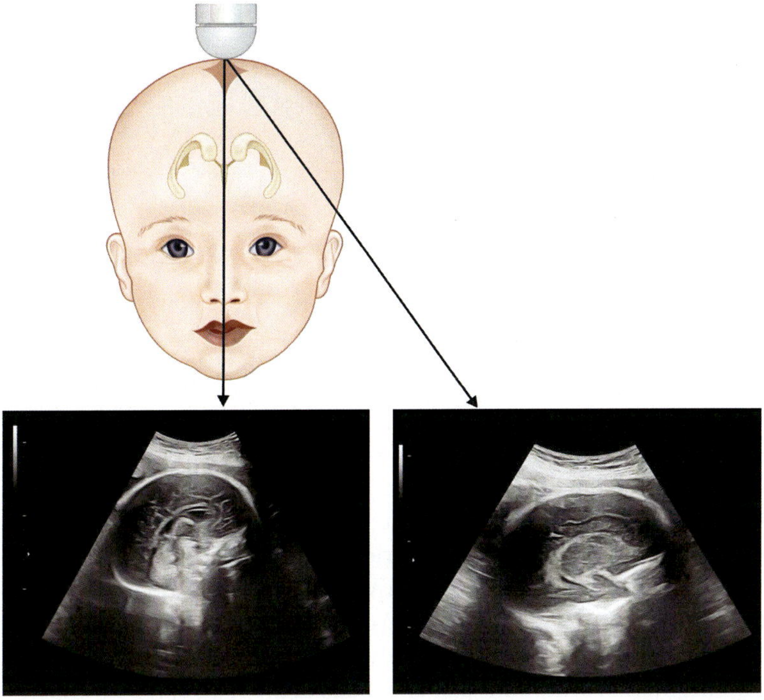

Fig. 2: Diagrammatic definition of midsagittal and parasagittal planes of the fetal head and their ultrasound images.

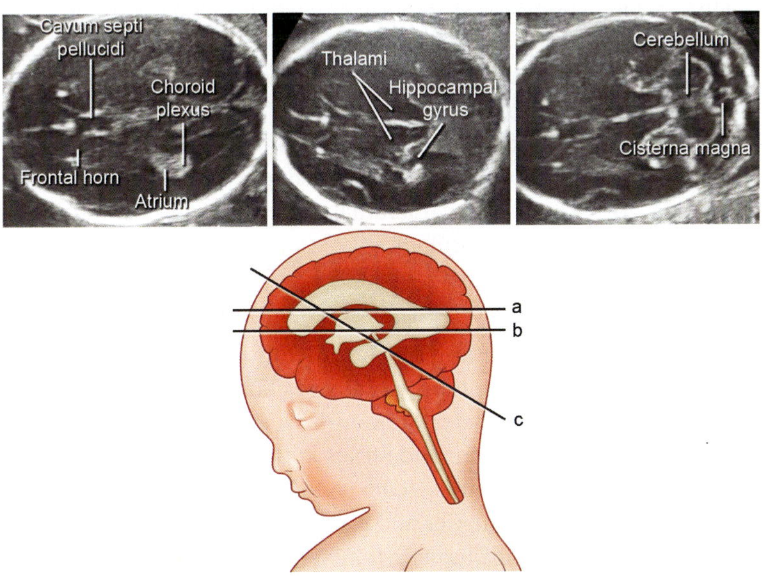

Fig. 3: Three axial planes of basic fetal neurosonogram and their diagrammatic representation: (a) Transventricular; (b) Transthalamic; and (c) Transcerebellar.

QUALITATIVE EXAMINATION OF THE HEAD

Transventricular Plane

- Head shape and calvarium
- Lateral ventricles
- Cavum septum pellucidum
- Thalami
- Cerebellum
- Cisterna magna

Head Shape and Calvarium

Normal shape of the calvarium is oval and the bone shows high echogenicity. The abnormalities that can be detected in calvarium are abnormalities of the shape of the calvarium, breech in the continuity of calvarium, and defective ossification of calvarial bone. Total absence of calvarial bone may be seen in anencephaly and acrania. Abnormal shapes of the calvarium can be brachycephaly-anteroposteriorly compressed calvarium (short occipitoparietal diameter). It is seen on Apert syndrome, Carpenter syndrome, Robert syndrome, trisomy 21, etc. Long calvarium/skull-long anteroposterior diameter of the skull is dolichocephaly and this is commonly seen in Crouzon syndrome, Marfan syndrome, etc. The shape of the skull may be compressed anteriorly and broader posteriorly and this is strawberry skull is commonly seen trisomy 18. Lemon skull where skull is compressed anteriorly with mild scalloping of frontal bones and this is seen in patients with open spinal canal defect in second trimester **(Figs. 4A to D)**.

Breech in the continuity of calvarium is associated with herniation of meninges or brain and is named as meningocele or encephalocele **(Figs. 5A and B)** and defective ossification of the skull bones occurs in abnormalities such as osteogenesis imperfecta, etc. Abnormal ossification is diagnosed by more clear visibility of the intracranial structures. This visualization is obscured by the dense bone normally.

Lateral Ventricles

Lateral ventricle consists of anterior horn (frontal horn), posterior horn (occipital horn), atrium—contains glomus of choroid plexus, and inferior (temporal horn). In first trimester, the ventricles are large and fill-up almost the whole cranial cavity with choroid plexus in the center. As the fetus grows the comparative size of the ventricles decreases. In second trimester, the lateral ventricles are seen only as anterior and posterior horns and atrium, which is partially occupied by choroid plexus. In transventricular section, the maximum normal ventricular diameter is 7.6 ± 0.6 and remains fairly constant in second and third trimester or may narrow down as gestational age (GA) advances.

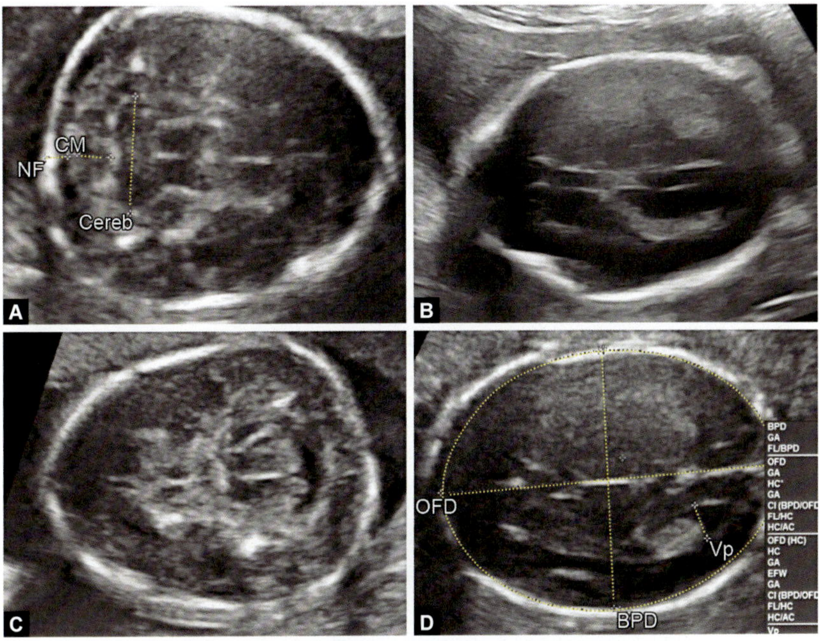

Figs. 4A to D: (A) Strawberry-shaped skull; (B) Lemon skull; (C) Brachycephaly; (D) Dolicocephaly.

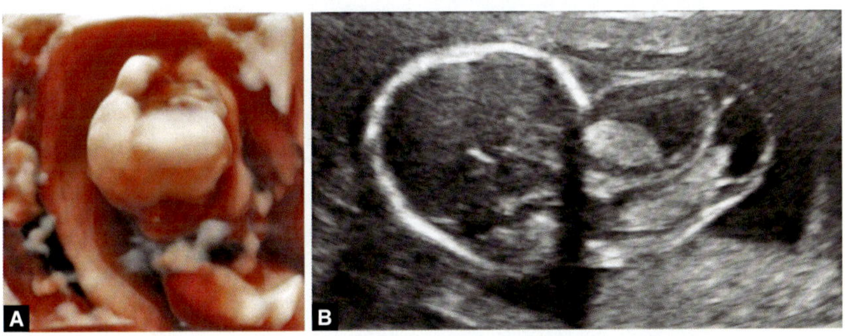

Figs. 5A and B: (A) Meningocoele seen on 3D ultrasound; (B) Large encephalocoele seen on 2D ultrasound.

This is because of compression of the ventricles by growing brain. Medial and lateral walls of ventricle are parallel to midline in second and third trimester.[3] The ventricular width is measured from inner to inner margin at the level of parieto-occipital sulcus. Parieto-occipital sulcus is identified as a diamond-shaped outline in the posterior half of the transventricular head section **(Fig. 6A)**. Anything more than 10 mm is termed as ventriculomegaly and ventricular size of more than 15 mm with increased intracranial pressure is hydrocephalus. Mild ventriculomegaly is often found in patients with chromosomal abnormalities, other brain abnormalities especially migration defects, fetal infections, etc. Whenever mild ventriculomegaly is seen, detailed assessment of fetus is done and amniocentesis to confirm chromosomal abnormalities or fetal infections with polymerase chain reaction is important. When no other abnormality is found, MRI should be suggested in third trimester to exclude migration defects.

The lateral ventricle to hemisphere width (measured as broadest perpendicular distance from falx to parietal bone of one side) ratio changes and decreases from 70% at 18–20 weeks to 30% at 28–29 weeks and remains steady thereafter. The ratio of anterior horn width to the hemisphere decreases from 60% at 14 weeks to 40% at 21 weeks.[4]

Dilatation of only posterior horn (tear-shaped ventricles) which is seen in agenesis of corpus callosum (CC), is known as colpocephaly **(Figs. 6A and B)**.

Choroid plexus normally fills the atrium **(Fig. 7A)**. Thinned out and hanging dangling choroid plexus is an indirect sign of ventricular dilatation.

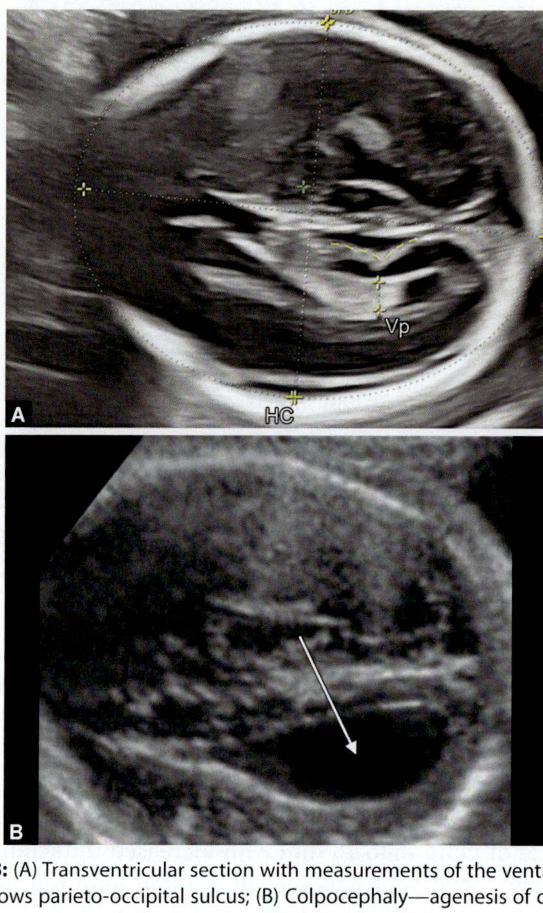

Figs. 6A and B: (A) Transventricular section with measurements of the ventricle atrium and dashed line shows parieto-occipital sulcus; (B) Colpocephaly—agenesis of corpus callosum (arrow).

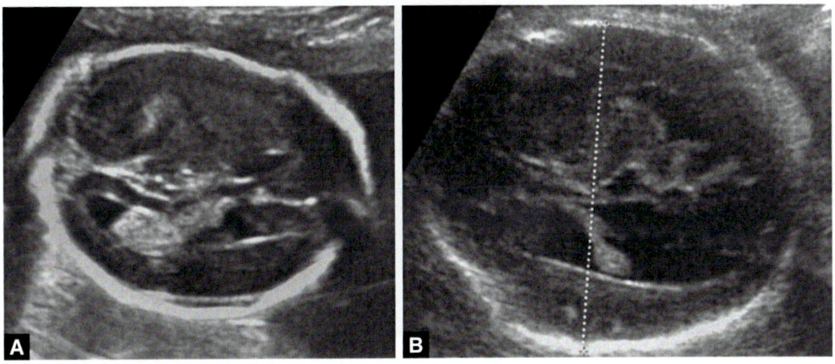

Figs. 7A and B: (A) Normal ventricle; (B) Ventriculomegaly.

An angle can also be drawn by a line along the median margin of the ventricle and posteromedial margin of the choroids plexus to assess the extent of ventriculomegaly **(Fig. 7B)**.

Most severe cerebral lesions are symmetrical and in basic examination symmetry of the brain is assumed, though most of the times the hemisphere on the near side is not visualized.

If the shape of the skull is symmetrically oval, then falx is seen in the midline, the symmetry is maintained, and unilateral lesion is not suspected.

Cavum Septum Pellucidum

Sonographically, it appears as two sheets of tissue extending from CC and separates the lateral ventricles from cavum. It becomes visible at 16 weeks and remains nearly steady throughout the second trimester, but obliterates near term. It must always be visualized between 18 and 37 weeks when biparietal diameter (BPD) is of between 44 and 88 mm. Septum cavum pellucidum is not seen in:

- Holoprosencephaly **(Fig. 8A)** with holoprosencephaly, falx is also completely or partially absent depending on whether it is alobar, semilobar or lobar holoprosencephaly.
- Agenesis of CC, other sign on the same plane is colpocephaly
- Severe hydrocephaly **(Fig. 8B)**
- Septo-optic dysplasia

Other Pathologies Diagnosed on this Plane (Figs. 9A to D)

- Arachnoid cyst
- *Porencephalic cyst:*
  - Vein of Galen aneurysm
  - Periventricular calcification (this occurs in fetal infections and tuberous sclerosis)

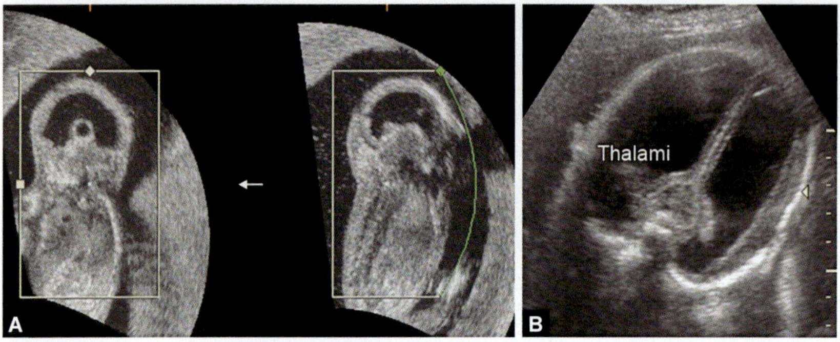

Figs. 8A and B: Holoprosencephaly and hydrocephaly.

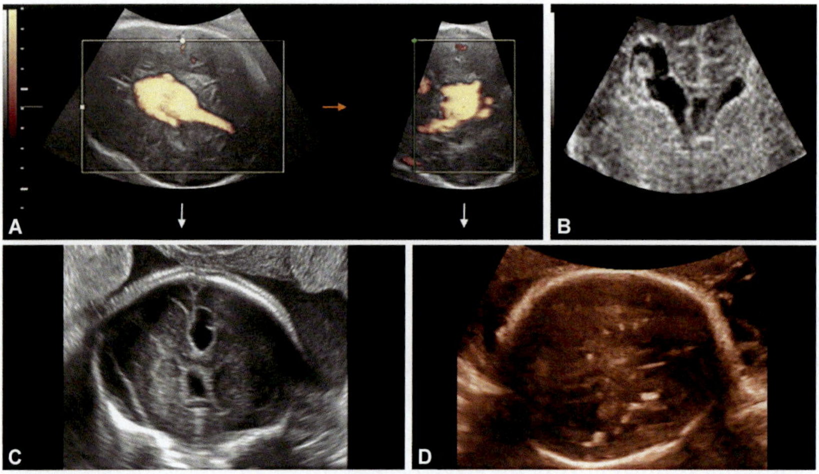

Figs. 9A to D: (A) Vein of Galen aneurysm; (B) Porencephalic cyst; (C) Arachnoid cyst; (D) Periventricular calcification.

Arachnoid cysts are more commonly seen in the fissures of the brain where there are folds of arachnoid membrane. These are usually rounded and if there are blood vessels around, these are displaced. Arachnoid cysts have a very good prognosis.

Porencephalic cysts are absolutely irregular cystic lesions in relation to the cortex and are a result of vascular insult to the brain. These have a very bad prognosis and may lead to intrauterine death or early fetal death.

Vein of Galen aneurysm is one of the most common intracranial vascular lesions. On B-mode it is seen as a round or oval cystic lesion in the midline in the posterior half of the transverse section of the head, more commonly in transthalamic section. On switching on Doppler, it fills up with color. Since it leads to hypercirculatory state, it may often be associated with cardiomegaly.

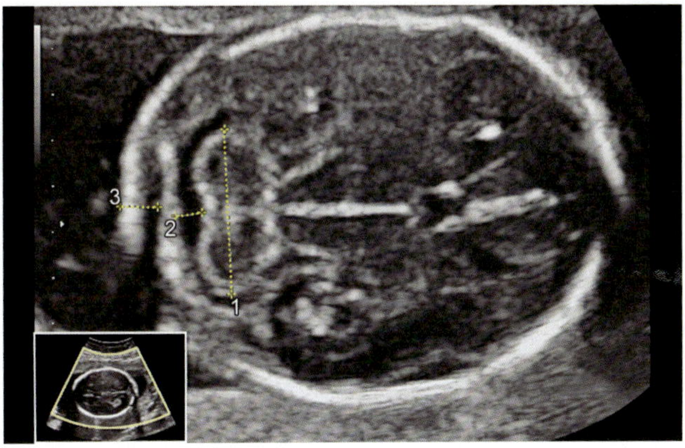

Fig. 10: Transcerebellar plane.

Transcerebellar Plane (Fig. 10)

It cuts through cerebellum and shows:

- Frontal horns of lateral ventricles
- Cavum septum pellucidum
- Thalami
- *Cerebellum:*
  - Two hemispheres
  - Vermis—after 20 weeks

Cerebellum which is seen as a B-shaped structure in the posterior fossa in second trimester and onward pregnancy becomes visible as early as 11–12 weeks. In second trimester, its diameter in millimeters corresponds to the number of weeks of gestation. It is measured from outer margin to outer margin at the broadest part, perpendicular to the midline. In late second and third trimester, sulci and gyri can also be appreciated on the cerebellar surface. Between the two cerebellar hemispheres, a thin solid structure is seen called vermis. Inferior vermis is seen at little lower level than superior vermis. There are two solid structures actually closely connected but separate—superior and inferior vermis. Superior vermis is "V" shaped and inferior vermis is "W" in shape. Inferior vermis is seen at little lower level than superior vermis. It is consistently visible after 18 weeks, but is absent in Dandy-Walker syndrome and variants and also be sometimes seen as isolated finding. When inferior vermis is absent the cisterna magna may or may not communicate with the 4th ventricle, and is seen as an open inverted "V" between cerebellar hemispheres **(Figs. 11A and B)**.

Cisterna Magna

This is the space between the cerebellum and the occipital bone and shows thin arachnoid septations as lines crossing the lucent space anteroposteriorly.

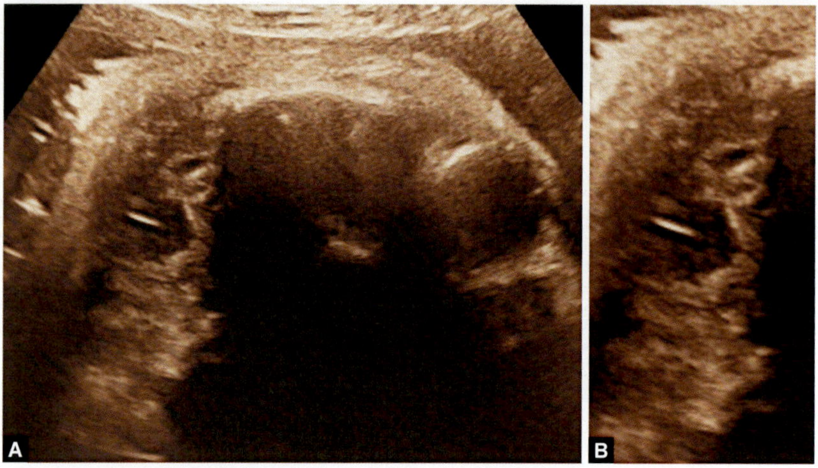

Figs. 11A and B: Absent inferior vermis—Dandy–Walker malformation.

Cisterna magna is enlarged in Dandy-Walker syndrome, Dandy-Walker variant mega cistern magna, Blake's pouch cyst, and any posterior fossa lesions. It is measured as the distance from posterior margin of vermis to anterior margin of occipital bone.

Dandy–Walker Malformation/Variation

About 32% of the fetuses having Dandy-Walker malformation have chromosomal anomalies, most commonly in trisomy 18 and 13.[3] Amongst the fetuses having Dandy-Walker variation also 53% have chromosomal anomalies. Cerebellar hypoplasia may also be associated with aneuploidies. The risk is higher when Dandy-Walker malformation or variation is detected at an early GA. An enlarged cisterna magna though may be seen with normal fetuses, especially in males and after 26 weeks.[4] It is likely to indicate trisomy 18 if seen in third trimester and is associated with polyhydramnios and intrauterine growth restriction (IUGR).

Dandy-Walker malformation is also seen in inheritable syndromes such as Ellis-van Creveld syndrome and Meckel-Gruber syndrome.

Transthalamic Plane (Fig. 12)

This plane is commonly known as biparietal plane and is easily reproducible in late pregnancy. But this plane is now not mandatory for detailed anomaly scan done in second trimester, because falx, cavum septi pellucidi (CSP), thalami, and lateral sulcus are all seen on other planes also. It shows:

- Frontal horns of lateral ventricles
- CSP
- Thalami

- Hippocampal gyrus
- Lateral sulcus (absence indicates lissencephaly)

STUDY OF THE CEREBRAL VASCULATURE

Cerebral circulation is first detectable at 8 weeks **(Fig. 13)** and can be seen in all the fetuses at 11 weeks. The circle of Willis which is formed by two posterior cerebral arteries, a posterior communicating artery, two middle cerebral arteries, two anterior cerebral arteries, and anterior communicating artery, is the landmark of fetal circulation **(Fig. 14)**.

This circle can be seen on axial plane and middle cerebral artery (MCA) is the most commonly interrogated vessel for fetal circulation. From

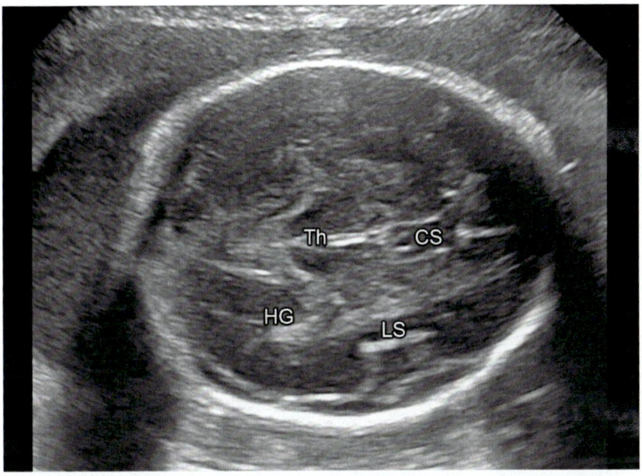

Fig. 12: Transthalamic plane (CS: cavum septi pellucidi; Th: thalami; HG: hippocampal gyrus; LS: lateral sulcus).

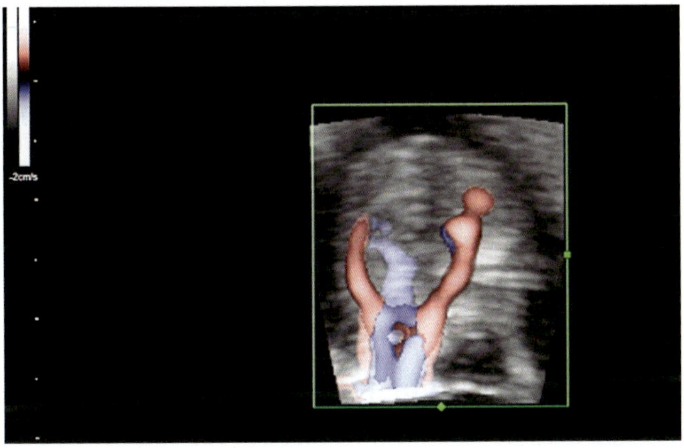

Fig. 13: Cerebral circulation in 8 weeks embryo.

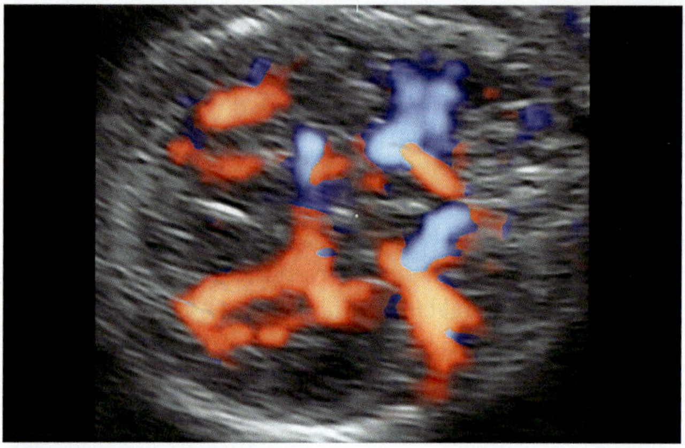

Fig. 14: Circle of Willis on power Doppler.

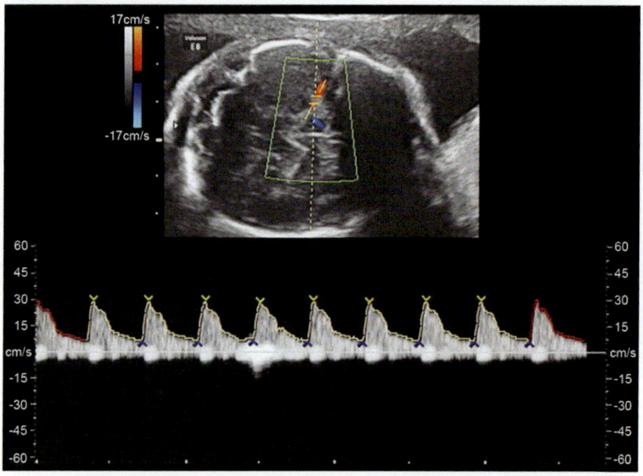

Fig. 15: Spectral Doppler of the middle cerebral artery.

transthalamic view, slight angulation of the probe towards skull base gives a star-shaped hyperechoic structure and placing Doppler there gives a good view of circle of Willis. From circle of Willis **(Fig. 15)**, vessel traveling towards the probe usually in Sylvian fissure is MCA. It has a high resistance flow in first trimester but with increasing GA the resistance decreases and peak systolic velocity in this vessel increases. MCA pulsatility index (PI) remains constant till 32 weeks and then falls.

QUALITATIVE EVALUATION OF FETAL SPINE

Full examination of spine with all projections is not a part of basic examination. This requires expertise and extra skill.

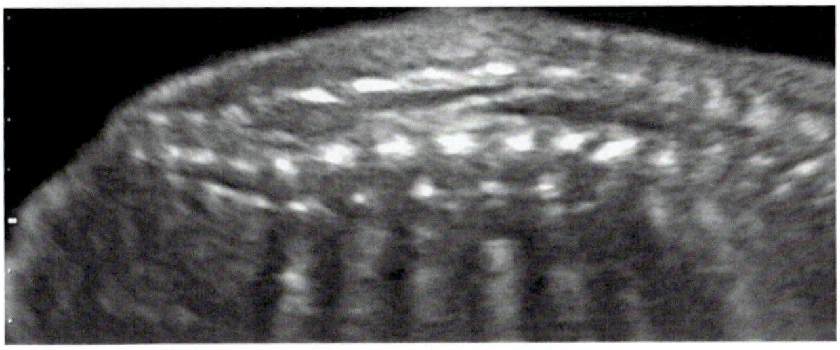

Fig. 16: Longitudinal spine.

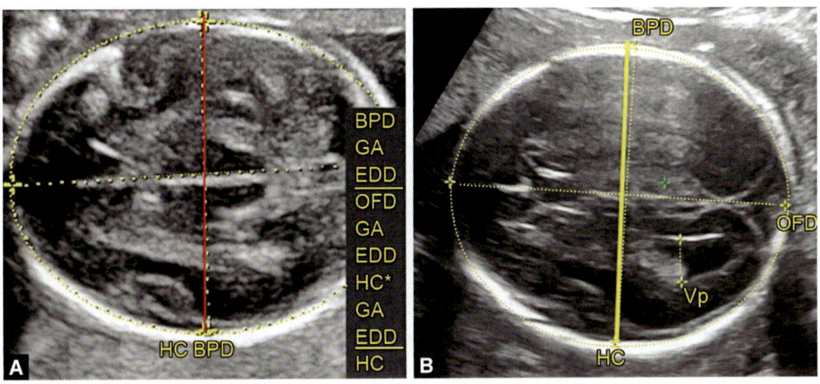

Figs. 17A and B: Biparietal diameter (BPD): (A) Transthalamic plane; (B) Transventricular plane.

Longitudinal section of spine is a must. After 14 weeks always three ossification centers are seen as three parallel lines. It is important to see intact overlying skin on long and transverse section **(Fig. 16)**.

QUANTITATIVE ASSESSMENT OF HEAD

Measurements include:
- Biparietal diameter
- Head circumference (HC)
- Internal diameter of the ventricular atrium
- Cerebellar transverse diameter
- Depth of cisterna magna

Biparietal Diameter

It has been a trend for many years to measure the BPD in transthalamic plane **(Fig. 17A)** and to measure it from outer to inner margin. The Fetal Medicine Foundation though prefers to measure it in transventricular plane **(Fig. 17B)** and measure it from outer to outer wall. As far as assessment of growth is the matter, it is essential that the same method and the same section are always used for this measurement. It is a reliable parameter for growth assessment of the fetus but is altered even when fetal growth is normal, but the head shape is altered.

Shape of the skull is represented by the ratio BPD/occipitofrontal diameter (OFD) (cephalic index) = 75–85%.

Breech presentations may show mild dolichocephaly where this ratio is decreased and in brachycephaly this ratio is increased.

Head Circumference

This is a more reliable parameter than the BPD, especially when the shape of the head is altered but the cephalic index is between 75 and 85%. It is measured from outside the skull bone echoes or may be calculated as HC = 1.62 (BPD + OFD).

Ventricular Atrium

It is measured at the level of parieto-occipital sulcus, perpendicular to the medial wall of lateral ventricle. Calipers are placed inside the ventricular walls **(Figs. 18 and 19)**. In second and third trimester it measures 6–8 mm, 8–10 mm is borderline ventriculomegaly and >10 mm is ventriculomegaly. Ventricular diameter of up to 10 mm is treated expectantly, if it is a solitary finding. Though it is considered as a soft marker for chromosomal abnormality. It is a marker of abnormal cerebral development. Ventricular diameter of 10–12 mm is ventriculomegaly and >15 mm with increased intracranial pressure is called hydrocephalus and may be associated thinning of skull vault and widening of sutures. This may require in utero or immediate postnatal treatment of the fetus.

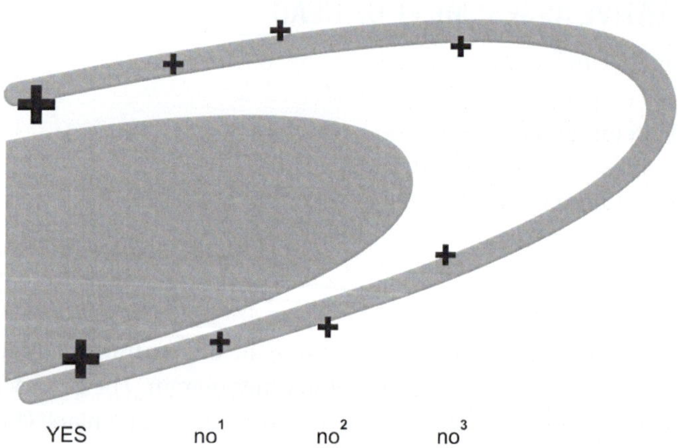

Fig. 18: Diagrammatic presentation of measuring ventricular width correct (larger cross) and incorrect methods.

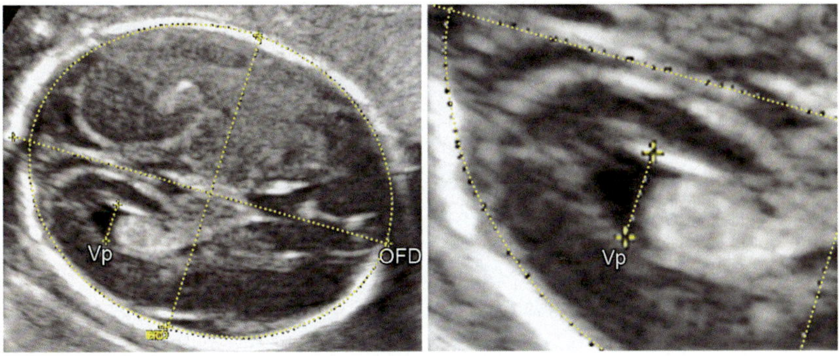

Fig. 19: Measuring ventricular width.

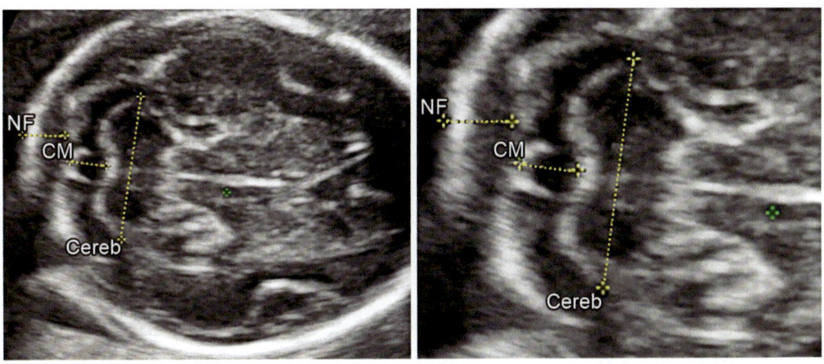

Fig. 20: Measuring cerebellar diameter (green) and cisterna magna (yellow).

Cerebellum

It is measured from outer to outer margin **(Fig. 20)** of the cerebellum on transcerebellar section. Transverse cerebellar diameter increases by 1 mm every week from 14 to 21 weeks. Diameter corresponds to the weeks of gestation in second trimester and is not affected by IUGR.

Cisterna Magna

It is measured from posterior margin of cerebellar vermis to the anterior margin of overlying occipital bone. Cistern magna is almost always traversed by thin septa of arachnoid membrane and this is a normal appearance. It measures 2–10 mm but is slightly more in dolichocephaly. It is enlarged in cerebellar pathologies, especially in vermian pathologies, like vermian hypoplasia, Dandy-Walker malformations or variants but in neural canal defects when cerebellum is pulled caudally, it is obliterated. This is known as "banana sign" of cerebellum **(Fig. 21A)**. This is also associated with collapsed

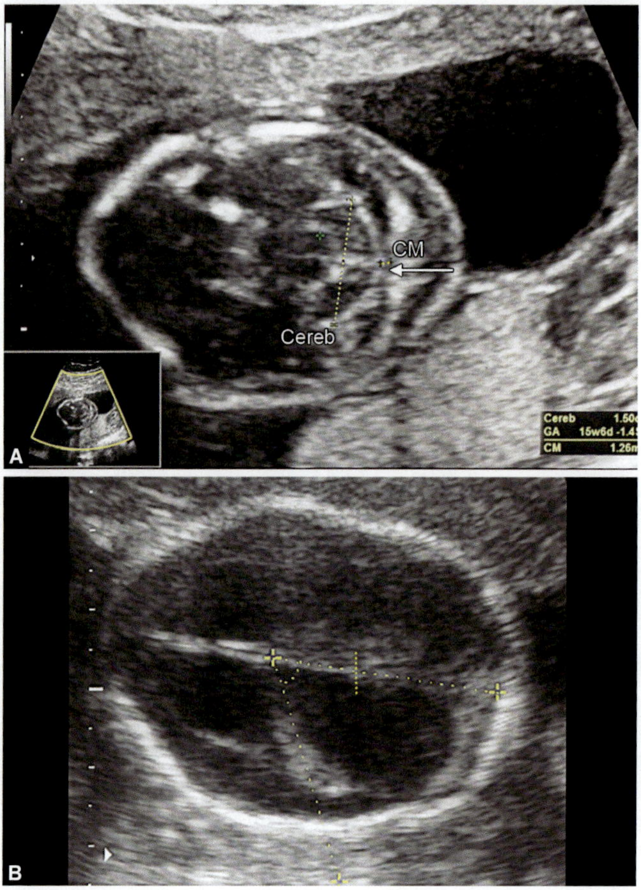

Figs. 21A and B: (A) Banana-shaped cerebellum (arrow); (B) Lemon skull sign.

frontal bones and makes the skull shape like a lemon and is called "lemon sign" **(Fig. 21B)**.

For patients with increased risk of CNS abnormalities and suspicious findings on basic examination, a detailed fetal neuroscan is required which includes the use of multiplanar and 3D US. It has a much greater diagnostic potential. Orthogonal planes—axial, sagittal, and coronal are obtained by aligning the transducer with sutures and fontanelles of fetal head.

Axial, coronal, and sagittal sections of the spine are also studied as a part of *detailed fetal neuroscan*.

Systematic evaluation of the head consists of detailed study of anatomical structures by:

- Four coronal planes
- Three sagittal planes
- Three axial planes

Coronal Planes (Fig. 22)

- Transfrontal plane (frontal 2 plane)
- Transcaudate plane (midcoronal 1 plane)
- Transthalamic plane (midcoronal 2 plane)
- Transcerebellar plane (occipital 1 and 2 plane)

Transfrontal plane **(Fig. 23)**: This plane cuts through anterior fontanelle and is rostral to the genu of CC. It shows midline hemispheric fissure, anterior horns of lateral ventricles, sphenoidal bone, and orbital plates.

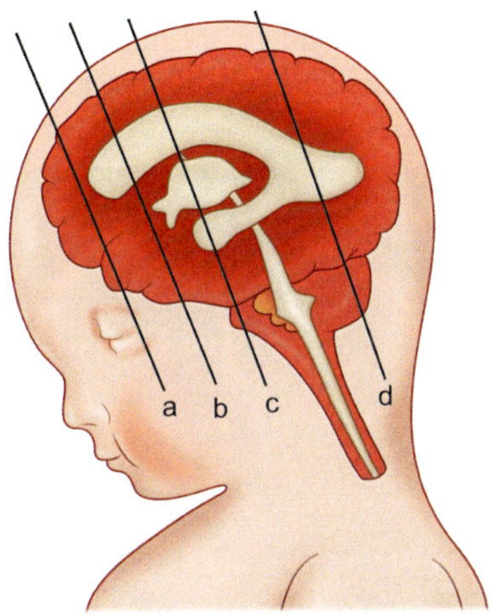

Fig. 22: Diagrammatic representation of coronal sections for detailed neurosonogram: (a) Transfrontal plane; (b) Transcaudate plane; (c) Transthalamic plane; and (d) Transcerebellar plane.

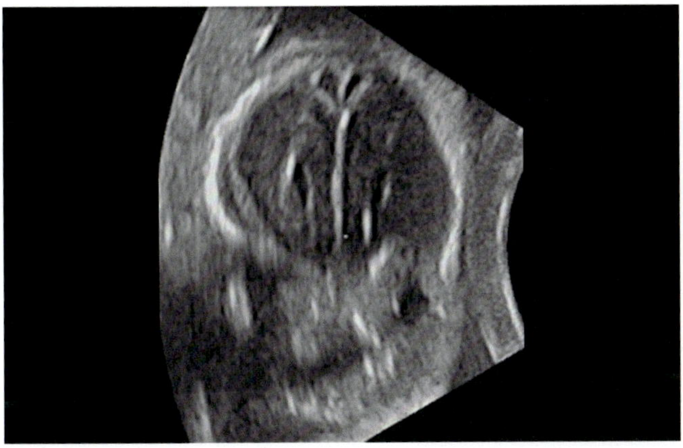

Fig. 23: Transfrontal coronal plane.

Transcaudate plane **(*Fig. 24*)***:* This section is at the level of caudate nuclei and cuts genu of CC. It shows CC in cut section, triangular cavum septum pellucidum, frontal horns of lateral ventricle, and sylvian fissures laterally.

Transthalamic plane **(*Fig. 25*)***:* This section cuts across the thalami which are seen closely apposed to each other on the sides of midline. Third ventricle is seen in midline. Third ventricle more than 5 mm is considered as dilated. This section also shows interventricular foramina and atria of lateral ventricles with choroid plexus, basal cistern containing vessels of circle of Willis and optic chiasma close to the skull base.

Transcerebellar plane **(*Fig. 26*)***:* This section is taken across the cerebellum, through posterior fontanelle. It shows occipital horns of lateral ventricle, interhemispheric fissure, cerebellar hemispheres, and vermis.

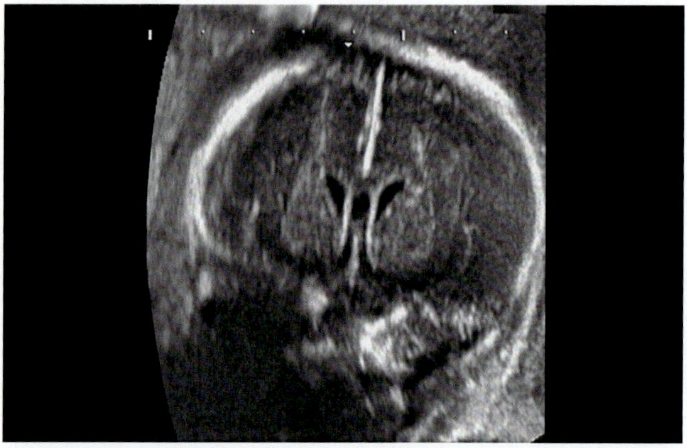

Fig. 24: Transcaudate coronal plane.

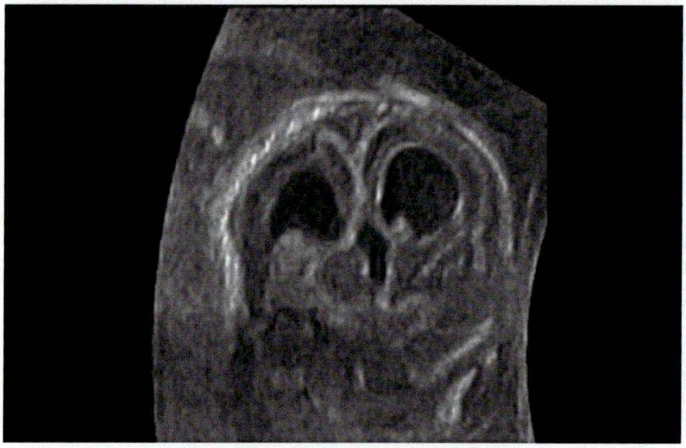

Fig. 25: Transthalamic coronal plane.

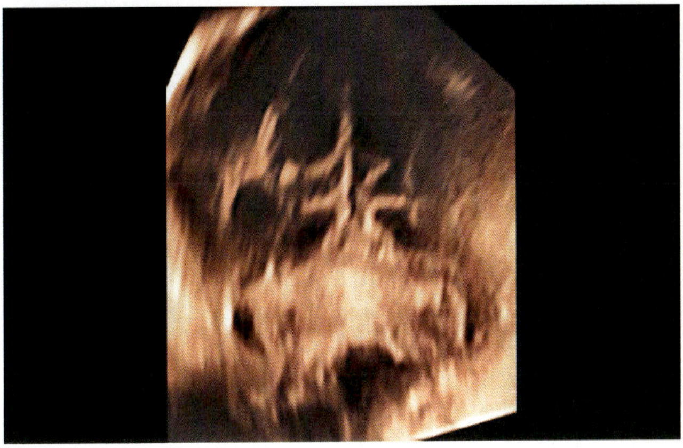

Fig. 26: Transcerebellar plane.

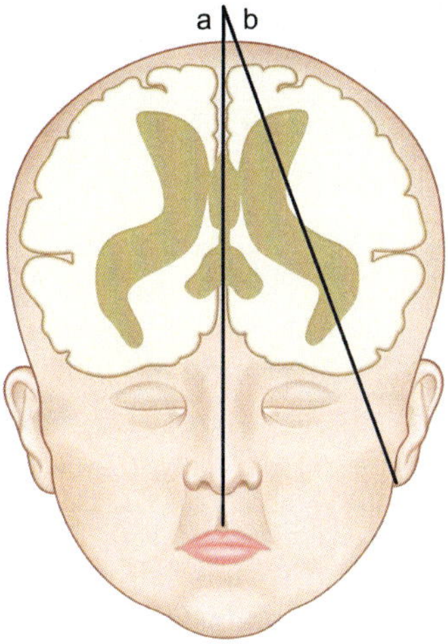

Fig. 27: Diagrammatic representation of sagittal sections of head for detailed neurosonogram: (a) Midsagittal and (b) Left parasagittal.

For vascular studies, amongst all coronal planes the midcoronal plane is most revealing. This shows MCA, ventriculostriate arteries, cross-section of pericallosal arteries, and superior sagittal sinus.

Sagittal Planes (Fig. 27)

- Midsagittal
- Right parasagittal
- Left parasagittal

Midsagittal plane ***(Figs. 28A and B):*** This section is in midline along the sagittal suture and shows CC and cavum septum pellucidum under it.

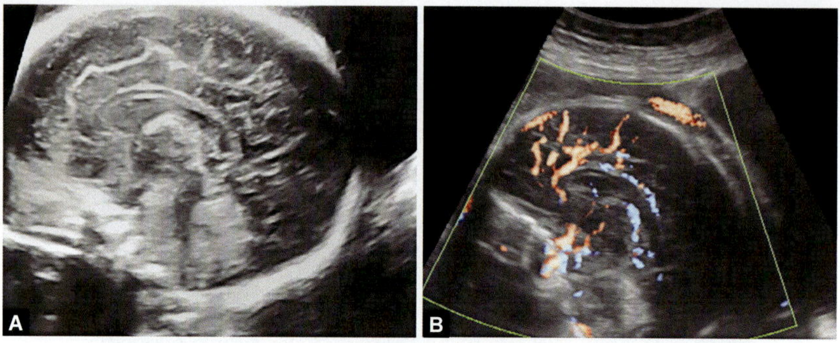

Figs. 28A and B: (A) Midsagittal plane showing corpus callosum; (B) Midsagittal plane of head shows pericallosal on Doppler.

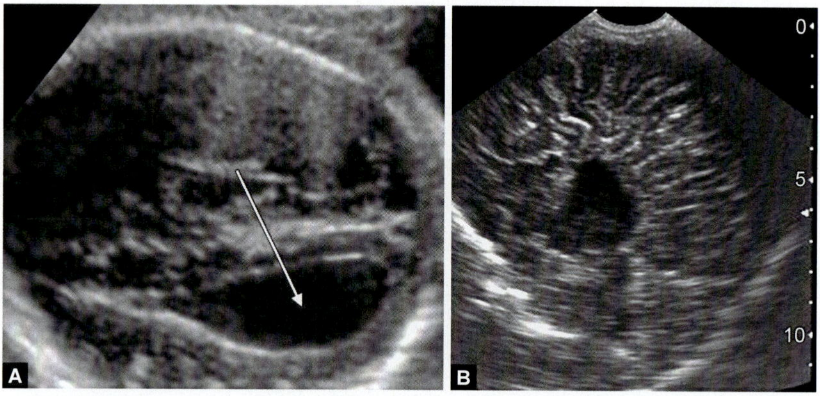

Figs. 29A and B: (A) Sunray pattern of sulci and gyri (arrow); (B) Colpocephaly, both are suggestive of absent corpus callosum.

In some cases cavum vergi and cavum veli interpositi may also be seen. Posterior part of the section shows brainstem, pons, vermis and 4th ventricle, possibly aqueduct also. Fourth ventricle is seen in median plane as a sonolucent triangle at the level of cerebellum.

Corpus callosum **(Fig. 28A)** starts forming at 12 weeks and is completed at 20–22 weeks. It can be seen only on sagittal section. Indirect sign of its presence is pericallosal artery **(Fig. 28B)**. Indirect sign of absent CC is tear-shaped ventriculomegaly/colpocephaly on axial section and directly upward pointing frontal horns on coronal section. But sagittal section shows absent CC with cortical sulci and gyri arising from single point instead of from coronal section **(Figs. 29A and B)**.

Cingulate gyrus and sulcus, the parieto-occipital fissure and calcarine fissure can be seen in this section. Both lateral and cingulate gyri appear between 22 and 24 weeks. Though this is pretty late than its anatomical appearance which is at 18 weeks. Maximum sulci and gyri appear between 28 and 30 weeks.

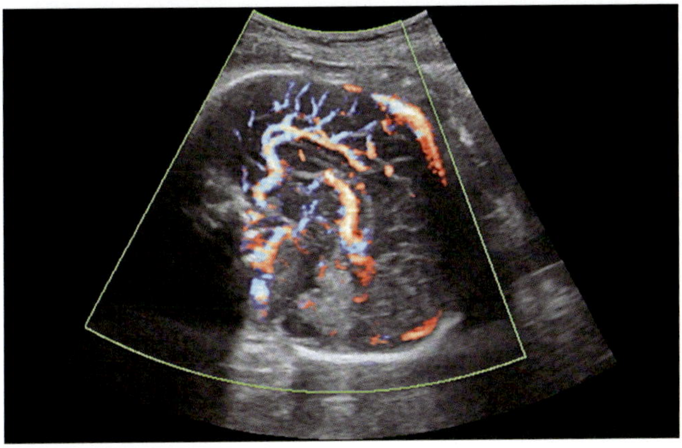

Fig. 30: Midline vessels on Doppler of midsagittal plane.

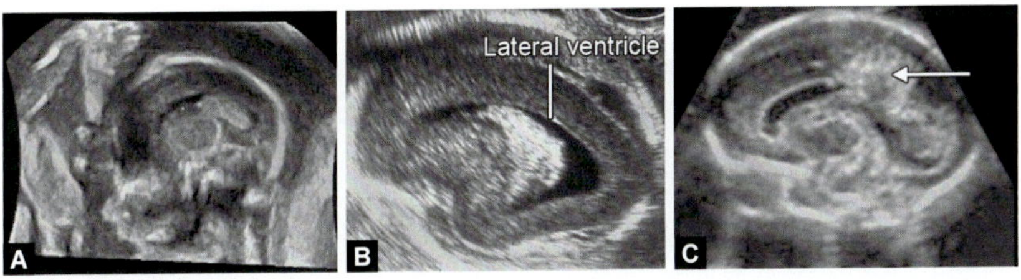

Figs. 31A to C: (A) Parasagittal plane showing thalamus; (B) Parasagittal plane showing lateral ventricle and choroid plexus; (C) Intraventricular hemorrhage (arrow).

Doppler studies in midsagittal section shows the branches of internal carotid artery **(Fig. 30)**. Its main branches are anterior and middle cerebral arteries and pericallosal artery. Superior sagittal sinus and vein of Galen can also be seen on this section.

Parasagittal or oblique plane shows entire lateral ventricle with choroid plexus, paraventricular tissue, and cortex **(Figs. 31A and B)**. This plane is for diagnosis of intraventricular hemorrhage **(Fig. 31C)**.

Parasagittal planes can show the protective layers of the brain such as scalp, skull periosteum, dura mater, arachnoid, and pia mater. Scalp is seen as outermost echogenic layer. Skull is the most echogenic covering, being a bone. A thin line can be seen just under the bone that is the periosteum. Under the periosteum a distinct echogenic layer is seen—the arachnoid membrane. Space between the later two is clear. This is a potential space and is more clearly seen only in presence of fluid collection. But under the arachnoid matter and above the echogenic covering of the brain, the pia mater, the space is seen traversed by several linear echogenecities (blood vessels), as seen on high resolution US. These planes are also used to study the subdural and subarachnoid pathologies such as hemorrhage.

FETAL SPINE EXAMINATION IN HIGH-RISK PATIENTS DEMANDS STUDY OF ALL THE THREE PLANES (FIGS. 32A TO C)

- Transverse/axial plane **(Fig. 32A)**
- Sagittal/longitudinal plane **(Fig. 32B)**
- Coronal plane **(Fig. 32C)**

Usually only two of these three planes can be examined in any fetus depending on its position but it is possible to assess all the three planes on B-mode US also in almost all cases and three-dimensional US (3D US) may be used if required to obtain all the three planes **(Fig. 33)**.

Transverse or axial plane of spine is obtained by sweeping the probe through the entire fetal length. When this is done the level of fetal spine must be kept in mind as vertebrae have different anatomy at different levels. Upper cervical vertebrae are quadrangular, thoracic and lumbar vertebrae are triangular, and sacral vertebrae are flat **(Figs. 34A to D)**.

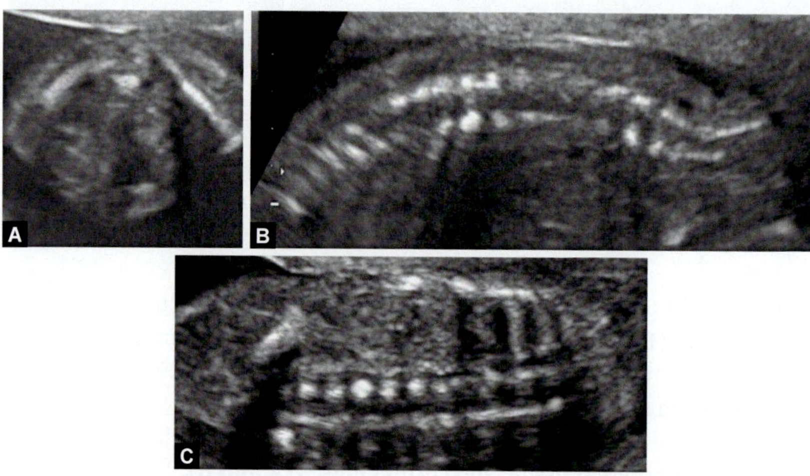

Figs. 32A to C: Transverse, sagittal, and coronal planes of spine.

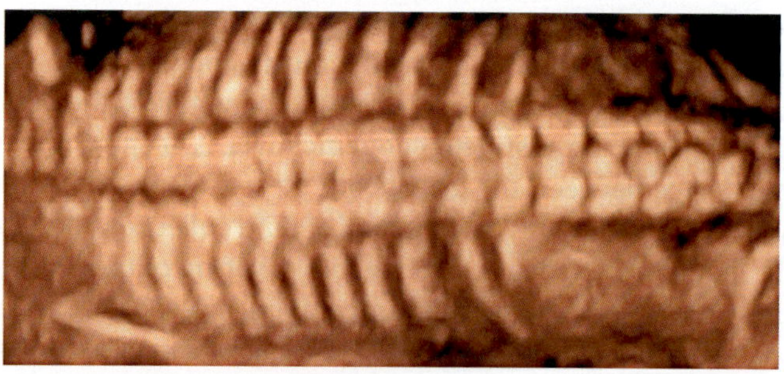

Fig. 33: Three-dimensional ultrasound of spine.

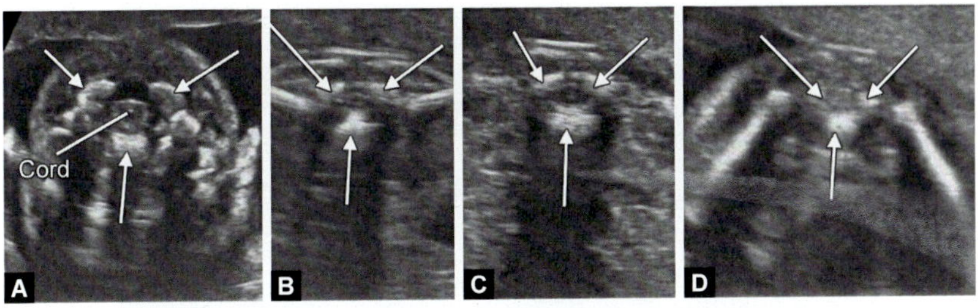

Figs. 34A to D: Spine in transverse sections at different levels.

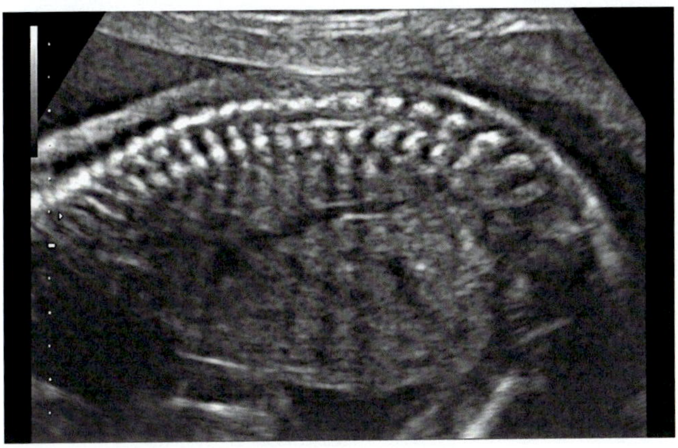

Fig. 35: Sagittal/longitudinal section of spine.

Sagittal Plane

The ossification centers of vertebral bodies and posterior arches form two parallel lines which converge at the sacrum. If spine is anterior, one can also see spinal canal and spinal cord through the unossified spinous processes.

Conus medullaris at L2–3 can be seen in second and third trimester as two thin lines converging in a point. It is essential to establish the integrity of the overlying skin also **(Fig. 35)**. Break or discontinuity in the skin overlying the spine can sometimes be the only clue to spinal canal defect **(Fig. 36)**.

Coronal Plane

This plane will show one, two or three parallel lines, depending on the section at the level of vertebral bodies or transverse process or spinous process **(Fig. 37)**. Regular and bilateral symmetrical disposition of ossification centers indicate integrity of the spine. Widening of the distance between these ossification centers indicate open spinal canal defect **(Figs. 38A to C)**. It is important to make a note here, that between 16 and 20 weeks of pregnancy the spinal canal appears wide in the lumbar region and this is normal at this GA and is known as physiological spina bifida.

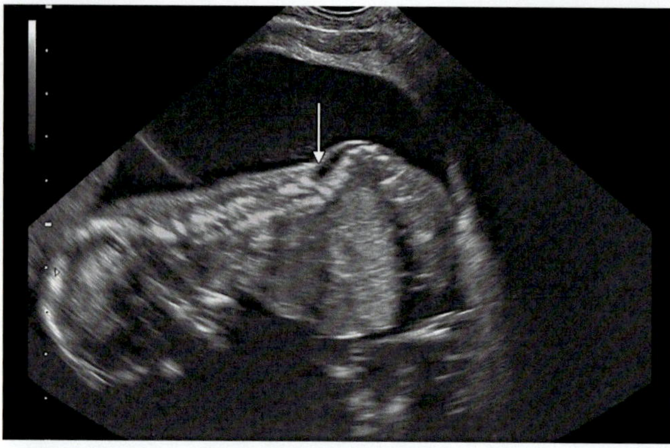

Fig. 36: Meningocele (arrow).

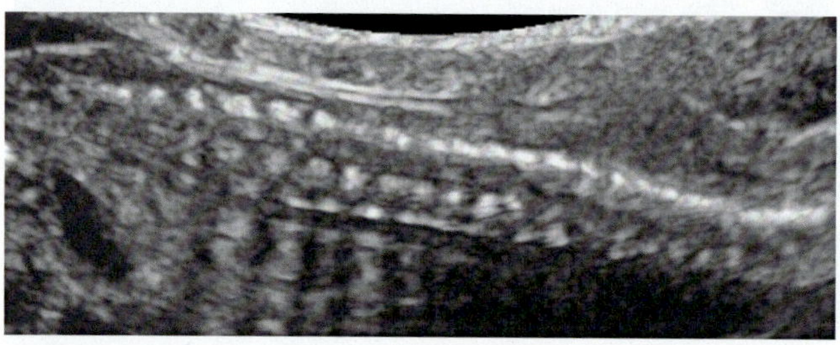

Fig. 37: Coronal spine.

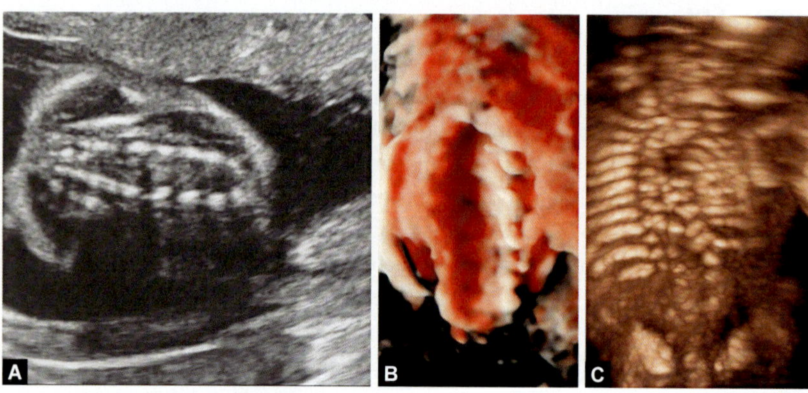

Figs. 38A to C: Open spinal canal defect.

Spinal abnormalities commonly seen are **(Figs. 39A to C)**:

- Hemivertebrae
- Open spinal canal
- *Spina bifida occulta:* When there is only mild widening of the spinal column with no herniation of neuronal tissue it is spina bifida occulta.

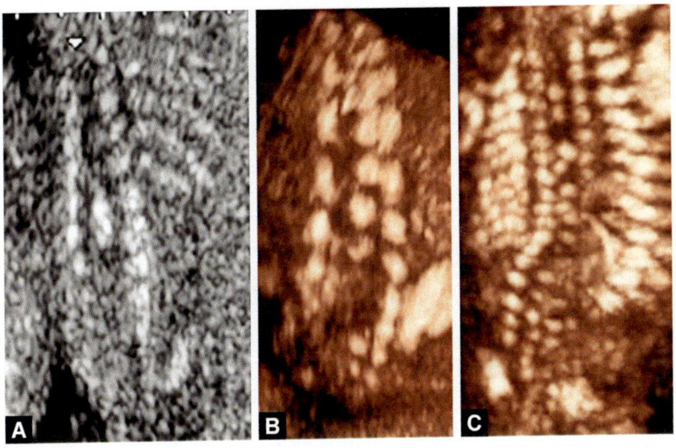

Figs. 39A to C: Spinal canal defects: Diastematomyelia, open spinal canal defect, and multiple spine abnormalities.

- *Platyspondyly:* Anteroposterior compression of the spinal column is platyspondyly.
- *Diastematomyelia:* Bony spur tethering the spinal cord within the margins of spinal column is diastematomyelia. This is identified on US as a bone piece between the two lines of ossification centers on coronal plane of the spine.
- Hemivertebra is identified by loss of parallelism between the ossification centers thus leading to abnormal curvature of fetal spine.
- Open spina bifida or open spinal canal defect is identified on US by undue widening of the distance between the ossification centers of two transverse processes. It is often associated with cranial abnormalities.

With advanced technologies now it is possible to make early diagnosis of cranial lesions **(Figs. 40A and B)**.

Brain development can be studied as early as in the first trimester. At 13 weeks, there is decrease in lateral ventricles dominance and choroid plexus, diencephalons, and posterior fossa structures appear. Till this GA the large part of the ventricle is filled by choroid plexus with falx in the center and the US appearance is described as "butterfly sign". As GA advances the ventricles become evidently smaller. Development of all other structures of brain follow.

Fetuses develop particular pattern of movement at particular GA and studying that would allow to assess the neurological development of the fetus. Fetal behavior can be correlated to the fetal brain maturation and therefore studying fetal behavior can indirectly assess the maturation of fetal brain. A systematic test was devised by professor Kurjak et al. to study the fetal behavior in later second trimester and third trimester and is named as Kurjak Antenatal Neurodevelopmental Test (KANET) test.[5,6]

Systematic assessment of the fetal movements, their types and frequency is done to derive a neurological score (KANET score) and this score is used to predict the neurological maturation of fetal brain.

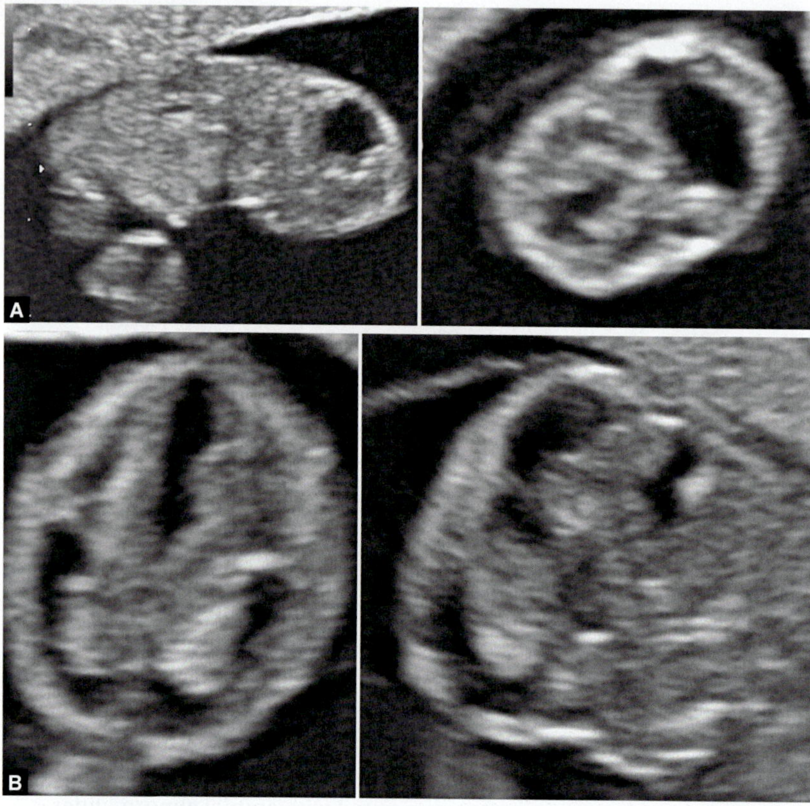

Figs. 40A and B: (A) *8 weeks:* Rhombencephalon; (B) *9 weeks:* Lateral ventricles.

It is the advancement in technology, 3D and 4D US that has made the detailed fetal neuroscan very easy, less time consuming, and a reproducible examination. Multiplanar mode, volume contrast imaging, and tomographic ultrasound imaging are the ones which have made it possible to study all the transverse, sagittal, and coronal planes of the head and spine from a single volume sweep **(Figs. 41A to C)**.

Sonography is an extremely informative imaging modality for study of fetal nervous system and is relatively inexpensive and definitely noninvasive. Better understanding of development and neuroanatomy makes detection of pathologies easier, especially by use of coronal and sagittal planes.

Though the facts to be remembered are that:

- Anomalies of neuronal proliferation such as microcephaly, tumors, and cortical malformations may remain undetected as brain continues to develop in the second half of gestation and in neonatal period.
- Moreover, some cerebral lesions may also develop due to acquired prenatal and perinatal insults and in these cases antenatal development has been normal.

But the inference is that at midgestation if:

- Normal transventricular and transcerebellar plane anatomy
- Normal BPD and HC
- Ventricular atria < 10 mm
- Cisterna magna 2–10 mm

  In a low-risk pregnancy, no further examination is indicated.

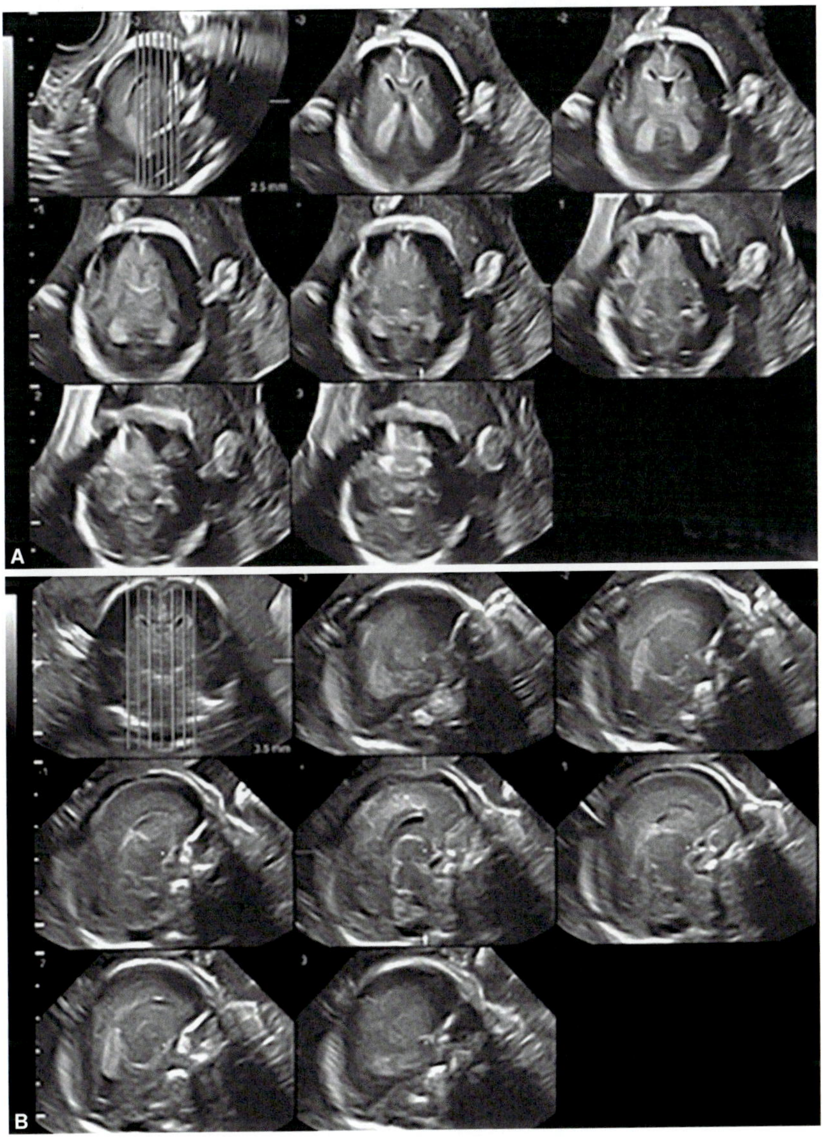

Figs. 41A and B

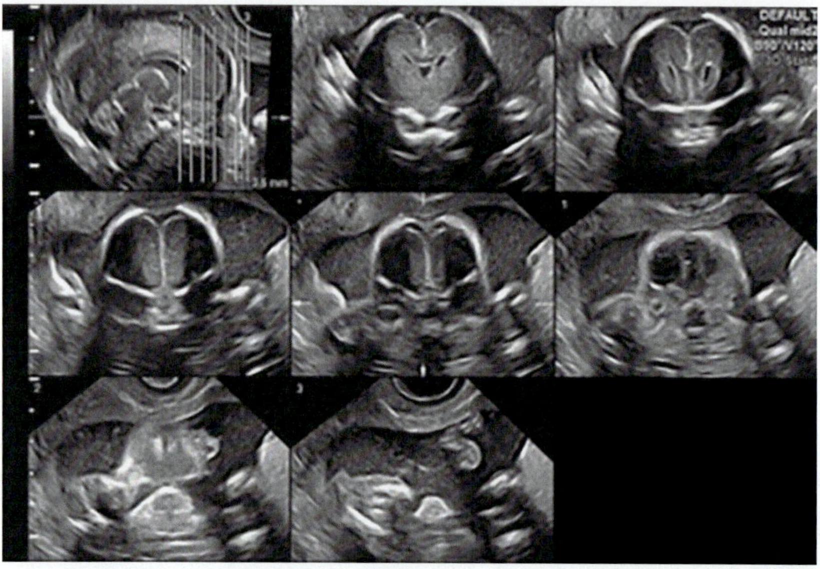

Fig. 41C

Figs. 41A to C: Tomographic ultrasound images of fetal head in transverse, sagittal, and coronal planes.

And even in expert hands some types of anomalies may be difficult or impossible to diagnose in utero, as they might have developed later during pregnancy or even in early neonatal life.

REFERENCES

1. Monteagudo A, Timor TI. Development of fetal Gyri, Sulci and fissures: a transvaginal sonographic study. Ultrasound Obstet Gynecol. 1997;9:422-8.
2. Malinger G, Ben-Sira L, Lev D, Ben-Aroya Z, Kidron D, Lerman-Sagie T. Fetal brain imaging: comparison between magnetic resonance imaging and dedicated neurosonography. Ultrasound Obstet Gynecol. 2004;23:333-40.
3. Cardoza JD, Goldstein RB, Filly RA. Exclusion of fetal ventriculomegaly with a single measurement: the width of the lateral ventricular atrium. Radiology. 1988;169:711-4.
4. Campbell S. Diagnosis of fetal abnormalities by ultrasound. In: Milunsky A (Ed). Genetic Disorders of Fetus. New York: Plenum Press; 1979.
5. Kurjak A, Miskovi B, Stanojevi M, Amiel-Tison C, Ahmed B, Azumendi G, et al. New scoring system for fetal neurobehavior assessed by three- and four-dimensional sonography. J Perinat Med. 2008;36:73-81.
6. Kurjak A, Abo-Yaqoub S, Stanojevic M, Yigiter AB, Vasilj O, Lebit D, et al. The potential of 4D sonography in the assessment of fetal neurobehavior—multicentric study in high-risk pregnancies. J Perinat Med. 2010;38:77-82.

CHAPTER 21

Fetal Echocardiography for Obstetrician

Sonal Panchal

INTRODUCTION

Cardiac anomalies are most common anomalies (one-third) found at birth. Its prevalence is 5 in 1,000 live births. 15% of abortions are due to cardiac anomalies. About 20% of neonatal deaths and 50% of infant deaths due to malformations are due to cardiac anomalies. Incidence of aneuploidy is 15–38% in fetuses with cardiac malformations and in live births also the incidence of aneuploidy is 11.8% in babies with congenital heart defects.[1] Congenital cardiac diseases thus is taking a larger toll of the newborn population than even the chromosomal anomalies. Therefore, diagnosis of cardiac diseases must not be missed in antenatal period. More so because many of these have good prognosis, if they are detected antenatally and can be treated immediately after birth. Screening for cardiac diseases by fetal echocardiography therefore must be included at least in the second trimester scan. Advancing technology and transvaginal approach now also allows fetal echocardiography with nuchal scan.

Risk factors for cardiac anomalies are:

- Family history of cardiac disease, e.g., Holt-Oram syndrome. Mother having congenital heart disease (CHD), risk to fetus of CHD is 5–10%,[2] though in fetuses who have fathers with CHD, the risk is lesser. Certain defects have higher (10–15%) recurrence rate, e.g., hypoplastic left heart, aortic stenosis, coarctation of aorta, 2–5% for septal and conotruncal anomalies and <5% for transposition of the great arteries (TGA), and single ventricle like abnormalities.
- *Maternal diseases*:
    - Diabetes mellitus [5% risk of CHD in fetus: ventricular septal defect (VSD), TGA, and coarctation and conotruncal abnormalities], phenylketonuria (VSD, coarctation of aorta, hypoplastic left heart, and Fallot's tetralogy)
    - Collagen disease [anti-Sjögren syndrome A or B antibodies (SS-A or SS-B)]—associated with myocarditis and heart blocks.
- *Teratogens*: *Drugs and infections*:
    - *Alcohol:* Patent ductus arteriosus (PDA) and septal defects: Up to 25% risk of CHD[3]
    - *Retinoic acid*: Conotruncal and great artery anomalies

- *Anticonvulsants*: Valproic acid, phenytoin, and trimethadione: PDA, aortic stenosis, Fallot's tetralogy, TGA, and coarctation of aorta
- *Thalidomide*: 5–10% incidence of CHD: Fallot's tetralogy, truncus arteriosus, and septal defects[4]
- *Lithium:* Ebstein's anomaly
- *Daunorubicin:* Myocardial necrosis
- *Rubella:* PDA, pulmonary stenosis, and septal defects
- *Parvovirus:* Damage to myocardial cell itself

▪ Chromosomal anomalies
▪ Extracardiac anomalies are present in 25–45% of fetuses with CHD and so whenever an abnormality is found anywhere in the body, the heart must be evaluated with care
▪ Monozygotic twins have double incidence of CHD and risk is much higher in conjoined twins
▪ *Arrhythmias*: Septal defects
▪ Nonimmune hydrops

The later two actually indicate that there is a possibility of CHD.

But it is important to know that as for trisomy 21, only 30% of cardiac anomalies are detected in high-risk group, whereas 70% are detected in the low-risk group. Therefore, screening for cardiac anomalies must be included for each fetus.

Till now screening meant looking at the four chambers of the heart and taking M-mode to look for arrhythmias. But four chamber view diagnoses only 50–60% of cardiac anomalies and including outflow tracts will diagnose up to 75% of cardiac anomalies if examined by trained and experienced person.[5]

Approximately 25% are still missed. A detailed fetal echocardiography is therefore essential. This must include gray scale, color Doppler, pulsed Doppler, and M-mode assessment all together.

EQUIPMENT SETTINGS

High resolution linear array, curved array or sector scanners can be used for this examination. 4–8 MHz is the preferred frequency range for this examination.

Settings for *2D imaging/grayscale* are set at high contrast. The angle of the scanning field should be wide enough to include the transverse section of the thorax. The focal depth is kept sufficient so the area of interest is seen in the center of the screen, and the focal point is adjusted at the level of the heart. Orient region of interest (ROI) collinear to beam. Select smallest possible angle of insonation. Zoom the image so that the heart is seen large enough to identify all the structures but not too large that the sharpness of the image is lost. Maternal abdominal fat or scars, anterior fetal spine or limbs may make the visualization of fetal heart difficult. Using harmonics, speckled reduction imaging (SRI) and compound resolution imaging (CRI) increases the sharpness of the image.

As heart has an anatomy to study and also the blood flows to be understood, cardiac examination cannot be complete without *color Doppler*. For color Doppler high wall filter, high pulse repetition frequency (PRF), low persistence, and low color sensitivity settings are done. The color box should be big enough only to include the heart. The gains and PRF are so set that chambers of the heart are adequately filled with color but there is no aliasing. The color balance is adjusted so that both the gray scale and color can be defined adequately at a time. Using B-mode and color dual display can be helpful to correlate the anatomy and the blood flows better.

Using *zoom and cine loop* examination can be very helpful with both gray scale and color Doppler.

For *pulsed Doppler* select small spectral sample volume to include the area of interest only with angle not more than 60°. PRF and wall filters should be high as for color Doppler. Sweep speed is set high. Remember angle corrections are required only for absolute values and not for study of waveform pattern or ratios. Spectral sample volume is placed just downstream of valve to study the flow through the valve. It is placed upstream to demonstrate regurgitation in outflow tracts. For tricuspid regurgitation (TR) the sample volume is placed across the valve. It may be placed by color Doppler guidance.

M-mode Study

Fetal echocardiography cannot be considered complete without M-mode evaluation. The M-mode cursor is aligned perpendicular to the interventricular (IV) septum at the level of atrioventricular (AV) valves **(Fig. 1)**.

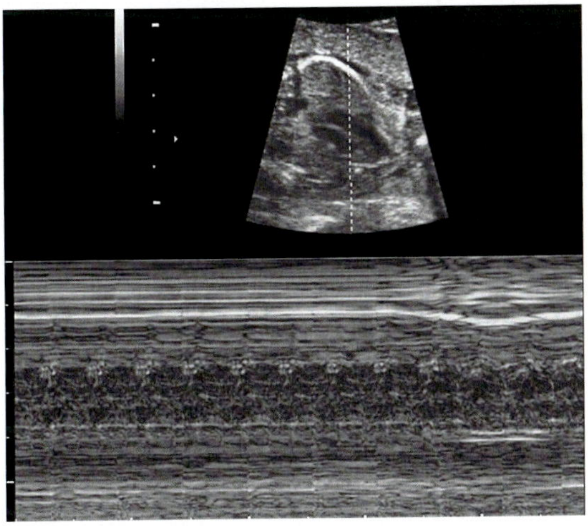

Fig. 1: M-mode study of fetal heart.

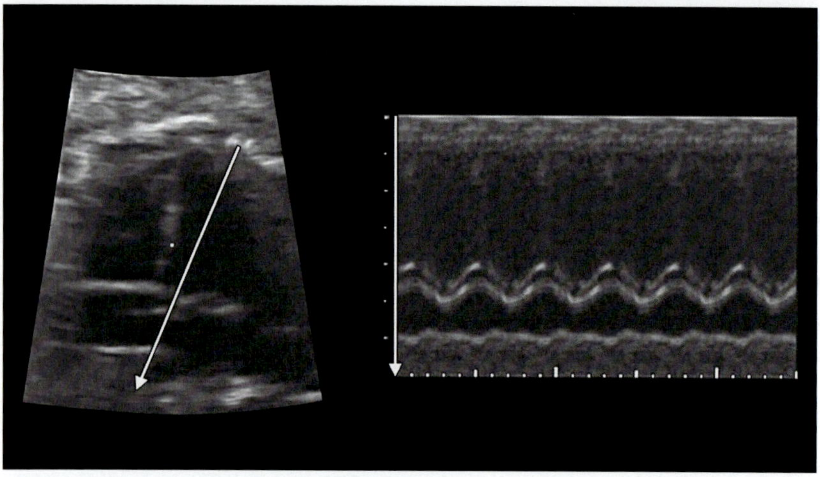

Fig. 2: Cursor placement on M-mode.

Interpreting M-mode correctly is based on identifying and correlating each line of M-mode with the anatomical structure on gray scale **(Fig. 2)**. Ventricular chamber size is measured at end diastole when ventricular size is the largest. Outer biventricular diameter is measured and right and left ventricular inner diameter is measured. Ventricular wall thickness and thickness of the IV septum are measured. Ventricular contractility is measured by measuring the systolic and diastolic outer dimensions and then subtracting systolic from diastolic measurement and then dividing it with diastolic measurement. Rhythm disturbances are assessed by correlating ventricular and atrial cycles when cursor passes through one atrium and one ventricle at 30° to the IV septum on four chamber view. M-mode can also be used with color Doppler to understand the regurge better **(Fig. 3)**.

B-mode scanning is the most important and color Doppler should be used only after B-mode diagnosis for demonstration and confirmation of a particular pathology. Color may be required sometimes for identification of anatomy only when evaluation of the heart is done at 11–14 weeks scan. Though with high resolution probes and improving technology, early fetal echocardiography can be done at 11–14 weeks with the nuchal scan with transvaginal probe with 5–9 MHz frequency range.

Cardiac evaluations have been made less time consuming and much easier with advancing technology. New four-dimensional ultrasound (4D US) technology with *spatial temporal imaging correlation (STIC)* can be used for offline 4D cardiac evaluation. After optimizing the two-dimensional (2D) image a single sweep is taken from the upper abdomen to the upper chest of the fetus in 7.5–15 seconds. Multiple B-mode images of the heart during different phases of cardiac cycle are captured and stored as a volume. This

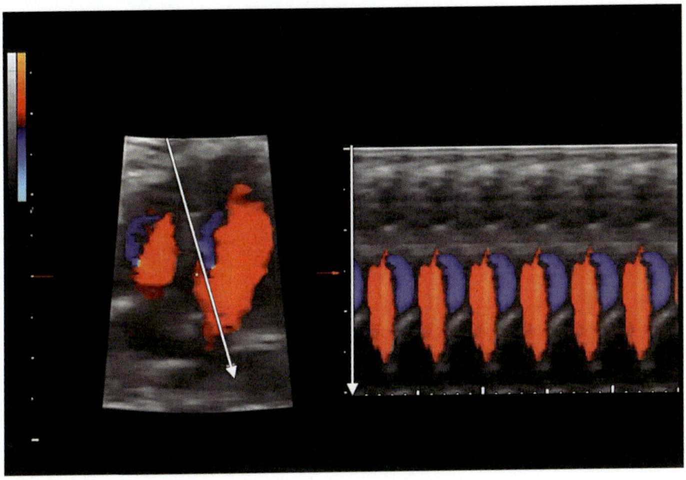
Fig. 3: M-mode tracing with color Doppler.

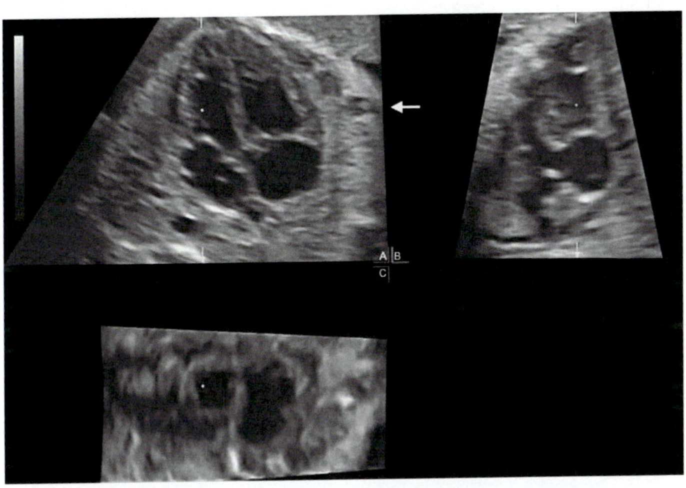

Fig. 4: Fetal heart with spatial temporal imaging correlation.

can be seen in all three planes—X, Y, and Z (sagittal, axial, and coronal) and can be run as a continuous cardiac cycle **(Fig. 4)**.

Walking through these sections give all the planes required for complete cardiac evaluation: four chamber heart, left ventricular outflow tract (LVOT), right ventricular outflow tract (RVOT), and three vessel-trachea view. Instead of walking through, all sections can be seen at a time, in all planes, using tomographic ultrasound imaging (TUI) on STIC acquired image **(Fig. 5)**. The image can also be seen as live three-dimensional (3D) by various rendering modes. Inversion mode of rendering can be an excellent tool to demonstrate septal defects and outflow tracts and great vessels. This mode shows all cavities

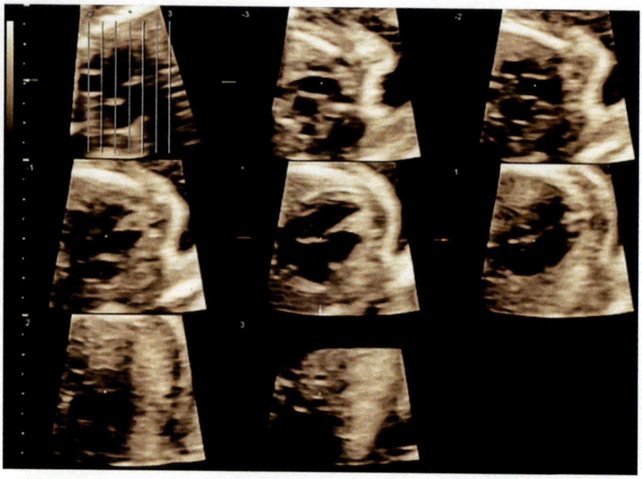

Fig. 5: Tomographic ultrasound imaging of spatial temporal imaging correlation.

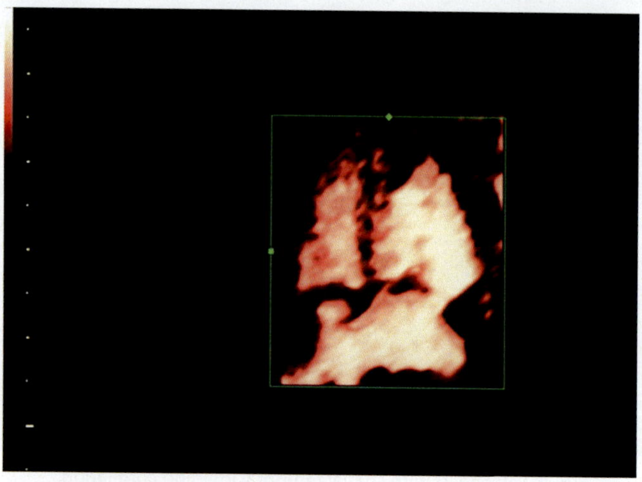

Fig. 6: Three-dimensional (3D) of four chamber heart view is rendered in inversion mode.

as solid structures **(Fig. 6)**. Rendering from different angles can give all those views of the heart which were never possible by any other modalities, e.g., basic view of the heart, which shows relationship of all the four valves **(Figs. 7A and B)**, which is very informative of outflow tract relationship, inflow tract abnormalities and important for surgeons. Using TUI may also help looking at the heart at different angles. Though standardization of stored images is necessary to understand and correctly interpret them.

The new scanners have now come up with still easier and more standardized techniques of storage and evaluation. This software is known

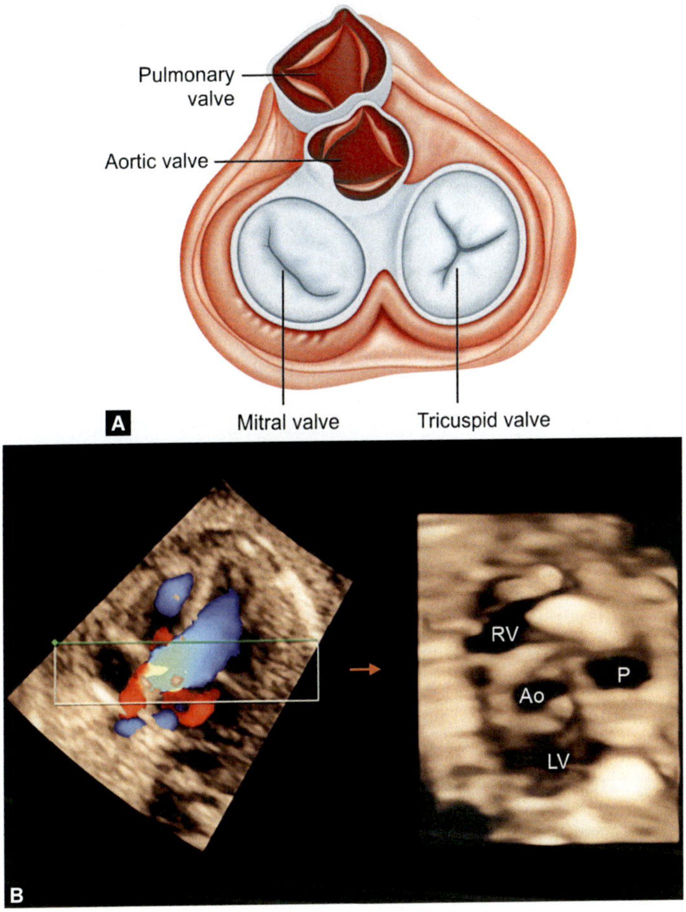

Figs. 7A and B: Basic view of the heart (Ao: aorta; LV: left ventricle; P: pulmonary; RV: right ventricle).

as *VCAD* **(Fig. 8)**. When working with this, the essential views of the heart are only a finger touch away. No manual rotations or walking through are also necessary. This makes cardiac evaluation much quicker both online and offline. Though detailed study of these techniques are out of scope of this chapter.

EVALUATION OF THE HEART

- *As a thoracic organ*:
  - Situs
  - Position
  - Axis

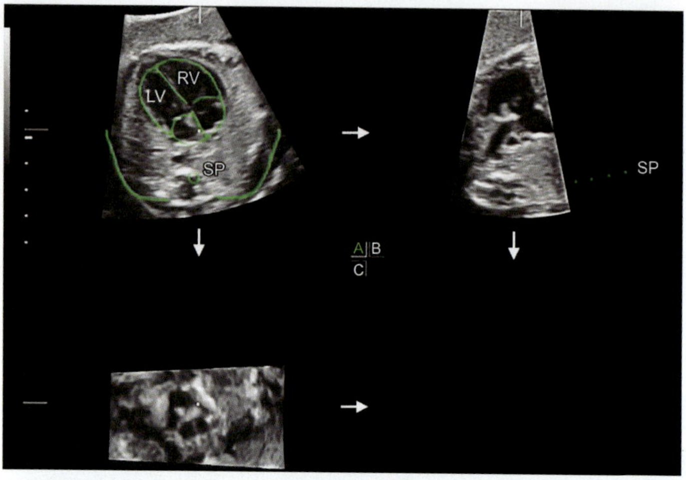

Fig. 8: VCAD software. Matching the diagram with acquired image (LV: left ventricle; RV: right ventricle; SP: spine).

- *Size:*
    - Transverse diameter
    - Cardiothoracic ratio
- Rate and rhythm

- Internal anatomy

Deciding the Cardiac Situs

Situs indicates sidedness of the heart in the chest, or may be decided as to which side the apex points. Do not depend on the stomach shadow to decide the situs.

First identify the position of the fetus: Vertex or breech and the position of the spine. Depending on this, decide the left side of the fetus. If imagining is difficult in the beginning one can use a doll model for the same. Once the left side of the fetus is decided, confirm the presence of heart and the stomach shadow on left side.

Another method which is easier and more practical is: See the fetus in its long axis on the screen and set the image so that the fetal head is seen to your right side on the screen. Turn the probe anticlockwise 90°. Consider transverse section of the thorax as a clock face and spine is at 12 o'clock and fetal left side is at 3 o'clock. Confirm stomach in abdominal section and heart in thoracic section on left side **(Figs. 9A and B)**.

Situs solitus which is a normal situs means that stomach is on left side and heart is on left with morphological right atrium (RA) on right side and morphological left atrium (LA) on left side. The apex of the heart points towards left and that is levocardia.

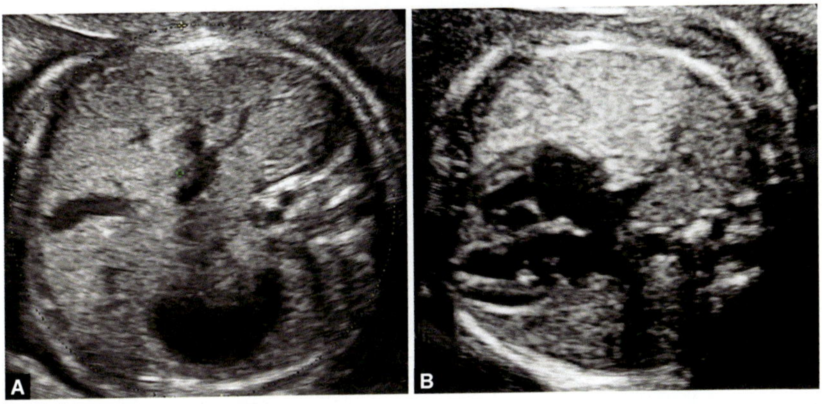

Figs. 9A and B: Transverse section of abdomen showing stomach and transverse section of thorax showing heart—both on same side.

Table 1: Incidence of cardiac abnormalities in different situs abnormalities.

Cardiac situs	*Incidence of congenital heart disease (CHD)*
Normal situs with levocardia	1%
Normal situs with dextrocardia	95%
Situs inversus with dextrocardia	5%
Situs inversus with levocardia	95%

Abnormal Cardiac Situs

- *Solitary dextrocardia:* With normal position of all other viscera, the heart is on right side (apex of the heart points towards right side).
- *Situs inversus*: All the viscera and the heart are on the opposite side like a mirror image.
- *Situs ambiguous:* Undetermined visceral situs, position of the stomach may be right or left, polysplenia (bilateral left) or asplenia (bilateral right), may be seen.

Situs abnormalities are commonly associated with structural cardiac anomalies **(Table 1)**.[6]

Cardiac Position (Fig. 10)

This means actual location of the heart in the chest. It is decided by point P. If a line is drawn along the IV septum on the four chamber heart view and is extended up to the posterior atrial wall, the point where this line intersects the posterior atrial wall is point P. It is almost at the center of the transverse section of the thorax. That means normally two-thirds of the heart is in left hemithorax and one-third of the heart is in right hemithorax. Any

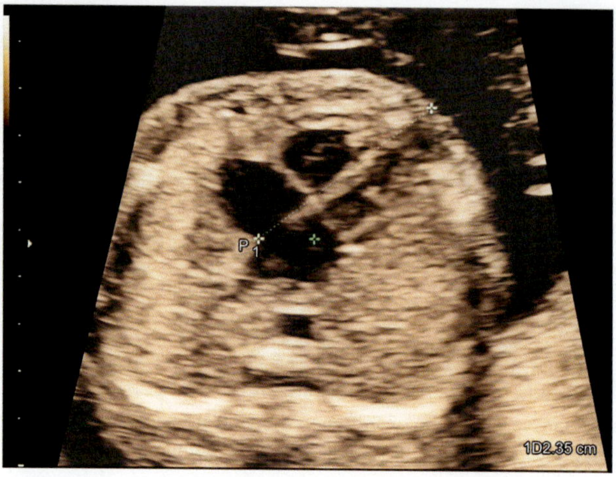

Fig. 10: Interventricular septal line continued to touch the posterior atrial wall point P—cardiac position.

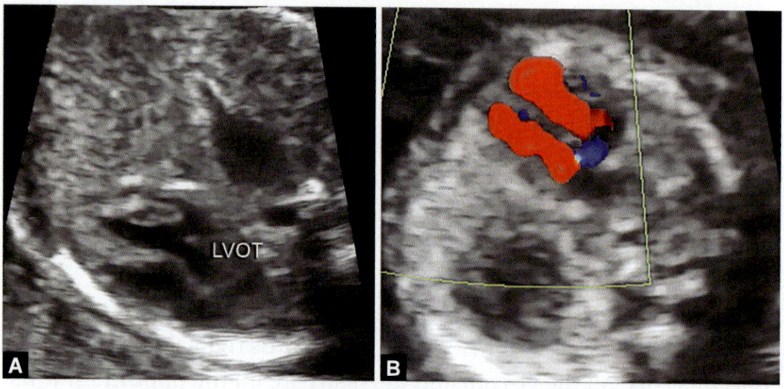

Figs. 11A and B: Altered cardiac position due to diaphragmatic hernia, though apex points towards left (LVOT: left ventricular outflow tract).

intrathoracic lesion, diaphragmatic hernia, lung hypoplasia, etc., will lead to abnormal cardiac position. A heart which is displaced towards right side is still a levocardia if the apex points towards left and a dextrocardia if the apex points towards right **(Figs. 11A and B)**.

Cardiac Axis

Draw one line passing through the IV septum on four chamber view of the heart and a second line passing from sternum to spine. The angle formed anteriorly between the two lines is cardiac axis. It is normally 25-65°. About 79.3% of fetuses with cardiac/intrathoracic defects had abnormal cardiac axis **(Fig. 12)**. Generally speaking when axis is >65° outflow tract abnormalities are more likely and when it is <25° inflow tract abnormalities are more likely.[7]

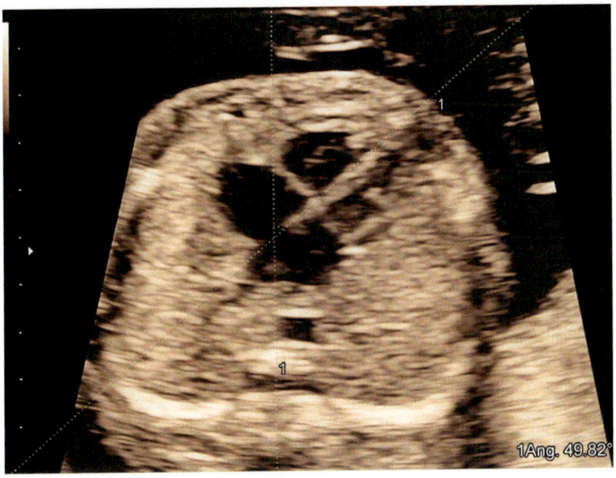

Fig. 12: Measuring cardiac axis.

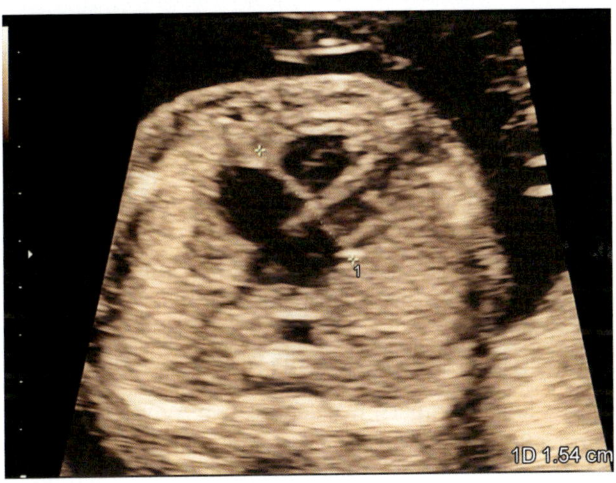

Fig. 13: Cardiac diameter.

Cardiac Size (Fig. 13)

Transverse diameter of the heart in millimeter on four chamber view is less than number of weeks of gestation, after 22 weeks. If this is more, cardiac area to thoracic area ratio is taken and up to 30% is considered as normal **(Fig. 14)**. Enlargement suggests failing heart.

Rate and Rhythm

Cardiac rate and rhythm are best assessed by M-mode. The method has already been described earlier. Normally at 5th week, cardiac activity is slow like peristalsis with a rate of 60–80 beats/min, at the end of 5th week it

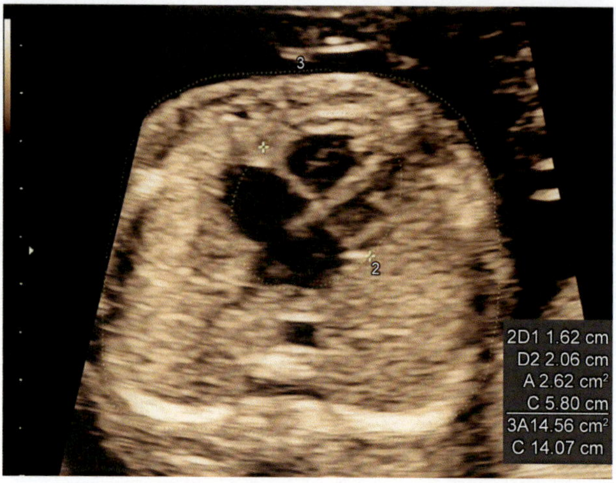

Fig. 14: Four chamber heart view showing measurement of transverse thoracic circumference and cardiac circumference.

reaches 100 beats/min, at the end of 6th week, it is 105–130 beats/min and at 9 weeks, it is 160–170 beats/min, and then settles down at 120–160 beats/min. It is called bradycardia when the rate is <100 beats/min, and most likely it is due to heart blocks. About 50% of fetuses with bradycardia have structural cardiac defects such as AV septal defects, ventricular inversion, heterotaxy syndromes, and corrected TGA.

It is tachycardia, if heart rate is >200 beats/min. Atrial or ventricular arrhythmias may lead to cardiac failure and hydrops.

STUDY OF INTERNAL CARDIAC ANATOMY

The heart shows four chambers, two septae, two AV valves and two outflow tract valves and inflow tracts into atria. Systematic study requires several views which would show anatomy and circulation of all these structures **(Fig. 15)**. These are:

- Four chamber view
- Left ventricular outflow tract
- Right ventricular outflow tract
- Three vessel view
- Short axis view
- Arch views

A transverse section of the thorax, at the level of 4th rib, gives a four chamber view. This can be done by rotating the probe transverse after seeing the thoracic spine or by moving the probe cephalad from the transverse section of the abdomen which shows a stomach bubble. A correct four chamber view will have only one rib in the transverse section of the heart **(Fig. 16)**.

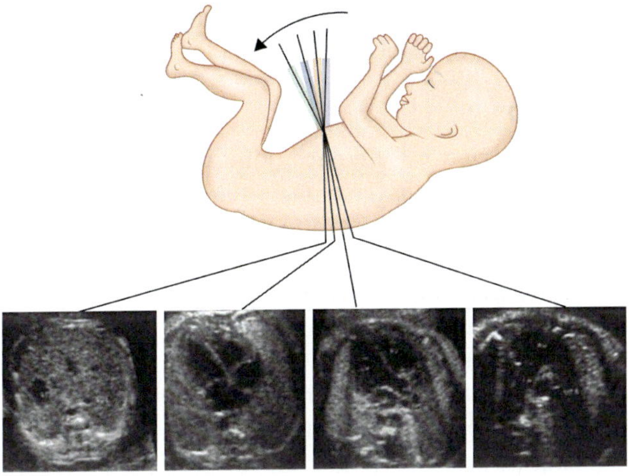

Fig. 15: Diagrammatic representation of probe position and movement and view of the heart achieved on fetal echocardiography.

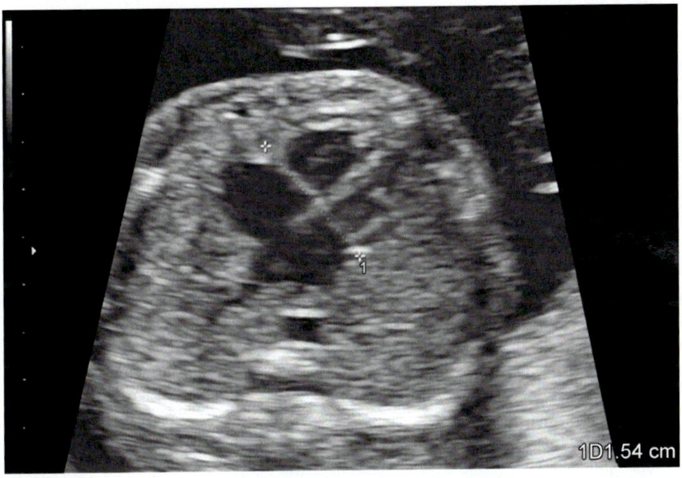

Fig. 16: Four chamber view of the heart on transverse thoracic section, with single rib seen on both the sides.

If one can see multiple rib ends it means it is an oblique section and will give erroneous calculation of cardiac size and axis and also erroneous impression about the symmetry of the cardiac chambers. All the other views can be achieved by systematic rotational or sliding movement of the probe from this view.

After several trials by several people, these movements of the probe have been systematized.

- *Cephalad sweep*: When fetus is supine or left side of the fetus is near the transducer.

- *Rotation towards left shoulder*: When IV septum is transverse or tangential.
- Five short axis views by Yagel et al.

Cephalad Sweep

Using four chamber view as reference point the US beam is directed—angulated cephalad in a transverse plane till the neck is imaged, which includes five imaging planes **(Figs. 17A to D)**.[8]

- *Level 1*: Four chamber view **(Fig. 17A)**
- *Level 2*: LVOT—ascending aorta **(Fig. 17B)**
- *Level 3*: RVOT—pulmonary trunk with its bifurcation running perpendicular to ascending aorta **(Fig. 17C)**
- *Level 4*: Ductus arteriosus originating from the pulmonary trunk bifurcation runs directly posterior and to the left of the spine to join the aorta. Rotating the probe 90° **(Fig. 17D)**
- *Level 5*: Transverse aortic arch—going from right side of the chest to descending aorta. Rotating the probe 90° at this level shows aortic arch with neck vessels.

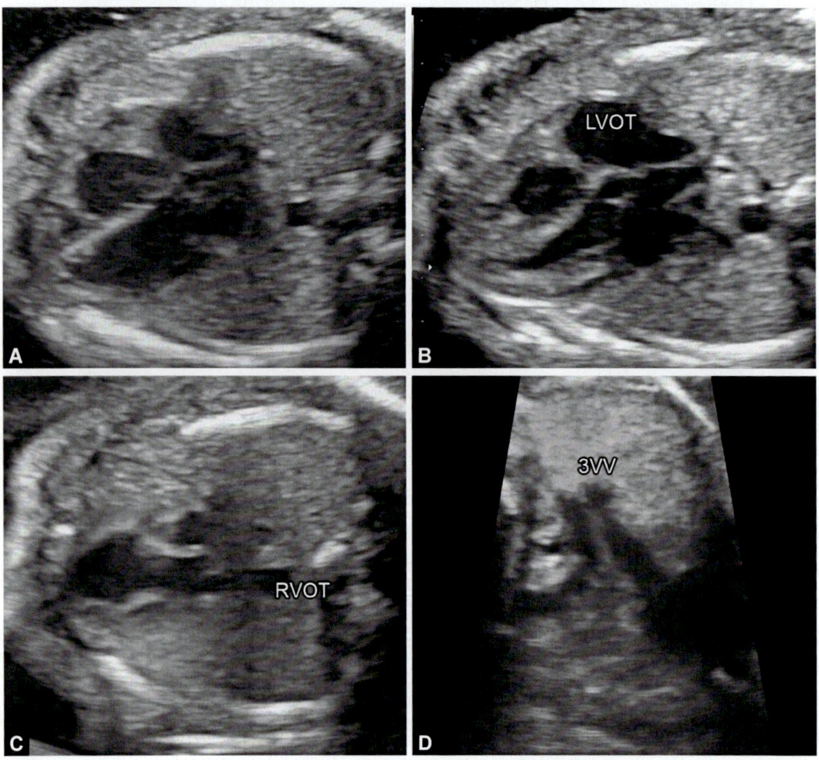

Figs. 17A to D: (A) Four chamber heart view; (B) Left ventricular outflow tract (LVOT); (C) Right ventricular outflow tract (RVOT); (D) Three vessels view (3VV).

Rotational Sweep

This has two variations:

1. *When IV septum is perpendicular to the beam*:[9] From four chamber view, rotate transducer 45° towards left shoulder of the fetus, so that beam bisects a plane between the left hip and right shoulder of the fetus. This shows LVOT—aorta and its curve as transverse part of the arch. Rocking the probe cephalad from this position shows RVOT—pulmonary trunk coursing perpendicular to the aorta.
2. *When IV septum is tangential to the US beam*: The angle of rotation increases or decreases depending on the angle of the IV septum, before the cephalad angulation.

Five Short Axis Views

These were first described by Yagel et al. and have been claimed to be simpler in few fetal positions.[10] First upper abdominal section is taken through stomach, second traditional four chamber, third five chamber, when aorta root is seen in the center of the four chamber view of the heart, fourth transverse view showing bifurcation of pulmonary trunk with aorta in the center which confirms the crossing over of great vessels, as aorta is seen in short axis and pulmonary trunk in long axis **(Figs. 18A and B)** and fifth showing three vessels and trachea.

We have seen that for any heart position, four chamber view is the baseline and only four chamber view diagnoses 50–60% of cardiac anomalies. So we shall first discuss four chamber view in detail and then the outflow tracts, short axis views, and arch views.

Now let us understand what all the different views show.

Four Chamber View

As name suggests it shows all four chambers of the heart in its long axis. This may be apical, basal, and lateral/oblique **(Figs. 19A to C)**. Apical when the

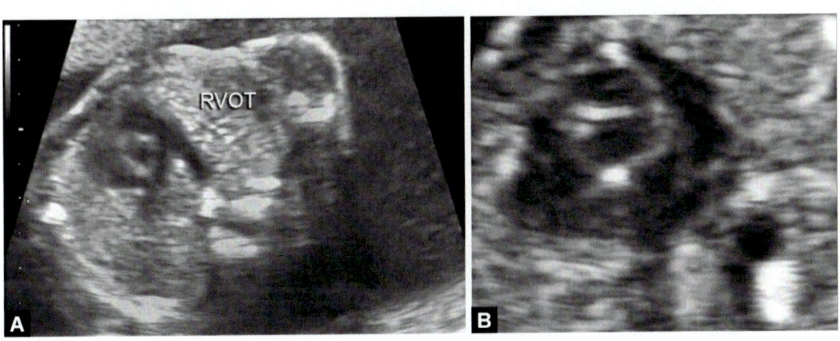

Figs. 18A and B: (A) Short axis view of the heart—right ventricular outflow tract (RVOT) encircling the aorta; (B) Short axis view of the heart.

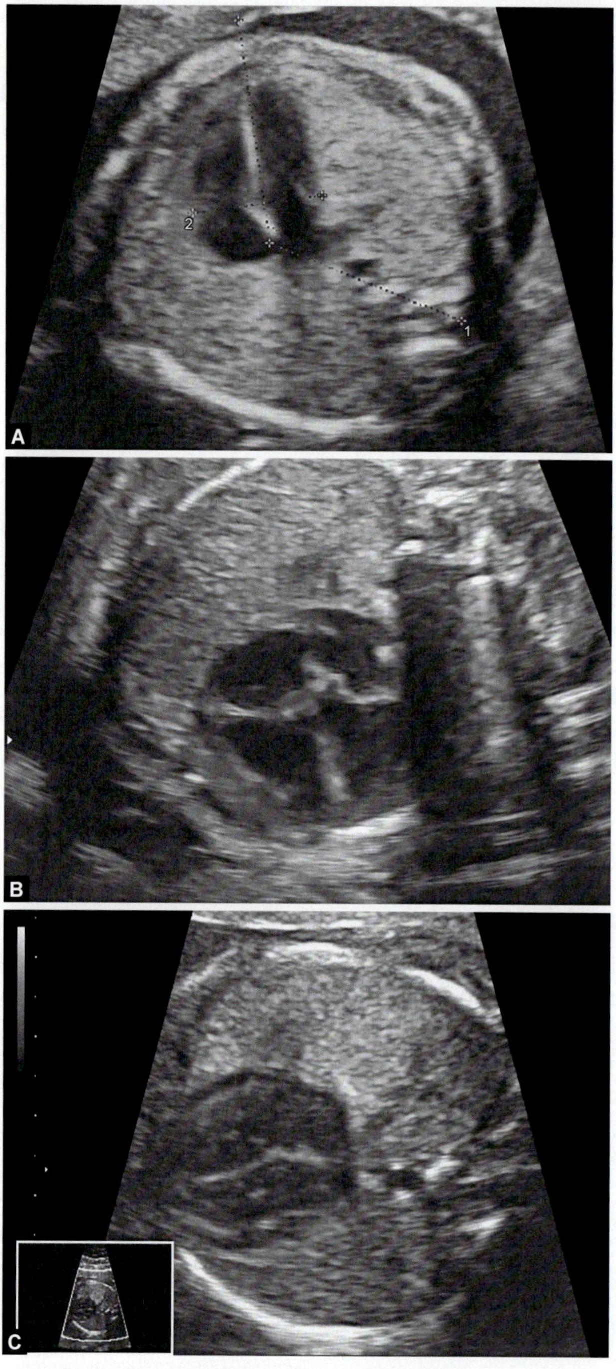

Figs. 19A to C: (A) Apical four chamber; (B) Basal four chamber; (C) Oblique four chamber view.

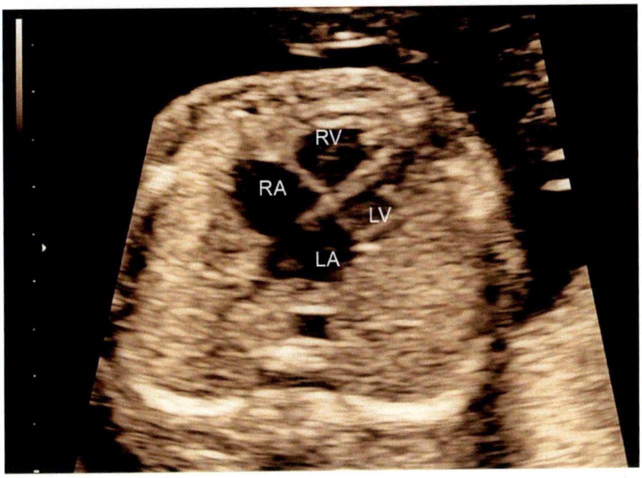

Fig. 20: Four chamber view of heart showing cardiac anatomy (LA: left atrium; LV: left ventricle; RA: right atrium; RV: right ventricle).

apex is towards the probe, basal when base of the heart is close to the probe, lateral when IV septum is perpendicular to the probe, and tangential when IV septum forms an angle with the US beam.

Structures to be identified on four chamber view:

- Cardiac size and axis
- Two ventricles
- Two atria
- Atrial and ventricular septae
- Atrioventricular valves
- Pulmonary veins draining to LA
- Atrioventricular concordance

On this view, the chamber closest to the spine should be the LA and the one closest to the anterior thoracic wall is right ventricle (RV) **(Fig. 20)**. Left ventricle forms the left heart border.

Features of Normal Four Chamber

- Cardiac area approximately one-third of thoracic area
- Cardiac axis 25–65°
- Both ventricles approximately same in size, ratio 1:1.1 to 1:1.2. Morphological RV is identified by thicker walls due to chordae tendineae/ moderator band and is close to the anterior thoracic wall.
- Both atria are approximately same in size. Morphological LA is the one in which the flap of foramen ovale opens and it is the chamber closest to the spine. RA may show eustachian valve lateral to foramen ovale and must not be mistaken for a mass.

Asymmetry of cardiac chambers is seen in almost all cardiac defects except:

- Fallot's tetralogy
- Double outlet RV
- Transposition of the great arteries.

- *Interatrial septum*: It shows foramen ovale in its mid part, the flap of which opens into morphological LA. The upper and lower third of the atrial septum is always seen as a thin line from posterior atrial wall and from the crux of the heart respectively. Normal diameter of foramen ovale is 75–100% of the aortic root diameter. On color Doppler it shows a peak systolic velocity (PSV) of approximately 45 cm/sec and flow is seen from RA to LA.
- *Interventricular septum*: It has three parts but only the muscular part is seen on four chamber view. Subpulmonary part is evaluated on short axis view and perimembranous part on long axis view. IV septum is best seen when it is perpendicular or tangential to the US beam that is in lateral or oblique four chamber view. The septum must be seen in its full width from side to side by sweeping the beam to stamp it as normal.
- *Atrioventricular valves*

  Mitral valve : Tricuspid valve = 1:1.1 to 1:1.2. Tricuspid valve is attached slightly more towards the apex than mitral at the IV septum and the attachment of the septal cusps of both the valves with the septum makes a cross which is known as crux of the heart.

  Color Doppler is required to detect stenosis or regurge of the AV valves.
- *Pulmonary venous (PV) drainage*: At least two pulmonary veins should be seen entering the LA which rules out total anomalous PV drainage. Partial anomalous PV drainage cannot be excluded on antenatal scan as it is difficult to see all the four pulmonary veins entering into the LA by routine B-mode and color Doppler techniques.
- *Atrioventricular concordance*: Concordance means the morphological RV is connected to the morphological RA with the tricuspid AV valve and vice versa for left side.

Four chamber alone can tell us about:

- Ventricular hypoplasias
- Inflow or outflow tract anomalies due to chamber asymmetry
- Atrioventricular valvular abnormalities
- Septal defects
- Myocardiopathies—thickened walls and decreased contractility.
- Arrhythmias—by visual impression though confirmation is always by M-mode.

Apical or basal four chamber view is good for inflow tracts and lateral four chamber view is required for evaluation of septae.

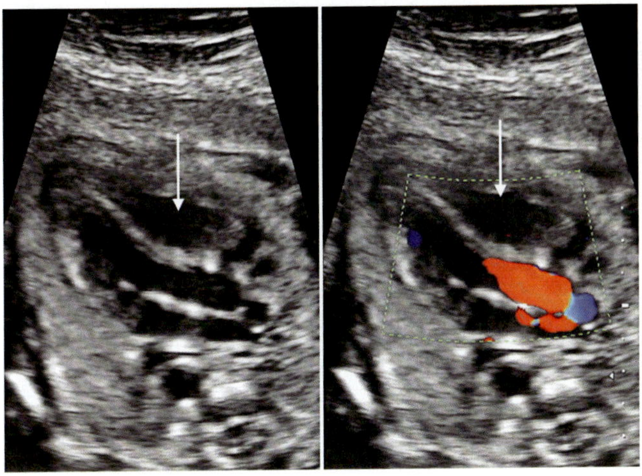

Fig. 21: Left ventricular outflow tract (arrows).

Left Ventricular Outflow Tract

This demonstrates the ascending aorta coming out of the left ventricle running anteriorly and to right from the ventricle **(Fig. 21)**. The crux seen on four chamber view is obliterated in this section and instead two parallel lines are seen, which is the aorta. The posterior wall of the aorta shows continuity with the anterior leaflet of mitral valve and anterior wall is contiguous with IV septum. This is the membranous part of the IV septum and VSDs of Fallot's tetralogy can be seen on this section.

Right Ventricular Outflow Tract

This shows pulmonary trunk coming out of the RV **(Fig. 22)**. Its direction is always perpendicular to the aorta and runs posteriorly and to right.

Both the vessels should be traced further to see the aorta curving round and pulmonary trunk bifurcating. It is also necessary to confirm that morphological RV gives out the pulmonary trunk and morphological left ventricle gives out the aorta. Confirming crossing over of two outflow tracts is very important.

Three Vessel View

Three vessels are seen running posteriorly and to left. From forward left to rear right pulmonary trunk and aorta are seen in long axis and superior vena cava (SVC) is seen in transverse/oblique section. The vessels show reducing caliber from pulmonary trunk to SVC. On color Doppler the direction of flow is same in aorta and pulmonary trunk in this view normally. Reversal of pulmonary trunk to aortic caliber ratio suggests pulmonary stenosis.

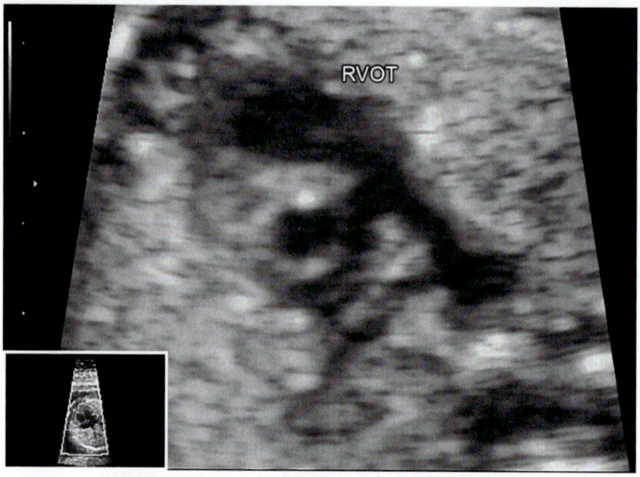

Fig. 22: Right ventricular outflow tract (RVOT).

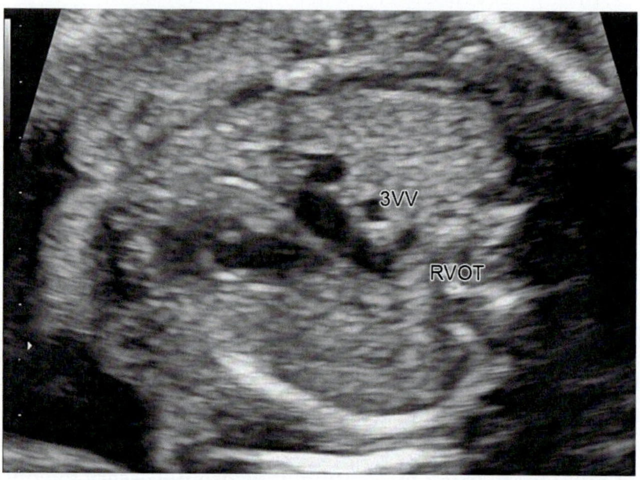

Fig. 23: Three vessel view (3VV). Aorta and pulmonary trunk are seen in long axis, forming a V towards the left of the spine. Superior vena cava (SVC) is seen in short axis (RVOT: right ventricular outflow tract).

Three vessel trachea section shows aorta and pulmonary trunk getting close to join by ductus arteriosus, forming a "V". Ductus arteriosus is seen as a vessel running posteriorly to the left of the spine from the bifurcation of the pulmonary trunk **(Fig. 23)**.

Slightly higher level also shows trachea, just anterior to the spine. Slight sweep of the transducer shows the right and the left pulmonary artery (PA).

Sliding the probe transverse further upwards shows aortic arch in transverse section with trachea in the concavity of "c". Slight caudal and left

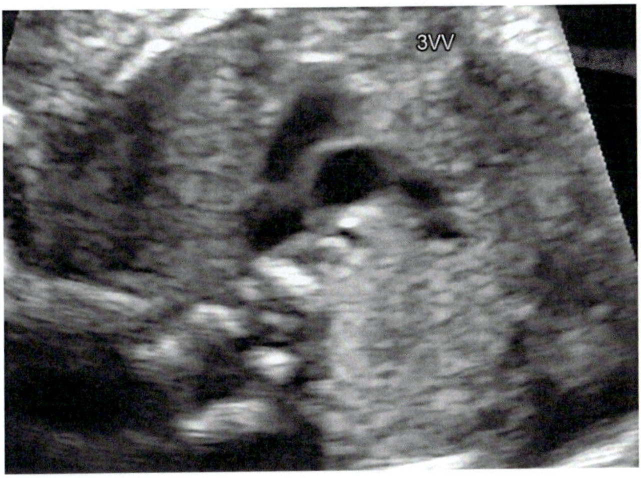

Fig. 24: Curve of aorta is seen with tiny anechoic trachea in its concavity (3VV: three vessel view).

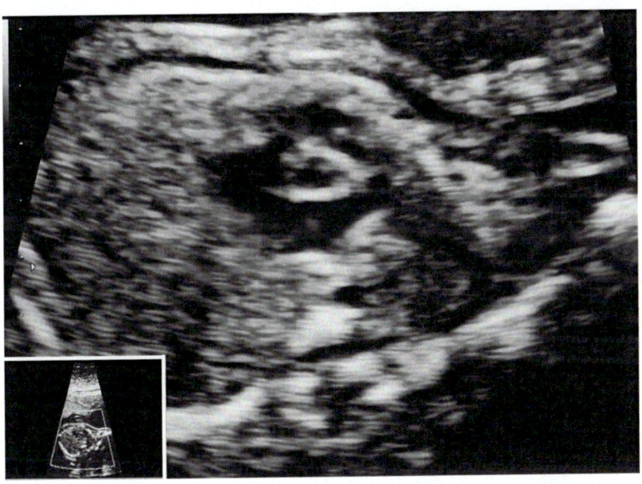

Fig. 25: Short axis view of the heart on inversion mode.

tilt from this shows aortic arch and duct together, with thymus anterior to the great vessels **(Fig. 24)**.

Short Axis View

As described in Yagel's technique it shows aorta in the center in transverse section and pulmonary trunk with bifurcation surrounding it which is also known as circle and sausage view **(Fig. 25)**. A section taken little inferior to this will show aortic root in the center protected by a complete circle

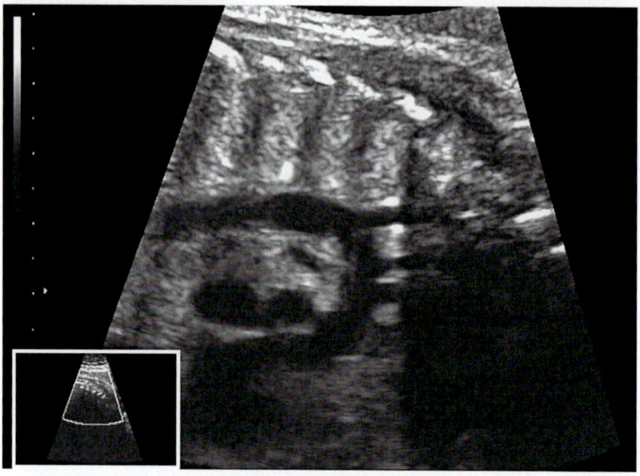

Fig. 26: Aortic arch.

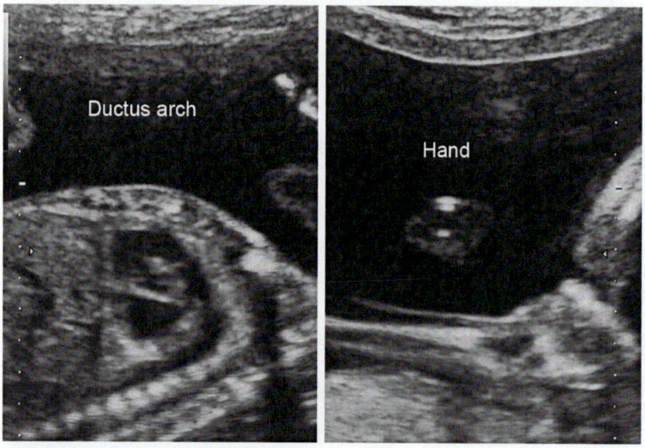

Fig. 27: Ductus arch.

formed by the right side of the heart. This view may be used for detection of subpulmonary VSD.

Arch/Longitudinal Views

- Aortic arch view can be achieved by rotating the probe 90° from the transverse aortic arch view **(Fig. 26)**.
- Ductal arch can be seen by rotating the probe 90° from ductus arteriosus in transverse view **(Fig. 27)**.

  On sagittal section of the fetus, heart is seen as a three chambered structure and aorta is seen arising from the middle chamber, the left ventricle, and is cane/"U" shaped. It gives off three neck vessels from the transverse part of

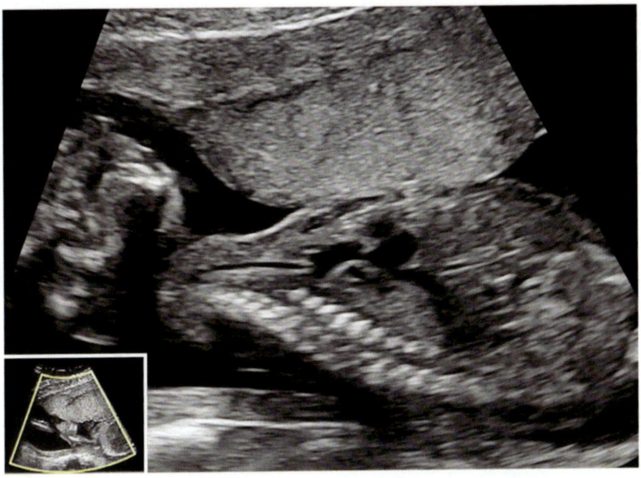

Fig. 28: Right atrial inflow tract view—inferior vena cava (IVC) and superior vena cava (SVC) are seen opening into right atrium on sagittal section.

the arch. Ductus arch is seen arising from the anterior most chamber, the RV of the heart and is "hockey shaped" or has a flat curve. Both the arches can be seen connecting to each other, forming a "Y" anterior to the spine.

- *RA inflow tracts*: Angulating the probe a little towards fetal right side from this *view shows SVC a*nd inferior vena cava (IVC) entering the RA **(Fig. 28)**.

Color Doppler is used for difficult to image patients when gray scale image quality is not very good and for diagnosis of flow abnormalities. It has also been used to potentiate the diagnosis made on gray scale. Color Doppler is especially useful for VSDs, stenosis, coarctation of aorta, ventricular hypoplasias, and ductus dependent diseases. Power Doppler is used to evaluate the septal defects when four chamber view is transverse. It also gives better edge definition.

Pulsed Doppler is used to find absolute velocities and to diagnose regurgitation or stenosis of the valves. Each vessel and each valve has a typical flow pattern. This can be seen as a typical waveform on pulsed Doppler.

To diagnose abnormalities in flow we need to know the normal waveform/ signature for that particular vessel and normal velocities. Normal flow velocities measures by pulsed Doppler in outflow tracts is 60–70 cm/s, and in ductus arteriosus it is 90–135 cm/s in systole and 15–25 cm/s in diastole.

Normal waveform through the AV valve is double peaked **(Fig. 29)** forward flow where the first one—E wave represents early diastolic filling of the ventricle and a wave represents filling of the ventricle by atrial contraction with no reverse flow throughout the cardiac cycle.

Outflow tracts show systolic single peaked forward flow due to ventricular systole. Studying and understanding these waveforms can also inform us about cardiac function **(Fig. 30)**.

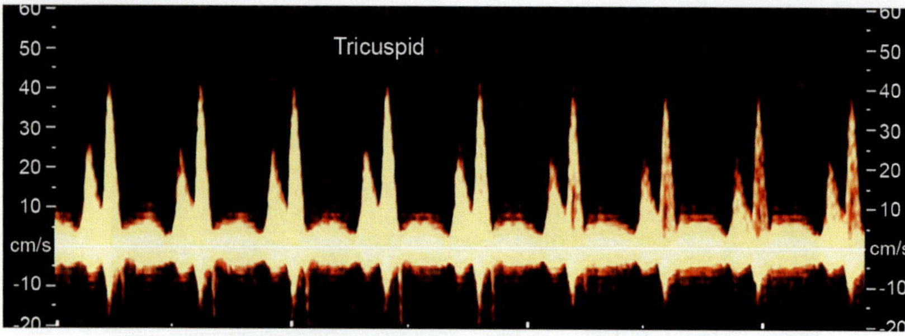

Fig. 29: Normal atrioventricular valve waveform.

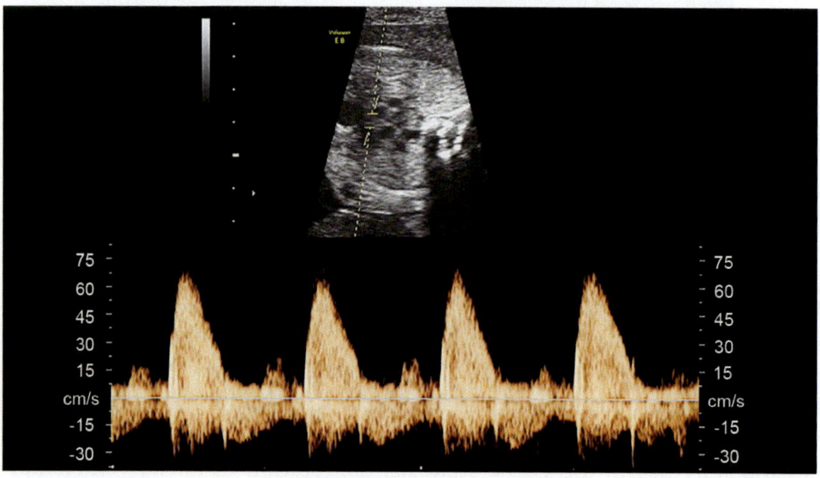

Fig. 30: Typical waveform pattern of ventricular outflow tracts.

M-mode

It is used to demonstrate arrhythmias, measure atrial and ventricular size and size of the outflow tracts.

Study of four chamber view can be considered complete only when it is assessed with gray scale, color and pulsed Doppler and M-mode.

Before discussing the abnormalities of the heart it is essential to understand the normal fetal circulation. This will help us to analyze the findings seen on fetal echocardiography and to arrive to a diagnosis.

Fetal Circulation (Fig. 31)

Inferior vena cava and SVC bring unsaturated blood from lower and upper part of the body respectively to RA. Saturated blood from umbilical vein enters ductus venosus. This is a trumpet shaped branchless vessel with the narrowest part only 2 mm in diameter and opens into the RA. The shape helps to create

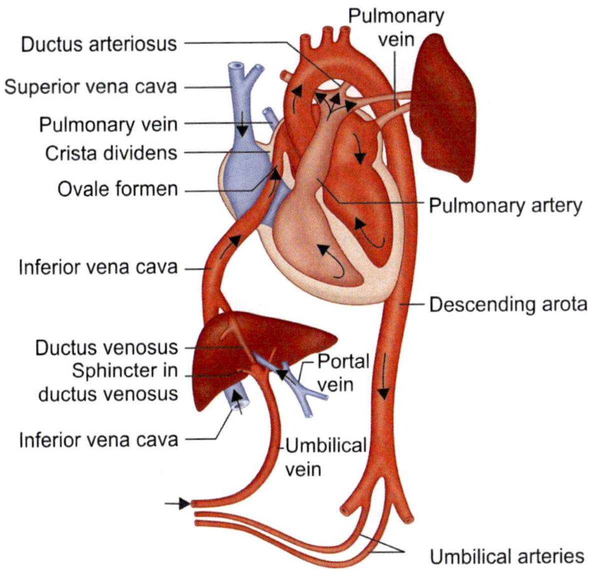

Fig. 31: Fetal circulation.

a high speed jet of blood, which is directed from the RA, through foramen ovale to LA, unmixed with the unsaturated blood. LA also receives blood from pulmonary veins. RV receives blood from RA and left ventricle from LA. RV gives out pulmonary trunk which apart from right and left PA also gives out a third branch—ductus arteriosus. Left ventricle gives out aorta, which gives out coronaries and neck vessels in turn and then through ductus arteriosus it is connected to pulmonary trunk. This causes mixture of blood from pulmonary trunk and aorta which is ultimately supplied to the unprivileged lower half of the fetal body. Because of any abnormalities in the heart the atrial changes precede the ventricular changes.

Cardiac diseases are of multiple types but classification according to the structure involved may make the understanding of these abnormalities simpler.

CLASSIFICATION OF CARDIAC DISEASES

- Septal defects
- Right heart abnormalities
- Left heart abnormalities
- Conotruncal defects
- Single ventricle defects
- Other cardiac abnormalities
- Arrhythmias

Septal Defects

- Ventricular septal defect (VSD)
- Atrial septal defect (ASD)
- Atrioventricular septal defect (AVSD)
- *Interventricular septal defects* are most common and consist of 30% of cardiac defects. They cause no hemodynamic disturbances in utero if not too large as in utero, pressures in both ventricles are similar and there is no significant shunting of blood. VSDs can be further classified according to their location in the ventricular septum.
    - *Muscular defects*: It is in muscular part of the septum. Lateral four chamber view is the best to diagnose these defects and shows drop out in septal shadow. But small defects are difficult to diagnose without color Doppler. On apical and basal four chamber view, the part of the septum close to the crux is often not seen. This must not be misinterpreted as septal defect. It is a defect only if the end of the septal line shows a thickened end otherwise it is an artifact **(Figs. 32A and B)**.

      Color Doppler may be used to define these defects. Even on color Doppler no turbulence will be seen as there is no pressure gradient between both chambers. The flow may be left to right or right to left **(Figs. 33 and 34)**.

      Three-dimensional US image rendered in inversion mode has been successfully used to demonstrate even small VSDs.
    - *Perimembranous defect*: This defect is in membranous part of the ventricular septum, below aortic valve and may extend into the muscular part. It is seen only in long axis view below the aortic

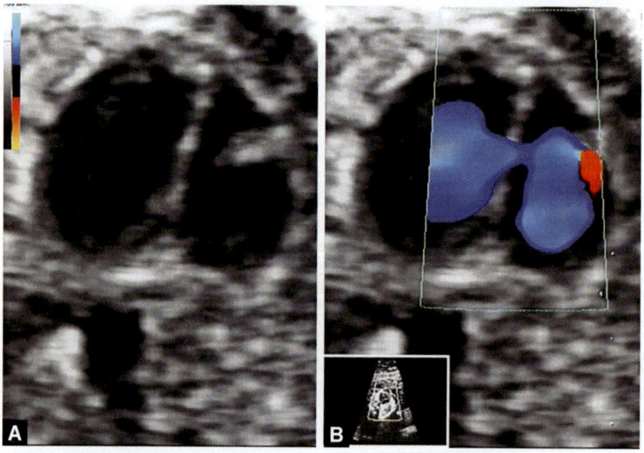

Figs. 32A and B: (A) Normal; (B) Ventricular septal defect.

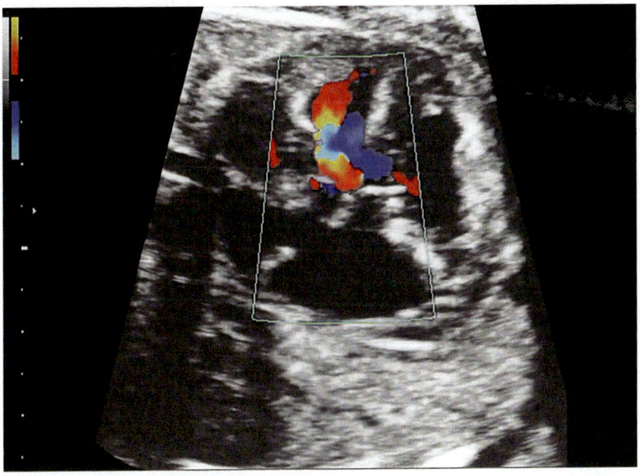

Fig. 33: Ventricular septal defect.

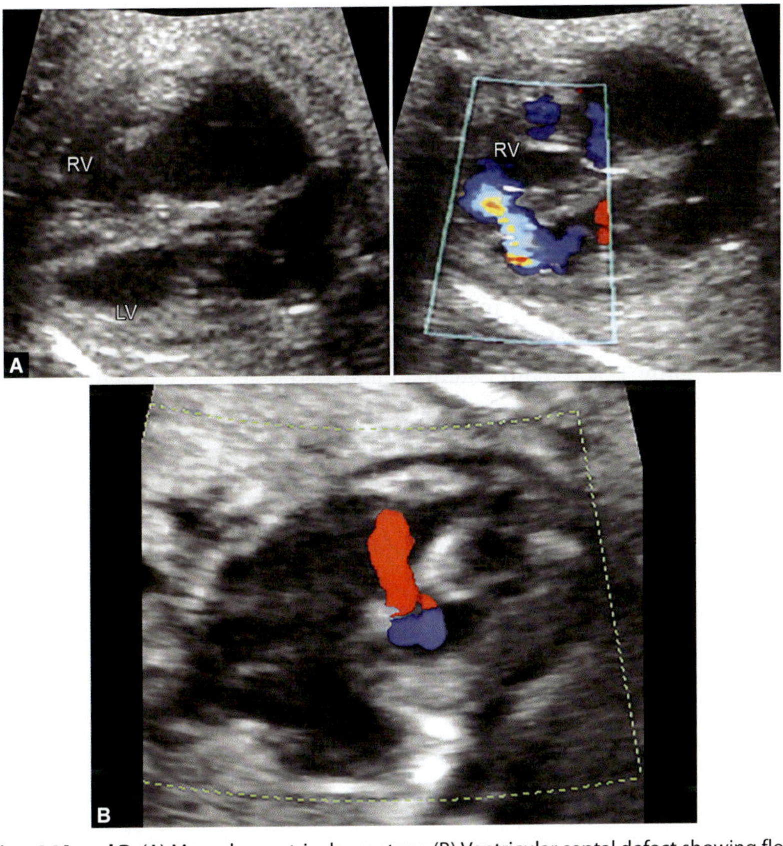

Figs. 34A and B: (A) Muscular ventricular septum; (B) Ventricular septal defect showing flow across the defect from one to another ventricle (LV: left ventricle; RV: right ventricle).

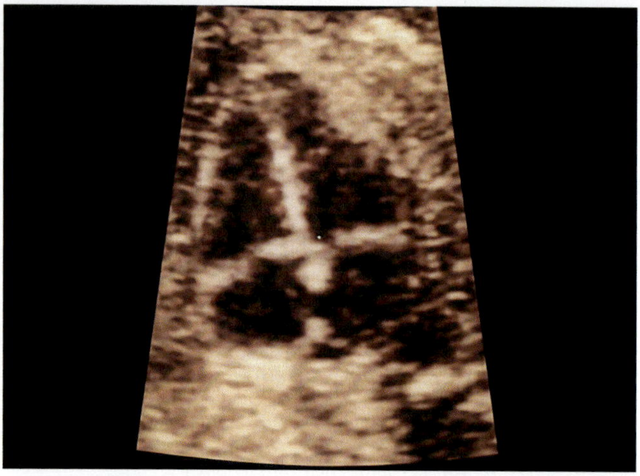

Fig. 35: Membranous ventricular septal defect.

valve. LVOT view may demonstrate this defect **(Fig. 35)**. These are malaligned if associated with conotruncal defects. If these are not malaligned the chance of spontaneous closure is significantly high.

- *Inlet defects*: This defect is in the inlet part of the septum, close to AV valves' septal insertion.
- *Subpulmonary defect*: This is seen at inflow part of the RV and affects implantation of septal chordae of tricuspid valve. It can be demonstrated only on short axis view below the pulmonary valve.

Small defects (<3 mm) may close spontaneously. About 46% of non-malaligned VSDs close in antenatal life and 23% during the first year of life. Only 31% remain patent. Malaligned defects are less likely to be corrected without surgery. Large muscular and large perimembranous defects and inlet and subpulmonary defects usually require surgery.

- *Atrial septum defects*: Consists of 8% of congenital cardiac defects. Defects can be at three locations—(1) secundum, (2) sinus venosus, and (3) primum.
  - Secundum defects are most common but cannot be diagnosed antenatally as are located at fossa ovalis. These may be isolated or with VSD/pulmonary valve stenosis. It is to be differentiated from foramen ovale thickening. Small defects may close spontaneously.
  - Redundancy of the foramen ovale flap is known as aneurysm of foramen ovale commonly associated with atrial arrhythmias **(Fig. 36)**.
  - Sinus venosus defects are difficult to diagnose. Only 5–10% of ASDs are sinus venosus defects, situated posterior to foramen ovale and inferior to SVC.
  - Primum defects are mostly a part of AV defect **(Fig. 37)**.

Atrial septal defects do not require alteration in obstetric care.

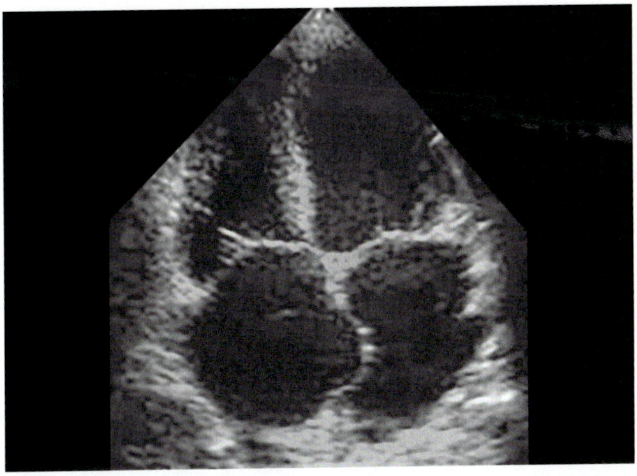

Fig. 36: Aneurysm of foramen ovale.

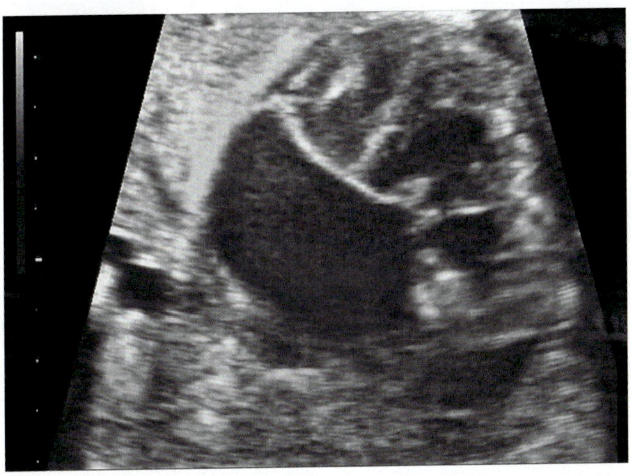

Fig. 37: Primum atrial septal defect, often a part of atrioventricular septal defect.

- *Atrioventricular septal defects*: These are the defects of endocardial cushion causing primum ASD with VSD. It may be associated with Fallot's tetralogy, double outlet RV, coarctation of aorta, ventricular hypoplasia subaortic or pulmonary valve stenosis. These defects are common with chromosomal abnormalities both aneuploidies and trisomies. The risk of recurrence is 7–17% in families with normal karyotype.[11] Isolated defects have 85–90% survival rates after surgical repair.

On US, complete AV septal defect will show single AV valve on four chamber view which is better demonstrated in diastole. In partial AVSD, both valves are attached at the same level to the septum instead of slight apical attachment of tricuspid valve normally **(Figs. 38A to F)**.

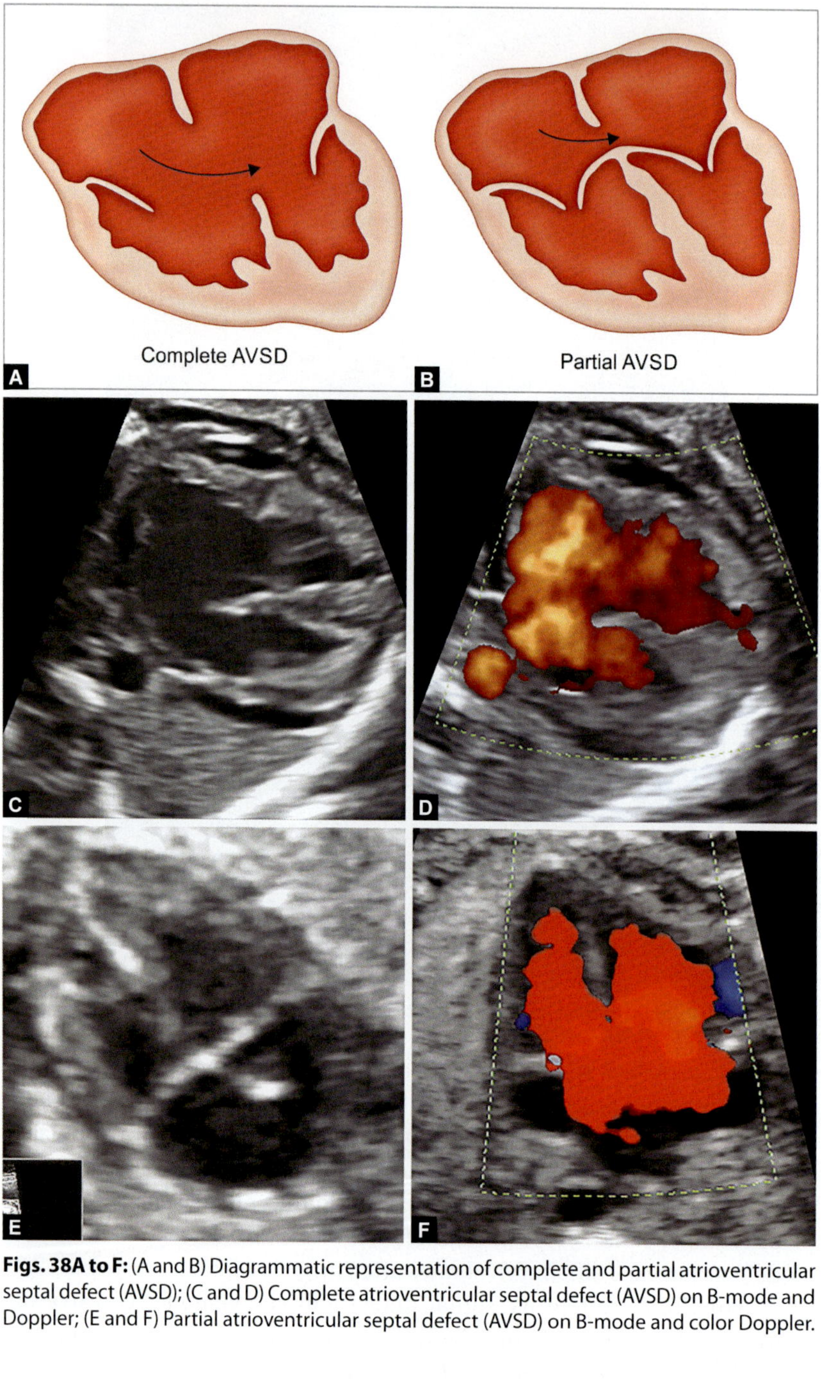

Figs. 38A to F: (A and B) Diagrammatic representation of complete and partial atrioventricular septal defect (AVSD); (C and D) Complete atrioventricular septal defect (AVSD) on B-mode and Doppler; (E and F) Partial atrioventricular septal defect (AVSD) on B-mode and color Doppler.

Color Doppler shows mixture of flow to ventricles. It is often associated with increased nuchal translucency. This anomaly can be diagnosed in late first trimester.

Right Heart Anomalies

- Tricuspid anomalies including Ebstein's anomaly
- Pulmonary valve atresia with intact ventricular septum-hypoplastic right heart
- Pulmonary stenosis
- *Tricuspid valve defects*:
    - *Ebstein's anomaly:* It is characterized by low placed tricuspid valve, its septal and posterior cusps. Due to this RA appears enlarged but actually it is atrialization of RV which is progressive in antenatal life. Color Doppler shows regurgitation into RA. Pulmonary trunk may be small/normal depending on the functional size of the RV.

      Severe right ventricular dysfunction may lead to severe pulmonary stenosis/atresia which is ductus dependent. Three vessel view shows reversal of pulmonary trunk to aortic ratio. It may often be associated with severe cardiac enlargement and lung hypoplasia. ASD may be associated with Ebstein's anomaly **(Figs. 39A to C)**.

      Other tricuspid valve abnormalities are:
        - Thick, dysplastic tricuspid valve
        - Unguarded tricuspid valve with almost no valvular tissue.[12]
- *Hypoplastic right heart/pulmonary valve atresia with intact septum*: Usually the RV is small and hypoplastic with decreased contractility even in early gestation but may be progressive and may appear normal till 20 weeks. IV septum is intact **(Figs. 40A to C)**.

  Occasionally RV may be enlarged and dysfunctional with dilated severely incompetent tricuspid valve. RA may be normal. On color Doppler no forward flow is seen through tricuspid and pulmonary valve as both are atretic. On three vessel view aorta and pulmonary trunk show flow in opposite directions with turbulence at ductus as pulmonary trunk is filled through ductus arteriosus.[13]

  Fetuses may develop cardiomegaly and hydrops due to cardiac decompensation. Termination should be offered for these fetuses.
- *Pulmonary stenosis:* There is thickening and doming of pulmonary valve. PA is small with increased Doppler velocities than in aorta causing turbulence. Reversed flow in ductus arteriosus is seen in ductus dependent disease, that is when pulmonary stenosis is critical.[14] Septal defects are common.

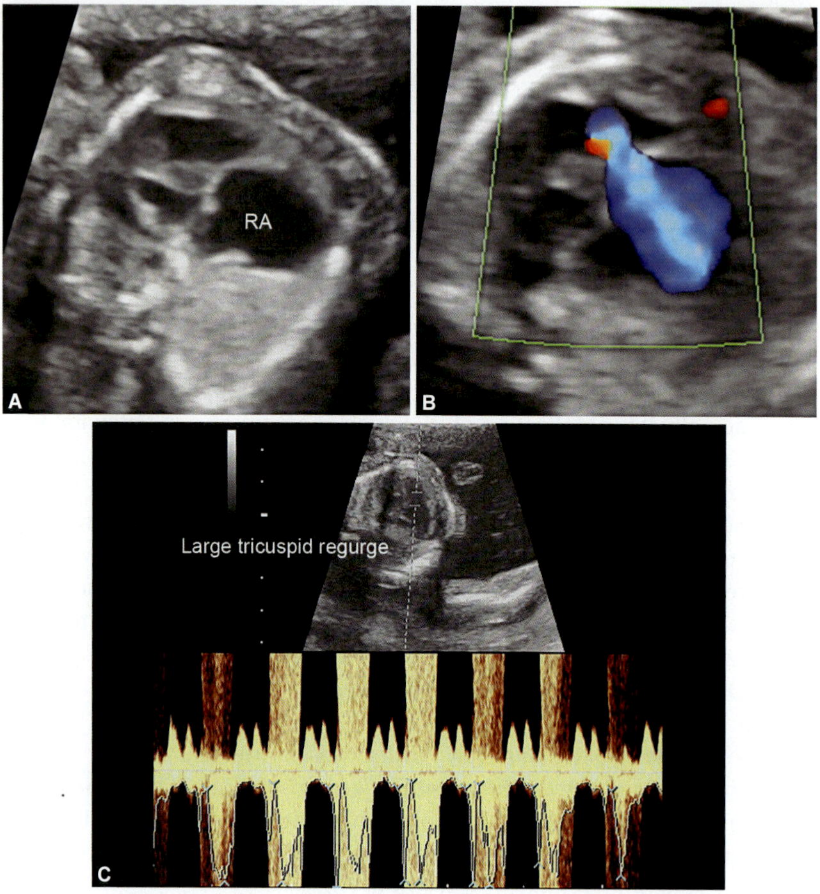

Figs. 39A to C: (A) Ebstein's anomaly; (B) Tricuspid regurgitation; (C) Tricuspid regurge (RA: right atrium).

Left Heart Anomalies

- *Aortic stenosis* may be progressive in utero and therefore often may not be diagnosed on early scan.

  Aortic valve is thickened and shows doming. Left ventricle may be hypertrophied and there may be asymmetric septal hypertrophy. Thickening of the ventricular septum may obstruct LVOT and cause subvalvular stenosis where valve may appear normal. These are not diagnosed in utero. Sometimes left ventricle may be dilated with decreased systolic function. Association with endocardial fibroelastosis is known.

  Color Doppler shows increased flow velocity through aortic valve with turbulence and reversed flow is seen in aortic arch.

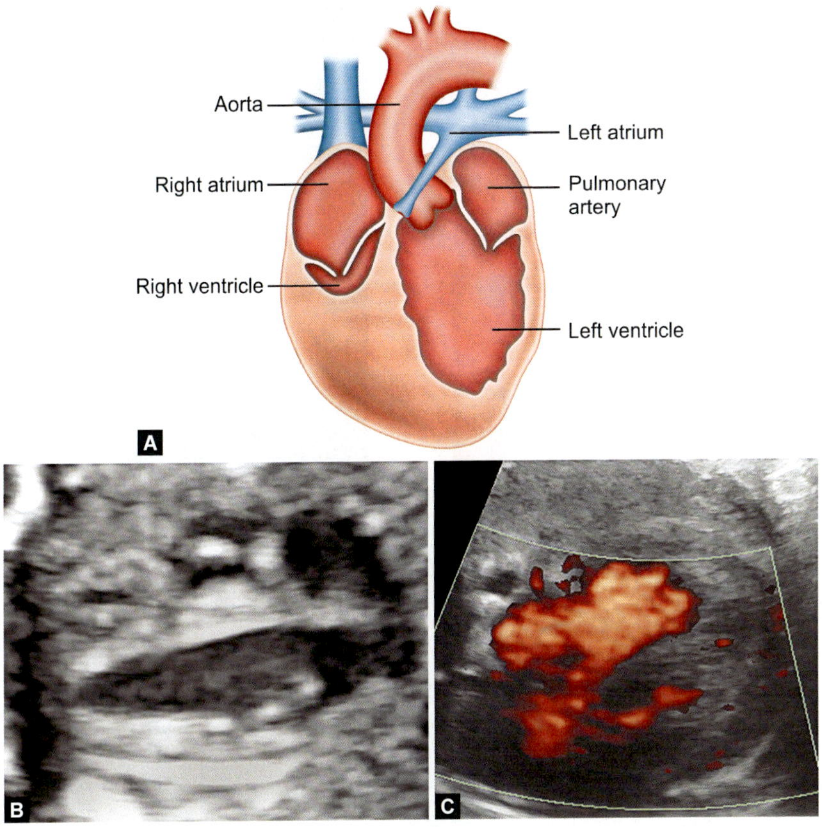

Figs. 40A to C: Right ventricular hypoplasia.

Decreased velocity in aorta in these cases is suggestive of left ventricular failure.[15] Mitral regurgitation is often present. Critical aortic stenosis is ductus dependent.

- *Coarctation of aorta*: Localized narrowing of the juxtaductal arch is known as coarctation of aorta. Most commonly this narrowing is between left subclavian artery and ductus arteriosus. Transverse arch and aortic isthmus appear small **(Figs. 41A and B)**. Aorta appears smaller than pulmonary trunk on three vessel view. There is relative right ventricular and pulmonary trunk enlargement without right heart disease.[16] On color Doppler there is high velocity flow in proximal descending aorta.
- *Interrupted aortic arch*: Aorta is not at all formed beyond the arch. The descending aorta is a continuation of ductal arch. This is a difficult diagnosis but the clue is straight ascending aorta on aortic arch view. Branches may or may not be present depending on the type of interruption **(Fig. 42)**.

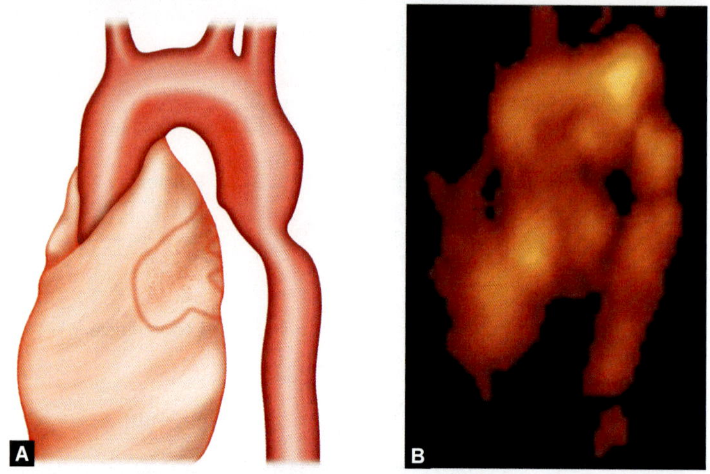

Figs. 41A and B: Coarctation of aorta—three-dimensional power Doppler.

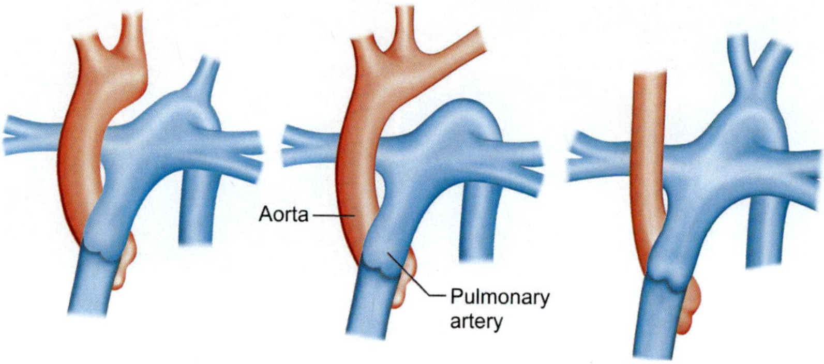

Fig. 42: Types of interrupted aortic arch.

- *Hypoplastic left heart syndrome*: Left ventricle is small on four chamber view with poor contractility. LA may be small or normal in size. There is no forward flow through mitral or aortic valve **(Figs. 43A and B)**. Aortic size and origin site are important for postnatal prognosis. Heart may appear normal at 16–18 weeks and disease may be progressive in utero. It is important to differentiate it from single ventricle by a septal ridge in the ventricle **(Figs. 44A and B)**.
- *Mitral valve defects*: Mitral valve defects are rare as isolated abnormalities. *Blood flow turbulences* on color Doppler are diagnostic.

Conotruncal Defects

These are commonly associated with deletion of chromosome 22q11.2 which can be diagnosed by fluorescence in situ hybridization (FISH). This anomaly

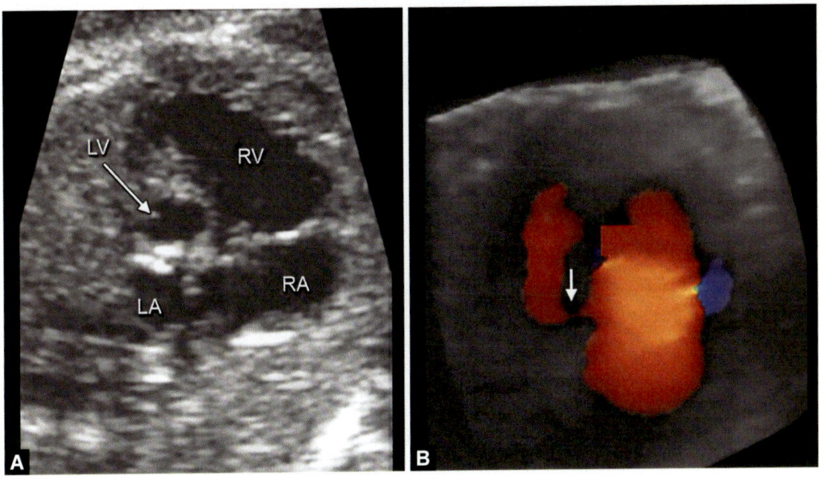

Figs. 43A and B: Left ventricular hypoplasia (LA: left atrium; LV: left ventricle; RA: right atrium; RV: right ventricle).

is associated with short stature, psychiatric problems, and mild-to-moderate learning difficulties.

- *Fallot's tetralogy:* It is the most common cyanotic heart defect and almost always missed if only four chamber view is obtained as cardiac screening. It has four components—(1) perimembranous VSD, (2) over-riding of aorta, (3) pulmonary stenosis, and (4) hypertrophic RV. But the last component always becomes evident only after birth. Obstetric management needs no change with isolated Fallot's tetralogy.

  On US, increased angle of cardiac axis is seen on four chamber view. Long axis view shows VSD in the membranous part, with large aortic root. RVOT view shows small PA. Three vessel view shows inverse PA/aorta ratio. Color Doppler shows increased velocity in PA due to RVOT obstruction and aorta is fed by two ventricles. Many a times only membranous VSD may be evident in early gestation **(Figs. 45A and B)**.[17]
- *Double outlet RV*: Both the great arteries arise from RV **(Figs. 46A to C)** and depending on the site of origin one of the two may show variable degree of stenosis. When both arteries are arising side by side, it is named as Taussig-Bing syndrome. Its differentiation from other outflow tract anomalies with large VSD may be difficult.

  On US, deviation of cardiac axis may be present but four chamber view is otherwise normal. Anterior angulation from four chamber view shows parallel great vessels instead of crossing over of great vessels and is known as Taussig-Bing heart. VSD may or may not be present but color Doppler is confirmatory.

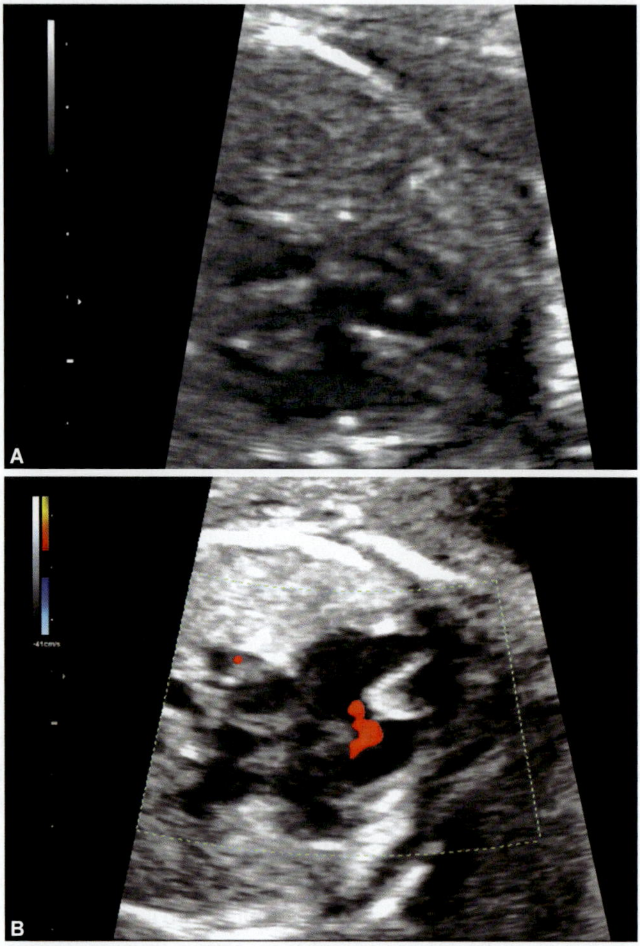

Figs. 44A and B: Small part of the ventricular septum seen at the apical region excludes single ventricle.

- *Truncus arteriosus*: Both the arteries arise as a single trunk from the ventricles. It is usually associated with a large VSD with the trunk over-riding the septum. Types of truncus have been shown in **Figure 47**.
  On US increased cardiac axis is seen on otherwise normal four chamber view. Malaligned large VSD is seen in outlet part of ventricular septum. Truncal root is seen arising from RV or over-riding the septum. Abnormal truncal valve may or may not be present. The origin of PA must be confirmed to exclude pulmonary stenosis.
  On color Doppler, VSD is seen with origin of truncus over-riding the septum. Origin of PA from the main trunk must be diagnosed. If dysplastic valve is present, it shows holodiastolic regurgitation on pulsed Doppler.

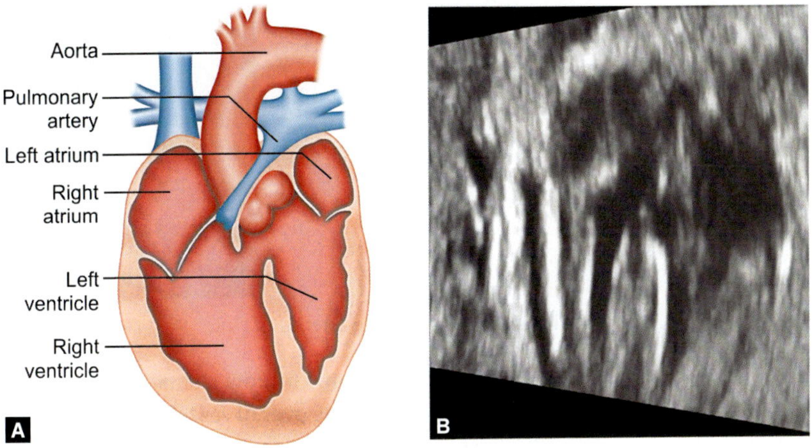

Figs. 45A and B: Fallot's tetralogy.

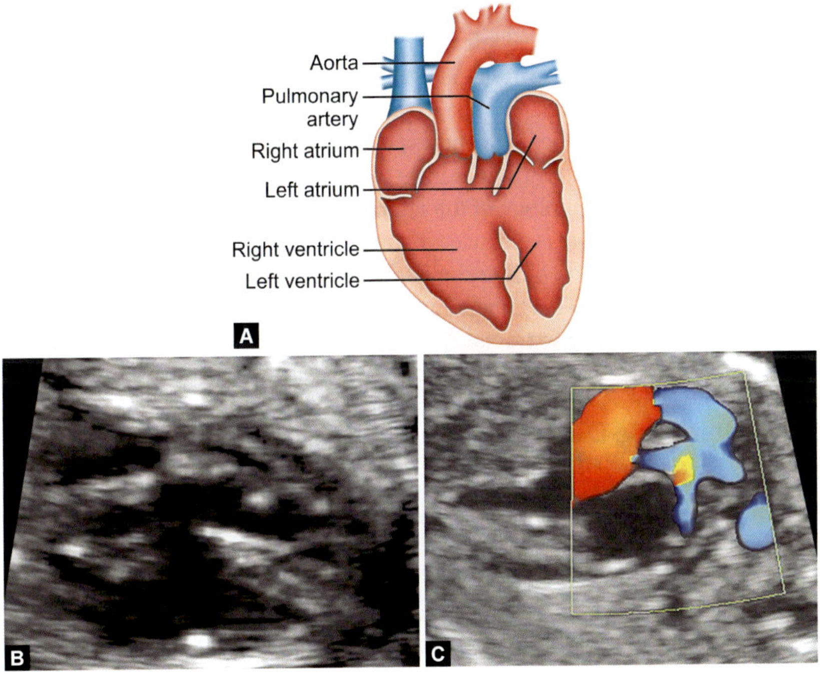

Figs. 46A to C: Double outlet right ventricle.

- *Complete transposition of great vessels*: Aorta arises from RV and lies anteriorly and to left of pulmonary trunk and pulmonary trunk arises from left ventricle. This means two great arteries arise side by side at the base of the heart instead of crossing over of great vessels.

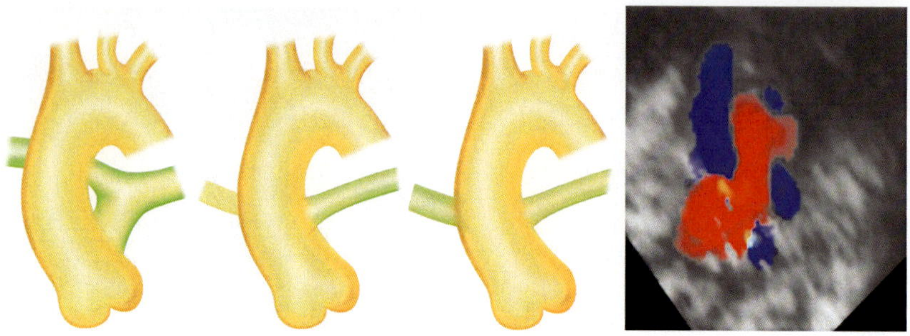

Fig. 47: Types of truncus arteriosus.

On US, normal four chamber view is seen. Outflow tracts show parallel great vessels at the roots. There is no crossing over of vessels. Vessel arising out of LV takes posterior course and bifurcates so is PA. Vessel arising out of RV takes long upward course and curves. This is aorta **(Figs. 48A to D)**. If associated with VSD and overriding, the diagnosis is difficult.

- *Corrected transposition of great vessels*: This is a very rare abnormality. RA opens into morphological left ventricle which gives out pulmonary trunk and LA opens into morphological RV and gives out aorta. These patients may have dextrocardia.

  On US, four chamber view shows deviated cardiac axis. Evidently normal looking heart shows ventricular inversion. AV discordance is confirmed by looking at the morphology of the chambers. Flap of foramen ovale opens in LA which opens in a ventricle which is morphologically right containing chordae tendinea and moderator band. Great vessels do not show crossing over, but are parallel. Ventriculoarterial discordance can be confirmed by tracing the outflow tracts. AV complete heart block may be seen on M-mode.[18]

Single Ventricle Defects

- Tricuspid atresia
- Single ventricle heart
- Heterotaxy syndromes

Tricuspid Atresia

This defect is commonly associated with transposition of great vessels but chromosomal defects are rare in such fetuses.

On US, single AV valve is seen. Tricuspid valve is absent/thick. RV is hypoplastic. The ventricle is sometimes so hypoplastic that it may be barely identified. RA is normal/large with restrictive ASD. Septal defects are common.

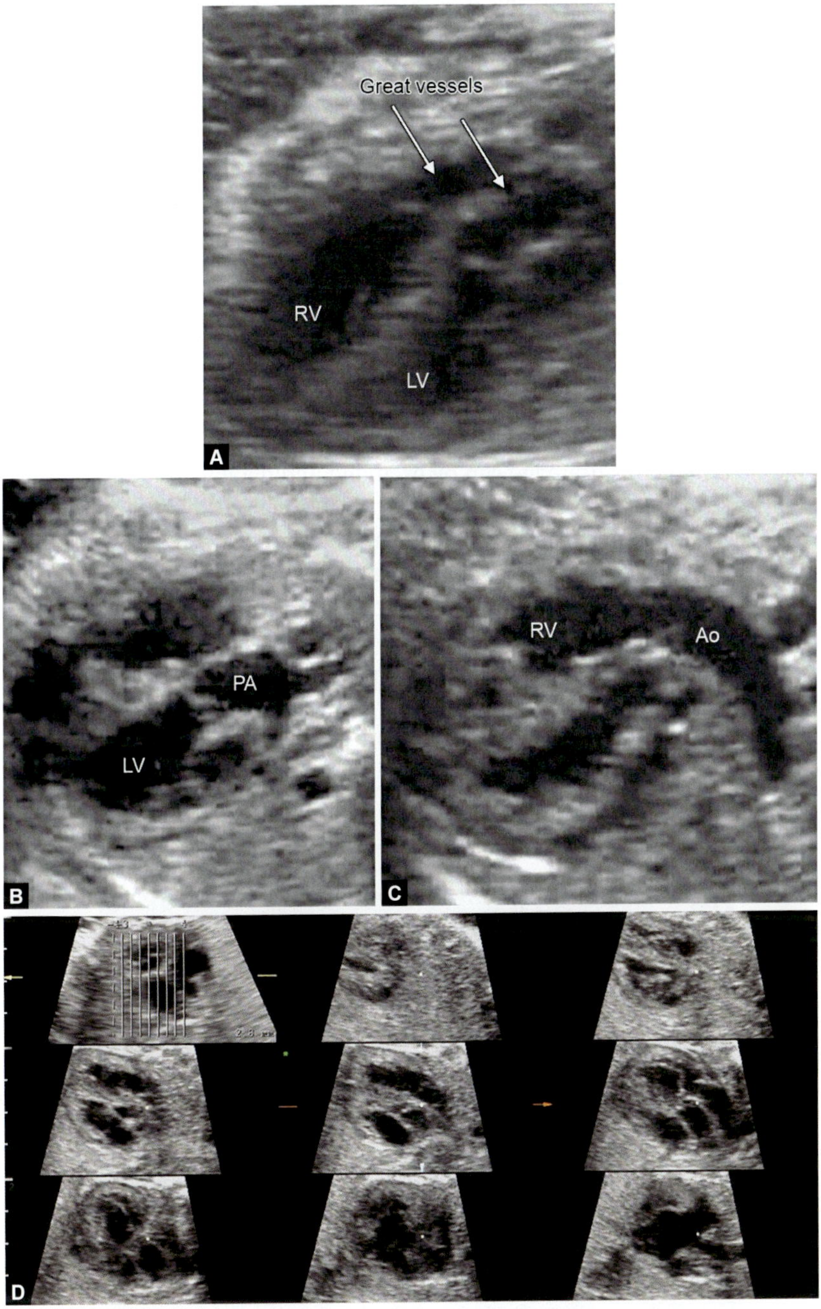

Figs. 48A to D: Complete transposition of great vessels (Ao: aorta; LV: left ventricle; PA: pulmonary artery; RV: right ventricle).

Heterotaxy Syndromes

These syndromes are rare. These should be suspected when there is abnormal disposition of thoracic and abdominal organs also. Descending aorta and IVC on same side. IVC is interrupted. Large azygos vein may open into SVC. Complex cardiac lesions are associated. Viscerocardiac heterotaxy may/may not be present. Fetal hydrops may develop and may have up to 100% in utero mortality with heart block.

Other Cardiac Defects

- *Abnormal PV drainage*: Normally two out of four pulmonary veins can be seen entering LA on four chamber view after 18 weeks. Anomalous PV drainage may affect one or more of these veins. If all the four are involved it is total anomalous PV drainage otherwise it is partial. Only total anomalous drainage can be excluded antenatally. Pulmonary veins instead of emptying into LA, may empty in RA or any other systemic veins. These may be portal-hepatic veins, innominate vein, SVC or coronary sinus. Total anomalous PV drainage has obligatory right to left atrial shunt.

  On US, no pulmonary veins seen on four chamber view entering the LA. PV confluence is seen behind the RA. RV is large, if total anomalous PV drainage is present, but enlargement is not seen if there is ASD or infradiaphragmatic drainage. Color Doppler may show the PV drainage precisely **(Fig. 49)**.
- *Ectopia cordis*:
  - *Thoracic type*: Heart protrudes out from the chest cavity with cephalic orientation of the cardiac apex.

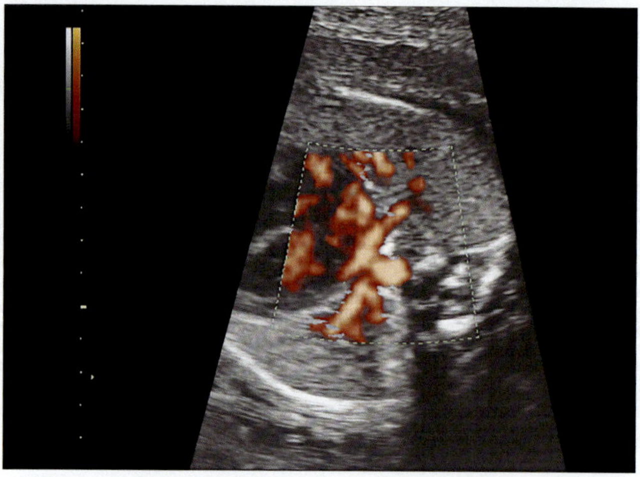

Fig. 49: Two pulmonary arteries are seen communicating with left atrium—normally seen on four chamber heart view.

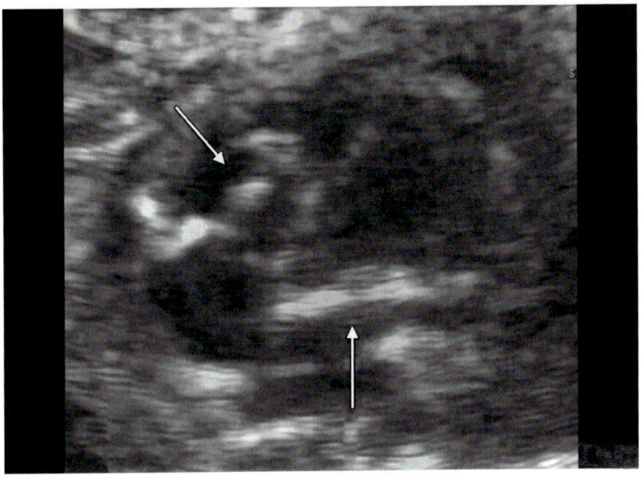

Fig. 50: Fibroelastosis—calcified echogenic walls (arrows).

- *Thoracoabdominal type*: Pericardium and diaphragmatic defects are present with heart displaced into the abdomen.

- *Myocardial diseases*:
  - *Hypertrophic cardiomyopathy*: Thickened less contractile heart. It is seen in diabetic mothers. May cause LVOT obstruction.
    In dilated cardiomyopathy there are dilated ventricles with decrease systolic function and leads to cardiac failure.[19]
  - *Fibroelastosis*: Thickening of ventricular endocardium with bright echogenic shadows are seen on US with decreased systolic function **(Fig. 50)**.
    - Both these conditions can lead to cardiac failure and hydrops.
    - *Obstructed foramen ovale*: Commonly associated with left heart obstructive defects. It may also be associated with mitral regurgitation, supraventricular tachycardia or fetal hydrops.

    This can lead to prenatal right heart failure, hydrops, and fetal death. Postnatally it leads to persistent fetal circulation, right heart failure, and death.
- *Cardiac tumors*: Rhabdomyomas are most common **(Fig. 51)**. They may be associated with tuberous sclerosis. May be multiple. Can be detected as early as 20 weeks of gestation and are progressive. They are seen as solid intracardiac tumors and show movements with cardiac cycle. Depending on size and position, these may cause obstructive defects, cardiac failure or arrhythmias. Others are fibromas, teratomas, myxomas, and hemangiomas. Fibromas are usually solitary and commonly arise from left ventricular apex. Though usually homogeneous may sometimes have cysts or calcifications.

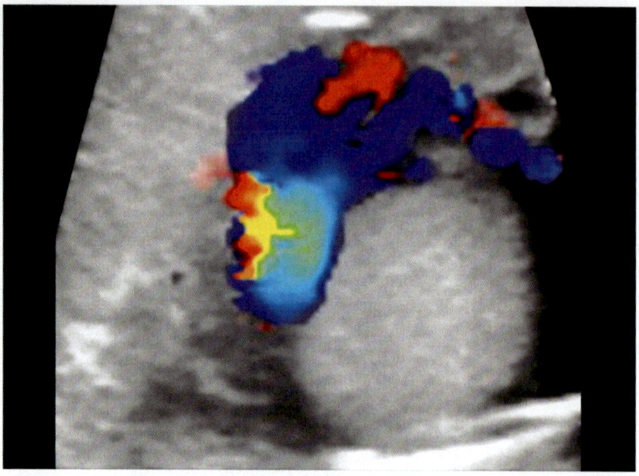

Fig. 51: Rhabdomyoma.

- *Premature constriction of ductus arteriosus*: Use of indomethacin may lead to ductal obstruction between 28 and 34 weeks. Evaluation for the same is to be done within 48–72 hours of starting indomethacin. Total ductal closure may be associated with fetal demise. Ductal arch patency must always be checked when doing a fetal echocardiography. Ductal obstruction will lead to RV enlargement, hypertrophy, RA enlargement and TR and ultimately may lead to right heart failure.

  On pulsed Doppler, normal velocity in ductus arteriosus is 150 cm/s (Sys), 40 cm/s (Dias). Its constriction causes higher systolic and diastolic velocities. Only high systolic velocity may be seen in last 4–6 weeks and in conditions with increased fetal cardiac output, but high diastolic velocity is diagnostic of ductal constriction.[20]
- *Obstructed foramen ovale*: Commonly associated with left heart obstructive defects. It may also be associated with mitral regurgitation, supraventricular tachycardia or fetal hydrops. Prenatal death may occur due to right heart failure, hydrops, and death.
- *Absence of ductus venosus*: Umbilical vein is connected to either IVC or renal vein leading to significant dilatation of IVC since midgestation. Umbilical vein takes an inferior course. A long aberrant vessel is seen from liver to right abdominal wall crossing the diaphragm.

Arrhythmias

It must be always confirmed by M-mode.

Tachycardia

Tachycardias are twice common than bradycardias. Tachycardias due to maternal fever, drugs, thyrotoxicosis, fetal distress or infection range from

180 to 200 beats/min. Those due to supraventricular tachycardia heart rates are 220–260 beats/min. Atrial flutter gives heart rate of >300 beats/min. Ventricular tachycardia may occur due to perinatal stress and hypoxia, cardiomyopathy, drug intoxication, electrolyte imbalance, and ventricular aneurysm.

Bradycardias are most likely due to heart blocks, which are often regular, 2:1 or variable. It is commonly associated with major cardiac defects or maternal anti-SS-A and anti-SS-B antibodies.

Irregular Rhythm

Arrhythmias are commonly associated with obstructed foramen ovale, cardiac tumors, cardiomyopathy, Ebstein's anomaly, and atrial septal aneurysm. It can occur due to maternal ingestion of caffeine, hydrazine, and nifedipine and are reversible after stopping drugs.

Fetal echocardiography must be included in the detailed structural scan in second trimester routinely and must be offered with nuchal scan or at least at 16–18 weeks for all the high-risk fetuses.

REFERENCES

1. Ferencz C, Rubin JD, Loffredo CA, Magee CA. Perspectives in pediatric cardiology. Congenital Heart Disease: The Baltimore-Washington Infant study 1981-1989. New York: Futura Publishing; 1993.
2. Nora JJ, Nora AH. Maternal transmission of congenital heart diseases: new recurrence risk figures and the questions of cytoplasmic inheritance and vulnerability to teratogens. Am J Cardiol. 1987;59:459-63.
3. Sandor GC, Smith DF, MacLeod PM. Cardiac malformations in the fetal alcohol syndrome. J Pediatr. 1981;98:771-3.
4. Copel JA, Pilu G, Kleinman CS. Congenital heart disease and extracardiac anomalies: associations and indications for fetal echocardiography. Am J Obstet Gynecol. 1986;154(5):1121-32.
5. McGahan JP. Sonography of the fetal heart: findings on four chamber view. Am J Roengenol. 1991;156:547-53.
6. McGahan JP, Benacerraf BR. Realtime examination of fetal heart. In: McGahan JP, Goldberg BB (Eds). Diagnostic Ultrasound: A Logical Approach. Philadelphia: Lippincott-Raven Publishers; 1998. pp. 257-81.
7. Crane JM, Ash K, Fink N, Desjardins C. Abnormal fetal cardiac axis in detection of intrathoracic anomalies and congenital heart disease. Ultrasound Obstet Gynecol. 1997;10:90-9.
8. Yoo SJ, Lee YH, Kim ES, Ryu HM, Kim MY, Choi HK, et al. Three-vessel view of the fetal upper mediastinum: an easy means of detecting abnormalities of the ventricular outflow tracts and detecting abnormalities of the ventricular outflow tracts and great arteries during obstetric screening. Ultrasound Obstet Gynecol. 1997;9:173-82.
9. DeVore GR. The aortic and pulmonary outflow tract and screening examination in the human fetus. J Ultrasound Med. 1992;11:345-8.
10. Yagel S, Cohen SM, Achiron R. Examination of the fetal heart by five short axis views: a proposed screening method for comprehensive cardiac evaluation. Ultrasound Obstet Gynecol. 2001;17:367-9.

11. Digilio MC, Marino B, Cicini MP, Giannotti A, Formigari R, Dallapiccola B. Risk of congenital heart defects in relatives of patients with atrioventricular canal. Am J Dis Child. 1993;147(12):1295-7.
12. Hornberger LK, Sahn DJ, Kleinman CS, Copel JA, Reed KL. Tricuspid valve disease with significant tricuspid insufficiency in the fetus: diagnosis and outcome. J Am Coll Cardiol. 1991;17(1):167-73.
13. Yagel S, Arbel R, Auteby EY, Raveh D, Achiron R. The three vessels and trachea view (3VT) in fetal cardiac scanning. Ultrasound Obstet Gynecol. 2002;20:360-5.
14. Berning RA, Silverman NH, Villegas M, Sahn DJ, Martin GR, Rice MJ. Reversed shunting across the ductus arteriosus or atrial septum in utero heralds severe congenital heart disease. J Am Coll Cardiol. 1996;27(2):481-6.
15. Jouk PS, Rambaud P. Prediction of outcome by prenatal Doppler analysis in a patient with aortic stenosis. Br Heart J. 1991;65(1):53-4.
16. Sharland GK, Chan KY, Allan LD. Coarctation of the aorta: difficulties in prenatal diagnosis. Br Heart J. 1994;71(1):70-5.
17. Lee W, Smith RS, Comstock CH, Kirk JS, Riggs T, Weinhouse E. Tetralogy of Fallot: prenatal diagnosis and postnatal survival. Obstet Gynecol. 1995;86:583-5.
18. Schmidt KG, Ulmer HE, Silverman NH. Perinatal outcome of fetal complete atrioventricular block: a multicenter experience. J Am Coll Cardiol. 1991;17(6):1360-6.
19. Schmidt KG, Birk E, Silverman NH, Scagnelli SA. Echocardiographic evaluation of dilated cardiomyopathy in human fetus. Am J Cardiol. 1989;63(9):599-605.
20. Huhta JC, Moise KJ, Fisher DJ, Sharif DS, Wasserstrum N, Martin C. Detection and quantitation of constriction of the fetal ductus arteriosus by Doppler echocardiography. Circulation. 1987;75(2):406-12.

CHAPTER 22

Role of Ultrasound in Diagnosis and Management of Fetal Growth Restriction

Sonal Panchal

DEFINITION

Fetal growth restriction (FGR) is suggested if gestational weeks determined by ultrasound (US) shows delay from the weeks determined by crown-rump length (CRL) or correct last menstrual period (LMP) in late second trimester or third trimester.

So, simply speaking, it is a process, which prevents the growth of the fetus up to the intrinsic fetal growth potential in utero. Though it must not be forgotten that the normal fetal growth is influenced by genetic predisposition, parental influence, ethnic differences,[1] environment (altitude), and fetal gender also. The biochemical changes associated with FGR fetuses are lower mean glucose and cholesterol ester concentrations,[2] higher nitrous oxide and total nitrite levels in fetal plasma and higher serum levels of inhibin and human chorionic gonadotropin (hCG).

Fetal growth restriction babies are different from low birth weight (LBW) babies, which are <2,500 g at birth, despite of their gestational age (GA) or small for gestational age (SGA) babies, which are smaller for their GA but not necessarily growth restricted.

Low birth weight babies may be prematurely delivered babies or SGA babies or truly FGR babies. SGA babies usually genetically have low growth potential or may have intrauterine infections or genetic disorders.

Most common causes for LBW babies are as follows:

- *Maternal*:
  - Pregnancy-induced hypertension (PIH)
  - Antiphospholipid antibody syndrome/prothrombotic states
  - Chronic hypertension
  - Severe diabetes mellitus
  - Collagen vascular disease
  - Cardiac or renal disease
  - Smoking and poor nutrition
  - Previous history of intrauterine growth restriction (IUGR) baby.
- *Uterine-placental*:
  - Uteroplacental dysfunction
  - Placental infarct

    - Chronic abruption
    - Multiple gestation—twin-to-twin transfusion
    - Confined placental mosaicism
    - Placental bleeding
    - Placental infections
    - Immunological causes
- *Fetal*:
    - Chromosomal abnormalities
    - Confined placental mosaicism
    - Major structural anomalies
    - Skeletal dysplasias
    - Multiple anomaly syndromes
    - Infections
    - Teratogens

Of all these, if the aneuploidies are excluded, the most common causes of LBW are PIH and uteroplacental vascular dysfunction. Those fetuses that have restricted growth due to circulatory abnormalities are FGR fetuses. The incidence of FGR varies from 1 to 12%.

The risk is higher in the females who had a history of IUGR or PIH or stillbirth in previous pregnancy or have hypertension are exposed to toxic substances such as alcohol or tobacco, or to infections such as cytomegalovirus (CMV) or rubella, etc., or have autoimmune, renal or vascular diseases. Approximately 20–30% of all SGA fetuses are true growth restricted fetuses.[3]

It is essential to diagnose FGR because these fetuses have lots of immediate and late consequences such as higher perinatal morbidity and mortality, perinatal asphyxia, hypothermia, persistent fetal circulation, hypoglycemia, polycythemia, and some neurological deficits and learning and behavioral problems.[4]

To decide whether the fetus is FGR or not, it is essential to first establish the correct GA and to assess the fetal growth by biometric measurements. The GA can be established by either LMP, which has a higher error rate, or by first trimester or possibly earliest ultrasonography (USG)–CRL measurement, which has lowest deviations from standard measurements. So earlier the fetus/embryo is measured, more accurate is its age assessment. If the dating is done in the second trimester it is not as reliable, because fetal growth then may be affected by several factors such as genetic causes, maternal diseases, fetal conditions, etc. The transcerebellar diameter[5] and the clavicular length[6] can be taken to more precisely assess the GA because these are the ones which show the GA most accurately and are not affected by IUGR.

Another simpler method of differentiating SGA from FGR fetuses is to plot the growth of these fetuses on the nomogram chart. If the growth curve of the fetus follows the curve of the nomogram, may be even lower than the nomogram curve, it is indicative of SGA fetus, but if the fetal growth curve crosses across the nomogram curve, it is indicative of FGR. It is therefore necessary to have serial measurements of biometric parameters at at least 2 weeks intervals, to diagnose growth abnormalities of the fetus.[7]

The fetal age is best decided between 9 and 11 weeks based on CRL. CRL is considered to be more reliable after it reaches 18–22 mm.[8]

CRL should be correctly measured. The CRL must be measures in the true midsagittal plane of the fetus, (confirmed by nonvisualization of the proximal parts of the limbs in that image planes), with the fetus in neutral position (neither extended, nor flexed, no rotation of the neck). Later in the pregnancy other biometric parameters such as biparietal diameter (BPD), head circumference (HC), femur length (FL), etc **(Figs. 1 and 2)**. Standardized

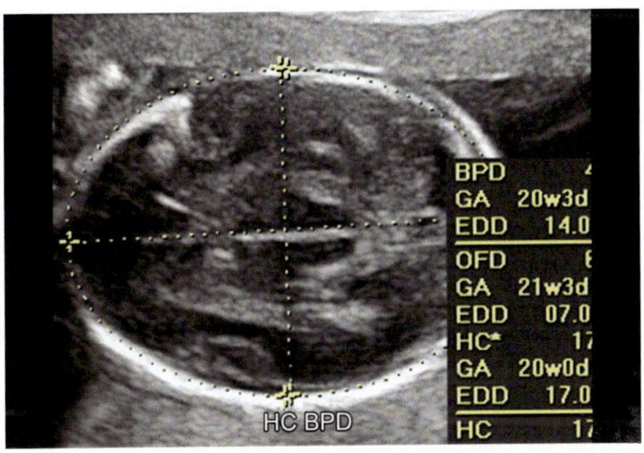

Fig. 1: *Head measurements:* Biparietal diameter (BPD) and head circumference (HC).

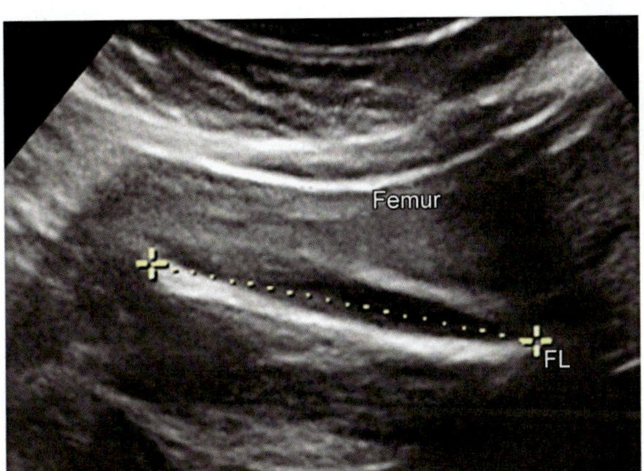

Fig. 2: Femoral length (FL) measurement.

planes/sections are achieved and standard methods are used to achieve correct measurements to assess the fetal age. The first scan done to assess the fetal age is known as pregnancy dating scan. When there is a discrepancy of 7 days or more in the first trimester between the GA calculated by LMP and GA calculated by US the dates are reassigned. From 14 to 20 weeks of GA, when the difference between the dates calculated according to LMP and US assigned GA is more than 10 days, the dates are reassigned according to the GA assigned by US. From 20 to 26 weeks the difference allowed is 14 days. Another method used to decide whether the dates need to be reassigned or not is by following the rule of 8%. Maximum 8% of discrepancy is acceptable during pregnancy between the gestational age calculated by LMP and that calculated by biometric parameters on US. If the difference between the GA calculated by LMP and by US is more than 8% of the US calculated age, the dates are reassigned. For example according to LMP the GA is 149 days and that according to US is 133 days. The difference between the two is 16 days. The expected margin of error 8% of 133 days is 10.64 days. Since 16 is more than 10.64, the dates will be reassigned according to the GA calculated by US, i.e., 133 days. Dates once assigned have to be followed throughout the pregnancy and have to be taken as a standard to further judge growth derangements. In spite of the fact that for the pregnancy dating head and long bone biometric parameters are considered more reliable, for the birth weight assessment and prediction of IUGR, abdominal circumference (AC) **(Fig. 3)** is considered to be more reliable. Estimated fetal weight (EFW) has a more stronger association with birth weight below 10th centile.[9] EFW could be assessed against birth weight and has a random error of 8%.[10]

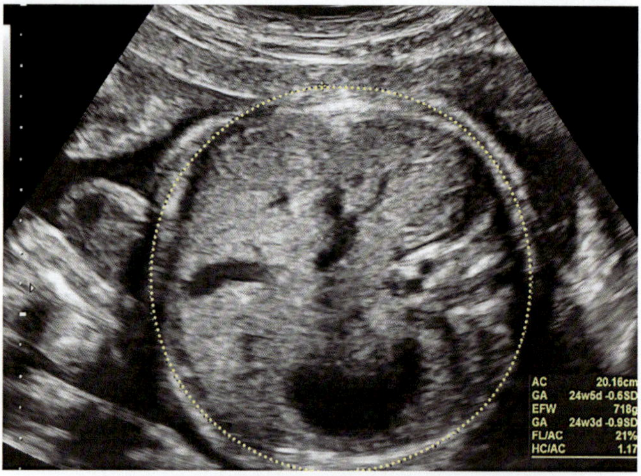

Fig. 3: Abdominal circumference (AC) measurement.

The growth assessed on the dating scan is plotted on the nomogram and the results of all the following scans are also entered on to the same graph. FGR is considered when the growth plotting done for a particular fetus, deviates from the normal curve instead of overlapping it or being parallel to it. It is important to remember that when the plotted graph remains below the 5th centile on the nomogram but is still parallel to it, it is not FGR **(Figs. 4A and B)**.

Associated B-mode finding is oligohydramnios. It may be measured as a single largest vertical measurement of fluid pouch, free of cord or fetal parts or as a sum of vertical depth of the deepest fluid pocket, free of cord loop or limbs, in all the four quadrants of the uterus, named as amniotic fluid index (AFI) **(Fig. 5)**. When a single pocket is considered <5 cm is considered abnormal and then AFI should be checked. When AFI is assessed it normally should be between 15 and 25 cm near term, but <10 cm is considered oligohydramnios.

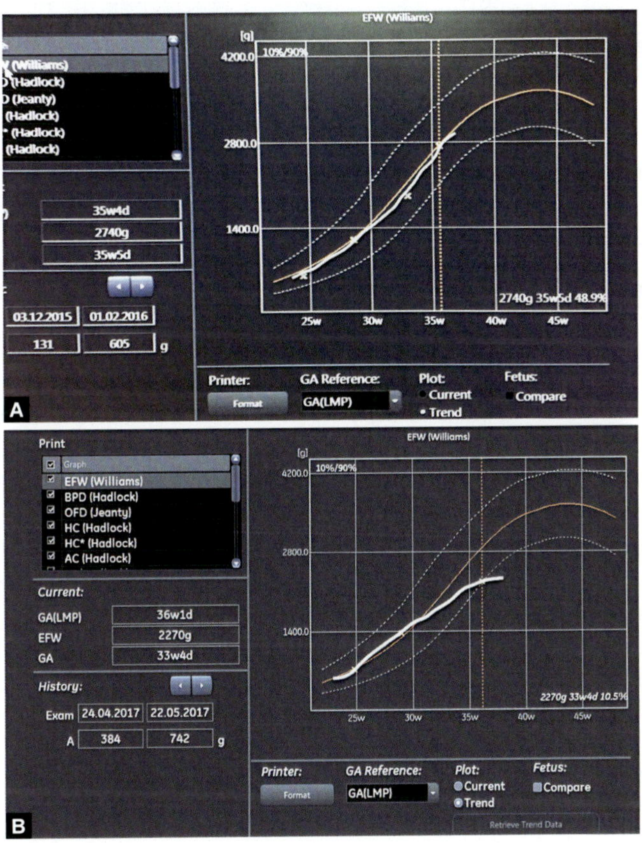

Figs. 4A and B: (A) Plotted growth curve follows that in the nomogram—normal growth; (B) Plotted growth curve deviates downwards from normal growth curve in nomogram—FGR.

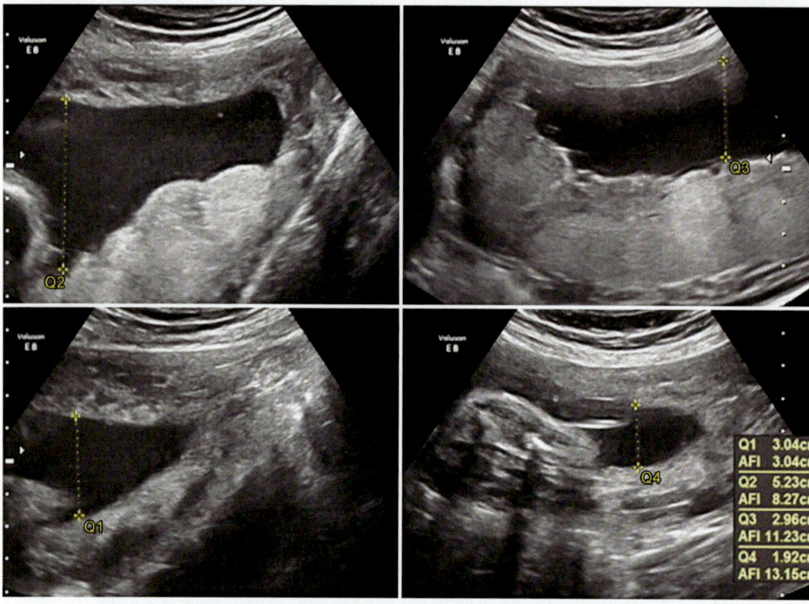

Fig. 5: Assessment of amniotic fluid index.

It is in IUGR fetuses that Doppler plays an important role for monitoring and management planning. This is so because IUGR is due to uteroplacental vascular dysfunction.

CLASSIFICATIONS

There are several classification documented earlier according to the cause and effects of FGR. But these are not used now. But still just to mention.

- *Campbell*:[11] First tried to classify IUGR based on BPD only and classified as *"early low profile"* IUGR or *"late flattening"* IUGR.
- Levi et al.[12] added a further dimension to this by taking HC/AC ratio into consideration and classified IUGR as *harmonious or proportionate and disharmonious or disproportionate.*
- Anglo Saxon specialists[13] then named these as *symmetrical/asymmetrical* and added a third entity as *symmetrical IUGR with femur sparing*. Naturally FL was also taken into classification here.
- Finally in 1976, *integrated classification* came in which took all the basic aspects of IUGR in consideration.

Integrated Classification[14]

- *Type I*: Intrinsic/harmonious/proportionate/symmetrical/early
- *Type II*: Extrinsic/disharmonious/disproportionate/asymmetrical/late
- *Type III*: Mixed/semiharmonious

RISK FACTORS FOR INTRAUTERINE GROWTH RESTRICTION

More than 50% of pregnancies are free of any associated conditions that would alert to the possibility of IUGR. Though the high-risk mothers are those who have:

- Previous history of LBW/IUGR babies
- Hypertension
- Autoimmune diseases
- Smokers

Diagnosis of FGR is based on clinical parameters and on B-mode US biometry, and amniotic fluid. Diagnosis of FGR was earlier based on certain clinical parameters such as:

- *Fundal height below 5th percentile based on the last date of menstrual period:* It is believed that patients whose fundal height falls below the 5th percentile are likely to have IUGR babies. Uterine volume may be more reliable than the height alone and is calculated as length × width × height × 0.523 = volume. IUGR based on uterine volume is diagnosed, when total uterine volume is ≤1.5 standard deviation (SD) of mean equivocal between +1.5 and –1.5. Errors are bound to occur due to oligohydramnios and polyhydramnios. It has a sensitivity of 60% and positive predictive value 30% for diagnosis of IUGR.
- *Date of quickening:* These methods are based on clinical judgment and have less reliability as compared to US measurement of fetal parts called biometry.

ULTRASOUND DIAGNOSIS OF INTRAUTERINE GROWTH RESTRICTION

Biometric parameters commonly used are:

- Biparietal diameter
- Head circumference and cerebral index (CI)
- Abdominal diameter and circumference
- Femur length
- Fetal organ biometry

Head Measurements (Fig. 1)

Biparietal Diameter, Head Circumference, and Cerebral Index

The BPD is measured on transthalamic plane. A correct transthalamic plane is a plane which shows frontal horns of lateral ventricles, cavum septum and falx anteriorly, thalami and third ventricle in the center and occipital horns of the lateral ventricles, Sylvian fissure, cisterna magna and insula posteriorly. The parietal bone should not be thicker than 3 mm, which confirms that the section is not oblique. Select the broadest part of the skull at this section and the measurement is taken from the outer table of the proximal parietal bone to the inner table of the distal parietal bone.

Though depending on the shape of the skull, BPD may be vary, but it is not much affected by placental insufficiency.

When BPD is lower than 5th percentile, FGR is confirmed in 68% of cases, but maximum errors are likely to occur when the values are between 5th and 10th percentile. FGR is suspected if growth rate is decreased (<5%) or the BPD is <10th percentile.

If CI is <70% or >85%, BPD is not considered to be of reliability and then one has to depend on HC for assessment of GA.

It can be either measured directly on the same section as BPD or can be calculated as [BPD + occipitofrontal diameter (OFD)] × 1.57. Its sensitivity for FGR is 52% and has a specificity of 80%. If the curve of cephalometric parameters deviates from and falls low, it is IUGR.

Femur Length (Fig. 2)

Long bones like femur and humerus are fairly accurate for estimation of GA. Femur has a typical "golf club" like appearance and a moderate curvature starts developing from 18 weeks onwards. Femoral length is measured from origin of the distal end of the shaft, from greater trochanter to the lateral condyle, excluding the femoral head, and the distal epiphysis in the measurement. Similarly while measuring the humerus length also, the head and the distal epiphysis are not included in the measurement. All long bones are measured on an image in which the bone is seen obliquely at 5–10° angle on the screen.

Femur length is not/little affected in FGR, but is affected in chromosomal abnormalities. The sensitivity of FL is 63% for FGR with a positive predictive value of 30% (independent of GA).

Though neither BPD, nor long bone lengths have been found to be useful in diagnosing early type II IUGR as both are the least affected FGR.

Abdominal Diameter and Circumference (Fig. 3)

Abdominal measurements represent nutrition of the fetus and reflect liver development and fetal fat deposition. It may also be affected by the level of diaphragm, depending on the extent of lung development.

Abdominal diameter and AC are measured at the level of stomach and bifurcation of the main portal vein into right and left branches in axial plane **(Fig. 3)**. Care must be taken to take a section which is most rounded, perpendicular to the spine, with the ribs symmetrically covering the AC, which confirms it is not an oblique section. It is best measured during fetal apnea and the smallest circumference is selected.

It has a linear rise till 36 weeks, beyond which it grows at a slower pace. AC is the single most sensitive measure of fetal growth and is affected much earlier than the head or femur measurements. It has 83% sensitivity and 87% specificity for diagnosis of IUGR. In both low-risk and high-risk subjects, AC below tenth percentile has the highest sensitivity and fetal weight has the highest odds ratio for diagnosis of IUGR.

Nutritional status of the fetus can also be assessed by thigh circumference of the fetus, but is not commonly used.

Rather than these biometric parameters individually there are certain ratios which may be more informative for suspecting FGR before the amniotic fluid decreases or the umbilical artery blood flow becomes abnormal.

Head Circumference/Abdominal Circumference Ratio

The normal values of HC/AC ratio are as follows:

- >1.2, 14–16 weeks
- >1 till 36 weeks
- =1 at 36 weeks
- <1 after 36 weeks

The HC/AC is the most reliable between 32 and 36 weeks for diagnosis and classification of IUGR. At 32 weeks, it has a sensitivity of 86.7% for FGR and at 35–36 weeks it has a sensitivity of 83% and a specificity of 79% for diagnosis of FGR.

Another ratio of importance is FL/AC. It has a sensitivity of 63% and is independent of GA.[15]

Apart from these routinely taken biometric measurements, fetal organs can also be measured for diagnosis and differentiation of certain pathologies.

Though it must be remembered that growth arrest in a high-risk fetus is an important sign of fetal distress and therefore a dynamic evaluation of the fetal growth is more reliable and relevant than the one time biometry when the fetal measurements are below 10th percentile. In low-risk fetuses, biometry may be repeated at longer intervals but in high-risk fetuses for FGR it is better to repeat biometry at least every 4 weeks beyond 20–22 weeks.

There are other measures also which can be used to assess a compromising fetus. These include the amniotic fluid levels, biophysical profile (BPP), cardiotocography (CTG), and the Doppler studies.

Assessment of the AFI is very essential when evaluating an FGR pregnancy. It is measured as largest vertical measurement of fluid pouch, free of cord or fetal parts in four quadrants of the uterus **(Fig. 5)**. It is essential in this case to keep the probe also absolutely vertical on patient's abdomen, not at right angle to the patient's abdominal surface.

A late-onset FGR with oligohydramnios indicates a chronic insult to the uteroplacental circulation leading to fetal hypoxia. Normal AFI suggests pathology of a more acute origin.

An early-onset FGR with polyhydramnios indicates a possibility of aneuploidy rather than of uteroplacental circulatory disorder origin, though triploidy and tetraploidy may show oligohydramnios.

Thus, diagnosis of IUGR is to be done by B-mode assessment of the fetus. It is the management that is dependent on Doppler findings.

PREDICTION OF PIH AND FGR

The first prediction of risk of FGR based on Doppler studies of the uterine and umbilical arteries can be done at 20–24 weeks.

- If a 20–24 weeks Doppler assessment shows high resistance flow in uterine arteries, there is 24-fold increased chances of PIH and FGR.
- Persistent early diastolic notch **(Fig. 6)** in the uterine artery was earlier thought to be a predictor of PIH and FGR. But the recent studies have shown that notch alone does not have a high predictive value unless it is associated with high uterine artery resistance.
- Mean pulsatility index (PI) of both the uterine arteries in the second trimester of >1.3 suggests a high risk for PIH.

Prediction of FGR

If predicted, pregnancies with FGR fetuses can be better managed. Uterine artery Doppler has an effective application for the same. Several workers have published on the importance and efficacy of biochemical markers along with uterine artery Doppler for prediction of FGR. First trimester high uterine artery resistance index (RI) (0.74) and bilateral uterine artery diastolic notch can be significant predictors for FGR. High uterine artery resistance at 11–14 weeks with low pregnancy-associated plasma protein A (PAPP-A) can provide early assessment of risk for uteroplacental insufficiency.[16]

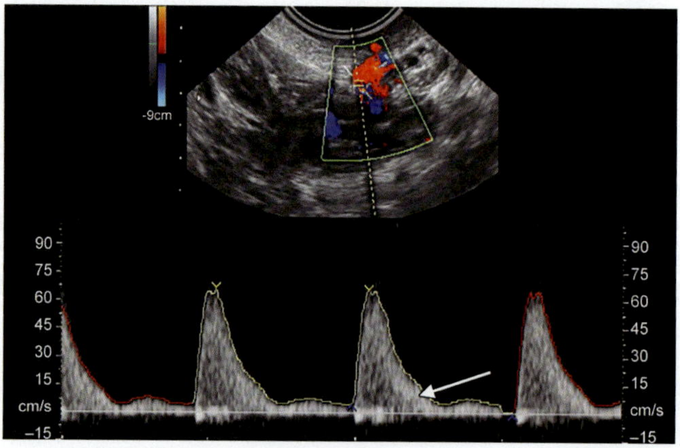

Fig. 6: Diastolic notch and high resistance uterine artery flow.

Uterine artery PI and PAPP-A have negative linear correlation. Low PAPP-A in first trimester in euploid fetus with growth restriction at 18–24 weeks predicts high chance of PIH, FGR, and preterm birth.[17] It has been shown that low placental growth factor (PlGF) and high uterine artery PI have a sensitivity of 89.5% and specificity of 95% for prediction of early-onset preeclampsia (PE) and IUGR.[18]

According to another study, combination of first trimester low placental protein 13 (PP13), high uterine artery PI, and uterine artery notch can be promising signs for prediction of PE in women with high a priori risk of PE.[19]

One more study shows that persistent early diastolic notch, increases predictive value from 4.3 to 23% for IUGR and 68-fold increased risk of developing PE.[20]

Low PAPP-A (<0.3 MoM), small placental size (<10 cm), and elevated alpha-fetoprotein (AFP) (>2.0 MoM) even in absence of abnormal uterine art indices (PI > 1.45), identify women with high risk of IUGR, extreme preterm delivery, and still birth.[21]

At 22–24 weeks if Doppler shows high resistance in uterine artery, 24-fold increased chances of PE and IUGR are estimated. It has an overall sensitivity of growth restriction of 16%. But its sensitivity for PE related or no PE growth restriction with risk of requiring delivery before 32 weeks is 93% and 56%, respectively with specificities of 95%.[22]

A systematic review with meta-analysis showed that uterine artery Doppler had limited accuracy in predicting IUGR and perinatal death.[23]

Combining all together, effective screening for early PE can be provided by a combination of maternal factors:

- Low PAPP-A
- Low PP13
- High Soluble endoglin
- Low placental growth factor
- Uterine artery resistance
- Uterine artery notch

Physiology

Normal umbilical artery flow velocity waveform (FVW) is the indicator of normal mother to fetus blood supply. On implantation of the embryo in the endometrium and development of the chorionic villi, the high resistance spiral vessels are converted into low resistance chorionic villous vessels. It is because of this conversion that the placental vessels have a low resistance flow. The key area in the placenta is intervillous space, filled with maternal blood, in which the tertiary villi are immersed and across these vessel walls there is exchange of blood, nutrients for the fetal nutrition. Any decrease in the blood supply to the placenta leads to decrease in oxygenated blood in intervillous space and therefore decrease oxygen supply to fetus. Normal umbilical artery FVW is the indicator of normal mother to fetus blood supply. Increase in umbilical artery flow velocities and decreased resistance are seen as the pregnancy advances normally and are due to:

- Continuous maturation of placental villi
- Widening of placental vessels
- Continuous rise in fetal cardiac output
- Continuous changes in vessel compliance
- Continuous rise in fetal blood pressure

This is because of conversion of spiral vessels, which are high resistance vessels into placental vessels, which are low resistance vessels **(Fig. 7)**. This conversion chiefly occurs in two phases, at 8–9 weeks of gestation and at 18–20 weeks of gestation. As a result of nonconversion of some of the spiral arteries and persistent high resistance circulation, more pressure is required for the large quantities of blood to be pushed through these vessels for fetal support, leading to uterine artery resistance and ultimately reduction in the umbilical artery flow **(Fig. 8)**.

This is inadequate placentation and it leads to:

- PIH and/or IUGR
- Inadequate trophoblastic invasion
- Absence of uterine vasodilatation
- Reduced placental perfusion
- Hampered villous microcirculation
- Umbilical hypoxemia
- Vascular changes for compensation

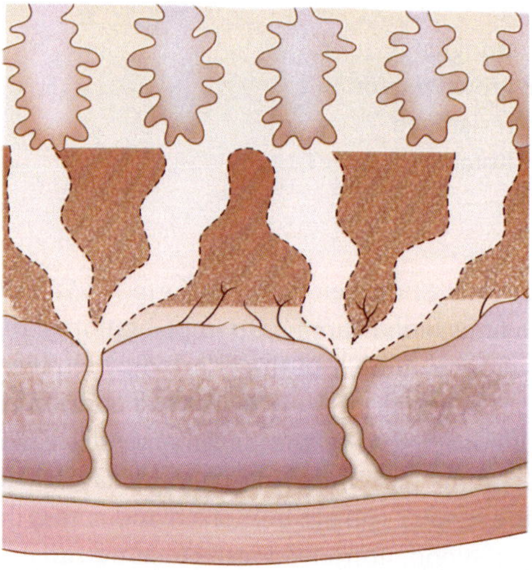

Fig. 7: Placental vasculature in normal cases.

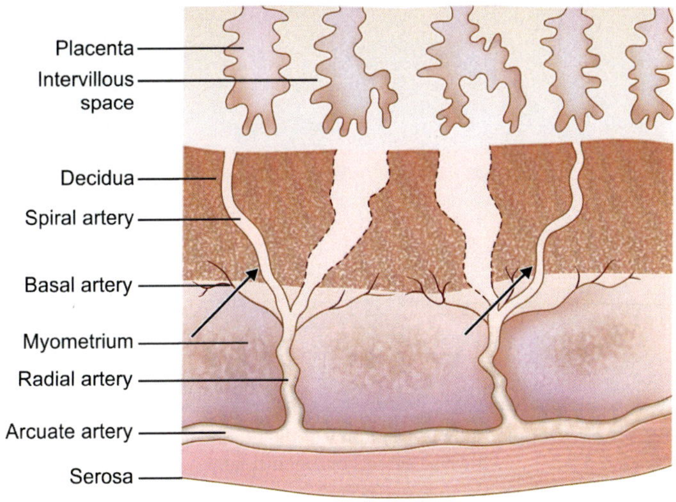

Fig. 8: Placental vasculature in pregnancy-induced hypertension.

So, primarily the flows in uterine and the umbilical arteries are to be assessed in IUGR fetuses. Uterine artery Doppler is the main screening method for prediction of IUGR. Normally the uterine artery and umbilical artery flow velocity increases in the normal pregnancy and resistance decreases as pregnancy advances.[24]

Abnormal umbilical artery Doppler correlates with histological evidence of placental vascular pathology. Therefore, umbilical artery Doppler indices correlate with the fetal levels of glucose, amino acids and blood gases.[25]

There is also a strong evidence to show that SGA fetuses with abnormal umbilical artery flow are at a higher risk of abnormal perinatal outcome.[26] And perinatal death with normal umbilical artery flow is very uncommon.[27]

Decreased umbilical vein flow is also documented in otherwise asymptomatic fetuses with decreased placental volume. But to study the oxygenation status of the fetus, it is essential to also evaluate the fetal vessels, and middle cerebral artery (MCA) is the one that is considered to be representing the fetal oxygenation status because the cerebral cortex reflects to hypoxia and MCA is the vessel that supplies more than 50% of the cerebral cortex.

Hypoxia leads to cellular dysfunction as the cells lose their ability for oxidative phosphorylation. This changes aerobic metabolism to anaerobic metabolism, accumulation of lactic acid and hydrogen ions, and decreased adenosine triphosphate (ATP) generation. This leads to failure of sodium-potassium pump and cellular edema. Activation of phospholipases also leads to accumulation of free fatty acids. All these lead to cell death and are the basis for neurological deficit in hypoxic fetuses.[28]

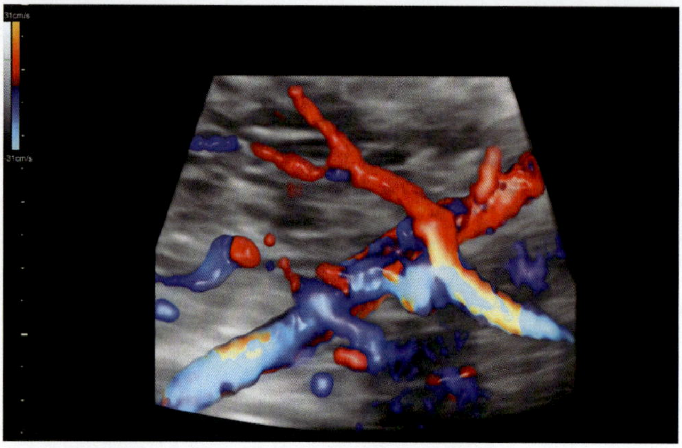

Fig. 9: Color Doppler showing anatomy of the uterine artery seen crossing the iliac vessels perpendicularly.

Technique of Doppler Assessment

Uterine Artery Doppler

- Uterine artery can be best located as it crosses the internal iliac vessels perpendicular to their path.
- Place the probe on the symphysis pubis and slide it laterally, holding vertically.
- Iliac artery and vein are seen as two easily recognizable vessels in their long axis.
- Switch on the color with pulse repetition frequency (PRF) of 0.6–0.9 and a low wall motion filter.
- Rotate the probe laterally and angulate medially and Doppler will show a pulsatile vessel crossing the iliac vessels perpendicularly. This is uterine artery **(Fig. 9)**.
- Sample volume should be 2 mm.
- Switch on the pulse Doppler and align the angle almost parallel to iliac vessels.
- Adjust the PRF to get a complete spectrum on one side of the baseline.
- Calculate PI of uterine artery.

Umbilical Artery Doppler (Fig. 10)

- In a free loop of umbilical cord
- On a zoomed image
- Pulsed Doppler sample volume of 1–2 mm
- Sample volume on one umbilical artery
- Adjust power Doppler scale to for velocity

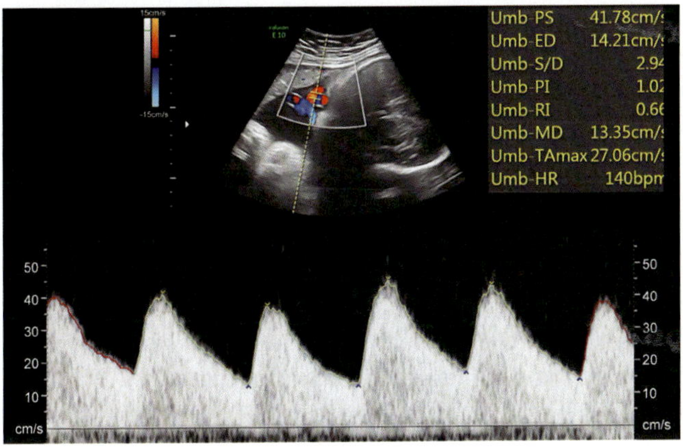

Fig. 10: Umbilical artery flow measured in the free loop of umbilical cord. Pulsed wave Doppler showing its normal flow pattern.

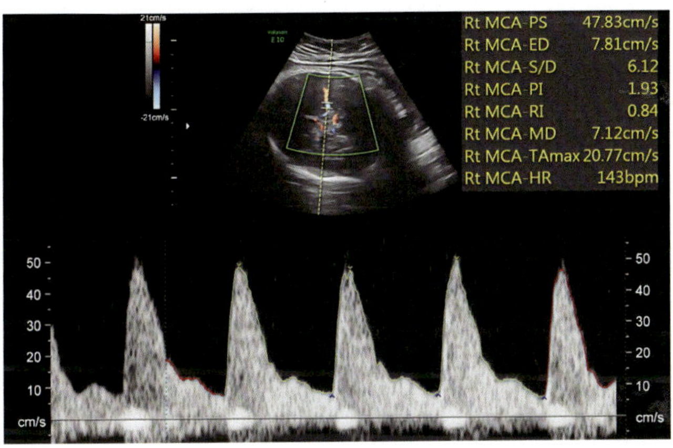

Fig. 11: Normal MCA flow on pulsed wave Doppler and on color Doppler showing circle of Willis.

- Obtain at least five waveforms for measurement of indices
- To be assessed when fetus is not breathing and not moving
- As low as reasonably achievable (ALARA) principle is followed.

Umbilical artery flow assessment is to monitor IUGR fetus but is not reliable screening tool for prediction of IUGR.[29]

Middle Cerebral Arterial Doppler (Fig. 11)

- Locate the MCA closest to the transducer on the circle of Willis section
- Magnify the image for MCA to occupy >50% of the image
- Pulse Doppler sample volume of 1–2 mm
- Sample volume is placed close to its origin

- Adjust pulse Doppler scale to fit the velocity
- Angle between US beam and blood flow should be smallest possible
- Obtain at least five waveforms
- Ensure no fetal movements or breathing
- Follow ALARA (as low as reasonably achievable) principle
- Take at least three traces and use the highest peak systolic velocity (PSV) and lowest RI for clinical care.

Intrauterine growth restriction can be divided into four periods of relatively well-defined hemodynamic, biophysical and biochemical changes and Doppler plays an important role in diagnosis of these different stages and decision making for the management of these fetuses.

Biochemically the different stages can be defined as stages of hypoxemia, hypoxia, and acidosis. While according to the vascular changes, these can be staged as a silent period of increased resistance, period of reduction in umbilical artery blood flow and centralization of fetal circulation and decentralization of fetal circulation.

SILENT PERIOD OF INCREASED RESISTANCE

Pathophysiology

Till decreased villous microcirculation up to 50%, no change is seen in the umbilical artery flow, if there is no defect in maternal supply.

During this stage no change is seen in the Doppler parameters of umbilical artery or MCA which are the most commonly interrogated vessels in mothers with PIH or fetuses with FGR. If growth parameters of the fetus are normal and umbilical artery waveform is normal, then no other Doppler studies are required.

Stage of Hypoxemia

There is fetal hypoxemia, with fetal partial pressure of oxygen (PO_2) 18–19 mm Hg and pH 7.20–7.25.

As primary compensatory mechanism to hypoxemia, there is reopening of the ductus venosus (DV) to divert blood from liver and increase in the MCA flow in the distal segment for better peripheral cerebral circulation.

Leading to decreased MCA PI in sector 2, the distal segment of MCA as compared to the proximal segment of MCA, M1/M2 >1 **(Fig. 12)** and increased velocity and low resistance in DV.

Reduction in circulatory oxygen level is sensed by peripheral chemoreceptors and leads to vagal stimulation of heart with preferential shift of cardiac circulation towards left ventricle (LV) leading to increased umbilical artery resistance and lower resistance MCA flow. But aortic and carotid chemoreceptors are mostly not affected.

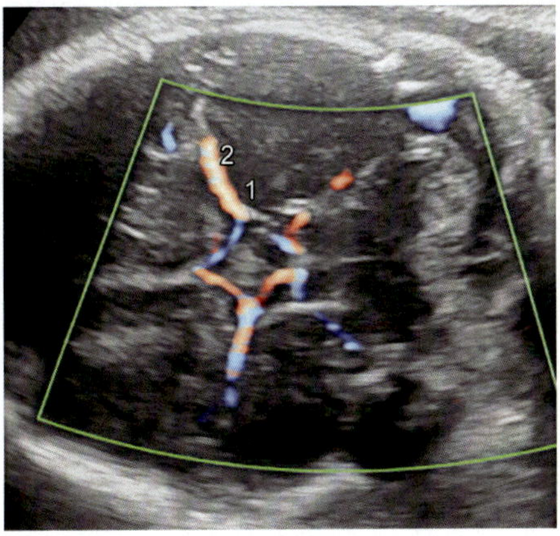

Fig. 12: HD flow image showing circle of Willis and location of MCA 1 and MCA 2 flow assessments to be done.

Mild increase in umbilical artery PI is the cause of hypoxemia, whereas lower resistance in MCA flow is the indication of the adaptation to hypoxemia. *The second phase is the phase of hypoxia*, which can be divided into:

- Initial phase
- Advanced phase
- Terminal phase

Initial Phase

Vascular changes during this period are:

- There is rise in umbilical artery PI but still positive flow is seen throughout the cardiac cycle in the umbilical artery **(Fig. 13A)**. Due to fall in resistance in the cerebral circulation, presence of end-diastolic flow in is seen at 32–34 weeks along with low MCA PI **(Fig. 13B)**. MCA PI/umbilical artery PI ratio [cerebroplacental ratio (CPR)] is the best indicator for fetal hypoxia. Prediction of the adverse outcome is improved using umbilical and cerebral parameters in combined ratio which is 70%. CPR is the single most sensitive parameter for assessment of the IUGR and has a single cut off value of one.[30]
- Biophysical profile may be unaltered at this stage and the biophysical score is usually less than 7. This phase lasts for 9–60 days, but its length is usually about 2–3 weeks.

Other progressive changes that occur during this period are:

- Reduced fetal respiratory and somatic movements
- Reduced AFI (5–8 cm)
- Raised aortic PI
- Raised renal artery PI

But these vessels are not routinely interrogated.

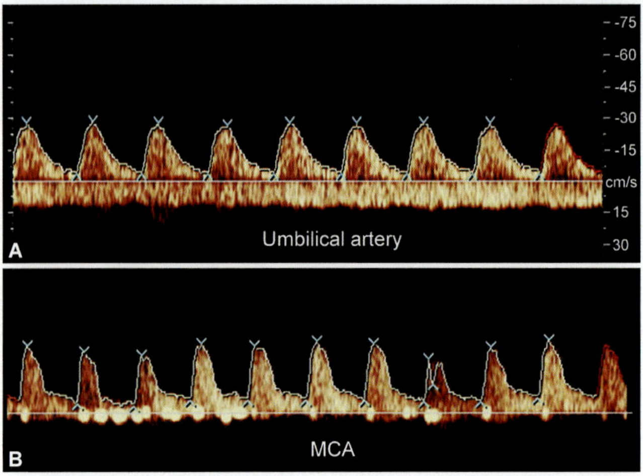

Figs. 13A and B: Doppler findings in initial phase of centralization. (A) Increasing umbilical artery resistance; (B) Minimal fall in middle cerebral artery (MCA) resistance.

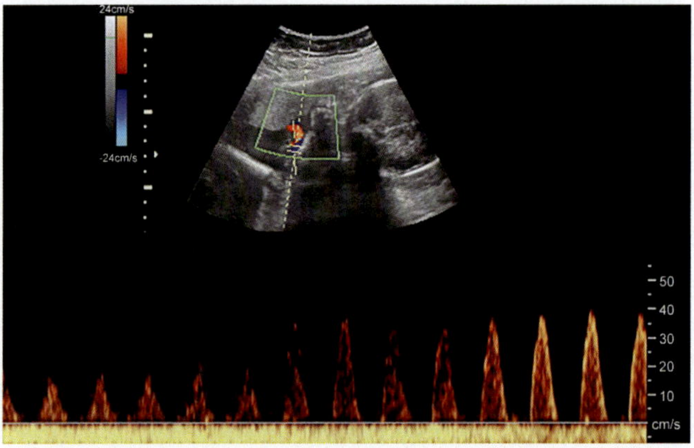

Fig. 14: Absent end-diastolic flow in umbilical artery.

Advanced Phase

When the placental villous circulation is compromised to about 80%, this is an advanced stage of fetal hypoxia. The vascular changes observed on Doppler at this stage are:

- Absent end-diastolic flow in umbilical artery **(Fig. 14)**. But it is to be remembered that, although umbilical artery waveform is a good reflector of placental resistance, it does not give any information as to fetus is coping up with the compromised blood supply or not.
- Absent end-diastolic flow in aorta is seen and this leads to significantly decreased circulation to the abdominal organs thus leading to high risk

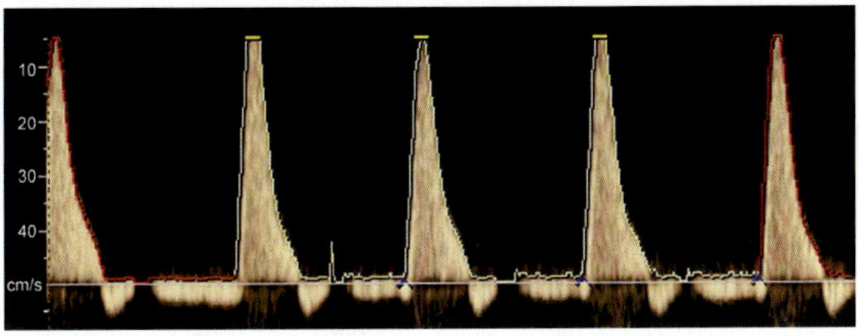

Fig. 15: Absent aortic end-diastolic flow.

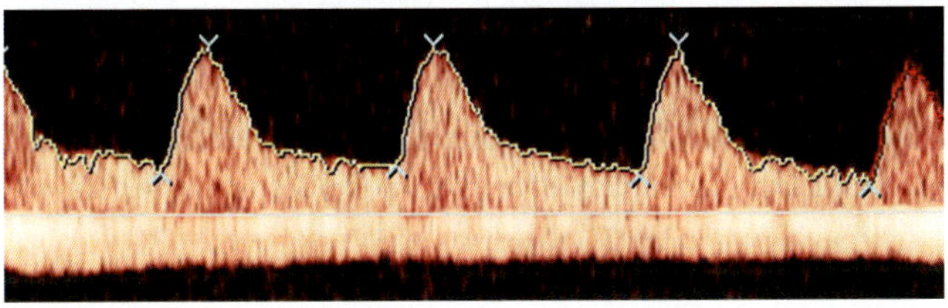

Fig. 16: *Low middle cerebral artery resistance:* Advance stage of centralization (hypoxia).

of necrotizing enterocolitis. Thus increasing the risk of morbidity and mortality **(Fig. 15)**.

- Low MCA PI values **(Fig. 16)** are seen as compensation to cerebral hypoxia by cerebral vasodilatation. But it must be kept in mind that prolonged cerebral vasodilatation and low MCA PI cannot be taken as a compensatory mechanism, as in the second phase of vasodilatation deoxygenated blood floods the brain and could lead to cerebral edema. There is also a higher risk of intracranial hemorrhages in the neonatal life in these cases. Fetus will also show loss of reactivity at this stage due to cerebral hypoxia.

Terminal Phase

This is a phase of acidosis. Doppler shows reversed end-diastolic flow in umbilical artery and aorta **(Fig. 17)**. MCA resistance may start rising due to cerebral edema. Severe hypoxia in the myocardium leads to failing of cardiac muscle and therefore marked reduction in ventricular ejection fraction. This leads to marked reduction in intracardiac flow velocities. To compensate for myocardial hypoxia there is dilatation of the coronary vessels, to the extent that sometimes blood flows in the coronaries may be documented. The dysfunction of the myocardium leads to decreased ventricular compliance, therefore incomplete emptying of the atrium and increasing preload reflecting as reversed flow or decreased telediastolic velocity values **(Fig. 18A)** in DV. But this stage precedes the stage when there is increase in the ductus venous PI **(Fig. 18B)**. Inferior vena cava (IVC) normally also shows negative flow during atrial contraction up to 10% but rises to up to 30% in terminal phase

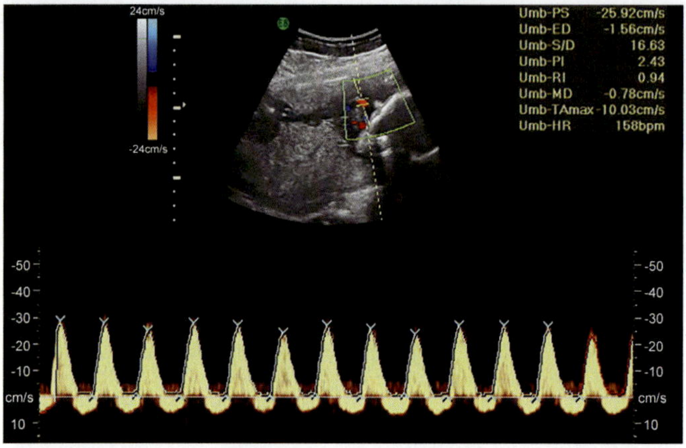

Fig. 17: Reversed end-diastolic flow of umbilical artery seen on pulsed wave Doppler.

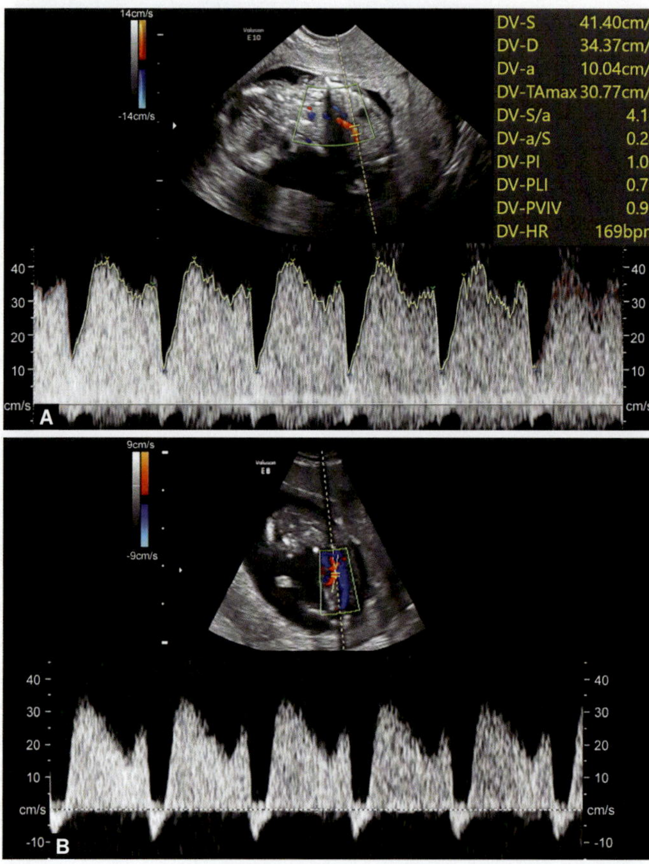

Figs. 18A and B: (A) Normal ductus venosus flow on pulsed wave Doppler; (B) Reversed A wave flow in ductus venosus (abnormal).

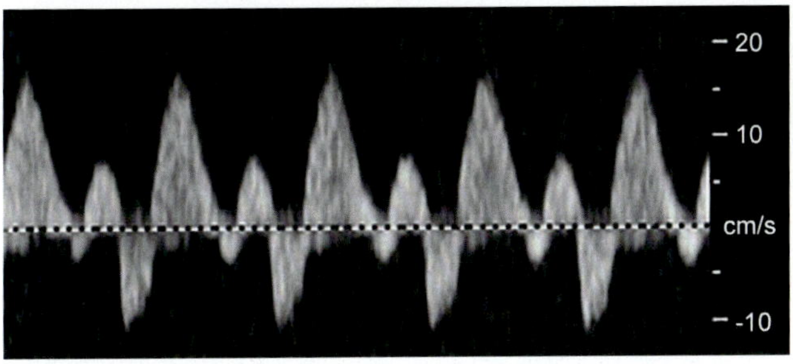

Fig. 19: Normal fetal IVC flow as seen on pulsed wave Doppler.

of centralization **(Fig. 19)**. Umbilical vein flow may also show pulsatility. Venous Doppler reflects the physiological status of right ventricle (RV) giving specific information regarding the ventricular preload, myocardial compliance, and right ventricular end-diastolic pressure.

These findings with reversed flow in hepatic vein and deceleration in heart rate are indicators of acidosis. Fetal acidemia reliably presents as very short-term and low value variations in fetal heart rate (FHR), and precedes intrauterine fetal death.

In about 90% of cases, DV flow also becomes abnormal only 48–72 hours before abnormal BPP.[31]

Longitudinal studies have demonstrated that AFI and FHR are the only two parameters that may change a little earlier in fetal compromise.

Abnormal DV flow may be seen as **(Figs. 20A to C)**:

- Deep "A" nadir (atrial contraction)
- Reduced second peak (diastole)
- Reduced diastolic flow
- Reversed diastolic flow
- PI 0.5 is normal, > 0.9 is very bad

Progressively increasing umbilical artery PI leads to impaired fetal cardiac performance, increased central venous pressure, and reduced diastolic flow in DV. Vasodilatation of DV diverts flow to the heart, further increasing the arterial pressure and leads to further decrease in DV flow during atrial contraction.

Aortic Isthmus Flow

Aortic isthmus is the part of aorta, just beyond the origin of brachiocephalic trunk **(Fig. 21A)**. The flow in this part of the aorta is usually a continuous positive flow with high velocity. Aortic isthmus flow represents the balance between right and left ventricular outputs. *In systolic phase, forward flow indicates LV output and reverse flow indicates RV output. Whereas in diastole,*

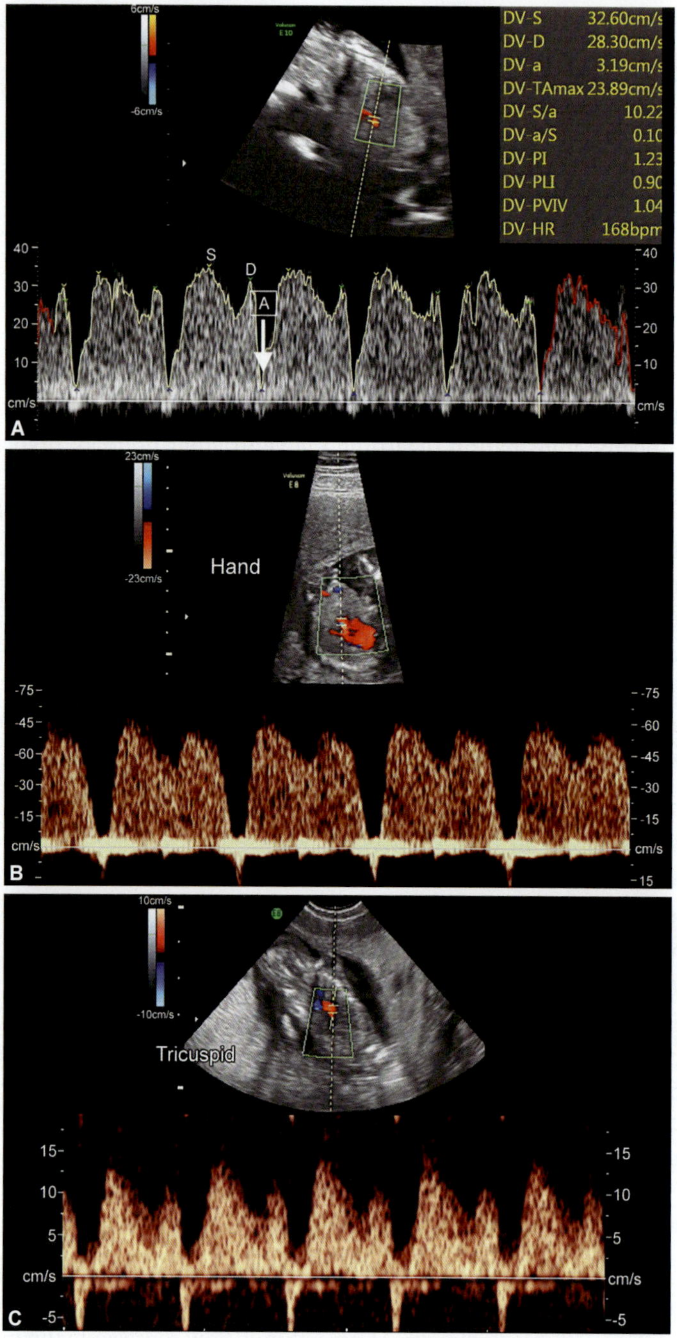

Figs. 20A to C: (A) Normal ductus venosus flow on pulsed wave Doppler; (B) Increased resistance (PI) due to deep A wave of ductus venosus; (C) Reversed A wave flow in ductus venosus (abnormal).

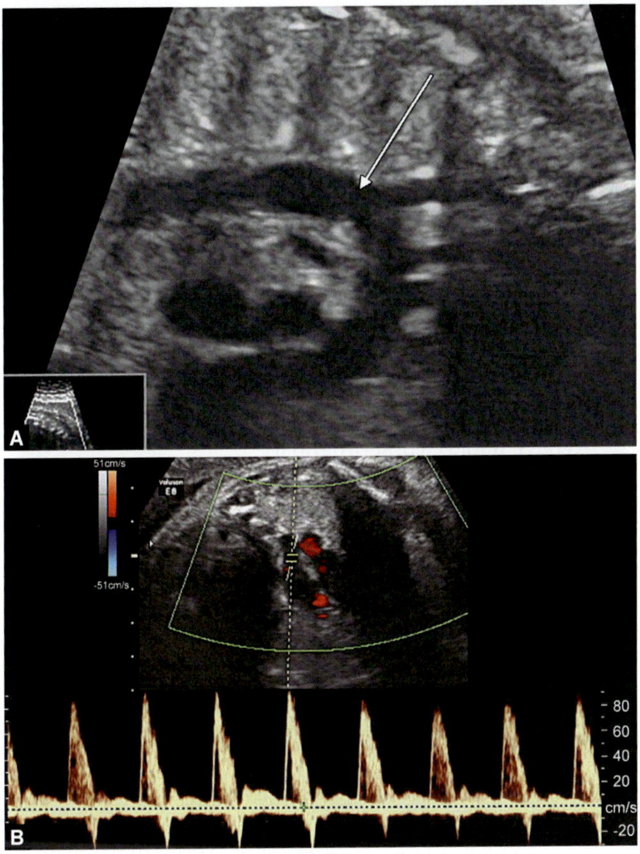

Figs. 21A and B: (A) Aortic isthmus on B-mode; (B) Aortic isthmic flow on spectral Doppler.

forward flow indicates upper body resistance and reverse flow indicates lower body resistance. Retrograde flow in the aortic isthmus represents increased right ventricular afterload and decreased left ventricular afterload. Though a small flow reversal in early diastole is normal in third trimester. Normal peak velocities in aortic isthmus is 30–100 cm/s from 11 weeks to term as compared to ductus arteriosus that is 40–120 cm/s. Low velocities and high resistance in aortic isthmic flow are seen in IUGR fetuses. Abnormality of this flow occurs about a week before the changes of hypoxia are seen in DV.[32]

Abnormal DV flow indicates high morbidity and mortality of the fetus. And therefore if delivery of the fetus is done after DV flow becomes abnormal the chances of fetal survival are very low. But, if the delivery of the fetus can be done before this stage, fetal survival and chances of its well-being can be improved significantly. Abnormal aortic isthmic flow impedance is an intermediate step between placental insufficiency-hypoxemia and cardiac decompensation. Retrograde flow in the aortic isthmus in growth restricted fetuses correlated strongly with adverse perinatal outcome.[33] Reversed diastolic flow in aortic isthmus clearly indicates poor neurological outcome. Abnormal aortic isthmus flow is a better marker than abnormal DV flow for predicting bad perinatal outcome, whereas abnormal DV flow is a better marker for predicting fetal mortality.

The aortic isthmic flow can be quantitatively rated by the isthmic flow index as follows:

- *Type 1:* IFI < 1: Antegrade systolic and diastolic flow
- *Type 2:* IFI = 1: Absent diastolic flow
- *Type 3:* IFI = 0–1: Predominant systolic but some reversed diastolic flow
- *Type 4:* IFI = 0: Some antegrade and some retrograde flow
- *Type 5:* IFI >1: Chiefly retrograde flow
- IFI type 3–5 have bad to worst prognosis

Applying this Knowledge for the Assessment of Fetal Well-being

These tests could be classified as chronic or acute. Chronic tests progressively become abnormal due to increasing hypoxemia and/or hypoxia. Whereas acute tests correlate with the acute changes occurring in advanced stages of fetal compromise due to severe hypoxia and metabolic acidosis.

Umbilical Artery

It is known that with the functional damage in the placental villi the umbilical artery resistance increases. But the placental histological changes cannot always be correlated with the severity of increased resistance in the umbilical artery. Though when the umbilical artery shows a reverse end-diastolic flow, it is considered that there is a severe placental damage and there is an increased risk of perinatal death. And this has a sensitivity and specificity of about 60%.[34]

Studies have shown that 80% of the fetuses have abnormal umbilical artery flow, 2 weeks before acute deterioration of fetal condition, and therefore this may be considered a chronic marker for fetal non-well-being. The same study has also shown that up to 1 week before fetal death the umbilical artery diastolic flow may be present.[35] Absent or reversed end-diastolic flow in the umbilical artery respectively has a relative risk of 4 and 10.6 for prediction of fetal morbidity and mortality and is also associated with long-term abnormal neurodevelopment.[36] A multicentric randomized trial on Growth Restriction Intervention Trial (GRIT) has concluded that early delivery for fetuses with reversed end-diastolic flow does not improve the outcome and 24–48 hours of interval after corticosteroids injection for lung maturation and then delivery should be planned.[37]

OBSTETRIC MANAGEMENT DEPENDING ON DOPPLER FINDINGS

Middle Cerebral Artery

In deteriorating FGR, MCA PI progressively becomes abnormal.[38] Up to 80% of fetuses have vasodilatation 2 weeks before acute deterioration in one study[35] and <50% in other.[37]

Moreover the paradoxical reversal of the MCA flow that is explained to be due to terminal cerebral edema has also not been documented in few other studies.[38] In near-term SGA fetuses, MCA could be useful to predict adverse outcome, independently of umbilical artery Doppler. But its value in overall SGA population is not proved in another study.[39]

Some studies have also shown that MCA vasodilatation may be a protective mechanism against hypoxia, but is associated with suboptimal neurological development.[40] And in one study its association is also shown with impaired visual function and visual motor capabilities at 11 years.[41] Brain sparing effect can also be considered a chronic marker of IUGR.

Ductus Venosus

Acidemia, acidosis, and abnormal venous Doppler are acute markers. Increasing PI in the DV may occur early but reversal of A wave represents the terminal changes. In preterm fetuses, a 3 SD cut-off optimize the sensitivity and specificity.[42] With absent or reversed A wave, perinatal mortality ranges from 60 to 100%.[42]

However its sensitivity for perinatal death is 40–70%. Abnormal venous flow may be DV or inferior vena cava or hepatic vein identifies about 90% of newborns with acidosis.[43] But in about 90% of cases, a DV flow shows reverse A wave only 48–72 hours before the BPP shows changes.[31]

Heart rate deceleration or loss of variability in heart rate is not a reliable guide to predict perinatal morbidity or mortality according to one study,[31] but other longitudinal studies have proved its potential role as acute marker.[38]

Intrauterine growth restriction can be divided into two types depending on the time of initiation of the manifestations. In some patients FGR sets in as early as 26–28 weeks of pregnancy and this is known as early-onset FGR, whereas when FGR sets in at about 32–33 weeks, it is late-onset FGR. It is important to differentiate between the two because the behavior of the fetus and deterioration pattern in the two situations is different. In the early-onset FGR, the fetal adaptation is better and in spite of redistribution of circulation, or marked circulatory changes, the fetus does survive the situation. But in late-onset IUGR the fetus does not get sufficient time to get adapted to the circulatory derangements and therefore the fetal deterioration is fast. In the early-onset FGR cases therefore one can wait even with absent umbilical artery diastolic flow and also at times till DV flow becomes abnormal. Because of fast deterioration in the late-onset cases, the entire cascade of vascular

Table 1: Management strategies for early- and late-onset intrauterine growth restriction (IUGR).[44,45]

Early-onset IUGR	***Late-onset IUGR***
Problem: Management	*Problem:* Diagnosis
Severe placental disease (abnormal umbilical artery, associated with preeclampsia)	Mild placental disease (normal umbilical artery Doppler, less associated with preeclampsia)
Hypoxia-systemic cardiovascular adaptation	Hypoxia may or may not be there, cardiovascular adaptation is central
Better fetal tolerance and adaptation to hypoxia	Lower fetal tolerance to hypoxia and poor adaptation
High morbidity and mortality; lower prevalence	Low mortality (but common cause of late stillbirth)

changes may not be followed and may result into unexplained fetal death. Unfortunately 70–80% of FGR fetuses are late-onset FGR.

The management strategies therefore in both the situations have to be different **(Table 1)**.

When and how often should these patients be monitored by Doppler?

It is very important to understand that a single Doppler assessment cannot be relied upon for decision making on the fetal oxygenation as well as obstetric management. One has to observe the trend of the vascular resistance in MCA and umbilical artery. Therefore a baseline Doppler at about 30–32 weeks will be helpful to serve as a guide for further Doppler changes in FGR fetuses. The follow-up would depend on GA at the onset of disease, severity of vascular changes at the primary examination, and presence of deterioration on subsequent assessment. The deterioration may be in the form of discrepancy in growth, reducing amount of liquor, abnormal nonstress test (NST), or worsening of Doppler parameters. The monitoring intervals may also vary depending on whether it is an early-onset FGR or a late-onset FGR.

For example, in an early-onset FGR even with umbilical showing absent end-diastolic flow, once a weekly Doppler follow-up may be maintained till the MCA flow and in turn the DV flow becomes abnormal, or fetus reaches 34 weeks or more of gestation or even with reversed end-diastolic flow in umbilical artery and DV PI > 95th centile, time can be bought to give steroids and plan a delivery. Whereas in late-onset FGR, even with umbilical artery PI > 95th centile or MCA PI < 5th centile, monitoring may be required much more often and any new development in Doppler finding is considered an emergency and especially when the fetus has already reached 34 weeks, no unnecessary delay in delivery is advisable. In short, in early-onset IUGR, the sequential changes that take about 7–10 days, in late-onset IUGR the same changes may occur in 7–24 hours.

- *IUGR with normal hemodynamic profile:* No immediate action and repeat Doppler and BPP every 2 weeks.
- *IUGR with hemodynamic redistribution 32–34 weeks:* Early stage of centralization, Doppler and BPP monitoring. With late stage of centralization and termination of pregnancy.
- If IUGR with hemodynamic redistribution is seen between 28 and 32 weeks, termination of pregnancy with advanced and terminal stages of centralization but expectant management with early stage of centralization with Doppler and BPP monitoring every 5 days.
- Same is true for the GA of <28 weeks. All chances are taken to allow the pregnancy to reach 30 weeks.

It was believed that as long as the fetal growth and the umbilical artery indices are normal, no further hemodynamic study is required. Though there are situations in which in spite of normal umbilical artery flow the fetal circulation is affected and reflects as abnormal MCA flow. This is especially common, when the causes for fetal hypoxia are nonplacental. Therefore, as a rule in all high risk cases for fetal hypoxia, MCA flow must be assessed with umbilical artery flow. Doppler findings must be evaluated in conjunction with GA fetal weight, liquor, BPP, fetal activity, and CTG. *Delivery must be considered if one of these parameters is persistently abnormal.*[38]

Role of Biophysical Profile

When used alone it has 50% false positive rate and so has a limited value clinically.[46] A meta-analysis has also not shown its significant benefit in high risk pregnancies. But both Doppler and BPP effectively stratifies IUGR into risk categories.[47]

Advances

The myocardial performance index (MPI) is a novel method in fetal medicine that assesses both systolic and diastolic functions by including the measurement of isovolumetrix and ejection times and would be useful in assessing the progressive hemodynamic deterioration. It has been reported to be associated with perinatal mortality in very preterm IUGR fetuses.[45]

It is essential to know that the abnormal Doppler findings correlate well with the onset of abnormal heart rate patterns. Fetal hypoxemia is always reflected by reduced heart rate variation and heart rate decelerations.[13] Fetal acidemia reliably presents as very short-term and low value variations in FHR, and precedes intrauterine death which corresponds with the increased DV PI, especially before 32 weeks and indicates more acute changes in the degree of abnormality. Delivery must be considered if one of these parameters is persistently abnormal.[38]

SUMMARY

Doppler is an important modality for predicting IUGR. It has an important role in deciding the progress and prognosis of the fetuses having IUGR and thus has an important role in taking management decisions. For long-term monitoring it is better than CTG. It warns for the potential of intrauterine oxygen deprivation. Though it is important to understand that definite cut-offs that may accurately predict the outcome of the patient is still not available. Association of abnormal intrafetal Doppler study and poor fetal outcome does not equate to cause. Our Doppler fetal tests do not measure the potential for damage. Damage to fetus may occur without gross alterations in hemodynamics.

REFERENCES

1. Alexander GR, Kogan MD, Hims JH, Mor JM, Goldenberg R. Racial differences in birth weight for gestational age and infant mortality in extremely low-risk US populations. Pediatr Perinat Epidemiol. 1999;13(2):129-43.
2. Spencer JA, Chang TC, Crook D, Proudler A, Felton CV, Robson SC, et al. Third trimester fetal growth and measures of carbohydrate and lipid metabolism in umbilical venous blood at term. Arch Dis Child Fetal Neonatal Ed. 1997;76(1):F21-5.
3. Wilcox AJ. Intrauterine growth retardation: beyond birth weight criteria. Early Hum Dev. 1983;8(3-4):189-93.
4. Spinillo A, Capuzzo E, Piazzi G, Baltaro F, Stratanati M, Ometto A. Significance of low birth weight for gestational age among very preterm infant. Br J Obstet Gynecol. 1997;104:668-73.
5. Altman DG, Chitty LS. New charts for ultrasound dating of pregnancy. Ultrasound Obstet Gynecol. 1997;10(3):174-91.
6. Stebbins B, Jaffe R. Fetal biometry and gestational age estimation. In: Jaffe R, Bui TH (Eds). Textbook of Fetal Ultrasound. New York: Parthenon Publishing; 1999. pp. 47-57.
7. Mongelli M, Ek S, Tambirajya R. Screening for fetal growth restriction: a mathematical model of the effect of time interval and ultrasound error. Obstet Gynecol. 1998;92(6):908-12.
8. Honemeyer U, Kurjak A, Monni G. Normal and abnormal early pregnancy. Donald School Textbook of Ultrasound in Obstetrics and Gynecology, 3rd edition. New Delhi: Jaypee Brothers Medical Publishers; 2011.
9. Chang TC, Robson SC, Boys RJ, Spencer JA. Prediction of the small for gestational age infant: Which ultrasonic measurement is best? Obstet Gynecol. 1992;80(6):1030-8.
10. Hadlock FP, Harrist RB, Sharman RS, Deter RL, Park SK. Estimation of fetal weight with the use of head, body and femur measurements: a prospective study. Am J Obstet Gynecol. 1985;151(3):333-7.
11. Campbell S, Dewhurst CJ. Diagnosis of small for dates fetus by serial ultrasonic cephalometry. Lancet. 1971;2:1002-15.
12. Levi S, Flamme P. Rlation entre divers parameters foeto-maternels et le diameter biparietal mesure par les ultrasons. Bruxelles: Fonds National de la recherche Scient. Med. Group de pernatologie; 1970. pp. 324-5.
13. Warsof SL, Cooper DJ, Little D, Campbell S. Routine ultrasound screening for antenatal detection of intrauterine growth retardation. Obstet Gynaecol. 1986;67:33-9.

14. Carrera JM, Devesa R, Serra B. Classification of intrauterine growth restriction. In: Kurjak A (Ed). Textbook of Perinatal Medicine. London: Parthenon Publishing; 1998. pp. 1192-200.
15. Benson CB, Doubilet PM, Saltzman DH, Jones TB. FL/AC ratio: poor predictor of intrauterine growth retardation. Invest Radiol. 1985;20:727-30.
16. Pilalis A, Souka AP, Antsaklis P, Daskalakis G, Papantoniou N, Mesogitis S, et al. Screening for pre-eclampsia and fetal growth restriction by uterine artery Doppler and PAPP-A at 11-14 weeks' gestation. Ultrasound Obstet Gynecol. 2007;29(2):135-40.
17. Fox NS, Shalom D, Chasen ST. Second-trimester fetal growth as a predictor of poor obstetric and neonatal outcome in patients with low first-trimester serum pregnancy-associated plasma protein-A and a euploid fetus. Ultrasound Obstet Gynecol. 2009;33:34-38.
18. Crispi F, Llurba E, Dominguez C, Martín-Gallán P, L Cabero, Gratacós E. Predictive value of angiogenic factors and uterine artery Doppler for early-versus late onset preeclampsia and uterine artery growth restriction. Ultrasound Obstet Gynecol. 2008;31:303-9.
19. Khalil A, Cowans NJ, Spencer K, Goichmans S, Meiri H, Hrrington K. First trimester markers for the prediction of pre-eclampsia in women with a-priori high risk. Ultrasound Obstet Gynecol. 2010;35:671:9.
20. Giguère Y, Charland M, Bujold E, Bernard N, Grenier S, Rousseau F, et al. Combining Biochemical and Ultrasonographic Markers in Predicting Preeclampsia: a Systematic Review. Clin Chem. 2010;56(3):361-75.
21. Proctor LK, Toal M, Keating S, Chitayat D, Okun N, Windrim RC, et al. Placental size and the prediction of severe early-onset intrauterine growth restriction in women with low pregnancy-associated plasma protein-A. Ultrasound Obstet Gynecol. 2009;34:274-82.
22. Papageorghiou AT, Yu CK, Bindra R, Pandis G, Nicolaides KH. Fetal Medicine Foundation Second Trimester Screening Group. Multicenter screening for preeclampsia and fetal growth restriction by transvaginal uterine artery Doppler at 23 weeks of gestation. Ultrasound Obstet Gynecol. 2001;18(5):441-9.
23. Chien PF, Arnott N, Gordon A, Owen P, Khan KS. How useful is uterine artery Doppler flow velocimetry in the prediction of pre-eclampsia, intrauterine growth retardation and perinatal death? An overview. BJOG. 2000;107(2):196-208.
24. Wherry KL, Dubinsky TJ, Waitches GM, Richardson ML, Reed S. Low resistance endometrial arterial flow in the exclusion of ectopic pregnancy revisited. J Ultrasound Med. 2001;20:335-42.
25. Nicolaides KH, Bilardo CM, Soothill PW, Campbell S. Absence end diastolic frequencies in umbilical artery: a sign of fetal hypoxia and acidosis. BMJ. 1988;297(6655):1026-7.
26. MoCowan LM, Harding JE, Stewart AW. Customized birth weight centiles predict SGA pregnancies with perinatal morbidity. BJOG. 2005;112(8):1026-33.
27. MoCowan LM, Harding JE, Stewart AW. Umbilical artery Doppler studies in small for gestational age babies reflect disease severity. BJOG. 2000;107(7):916-25.
28. Trudinger BJ, Cook CM, Giles WB, Ng S, Fong E, Connelly A, et al. Fetal umbilical artery velocity waveforms and subsequent neonatal outcome. Br J Obstet Gynecol. 1991;98(4):378-84.
29. Society for Maternal Fetal Medicine Publications Committee, Berkley E, Chauhan SP, Abuahmad A. Doppler assesment of the fetus with intrauterine growth restriction. AJOG. 2012;206:300-8.
30. Odibo AO, Riddick C, Pare E, Stamilio DM, Macones GA. Cerebroplacental Doppler ratio and adverse perinatal outcomes in intrauterine growth restriction: evaluating the impact of using gestational age-specific reference values. J Ultrasound Med. 2005;24(9):1223-8.

31. Baschat AA, Gembruch U, Harman CR. The sequence of changes in Doppler and biophysical parameters as severe fetal growth restriction worsens. Ultrasound Obstet Gynecol. 2001;18(6):571-7.
32. Figueras F, Benavides A, Del Rio M, Crispi F, Eixarch E, Martinez JM, et al. Monitoring of fetuses with intrauterine growth restriction: longitudinal changes in ductus venosus and aortic isthmus flow. Ultrasound Obstet Gyneol. 2009;33(1):39-43.
33. Del Rio M, Martinez JM, Figueras F, et al. Doppler assessment of the aortic isthmus and perinatal outcome in prenatal fetuses with severe intrauterine growth restriction. Ultrasound Obstet Gynecol. 2008;31(1):41-7.
34. Sebire NJ. Umbilical artery Doppler revisited: pathophysiology of changes of intrauterine growth restriction revealed. Ultrasound Obstet Gynecol. 2003;21(5):419-22.
35. Ferrazzi E, Bozzo M, Rigano S, Bellotti M, Morabito A, Pardi G, et al. Temporal sequence of abnormal Doppler changes in the peripheral and central circulatory systems of severely growth-restricted fetus. Ultrasound Obstet Gynecol. 2002;19(2):140-6.
36. Cosmi E, Ambrosini G, D'Antona D, Saccardi C, Mari G. Doppler cardiotocography and biophysical profile changes in growth-restricted fetuses. Obstet Gynecol. 2005;106(6):1240-5.
37. Thornton JG, Hornbuckle J, Vail A, Spiegelhalter DJ, Levene M, GRIT study group. Infant wellbeing at 2 years of age in growth restriction intervention trial (GRIT): Multicentred randomized controlled trial. Lancet. 2004;18(6):571-7.
38. Hecher K, Bilardo CM, Stigter RH, Ville Y, Hackelöer BJ, Kok HJ, et al. Monitoring of fetuses with intrauterine growth restriction: a longitudinal study. Ultrasound Obstet Gynecol. 2001;18(6):564-70.
39. To WW, Chan Am, Mok KM. Use of umbilical-cerebral Doppler ratios in predicting fetal growth restriction in near-term fetuses. Aust NJ Obstet Gynecol. 2005;45(2):130-6.
40. Scherjon S, Briet J, Oosting H, Kok J. The discrepancy between maturation of visual evoked potentials and cognitive outcome at five years in very preterm infants with and without hemodynamic signs of fetal brain-sparing. Pediatrics. 2000;105(2):385-91.
41. Kok JH, Prick L, Merckel E, Everhard Y, Verkerk GJQ, Scherjon SA. Visual function at 11 years of age in preterm-born children with and without fetal brain sparing. Pediatrics. 2007;119(6):e1342-50.
42. Bilardo CM, Wolf H, Stigter RH, Ville Y, Baez E, Visser GHA. Relationship between monitoring parameters and perinatal outcome in severe, early intrauterine growth restriction. Ultrasound Obstet Gynecol. 2004;23(2):119-25.
43. Baschat AA, Cosmi E, Bilardo CM, Wolf H, Berg C, Rigano S, et al. Predictors of neonatal outcome in early-onset placental dysfunction. Obstet Gynecol. 2007;109(2 Pt 1):253-61.
44. Muresan D, Rotar IC, Stamatian F. The usefulness of fetal Doppler evaluation in early versus late onset intrauterine growth restriction. Review of literature. Med Ultrason. 2016;18(1):103-9.
45. Miller DA, Rabello YA, Paul RH. The modified biophysical profile: antepartum testing in the 1990s. Am J Obstet Gynecol. 1996;174(3):812-7.
46. Baschat AA, Galan HL, Bhide A, Berg C, Kush ML, Oepkes D, et al. Doppler and biophysical assessment in growth restricted fetuses: distribution of test results. Ultrasound Obstet Gynecol. 2006;27(1):41-7.
47. Hernandez-Andrade E, Crispi F, Benavides-Serralde A, Plasencia W, Diesel HF, Eixarch E, et al. Contribution of the modified myocardial performance index and aortic isthmus blood flow index to refine prediction of mortality in preterm intrauterine growth restricted fetuses. Ultrasound Obstet Gynecol. 2009;34(4):430-6.

CHAPTER 23

Ultrasonography in Male Infertility

Sonal Panchal

INTRODUCTION

Male factor is the primary cause of infertility in 20–30% of couples and a contributing factor in other 20–25%. The male reproductive system consists of testes, epididymis, vas deferens, ejaculatory ducts, and accessory glands such as prostate, seminal vesicles, bulbourethral glands, and penis. The disorders that cause male infertility interfere with either production or transport of the normal sperms.

There are many possible etiologies for male infertility. It may be defective sperm production, storage and maturation, transport, secretions of accessory organs, and delivery.

- *Defective production*: Testicular dysfunction—abnormal number/ abnormal function
- *Defective transport*: Obstruction in epididymis, vas deferens or ejaculatory ducts
- *Defective secretions*: Disease of prostate or seminal vesicles
- *Defective delivery*: Stricture urethra

Apart from these structural causes, there may also be endocrine, genetic or immunological factors also and a retrograde ejaculation also in some. A physical cause can be identified in one-third of these patients[1] and it is idiopathic in the rest. A systematic, logical, and thorough evaluation of the infertile male patients is therefore mandatory. It helps to distinguish patients with surgically correctable from uncorrectable abnormalities.

Ultrasound (US) is safe and effective method of demonstrating and differentiating these abnormalities. Scrotum and penis can be studied well by a small part US probe, while transrectal sonography may be required to study the distal male reproductive system that helps to identify patients appropriate for surgical or radiological intervention. Penile US helps to evaluate erectile disorders.

SCROTAL ULTRASOUND

Scrotal ultrasound is done with high frequency (7–12 MHz) linear probe. Wider footprint is better so that the entire testis is seen in a single image. It is always preceded by a detailed abdominal scan. Scrotum is supported by a towel between the two thighs and penis is retracted over the abdomen and also covered with towel. Each testis and epididymis should be examined separately in longitudinal and transverse planes. Study is done using grayscale, color, and spectral Doppler techniques.

Normal Appearances on Ultrasound: Grayscale

Testis is homogeneous intermediately echogenic ovoid organ, measuring 5 × 3 × 2 cm **(Fig. 1A)**. One testis lies on each side of the central fibromuscular septum of the scrotum. Each testis is assessed in longitudinal and transverse sections. Three orthogonal diameters are taken—longitudinal, transverse, and anteroposterior (AP) on two orthogonal planes. Volume is calculated as length × width × height × 0.523. Normal volume of each testis is 12–15 mL.[2]

The size of the testis gradually decreases with increasing age. It shows an echogenic vertical line—the mediastinum testis, which is seen only after puberty. The rete testis at the mediastinum testis is sometimes seen as a hypoechoic area in the posterosuperior aspect of the testis in transverse section. Epididymis is isoechoic or slightly hyperechoic to testis and is seen on the lateral aspect of the testis, extending to the cephalic end of the testis and widening there to make the head of the epididymis (10–12 mm in diameter). The part on the lateral aspect is the body of the epididymis, which tapers close to the caudal end of the testis and is called tail of epididymis. Spermatic cord is seen as a predominantly echogenic heterogeneous structure arising near the head of the epididymis.

On color Doppler study, fine vessels coursing through the normal testis is seen and normal intratesticular flow is symmetrical on both sides **(Fig. 1B)**. Normally, there is very minimal flow or no flow in the epididymis testicular artery and intratesticular arteries usually show a moderate resistance flow with resistance index (RI) of 0.64 (±0.14).

VARICOCELE

Varicocele is a pathological dilatation of veins of the pampiniform plexus in the spermatic cord.[3] Varicoceles develop from a reversal of blood flow within the internal spermatic and cremasteric veins.[4] Because of anatomical reasons; varicocele is more common on left side. This is because right testicular vein drains directly into inferior vena cava (IVC) and drains into the left renal vein at right angle and so there is more hydrostatic pressure in the veins of left testis. This may also be due to compression of the renal vein between aorta and superior mesenteric artery.[5] Approximately 15% of all men in the general population have a clinical varicocele. In contrast, between 19% and 41% of men evaluated for infertility are found to have varicoceles.[5] It is more common in men with secondary infertility and may reach almost up to 70%.[6]

Solitary right-sided varicocele may be due to aging, retroperitoneal mass, hepatic enlargement or hydronephrosis. Approximately 50% of men with

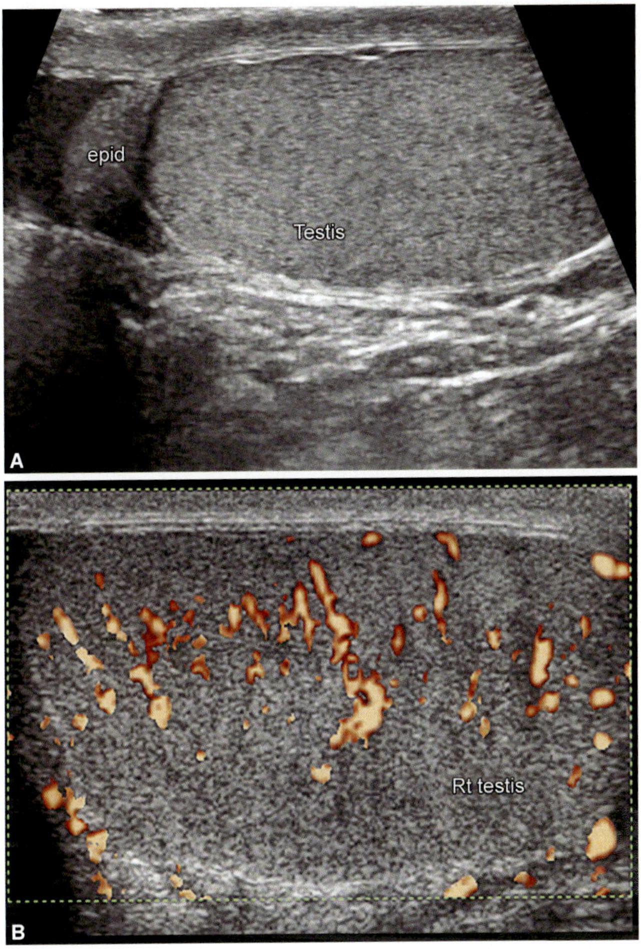

Figs. 1A and B: (A) B-mode image of normal testis and epididymis; (B) Power Doppler image showing normal testicular vascularity.

varicocele show improvement in seminal parameters after surgery. Therefore varicocele must be operated only if it is grade II or more and only if sperm count and motility are variable.

Theories Why Varicocele is Responsible for Male Infertility[7-9]

- Increased testicular temperature due to increased venous flow leading to abnormal spermatogenesis.
- Reflux of spermatotoxic metabolites from the kidneys and adrenal along with the reflux of the venous blood.
- Hormonal cause due to alteration in the hypothalamic-pituitary-gonadal axis.

- Venous dilatation causing stagnation of the blood flow and testicular hypoxia.

Most patients are asymptomatic, but some may present with scrotal, swelling, pain, and discomfort especially after standing for long time.

Clinical examination for varicocele is done in erect position, in resting state, and with Valsalva maneuver. It is felt as a bag of worms and increase in caliber with Valsalva maneuver. Clinical diagnosis may be difficult when patient also has hydrocele, obesity, cremasteric contraction, and hernia.

Technique

The patient is examined in supine and erect positions, in resting state, and with Valsalva maneuver. Study is performed with grayscale and repeated with color and spectral Doppler. The pulse repetition frequency (PRF) is kept low since venous flow is studied but it should be high enough to avoid movement artifact due to Valsalva maneuver.

Clinical Grading[10-12]

- *Grade 1*: Palpable only during Valsalva
- *Grade 2*: Palpable without Valsalva
- *Grade 3*: Dilated veins palpable and seen on inspection

Ultrasound Findings

On B-mode, varicocele appears as multiple serpiginous, tubular vascular structures measuring over 2.5 mm in diameter, more on the superolateral aspect of testis **(Fig. 2A)**. The caliber of the vein increases with Valsalva maneuver. On color Doppler study, there is usually no flow seen in resting state. On Valsalva maneuver, there is reflux of flow in the veins. As the veins are tortuous, there may be mix of colors on Doppler **(Fig. 2B)**. On spectral Doppler, may be done to elicit the reflux.

But a more recent work has suggested to define varicocele on the basis of US findings such as extension, size and number of dilated veins, affected side, duration of retrograde flow during Valsalva maneuver, presence of spontaneous retrograde flow in the upright position, volume and echotexture of the affected testicle (in comparison to the contralateral), and demonstration of retrograde flow in the inguinal canal of the affected side.

Ultrasound Grading (Table 1)

Isidori and Lenzi[13] have proposed a revised integrated classification of varicocele that offers a comparison between the clinical (Dubin) and US classifications.

Urology on male infertility (2016) has described the following recommendations for management of varicocele:

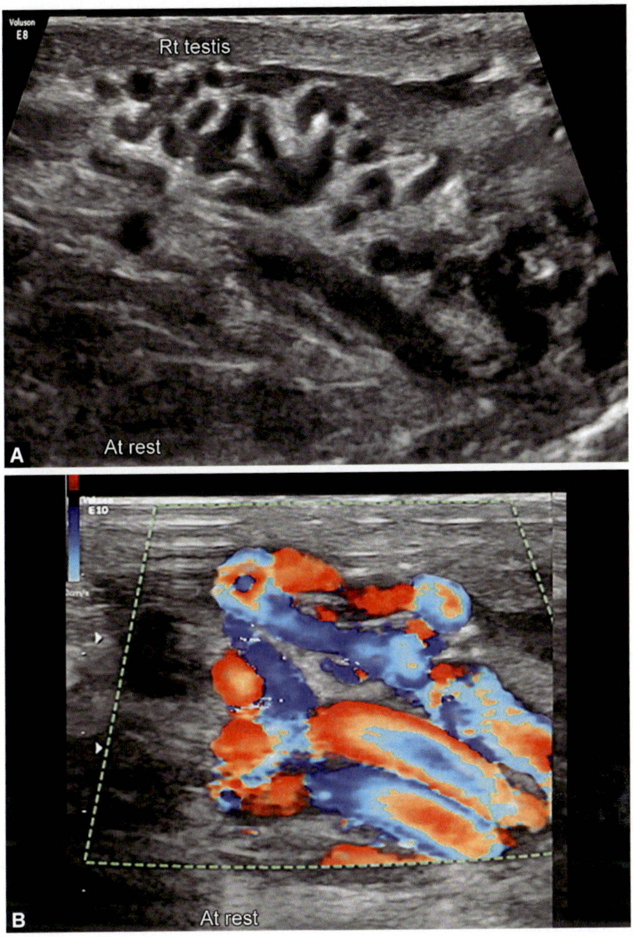

Figs. 2A and B: (A) B-mode image showing peritesticular veins of varicocele; (B) Color Doppler image of varicocele showing turbulent flow in dilated vessels.

- Treat varicoceles in adolescents with progressive failure of testicular development documented by serial clinical examination.
- Do not treat varicoceles in infertile men who have normal semen analysis and in men with a subclinical varicocele.
- Treat varicoceles in men with a clinical varicocele, oligospermia, and otherwise unexplained infertility in the couple.

COMMON TESTICULAR ABNORMALITIES

Cryptorchidism (Undescended Testis)

The testis develops intra-abdominally and moves toward the scrotum during fetal development. Normally, the descent of testis into the scrotum occurs by

Table 1: Ultrasound grading of varicocoele.

Grade	*B-mode*	*Doppler*
Grade 1	Vessels >2.5 mm in inguinal region only	Inguinal reflux for 2–3 sec on Valsalva
Grade 2	Supratesticular vessels >3 mm	Supratesticular reflux on Valsalva for >3 sec
Grade 3	Supra- and peritesticular vessel dilatation >3 mm	Reflux in these vessels on Valsalva for >3 sec **(Fig. 3A)**
Grade 4	Peritesticular vessel dilatation with further dilatation on Valsalva, testicular hypotrophy	Reflux at rest which may or may not increase during Valsalva **(Fig. 3B)**
Grade 5	Peritesticular vessel dilatation does not increase on Valsalva	Reflux that increases on Valsalva with filling of intratesticular vessels also **(Fig. 3C)**

the ninth month of gestational age or a few weeks of postnatal life. The descent may be arrested at any level along the path from the retroperitoneum to the scrotum. In undescended testis, scrotal sac is empty. Progressive germ cell damage occurs in undescended testis secondary to increased temperature at its extra scrotal location and untreated postpubertal undescended testis may be completely devoid of germ cells. In bilateral cryptorchidism, the rate of paternity is approximately 50% but unilateral condition results in little, if any, impairment of fertility.[14] Other complications are testicular malignancy, torsion, and inguinal hernia.

Small hypoechoic testis may be located anywhere in the path of descent of the testis. Transabdominal scan is required and it is difficult to find these testes as these are small and hypoechoic as these are atrophic **(Figs. 4A and B)**, and therefore was very difficult to locate these testis.[15,16] Tracking the spermatic cord is a new technique to locate the testis.[17] It can be seen in the inguinal canal, anteromedial to femoral vessels, with high-resolution US as oval echogenic structure in transverse section, around which few hypoechoic round areas are seen. These are vas deferens and vessels. Undescended testis can also be away from the path of its descent. It can be in superficial inguinal pouch, anterior abdominal wall, prepenile region, perineal region, etc. It is for these locations that tracking the spermatic cord is really useful. At times both testes may also be seen in the same hemiscrotum.

It needs to be differentiated from ascended or retractile testis and this can be confirmed by looping of the spermatic cord.

Testicular Atrophy

Testicular atrophy refers to small hypoechoic testis with less vascularity but normal epididymis. It may result from inflammation, nondescent, trauma,

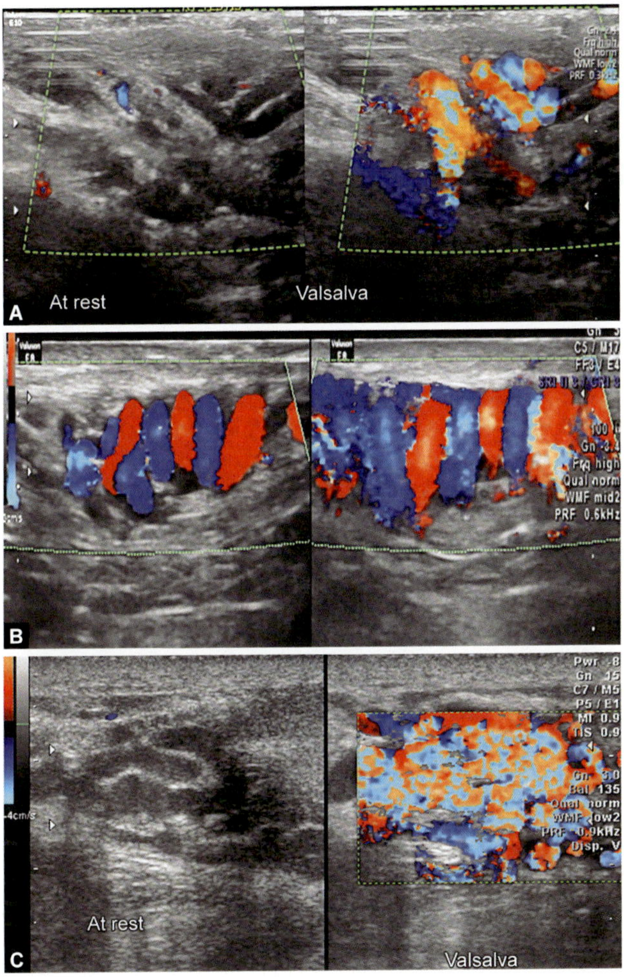

Figs. 3A to C: (A) B-mode and Doppler image showing reflux in dilated peritesticular vessels on Valsalva; (B) B-mode and Doppler image showing reflux at rest which minimally increased during Valsalva; (C) B-mode and Doppler image showing reflux that increases on Valsalva with filling of intratesticular vessels also.

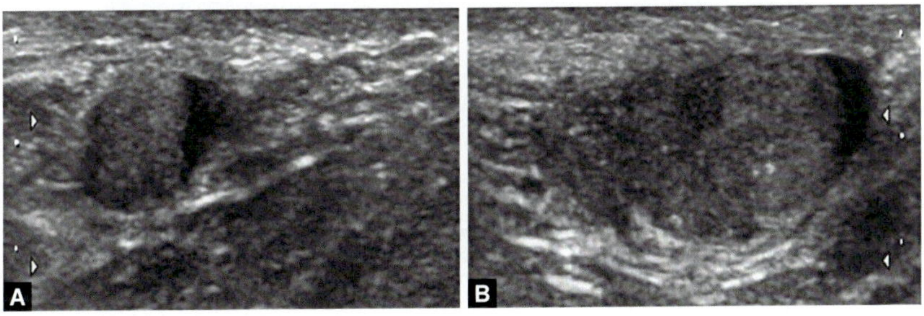

Figs. 4A and B: B-mode images showing small heterogeneous testis—atrophy.

torsion, cirrhosis, estrogen therapy, hypopituitary disorders, Klinefelter's syndrome, and Y-chromosome deletion. With very small or hardly identifiable testis, it is essential to track the spermatic cord to the scrotal sac and document absence of normal testis.

Testicular Neoplasms

Testicular neoplasms are commonly malignant and are diagnosed by heterogeneous localized mass with gross increased vascularity.

Orchitis

Chronic inflammatory conditions of the testes disrupt spermatogenesis and irreversibly alter both the quantity and quality of sperm.[18] Mumps is a one of the common causes for the same. Apart from clinical presentation, hypoechoic or heterogeneous testis with hypoechoic focal areas and increased low resistance vascularity may be diagnostic features **(Fig. 5)**.

Microlithiasis

Tiny multiple hyperechoic areas in the testis are seen on US. It may be due to chronic inflammation or any other insult to testicular parenchyma. Its direct relation to spermatogenesis is not yet established.

Testicular Torsion

Testicular torsion refers as hypoechoic hypovascular testis. Whirlpool sign, if present is diagnostic.

Testicular Infarction

In testicular infarction, wedge-shaped hypoechoic area is seen in the testis with base on the surface of the testis. This localized area shows loss of signals on Doppler due to no vascularity.

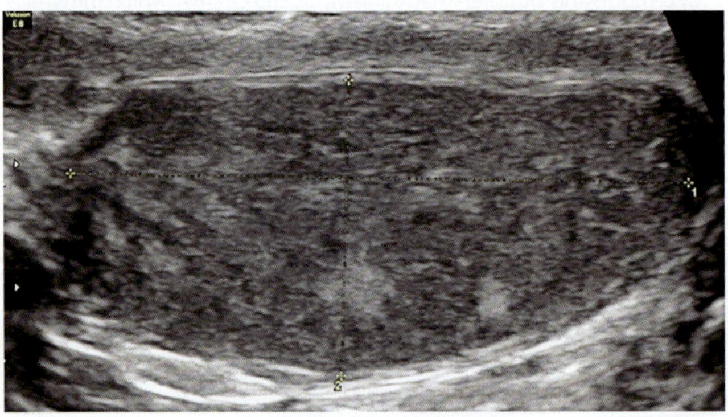

Fig. 5: B-mode image of hypoechoic heterogeneous testis—orchitis.

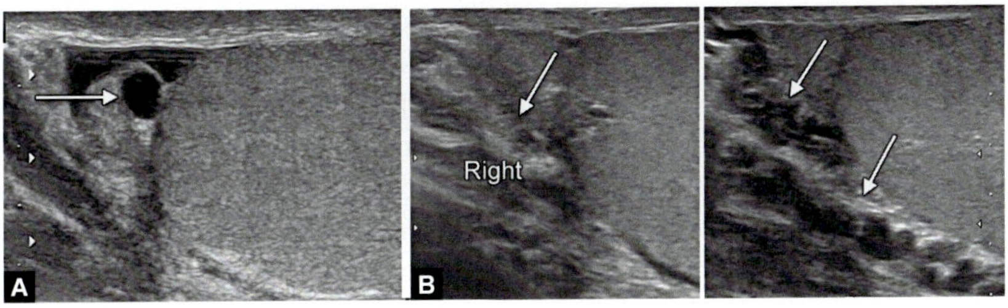

Figs. 6A and B: (A) B-mode image showing epididymal cyst by arrow; (B) B-mode images of epididymal ductal ectasia.

Testicular Trauma

In testicular trauma, capsular tear may be seen. Testicular contusion may be seen as irregular hypoechoic areas in relation to capsular tear. It may be associated with scrotal hematoma also.

Epididymal Lesions

Epididymal lesions may be a cause of obstructive azoospermia. As a result of obstruction of the epididymal ducts and their resulting proximal dilatation epididymis may show a single cystic lesion of variable size or multiple small cystic lesions **(Fig. 6A)**. Acute epididymitis is often associated with acute orchitis. Chronic epididymis is seen as a small head size of epididymis. Filariasis may be seen as dilated epididymal ducts due to distal obstruction **(Fig. 6B)**. This also leads to obstruction of the lumen and thus severe oligo- or azoospermia.

TRANSRECTAL ULTRASOUND

This is essential for the adequate study of prostate and distal male genital tract. Transrectal ultrasound (TRUS) is especially indicated in patients with azoospermia or severe oligozoospermia with a semen volume of <1.0 mL, because these patients, usually have obstructive azoospermia, and in patients with semen volume of >1 mL when vas is not felt on physical examination.

Transrectal ultrasound is useful for systematic evaluation of the terminal vas deferens, seminal vesicles, ejaculatory ducts, and prostate can be carried out in both axial and sagittal planes and to differentiate the surgically correctable lesions (obstructive) from the surgically noncorrectable (nonobstructive) lesions. Most common causes of obstruction are bilateral congenital absence of vas deferens (CABVD), absent seminal vesicles, ejaculatory ducts, obstructing cysts, and calculi.

It is done with high frequency (6–10 MHz) endocavitary—rectal probe. Patient should empty the bladder first. Patient should lie in left lateral decubitus position with flexion of his right hip and knee. A sterile cover with gel inside it is placed over the probe. Gel is applied over the sterile cover. The probe is inserted gently into the rectum through the anus to relax the sphincter. Systematic survey of prostate, seminal vesicle, and vas deferens has to be done in axial, sagittal, and oblique planes. On sagittal plane, base and apex of prostate, urethra, seminal vesicles, and ejaculatory ducts are assessed. On transverse plane, prostate gland, lateral gland margin, neurovascular bundle, and seminal vesicles are assessed. Oblique scan is done mainly to visualize the long axis of the vas deferens and seminal vesicles.

Normal prostate is a symmetric triangular and ellipsoid structure with homogeneous echogenicity. Normal prostate measures 4.0–4.5 × 2.5–3.0 × 3.0–4.0 cm and is homogeneous in echogenicity **(Fig. 7A)**. Normal seminal vesicles are paired, well-defined, saccular, elongated hypoechoic organs situated cranial to the prostate, and posterior to urinary bladder with bow-tie appearance on axial images. Seminal vesicles diverge in the perivesical fat and medially converge to join with the ampulla and form the ejaculatory ducts at the level of the prostatic capsule, producing a typical "bow-tie" appearance on axial TRUS **(Fig. 7B)**. They measure 5–10 cm in length and 2–5 cm in width with a mean volume of 15 mL. On axial TRUS imaging, the distal portion of the vas is seen passing posteromedial to the ipsilateral seminal vesicles and has a mean diameter of 3–5 mm. The ampulla is a dilated terminal 5 mm of each vas, with external diameter of 5–8 mm **(Fig. 7C)**. The intraprostatic part of the ejaculatory duct is seen as a fine hypoechoic curvilinear structure with the lumen not exceeding 2 mm in its maximum diameter. On sagittal scan, it can be seen up to the verumontanum, which is a focal area if hyperechogenicity, with small echogenic concretions **(Fig. 7D)**.

Vas Deferens

Congenital absence or agenesis (bilateral) is seen in 1–2.5% of infertile men and accounts for 4.4–17% of azospermia.[19] The condition is typically associated with low ejaculatory volumes. Agenesis may be partial or complete and unilateral or bilateral. It is often (30%) associated with absent or hypoplastic distal two-thirds of epididymis and absent ipsilateral ejaculatory duct. Testis size and consistency are typically normal. True vasal agenesis is associated with ipsilateral seminal vesicle anomaly. About 16–43% of patients with vasal agenesis is associated with congenital renal anomalies, more commonly affecting the left side.[19] Bilateral vasal agenesis is commonly associated with detectable cystic fibrosis gene mutation (82%), though the disease may not be presenting in majority of them. This gene mutation is not seen in patients with associated renal anomalies. CABVD on transrectal ultrasonography shows absence of the ampulla of the vas deferens. It is associated with abnormalities of seminal vesicles and congenital renal abnormalities.

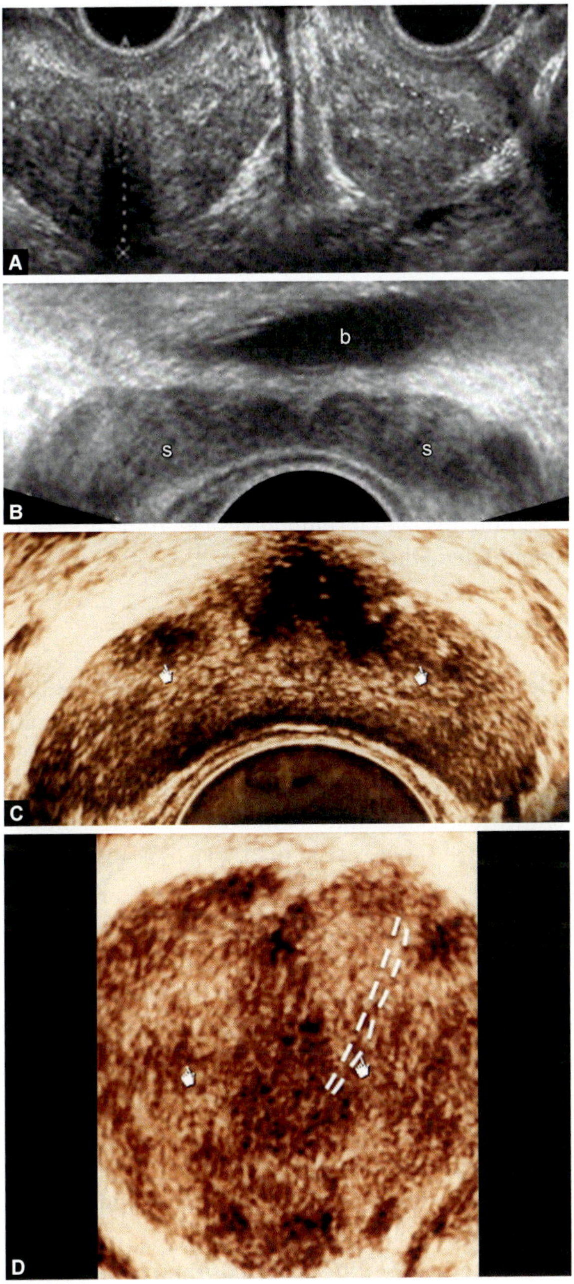

Figs. 7A to D: (A) B-mode image of normal prostate on transverse section by transrectal ultrasound (TRUS); (B) B-mode image of seminal vesicles transverse image by TRUS; (C) Three-dimensional ultrasound image showing vas deferens on coronal plane; (D) Coronal image of the prostate showing thin linear hypoechoic structures on each side of urethra—ejaculatory ducts.

Obstruction of vas is commonly associated with dilatation of epididymal ducts, seen as ductal ectasia in epididymis **(Fig. 8A)**. Epididymis may be seen abruptly stopping at the junction of body and tail.

In partial absence, the persistent vestigial remnant may be seen as a hyperechoic or isoechoic oval structure of approximately 3 mm posterior to the bladder. Hypoplastic vas may be seen as a small vas on TRUS.

Rarely vasal atrophy may be secondary to infection or obstruction. In these cases the distal vas and the ampulla may be absent on US but the proximal vas is palpable clinically and the ipsilateral seminal vesicle is normal. In these cases, dilated vas may be seen on TRUS with epididymal ductal ectasia on scrotal scan.

Other anomalies of the vas are occlusion of vas by fibrosis or calcification, which may be seen as subtle alteration in echogenicity to calcification, with or without similar changes in seminal vesicles and ejaculatory ducts. Cysts or calculi of vas are most common in the ampulla, and cause dilatation of the proximal vas and the ipsilateral seminal vesicle. If the cyst is too large may obstruct the contralateral ducts also.

Seminal Vesicles

Seminal vesicles may be absent, atrophic or hypoplastic (<30% the normal volume). Normal seminal vesicles are >25 mm, hypoplastic are 16–25 mm and atrophic are <16 mm in length. Sometimes only a rudimentary fibrotic vestige may be seen posterior to the bladder. In case of absence of seminal vesicle, the empty fossa is seen to be filled with vessels on color Doppler. Congenital unilateral absence is seen in up to 0.07% and bilateral absence is seen in 1% of males.

Fibrosis and calcification may be congenital or secondary to chronic seminal vesiculitis (which may also be due to calculi formation due to static fluid and cellular debris). Tuberculosis causes solid-looking seminal vesicles with or without calcifications. Both show mildly increased echogenicity with loss of internal convolutions with mild increase or decrease in size. Vas and contralateral ductal system may show similar changes.

Seminal vesiculitis is seen as cystic dilatation of the seminal vesicle **(Fig. 8B)** with multiple homogeneous echoes, with or without edema. Tubercular vesiculitis may be seen as dilated vesicles with multiple echogenic septae and low level echocollection.

Seminal vesicle cysts are due to discontinuity between the seminal vesicle and the ejaculatory duct, mostly congenital and associated with renal, ureteric or bladder trigone anomalies. This may be associated with bilateral adult polycystic kidneys, especially if bilateral. Cysts must be differentiated from the cystic dilatation due to obstruction of the ejaculatory duct as cyst

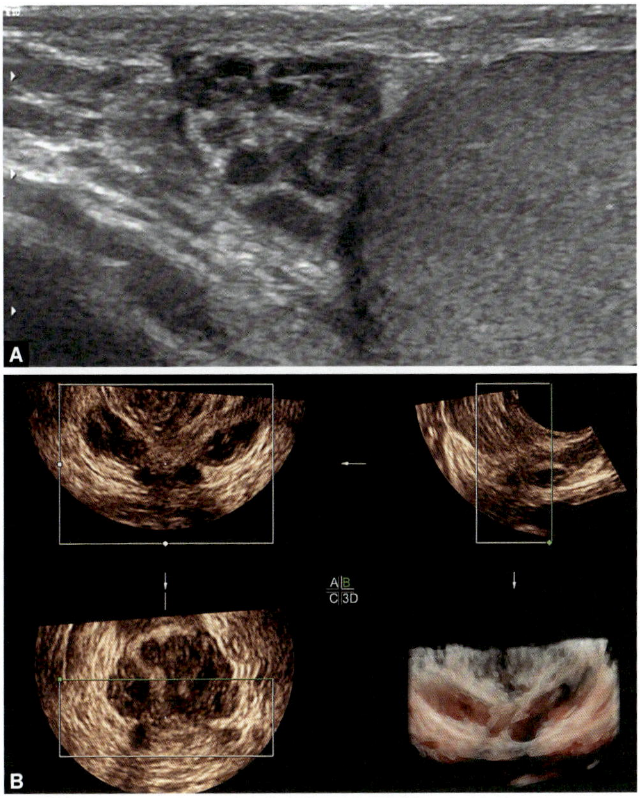

Figs. 8A and B: (A) Epididymal ductal ectasia as a result of vas obstruction; (B) Three-dimensional image of seminal vesicles showing dilated tubules in vesicles.

may require only percutaneous aspiration, while the cystic dilatation may require transurethral resection.

Ejaculatory Ducts

Ejaculatory ducts are best studied in sagittal sections of TRUS. Obstruction of the ejaculatory duct may be extrinsic or intrinsic. Extrinsic, due to compression of the duct by periurethral and prostatic cysts.

It is difficult to differentiate the cyst of prostatic utricle and ejaculatory duct cyst, since both are seen as pyriform cysts in midline—even though the latter can be paramedical and become very large extending beyond the prostate.

Ejaculatory duct cysts are prostatic cysts derived from the Wolffian duct and urogenital sinus, into which the ejaculatory ducts empty, and therefore these cysts will contain sperms. Corrective surgery of the same can lead to nearly normal sperm count in ejaculate. Intrinsic causes of obstruction are calcification, fibrosis, calculi, agenesis or hypoplasia. Except for agenesis, atrophy and hypoplasia, which are all associated with similar changes in vas and seminal vesicles, the obstruction of the ejaculatory duct is associated with dilatation of proximal ejaculatory duct, seminal vesicles and vas. Echogenic foci in the prostate and adjacent to the ejaculatory duct may lead to ejaculatory duct obstruction. Iatrogenic causes include surgery to the base of the bladder and infections acquired following catheterization.[14]

Prostatic and Periurethral Cysts

These cysts cause obstruction of the ductal system leading to infertility. If tense, this cyst may cause obstruction of the ejaculatory duct. Persistent large ejaculatory ducts may be associated with various congenital anomalies such as proximal hypospadias, posterior urethral valves, prune belly syndrome, imperforate anus, and Down syndrome.[20] Midline cysts with sperms are mostly ejaculatory duct cysts. These are actually paramedian, but may appear as midline on TRUS. Laterally situated ones contain no sperms and are mostly degenerative prostatic cysts or retention cysts **(Fig. 9)**. They rarely enlarge enough to block the ejaculatory duct. These are seen in both normal and infertile males though more common in the later. These cysts are well seen on US but difficult to classify by US only. They can be differentiated from dilated ejaculatory ducts which are oval.

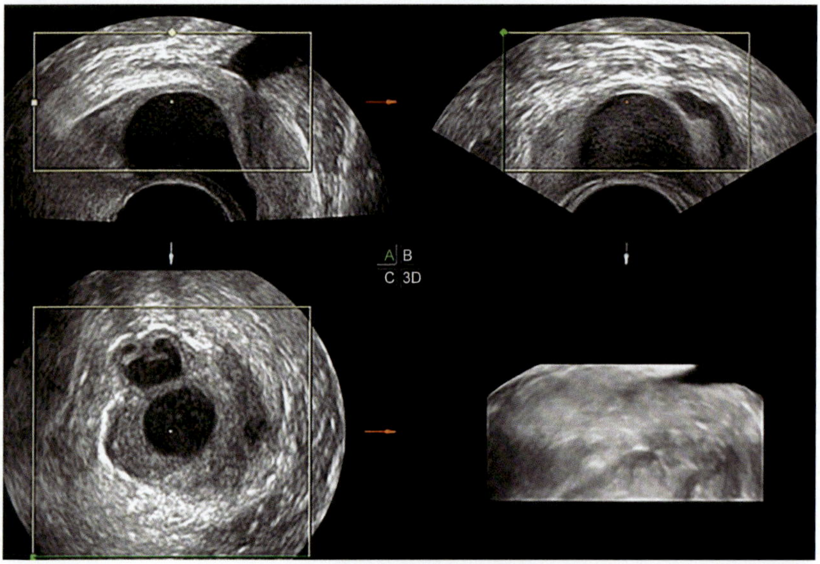

Fig. 9: Large cystic lesions in prostate seen in midline on three-dimensional (3D) image—prostatic cysts.

Prostatic Inflammation

Prostatic inflammation may be acute or chronic. Acute prostatitis may be localized or generalized. It appears as ill-defined hypoechoic area with increased vascularity on color Doppler as acute inflammation anywhere else. Chronic prostatitis may appear heterogeneous with or without dystrophic calcifications and may be difficult to differentiate from a neoplasm. At times, even abscess may develop which appears as thick-walled anechoic area or an area with low level echoes, with peripheral vascularity.

Genital Tuberculosis

Primary site for genital tract tuberculosis in men is epididymis, and from there may spread to neighboring organs by direct extension or hematogenous spread. It more commonly affects its tail because it is rich in blood supply. Tuberculous epididymitis appears as a diffusely enlarged heterogeneously hypoechoic epididymis or more focally with nodular heterogeneous hypoechoic lesions in epididymis but rarely enlarged epididymis may show homogeneous echogenicity or rarely an abscess formation (cystic lesion with thick hypoechoic fluid) may be seen.[21,22]

The scrotal skin may become thickened, a hydrocele may form, or the patient may develop calcification of the epididymis and tunica vaginalis.[23,24] Tuberculous lesions typically show less vascularity.

Tuberculous orchitis shows enlarged testis with multiple small and hypoechoic nodules or rarely diffuse enlargement of the testis with a homogeneous or heterogeneous hypoechoic texture. Separation between the testis and epididymis may be blurred.[23,25,26]

Fibrosis of ejaculatory ducts may lead to dilatation of tubules in seminal vesicles and in epididymis. Rarely, there may be prostatic tubercular abscess.

Occasionally, focal areas of decreased echogenicity can be seen, as areas of dystrophic calcification.[27,28] Transrectal ultrasonography reveals small solid seminal vesicles with or without calcifications. There may be single or multiple hypoechoic masses in the vas within the spermatic cord and possible calcification of the vas deferens. Fibrosis or atrophy of the seminal vesicles may be seen.

Stricture Urethra

The patient will usually have urinary symptoms. US gel urethrogram is an excellent method to study the urethra. Sterile US gel is pushed into the urethra with a blunt cannula at the meatus. The gel distended urethra is well seen on sonography. The luminal narrowing caused by the stricture is well seen. The length and the amount of narrowing can be measured.

Thus, US with the use of color Doppler and three-dimensional (3D) and four-dimensional (4D) US is now the primarily indispensable and decisive investigation for the male patients with abnormal seminal parameters. The total assessment includes scrotal US with Doppler and transrectal US with Doppler. Scrotal US is used for diagnosis of testicular and epididymal pathologies including varicocele. TRUS is for evaluation of prostate, seminal vesicles, vas deferens, and ejaculatory ducts and must always be done with scrotal US. Penile US can be discussed in detail for the differential diagnosis of causes of erectile disorders, though was not in scope of this chapter.

REFERENCES

1. Edey AJ, Sidhu PS. Male infertility: role of imaging in the diagnosis and management. Imaging. 2008;20:139-46.
2. Sidhu PS. Diseases of the testis and epididymis. In: Baxter GM, Sidhu PS (Eds). Ultrasound of the Urogenital System, 1st edition. Stuttgart, Germany: Thieme; 2006. pp. 153-80.
3. Nöske HD, Weidner W. Varicocele: a historical perspective. World J Urol. 1999;17(3):151-7.
4. Marmar JL. The pathophysiology of varicoceles in the light of current molecular and genetic information. Hum Reprod Update. 2001;7(5):461-72.
5. Naughton CK, Nangia AK, Agarwal A. Pathophysiology of varicoceles in male infertility. Hum Reprod Update. 2001;7(5):473-81.
6. Witt MA, Lipshultz LI. Varicocele: a progressive or static lesion? Urology. 1993;42(5):541-3.
7. Schoor RA, Elhanbly SM, Niederberger C. The pathophysiology of varicocele-associated male infertility. Curr Urol Rep. 2001;2(6):432-6.
8. Benoff S, Gilbert BR. Varicocele and male infertility: part I. Preface. Hum Reprod Update. 2001;7(1):47-54.
9. Benoff S, Marmar JL, Hurley IR. Molecular and other predictors for infertility in patients with varicoceles. Front Biosci. 2009;14:3641-72.
10. Dubin L, Amelar RD. Varicocele size and results of varicocelectomy in selected subfertile men with varicocele. Fertil Steril. 1970;21(8):606-9.
11. Beddy P, Geoghegan T, Browne RF, Torreggiani WC. Testicular varicoceles. Clin Radiol. 2005;60(12):1248-55.
12. Cornud F, Belin X, Amar E, Delafontaine D, O Hélénon, Moreau JF. Varicocele: strategies in diagnosis and treatment. Eur Radiol. 1999;9(3):536-45.
13. Isidori AM, Lenzi A. Scrotal ultrasound: morphological and functional atlas. Genova: Forum Service; 2008.
14. Jarow JP. Role of Ultrasonography in the evaluation of infertile male. Semin Urol. 1994;12:274-82.
15. Cain MP, Garra B, Gibbons MD. Scrotal-inguinal ultrasonography: a technique for identifying the nonpalpable inguinal testis without laparoscopy. J Urol. 1996;156(2 Pt 2):791-4.
16. Nijs SM, Eijsbouts SW, Madern GC, Leyman PM, Lequin MH, Hazebroek FW. Nonpalpable testes: is there a relationship between ultrasonographic and operative findings? Pediatr Radiol. 2007;37(4):374-9.
17. Vijayaraghavan SB. Sonographic localization of nonpalpable testis: tracking the cord technique. Indian J Radiol Imaging. 2011;21(2):134-41.

18. Schuppe HC, Pilatz A, Hossain H, Meinhardt A, M Bergmann, G Haidl, et al. Orchitis and male infertility. Urologe A. 2010;49(5):629-35.
19. Levine LA, Coogan CL. Penile vascular assessment using color duplex sonography in men with Peyronie's disease. J Urol. 1996;155:1270-3.
20. Kuligowoska E, Baker CE, Oates RD. Male infertility: Role of transrectal ultrasound in diagnosis and management. Radiology. 1992;185:353-60.
21. Hill GS, Billey-Kijner C. Paratesticular structures: nontumorous conditions. In: Hill GS (Ed). Uropathology. New York: Churchill Livingstone; 1989.
22. Kim SH. Genitourinary tuberculosis. In: Pollack HM, McClennan BL (Eds). Clinical Urolography, 2nd edition. Philadelphia: WB Saunders Company; 2000. pp. 1193-228.
23. Kim SH, Pollack HM, Cho KS, Pollack MS, Han MC. Tuberculous epididymitis and epididymo-orchitis: sonographic findings. J Urol. 1993;150(1):81-4.
24. Muttarak M, Peh WC, Lojanapiwat B, Chaiwun B. Tuberculous epididymitis and epididymo-orchitis: sonographic appearances. Am J Roentgenol. 2001;176(6): 1459-66.
25. Drudi FM, Laghi A, Iannicelli E, Di Nardo R, Occhiato R, Poggi R, et al. Tubercular epididymitis and orchitis: US patterns. Eur Radiol. 1997;7(7):1076-8.
26. Heaton ND, Hogan B, Michell M, Thompson P, Yates-Bell AJ. Tuberculous epididymo-orchitis: clinical and ultrasound observations. Br J Urol. 1989;64(3):305-9.
27. Hamrick-Turner J, Abbitt PL, Ros PR. Tuberculosis of the lower genitourinary tract: findings on sonography and MR. Am J Roentgenol. 1992;158(4):919.
28. Wolf LE. Tuberculous abscess of the prostate in AIDS. Ann Intern Med. 1996;125(2):156.

CHAPTER 24

3D and 4D Ultrasound in Obstetrics and Gynecology

Sonal Panchal

INTRODUCTION

Invention of three-dimensional (3D) and four-dimensional (4D) ultrasound (US) has made a dramatic improvement in fetal imaging. On 3D US, multiple two-dimensional (2D) US sections are taken very closely placed to each other and they are all put together to construct a 3D image. That means we have a whole block of information instead of just a thin slice of a 2D US. 4D US is a live 3D, where 3D reconstruction is so fast, 16–32 frames/min, that it appears real time. 3D and 4D US is, therefore, a volume US **(Fig. 1)**.

The volume data can be viewed as a 3D object and in multiplanar mode in three orthogonal planes—sagittal, coronal, and axial **(Fig. 2)**. All can be correlated to each other by the reference point which is represented as a dot on all three images. This dot is actually an intersecting point of two lines seen on all three images and it is actually an intersection of x, y, and z axis. This dot represents the same structure on all three planes **(Fig. 3)**.

The volume can be seen as rendered image. Rendered image means watching the whole volume as a whole block of tissue. The rendering direction can also be selected. Which means one can select to see the volume from above, below, right, left, front or back.

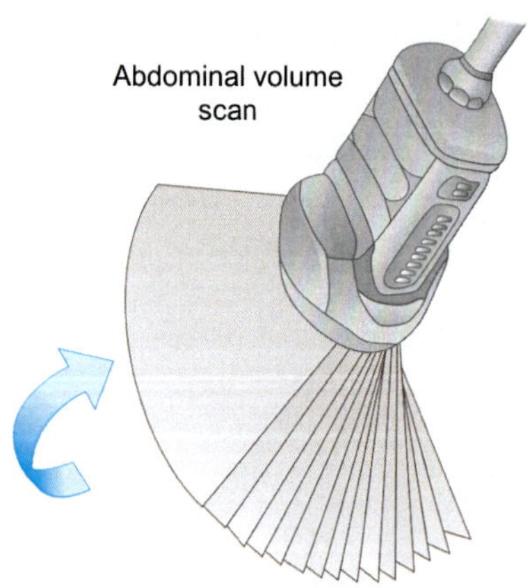

Fig. 1: Diagrammatic representation of how three-dimensional volume data acquired. (*Source:* GE Healthcare)

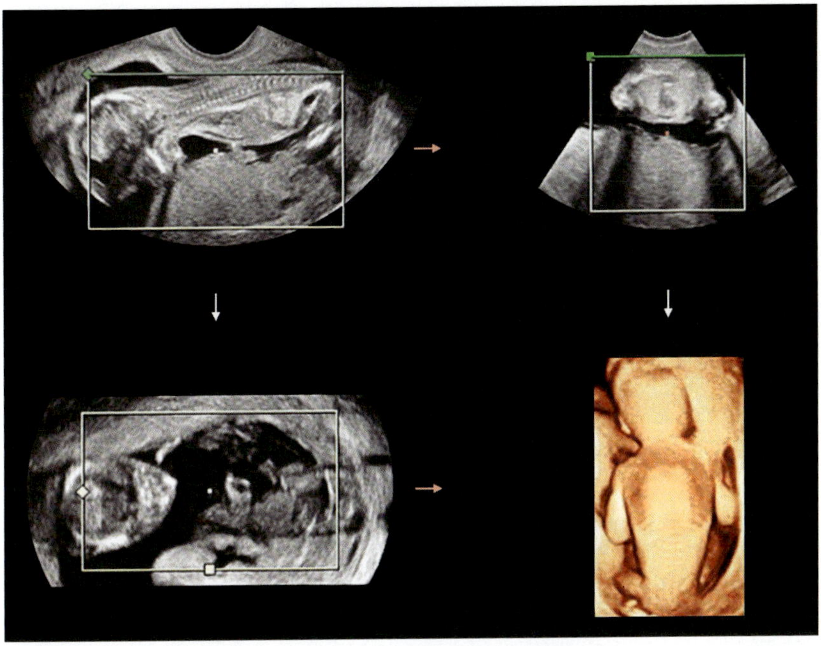

Fig. 2: Acquired volume data in longitudinal, transverse, sagittal planes, and rendered image.

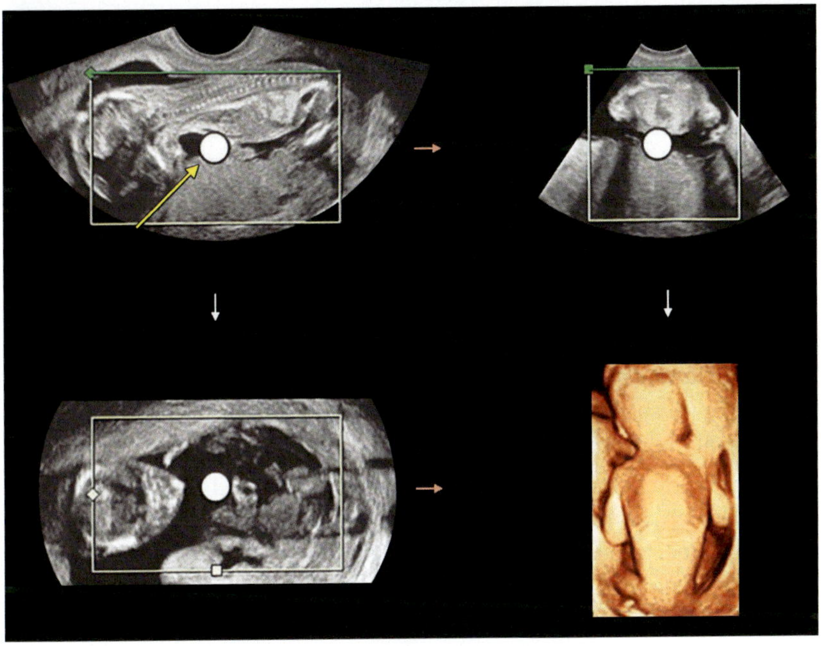

Fig. 3: Multiplanar and rendering mode of 13 weeks, fetus on three-dimensional ultrasonography.

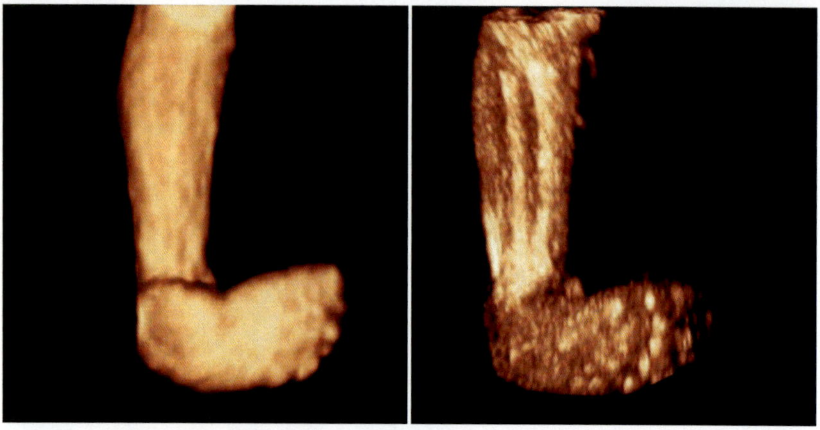

Fig. 4: Surface and transparent modes rendered on the same volume.

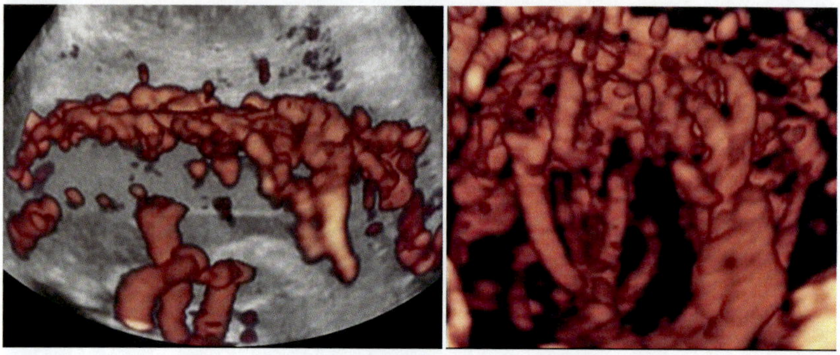

Fig. 5: Normal placental vasculature on angiomode.

Various modes of rendering can be selected singularly or combined to optimize the visualization of soft tissues, bony structures or vessels. Face watching is the most popular use of volume US. This is surface rendering. It is used to see the face and limbs of the fetus. Rendering by transparent modes show the internal organs of the fetus and bones in the same acquired volume depending on selection of rendering mode transparent minimum, X-ray or transparent maximum **(Fig. 4)**.

Angiomode can be applied on a volume acquired with power/color Doppler which shows the vasculature in the given volume such as angiography. One can select to see the blood vessels in reference with the surrounding tissues by glass body rendering or only the blood vessels by angiomode **(Fig. 5)**. This is like doing an angiography, where only the contrast-enhanced blood vessels will be seen. The advantage here is that no contrast or invasive procedure is required.

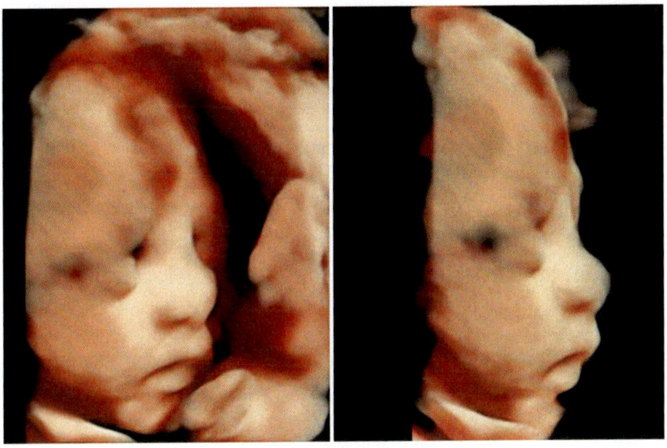

Fig. 6: Magicut.

Magicut is an electronic scalpel. This is used to cutoff the unwanted tissue information from the rendered image. Tissues can be cutoff in whole thickness or up to variable depth **(Fig. 6)**.

Tomographic ultrasound imaging (TUI) allows simultaneous visualization of multiple parallel slices in one of three orthogonal planes at a time, such as computed tomography (CT) or magnetic resonance imaging (MRI). This is very important for the understanding of fetal anatomy and diagnosing abnormalities such as posterior urethral valve, tracheoesophageal fistula, diaphragmatic hernia, cleft palate, fetal mass lesions, cranial and spinal abnormalities, etc. **(Fig. 7)**.

Omniview or a single view is a tool that allows the visualization of any scanned structure/lesion in coronal plane, that means in a plane that is perpendicular to the scanning plane. This can be done in real time as well as on acquired image also. It is very useful again for spine and corpus callosal defects, etc. **(Figs. 8A to C)**. Volume contrast imaging (VCI) allows thicker slices to be examined in real time. These slices can be done in A plane—the plane of acquisition and in C plane—coronal plane. Thicker slices help to improve the contrast and, therefore is an excellent tool to demonstrate subtle lesions **(Fig. 8C)**.

Volume calculations by 3D using virtual organ computer-aided analysis (VOCAL) software are much more accurate than 2D volume calculations for lung, liver, cerebellum, ventricles, follicles, endometrium, etc. **(Fig. 9)**.

Spatial temporal imaging correlation (STIC) is offline 4D US and has proved to be extremely useful for evaluation of the heart.

All these together ultimately help to understand the complex anatomy better with surface analysis of minor defects, volume measurements, and vascular studies.

In gynecology, it has a major role in diagnosis of congenital uterine anomalies, diseases of the endometrium and evaluation of adnexal masses, and also for assessment of follicle and endometrium in infertility cases.

VOLUME ULTRASOUND IN OBSTETRICS

In early pregnancy, 3D sonography is absolutely superior to the standard 2D sonography in assessment of first trimester of pregnancy. It has moved the embryology from specimen studies to in vivo. Development of the embryo

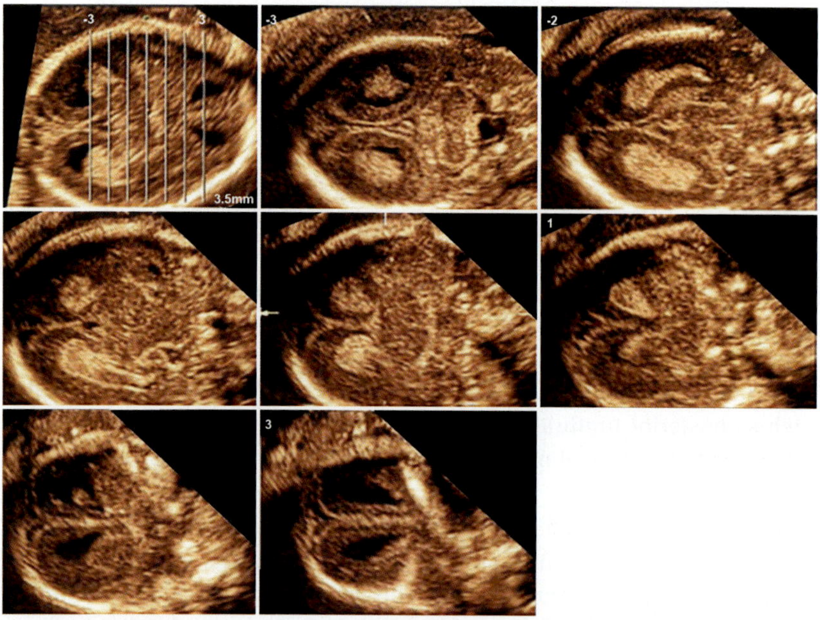

Fig. 7: Tomographic ultrasound imaging for sectional anatomy.

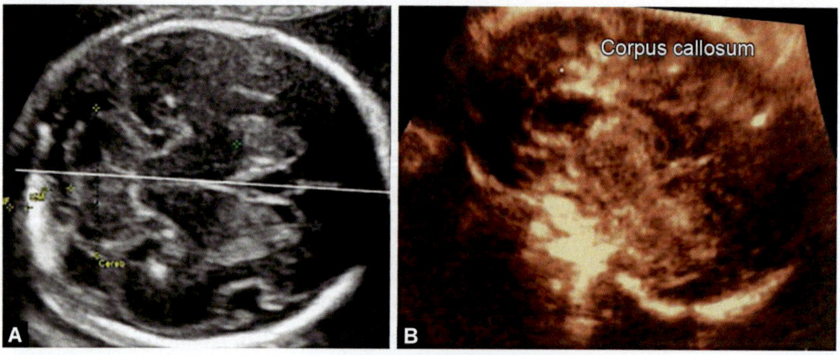

Figs. 8A and B

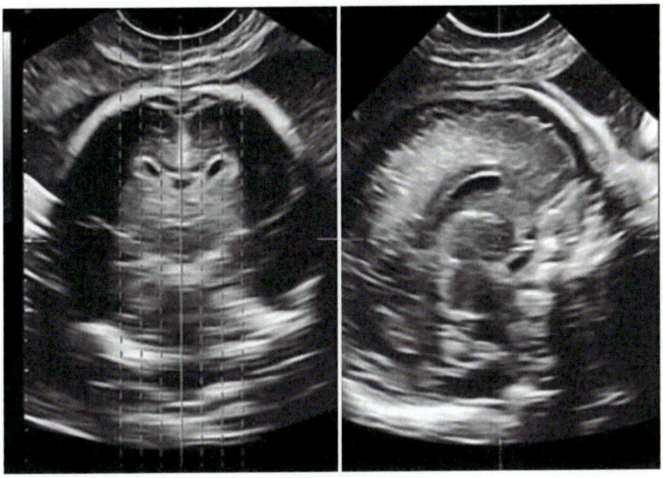

Fig. 8C

Figs. 8A to C: (A) Transthalamic section of head on B-mode with line for Omniview; (B) Corpus callosum seen on Omniview; (C) Using volume contrast imaging (VCI) gives better contrast and visibility of corpus callosum.

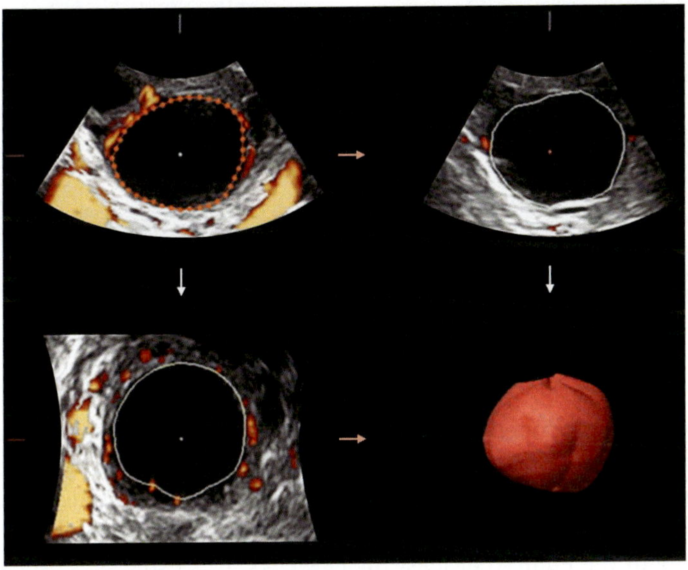

Fig. 9: Virtual organ computer-aided analysis (VOCAL).

can be studied in detail by transvaginal 6–9 MHz volume probe. This is known as sonoembryology **(Fig. 10)**.

Using 3D power Doppler (PD) hemodynamic changes occurring during early placentation can be studied. Moreover, this accuracy can be achieved with even a shorter examination time. 3D orientation and multiplanar

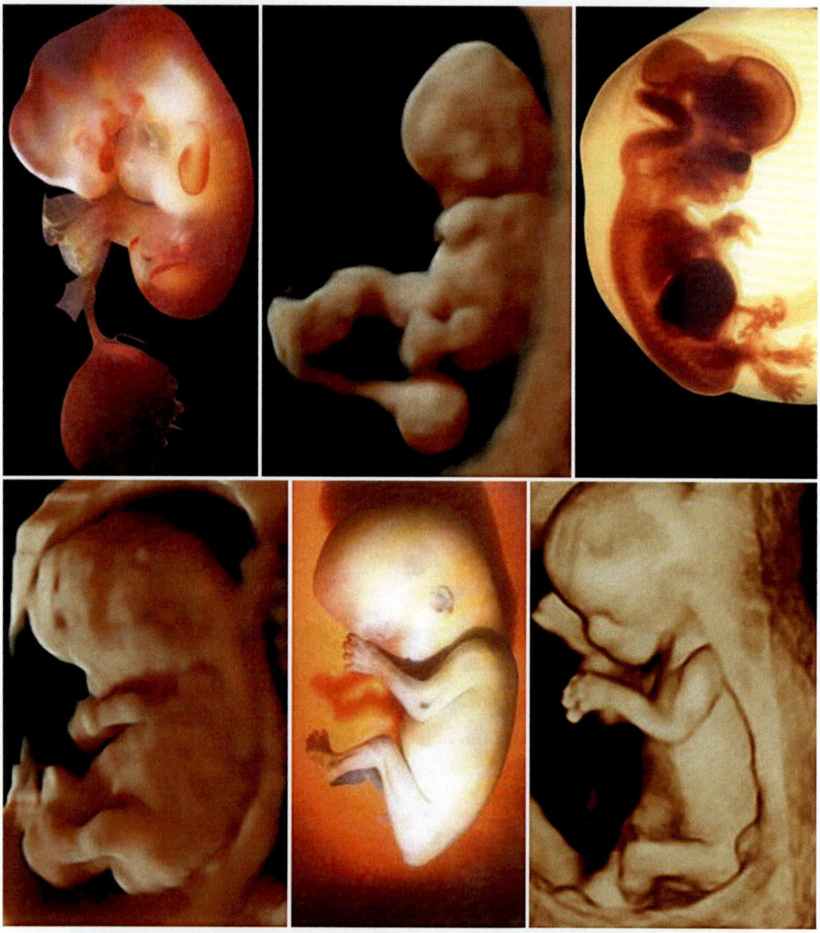

Fig. 10: *7, 11, and 13 weeks gestation:* Embryological picture and volume sonography comparison.

imaging gives unlimited tomograms, with only limited probe manipulation and minimizes the fetal exposure to US waves. Acquire a single sweep of the complete fetus in up to 5 seconds maximum. Using surface rendering and maximum mode multiplanar mode and TUI shows a complete detailed anatomy of the embryo at least till 12 weeks. It is especially useful with unfavorable fetal position.

NUCHAL SCAN

Nuchal scan is done between 11 and 14 weeks of pregnancy to exclude chromosomal malformations. This includes measuring nuchal translucency, nasal bone, ductus venosus flow, looking for tricuspid regurge, measuring

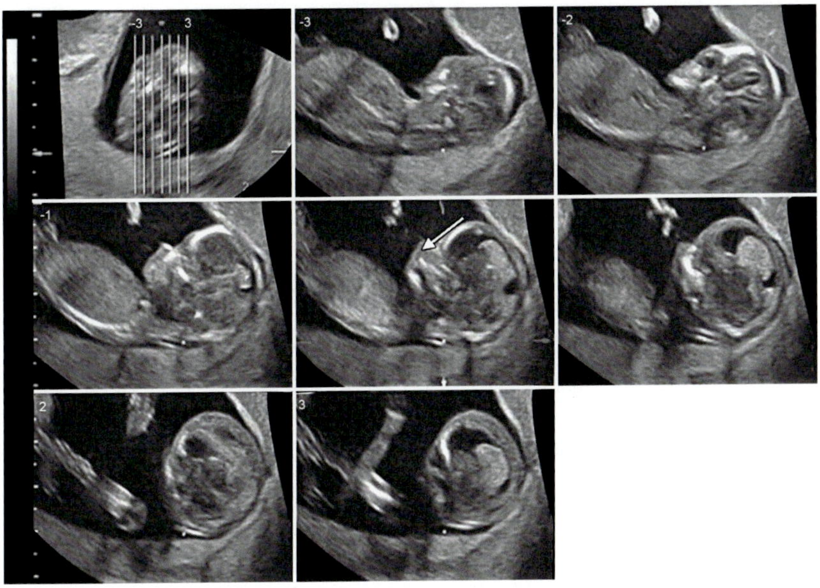

Fig. 11: Nuchal translucency seen multiplanar view.

facial angle, looking for omphalocele, renal pyelectasis, etc. Assessing for nuchal translucency, nasal bone, and facial angle require a true midsagittal section. This may always not be easy whether abdominal or vaginal route is selected. A study by Kurjak et al. has shown that using 3D US, midsagittal plane of the fetus can be visualized successfully 100% of the times versus 80% of the times with 2D technique.[1] A study by Eppel et al. shows that 3D transvaginal technique offers a shorter examination time and higher success rate for measuring nuchal translucency though it results in slight but significant underestimation of the measurement **(Fig. 11)**.[2] This probably may be due to the transvaginal approach instead of transabdominal.

When the starting section is transverse or coronal it is very difficult to find out nasal bone in midsagittal plane by 2D US. 3D US can be a useful tool to find out and measure the nasal bone. But if the angle between US transducer and imaginary line passing through fetal face profile is <30° or >60°, that is if fetal head is hyperextended or flexed, 3D cannot help over 2D technique to see the nasal bone. Using multiplanar mode Peralta et al. have described a gap between the nasal bones on axial plane in 20% of fetuses and in about 40% of these fetuses in midsagittal plane, nasal bone may be erroneously considered absent on 2D US.[3] So, 3D US can demonstrate absent nasal bone in axial plane, reducing the false positives. In second trimester, screening on maximum transparent rendering mode is preferred to multiplanar to show unilateral or bilateral absence of nasal bone.

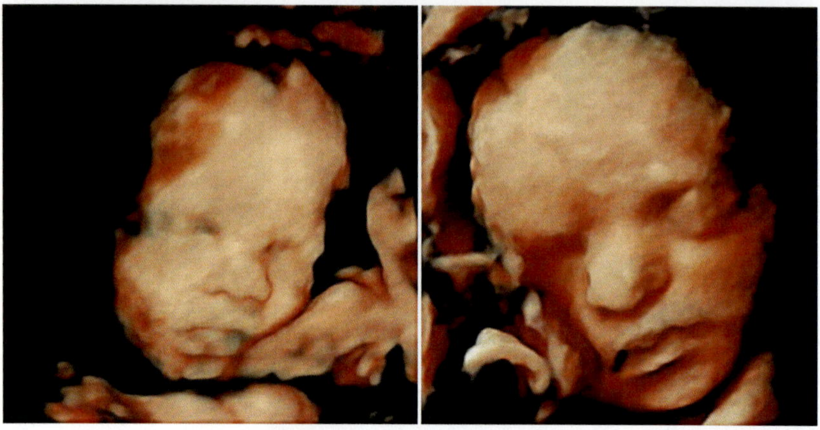

Fig. 12: Fetal faces between 20 and 25 weeks.

Genetic syndromes are often diagnosed by craniofacial dysmorphism. Three-dimensional US has remarkably improved the detection rate of facial anomalies and thus, helped in diagnosis of genetic syndromes.

Facial Abnormalities

Three-dimensional US has improved the detection rate of facial anomalies. In 90% of cases, correct and reproducible face images can be produced in second trimester **(Fig. 12)**. Best time to see the facial details is between 23 and 30 weeks but proper fetal position and fluid pocket are essential. To get a proper position pressing mother's abdomen repeatedly, turning mother to one or another side or reexamining after a few minutes would help when fetus is not in a favorable position to see the fetal face.

Though this reduces to only 30% after 34 weeks due to the obligatory position that the fetus has to attain with its growing size.

Merz et al. have reported well-defined facial images as early as ninth week of pregnancy.[4] 3D US has an important role in diagnosis of facial cleft, micrognathia, nasal abnormalities, and eye abnormalities.

Diagnosis of cleft lip and palate is almost 100%, including the cleft of soft palate also **(Fig. 13)**.[5-7] Cleft palate can be diagnosed by TUI **(Figs. 14A and B)**, by mixture of light and surface rendering.

Three-dimensional US can also pick up isolated soft palate defects as shown by studies by Pilu et al.[6] Another technique to detect the cleft palate is the 3D "reverse face" view[8] **(Fig. 15)**. After acquiring the face volume, the viewing direction is changed to back, so that you see the facial bones from inside the skull. Maxilla and palate can be reliably studied as early as 11 weeks. Early diagnosis of median cleft syndrome is possible in which the

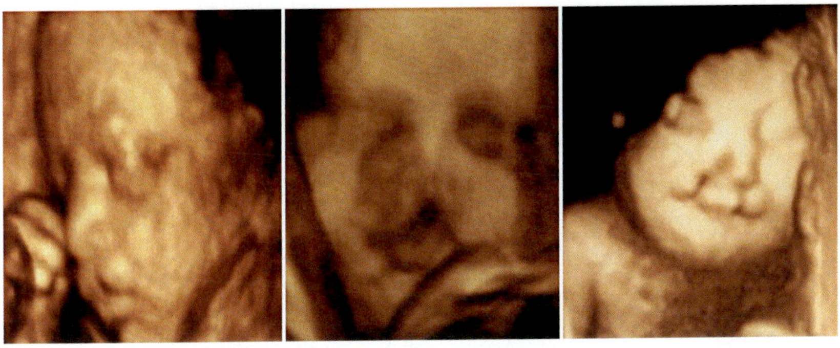

Fig. 13: Cleft lip and palate by rendering mode.

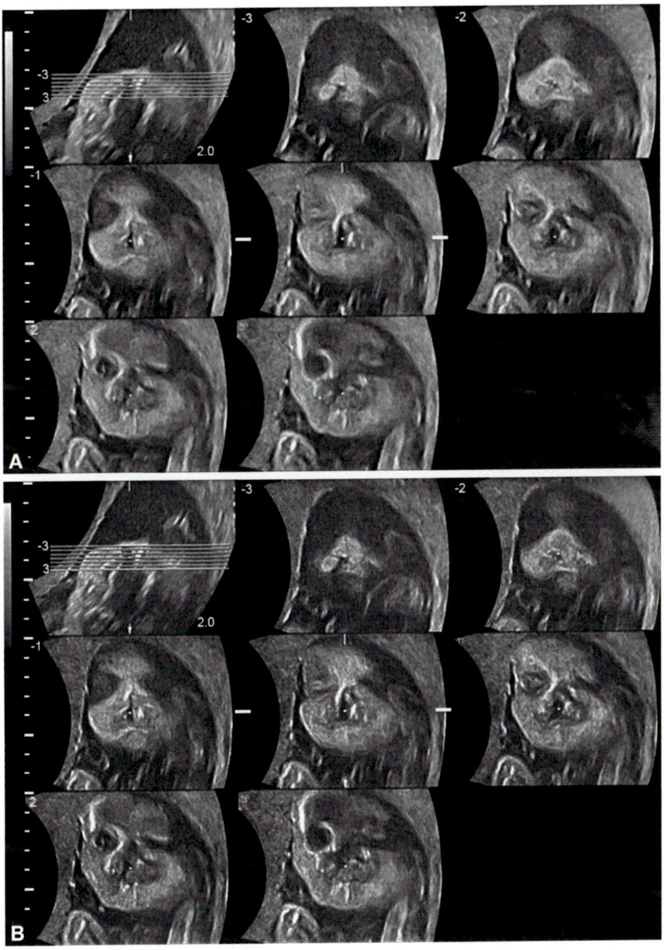

Figs. 14A and B: Cleft palate seen by tomographic ultrasound imaging (TUI).

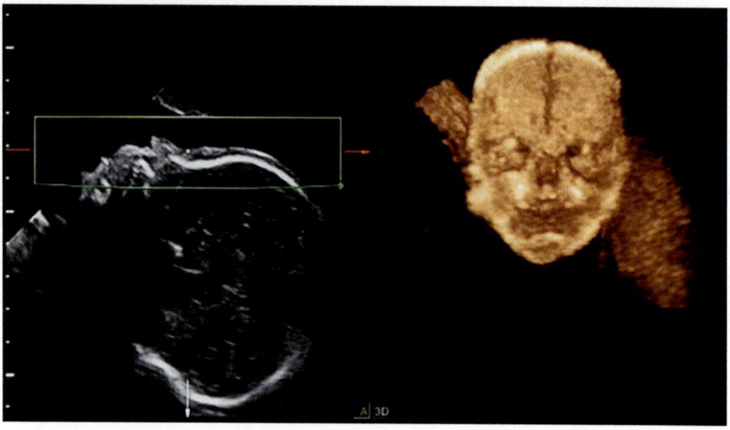

Fig. 15: Reverse face view and reverse viewing direction.

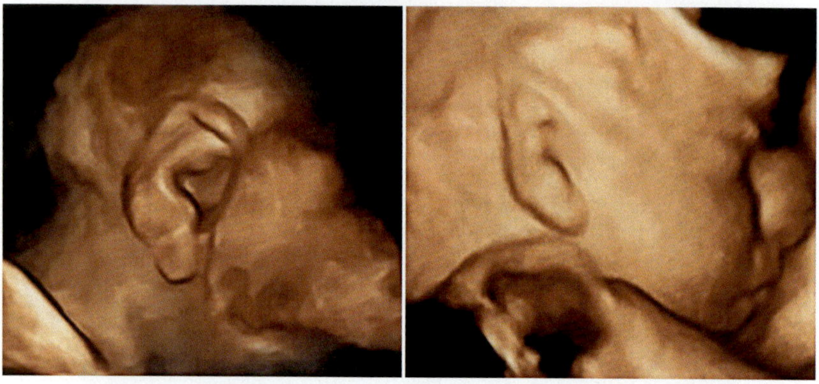

Fig. 16: Ear as seen on 3D surface rendering.

frontal bones and nasal bones are largely separated with hypertelorism, flat nasal bridge, rudimentary nostrils, and other facial abnormalities.[9]

Size, morphology, and placement of the ear are important for diagnosis of chromosomal abnormalities **(Fig. 16)**. About 70% of trisomy 21 babies have helix-lobe lengths more than 2 standard deviation from mean. Detection of ear appendices may be a marker of renal malformation.

The important features of fetal dysmorphism diagnosed by 3D US are:

- Flattening or prominence of occipital bones
- Early closure of sutures
- Hypo/hypertelorism/microphthalmia
- *Retro or micrognathia and jaw index*: Anteroposterior (AP) diameter of mandible/biparietal diameter (BPD) (<0.23 is micrognathia)[10]
- Low placed or abnormal shape of ears, ear appendices
- Asymmetry of face

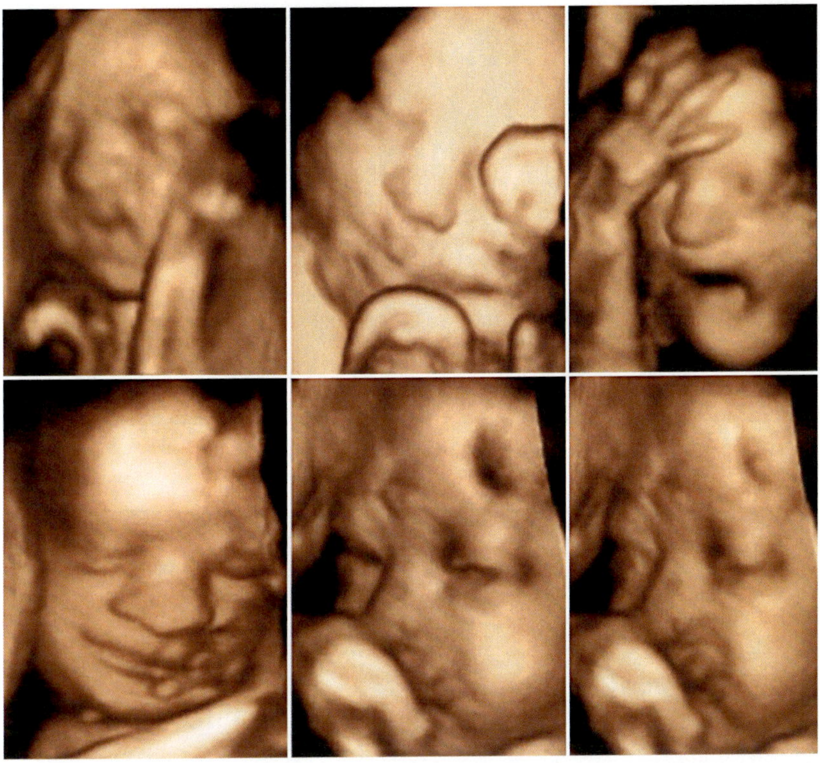

Fig. 17: Fetal expressions—grimacing, mouthing, yawning, smiling, and opening eyes (eyelid movements).

- Altered facial angles—superior or inferior
- Cleft lip/palate

Apart from the defects or anatomical variations, 3D and 4D US can also show the fetal expressions which express the fetal behavior. The expressions recorded so far are **(Fig. 17)**:

- Yawning
- Smiling
- Swallowing
- Sucking
- Blinking
- Grimacing
- Mouthing
- Tongue expulsion

Cranial Abnormalities

Skull bones and sutures can be identified by 3D US, which is difficult with 2D US due to natural curve of the skull. Maximum transparency mode is used

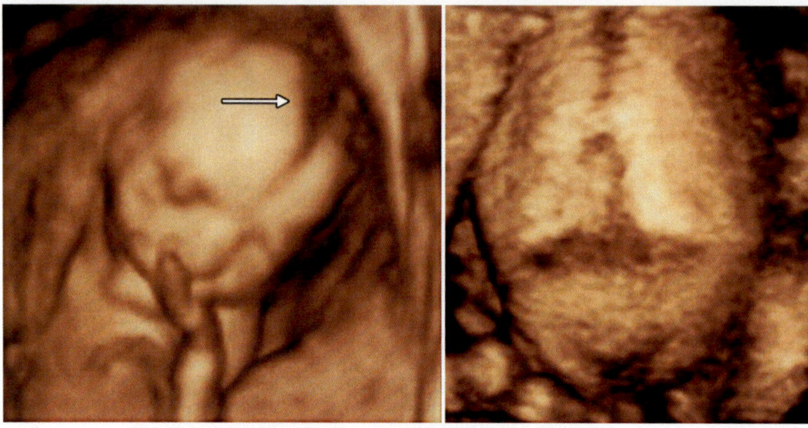

Fig. 18: Cranial sutures (arrow).

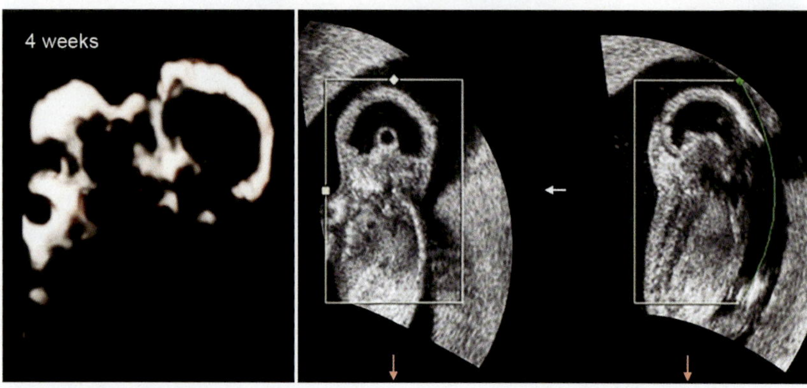

Fig. 19: *Neural canal inversion mode:* 9–10 weeks and holoprosencephaly.

for this **(Fig. 18)**. Excessive diastases of the sutures can be seen in cranium bifidum occultum and premature closure can diagnose craniostenosis and microcephaly early.[11] By 3D multiplanar display diagnosis of acrania and exencephaly can be rather easy depicting correct sagittal and coronal sections.

Central Nervous System

Development of diencephalon, mesencephalon, and rhombencephalon can be studied from 9 weeks of gestation. Diagnosis of alobar holoprosencephaly is possible as early as 10 weeks by absence of central cleft **(Fig. 19)**.[12]

In late second and third trimester, if fetus is in cephalic presentation, transvaginal approach can be a better approach to study fetal brain. Placenta and thick skull bones may be obstructing the vision on transabdominal

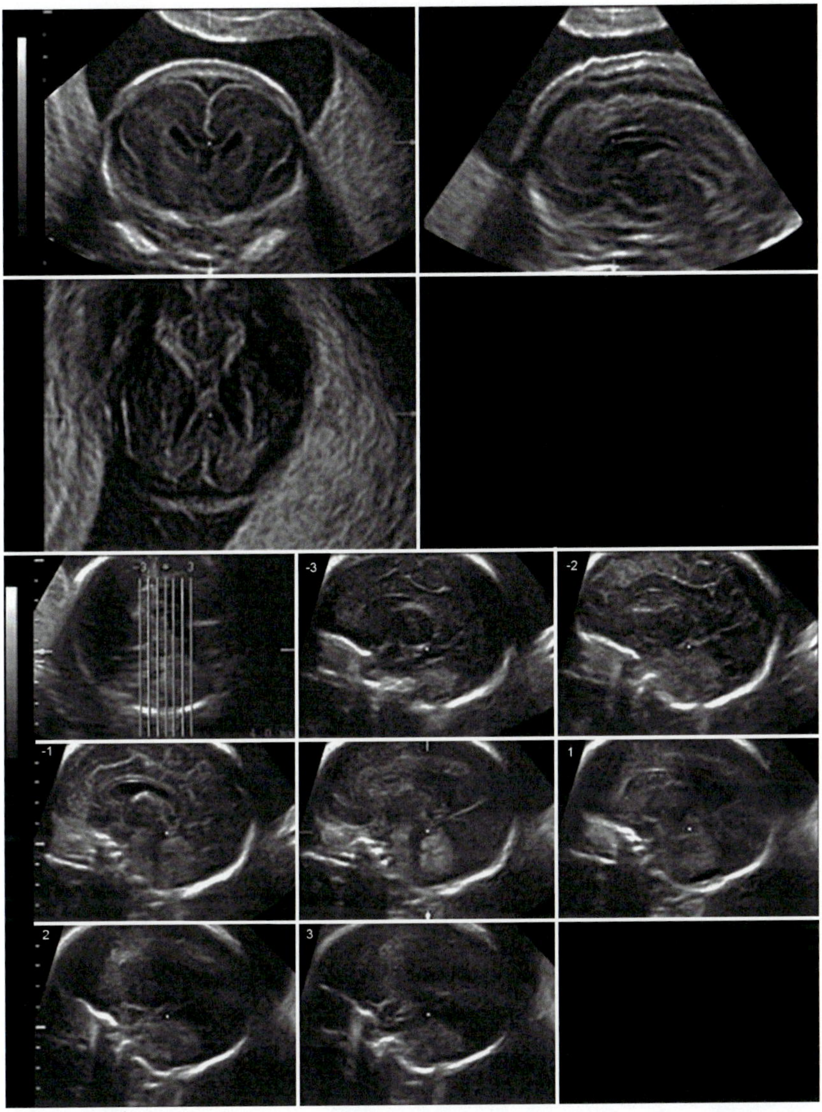

Fig. 20: Brain on multiplanar mode and tomographic ultrasound imaging (TUI).

approach. Once the fetal brain has been scanned, it is then possible to navigate in the stored volume. By multiplanar display, the brain anatomy can be studied in detail **(Fig. 20)**.

Using TUI in all the three orthogonal planes all the coronal, sagittal, and axial sections required for a detailed neurosonogram can be achieved by one single sweep of the fetal head. This has been discussed in detail in the chapter dedicated to fetal central nervous system (CNS).

Omniview with VCI in coronal plane depicts the midline structures such as corpus callosum, optic chiasma, and cerebellar vermis **(Fig. 8)**. Agenesis of corpus callosum and cerebellar vermian hypoplasia—Dandy-Walker syndrome can be diagnosed by this method. Normal corpus callosum and cerebellar vermis with ventriculomegaly is most likely due to aqueduct stenosis. Paladini and Volpe[13] have suggested tentorovermian angle, tentoroclivus angle, clivovermian angle, etc. to diagnose vermian abnormalities. Skull-base development can be studied by measurement of anterior skull-base length and posterior cranial fossa length and skull-base angle. Brain growth leads to higher increment in posterior cranial fossa length leading to 6° flexion in the skull-base angle.[14] Craniofacial variability index (CVI) can assist in fetal facial anatomy to study craniofacial development.[15] This can be all measured on TUI and multiplanar mode. This technique has proved to be almost as sensitive as CT scan or MRI for study of expansive brain lesions. 3D US may be applied to every CNS abnormality diagnosed with traditional 2D technique and may offer further information helpful to arrive to correct diagnosis. It can delineate the exact nature and anatomic level of anomaly. Three-dimensional PD also delineates the cerebral vasculature and its abnormalities **(Fig. 21)**.

Study of *fetal motorial and behavioral pattern* is essential for complete evaluation or functional integrity of fetal CNS. 4D US allows the evaluation of fetal motorial and behavioral patterns. With 4D US, it is possible to better define the degree of normality and pathology of fetal neurological functions in utero and to find out which fetuses are at risk of bad neurological outcome. Kurjak et al. have described patterns of neurodevelopmental behavior during the three trimesters of pregnancy using 4D US **(Figs. 22A and B)**.[16] The changes in the motorial pattern expresses the evolution of the maturative process of

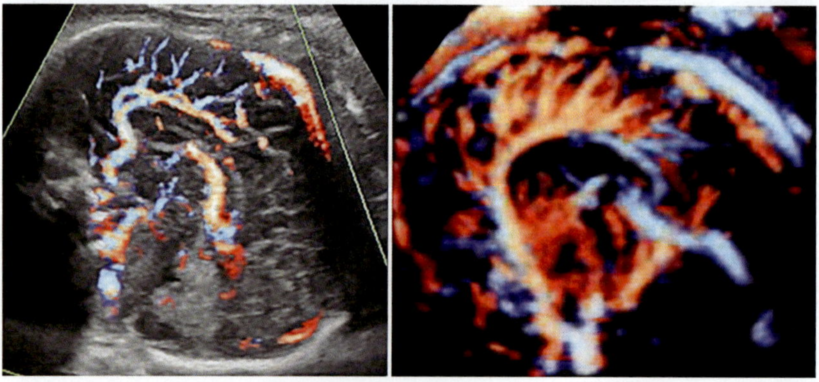

Fig. 21: Cerebral vasculature on 2D HD flow and on 3D HD flow rendered with angiomode.

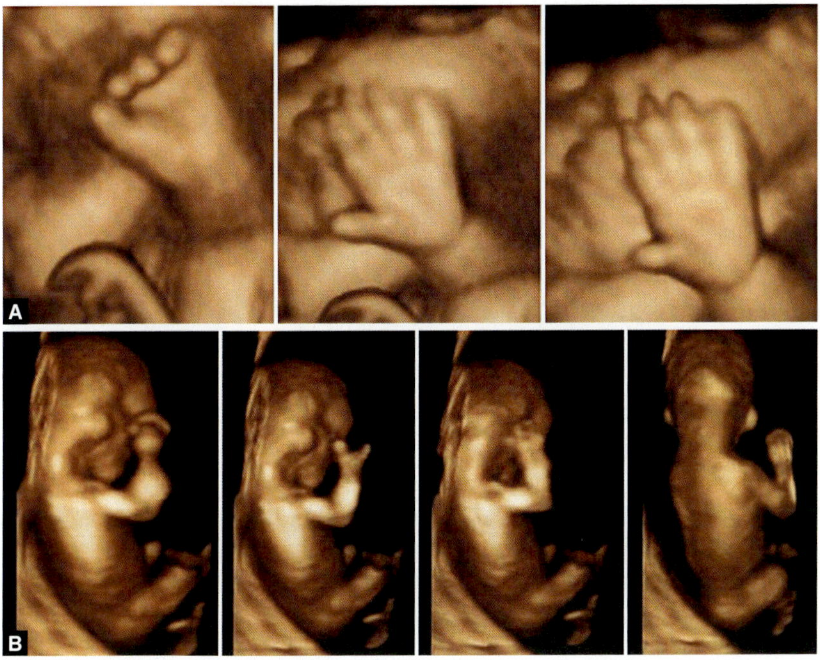

Figs. 22A and B: (A) Movements of hand; (B) Fetus scratching the ear.

CNS during intrauterine life. These fetal behavior and movements can help diagnosis of motoric development failure at the end of the first trimester. Delayed motoric development is seen in fetuses of diabetic mothers.

Fetuses with arthrogryposis show early disturbances in motoric development with absent limb movement and joint contractures.

Spinal Abnormalities

Evaluation of spine in sagittal, coronal, and axial all three planes are essential to diagnose spinal abnormalities correctly. All the three views cannot be achieved in one fetal position on 2D US. Three-dimensional US saves examination time and clearly can show all the three views at a time on multiplanar view along with the overlying skin surface by using maximum mode transparent rendering and surface rendering. Using 4D VCI C can also show coronal view even when on 2D US only axial section is seen **(Fig. 23)**.

Using Magicut and 3D rotation, it is also possible to see each vertebra separately and to define the extent of lesion especially in cases of open spinal canal defects **(Fig. 24)**. 3D–4D US have almost 100% sensitivity and very high specificity for diagnosis of spinal abnormalities. Longitudinal scan of the fetus is used with maximum mode to evaluate the thoracic cage, clavicle, and scapulae. Absent 12th rib is a marker for trisomy 21.

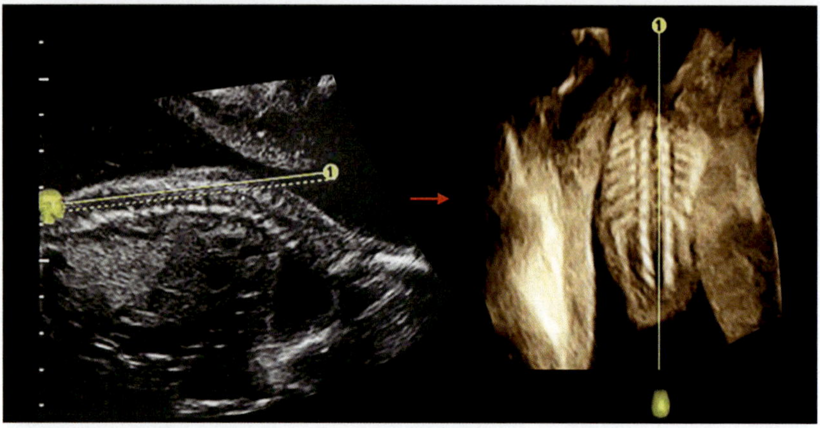

Fig. 23: *Normal spine:* Volume contrast imaging (VCI).

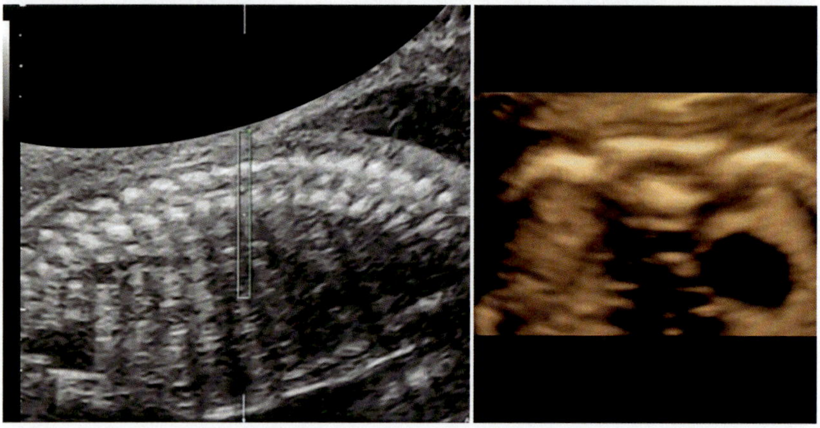

Fig. 24: Spine vertebra—transverse section.

Chest

Multiplanar mode and TUI allows to study the spatial relationship between lungs, heart, esophagus, and diaphragm.[17] Trachea and esophagus morphology can be studied thus, helping to diagnose tracheoesophageal fistulae early and decide the type in utero **(Fig. 25)**. VOCAL and 3D-4D multiplanar mode is useful for assessment of fetal lung volume and thymus volume.

Diaphragmatic hernia can be easily diagnosed by 2D US also but the role of 3D US here is to assess the amount of lung compression and calculate the exact lung volume which is very important for deciding the prognosis.

Ruano et al. have evaluated the potential of 3D PD to predict neonatal outcome and pulmonary arterial hypertension in fetuses with congenital diaphragmatic hernia.

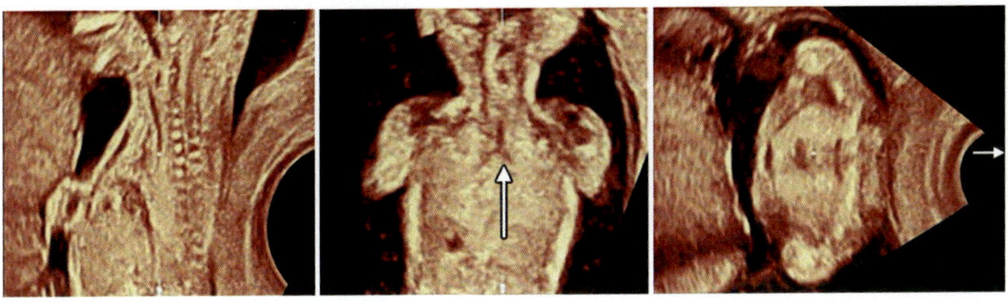

Fig. 25: *Chest—multiplanar mode:* Tracheal bifurcation.

Abdomen

Using transparent mode and multiplanar mode, the abdominal organs can be very well-defined with definition of all tissue planes. 3D US is an effective tool for diagnosis of gastrointestinal malformations and gives additional information over 2D US for pediatric surgeons for surgical planning and for counseling with parents. All abdominal masses may be better evaluated by multiplanar mode to evaluate the origin and extension. Inversion mode helps to define cystic lesions and can be best used to confirm the diagnosis of pyloric stenosis, duodenal atresia, posterior urethral valves, obstructive uropathy, etc. **(Figs. 26A and B)**. Surface rendering allows clear visualization of genitals. Hypospadias is seen as "Tulip sign"[18] and clitoral hypertrophy can be diagnosed in third trimester.

Anterior abdominal wall defects are well demonstrated on volume US. 3D is very useful to differentiate the bowel containing from the liver containing omphalocele. Use of 3D multiplanar display is more accurate than the use of 2D US for measuring the size of omphalocele. Congenital anomalies of the abdomen such as omphalocele and gastroschisis can be clearly evaluated through 3D US **(Fig. 27)**.

Role of 3D–4D US in fetal echocardiography is discussed in the Chapter 21.

Limb Abnormalities

Accurate analysis of majority of bony structures can be done using maximum mode rendering of 3D US. Phocomelia and sirenomelia like abnormalities can be diagnosed as early as 11–12 weeks. 3D–4D US enables detailed examination of fingers and toes with almost 100% certainty of detecting club feet **(Fig. 28)**, agenesis and extra digits **(Figs. 29 and 30)**. Motor abnormalities and abnormal attitude of fingers, toes or hands, and legs such as club feet, overriding of fingers or thumb in the fist may be a manifestation of chromosomal or neurological abnormality **(Fig. 31)**.

Placenta

It is known that pregnancy-induced hypertension (PIH) occurs only after at least 70% of the placental vasculature is obliterated. 3D PD with angiomode

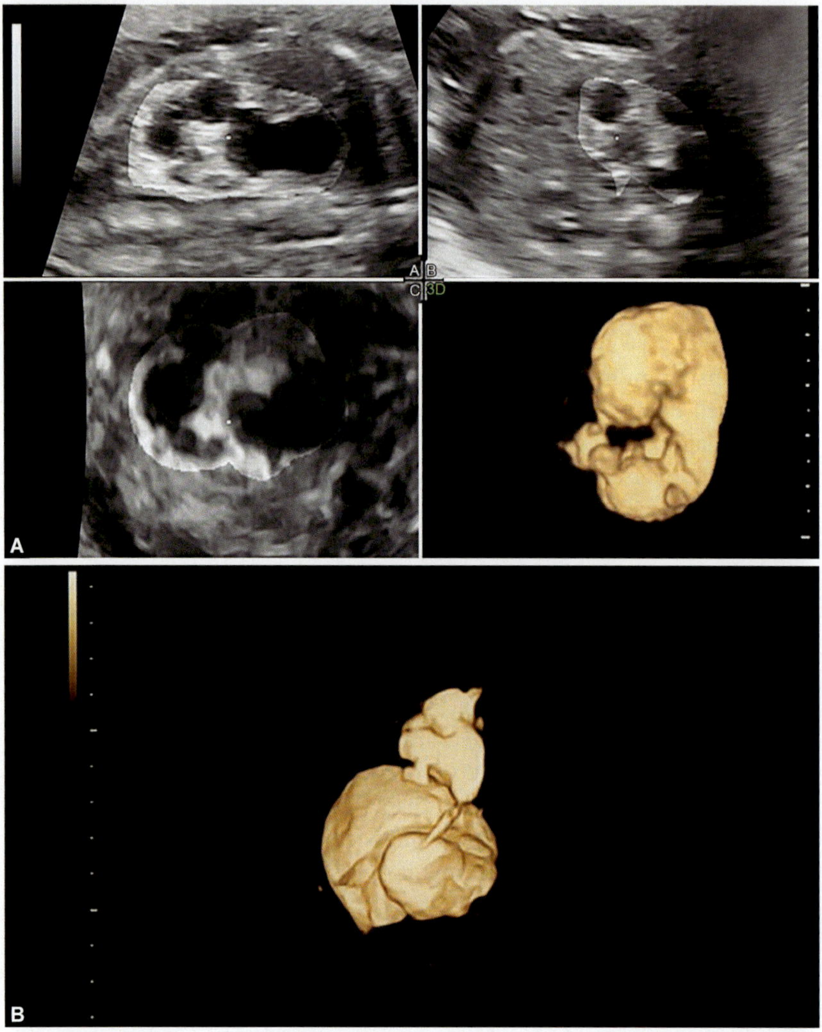

Figs. 26A and B: (A) Dilated stomach and duodenum is seen on the sectional planes in fetal abdomen as multiple anechoic bubbles and on inversion mode-rendered image, stomach and duodenal cap is seen suggesting duodenal atresia; (B) Inversion mode showing distended renal pelvicalyceal system, ureter, and bladder.

of the placental vasculature may show obliteration of the placental vessels and help to predict PIH much earlier.

HD live is an absolute novel rendering mode. This allows editing the direction of light falling on the rendered image. It is very useful for sonoembryology, for detection of subtle facial defects such as slanting eyelids in Down syndrome, etc **(Fig. 32)**. Silhoutte mode has added the transparency to this thus allowing to see not only the surface but also the deep lying

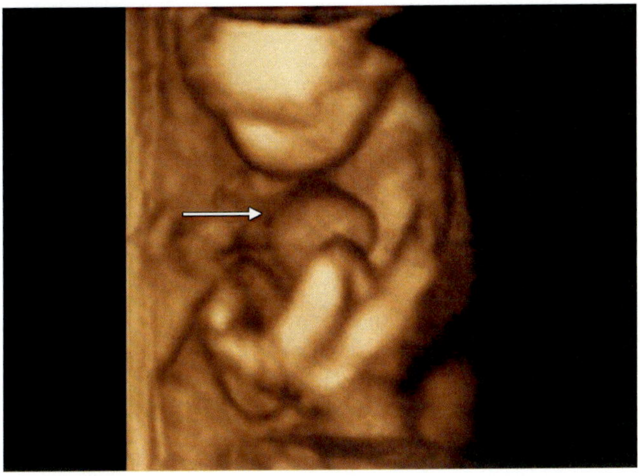

Fig. 27: Omphalocele three-dimensional ultrasound (arrow).

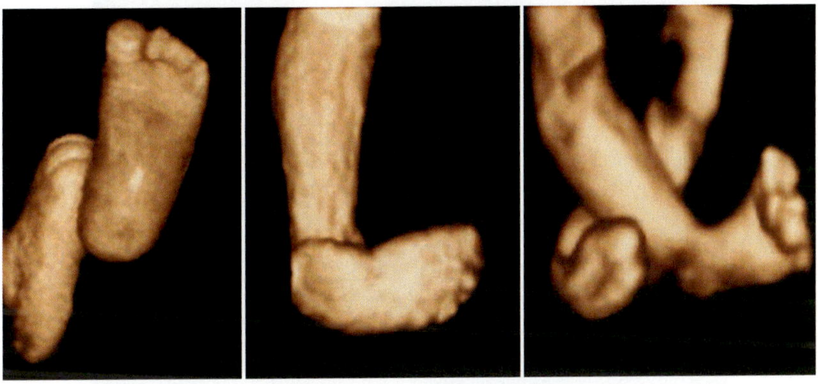

Fig. 28: Normal feet and club feet.

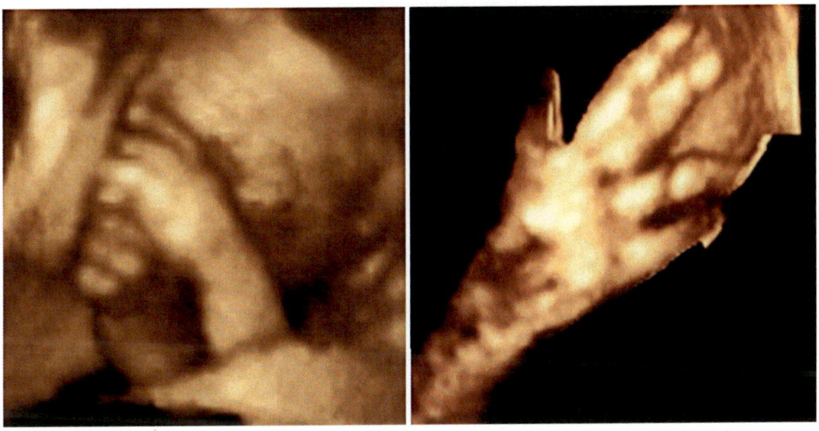

Fig. 29: Normal hands and fingers.

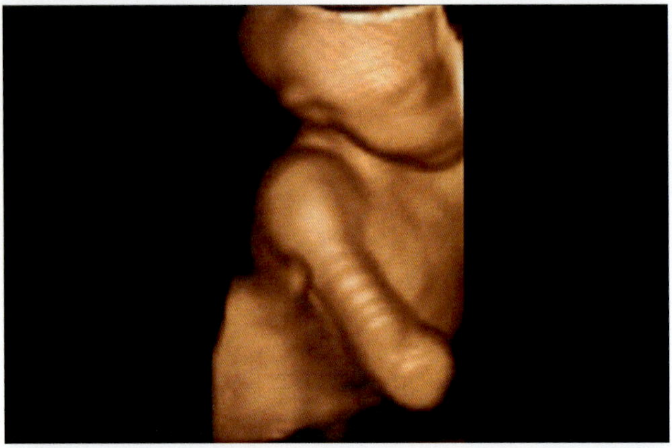

Fig. 30: Absent forearm.

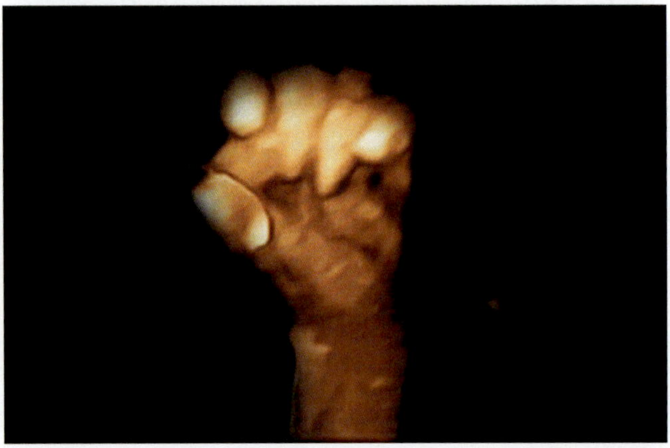

Fig. 31: Infolding of the thumb in the fist is seen on 3D rendered image—neurological thumb.

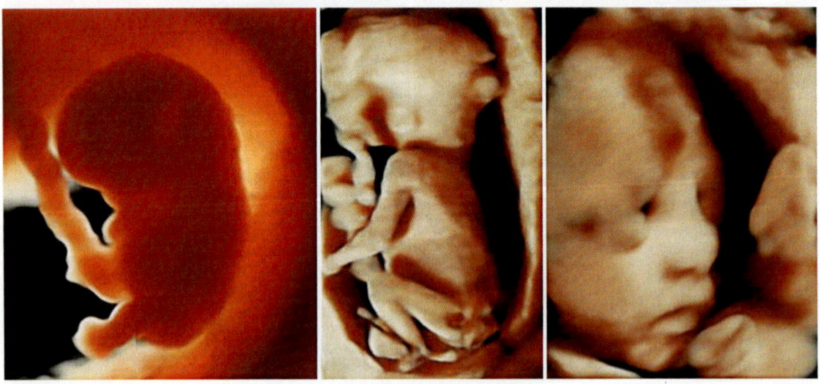

Fig. 32: HD live.

anechoic areas thus playing a very important role in assessment of cerebral ventricles, stomach, bladder, hydronephrosis, neural canal, etc.

Benacerraf et al.[19] have described a novel use of 3D US in offline fetal evaluation. According to her study, five volume sweeps should be taken of every fetus, and these are examined offline. This method has proved to be successful in detailed evaluation of fetal anatomy and very sensitive for diagnosing fetal anomalies. These sweeps are axial section of fetal head, axial section of fetal thorax, axial section of fetal abdomen, longitudinal sweep of lower limbs, and longitudinal section of head.

Limitations of 3D–4D Ultrasound

As for 2D US maternal obesity, maternal scar, maternal movements, excessive fetal movements, that come in way of sound propagation are obstacles for 3D US also. Oligohydramnios does not permit sufficient fluid interface for rendering and so, is not a favorable factor for reconstruction and surface rendering.

Conjoined Twins

In conjoined twins **(Fig. 33)**, practicability and the consequent morbidity of the fetuses after separation depend on the degree of codivision of organs and vascular structures. Therefore, detailed and accurate anatomic and vascular map is fundamental for evaluation of joined organs in conjoined fetuses is of fundamental importance to decide the line of treatment. Moreover, defects such as orofacial cleft, diaphragmatic hernia, imperforate anus, and neural tube defects are also common. Bega et al. have reported that combining multiplanar display and surface rendering can assess these fetuses fairly

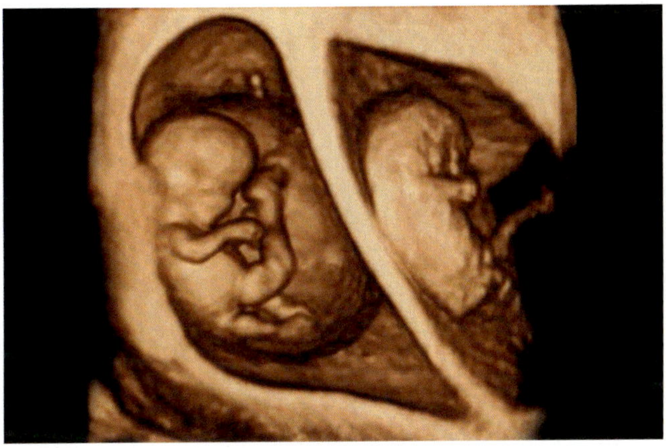

Fig. 33: Dichorionic–diamniotic twins.

reliably, as early as 10 weeks.[20] 3D US can be of great help in classifying more accurately the type of conjoined twins and color Doppler may be of further help. Apart from rendering, multiplanar imaging is also useful to define the anatomy and organ sharing in conjoined twins.

Four-dimensional US is also useful to observe and analyze interfetal behavior.

Ectopic Pregnancy

Three-dimensional US with rendered image in coronal plane plays an important role for the diagnosis of cornual or interstitial pregnancy **(Fig. 34)**. We have used 3D PD for monitoring the vascularity of ectopic pregnancy which is treated conservatively. Decreasing vascularity indicates a regressing pregnancy.

Gynecology

Three-dimensional US in gynecology has one great advantage and that is coronal view of uterus. This has made 3D US as effective a tool as magnetic resonance (MR) for diagnosis of uterine abnormalities. Most commonly used tools in gynecology are surface texture rendering, at times mixed with smooth surface mode, multiplanar mode, and TUI in coronal section. The rendering direction is most commonly from above, as if you are looking at the uterus from the top. Transvaginal is the approach always selected.

Congenital uterine abnormalities 3D US is a very sensitive tool for the diagnosis of congenital uterine anomalies **(Fig. 35)**. It is known as virtual hysteroscopy. This is discussed in detail in Chapter 14.

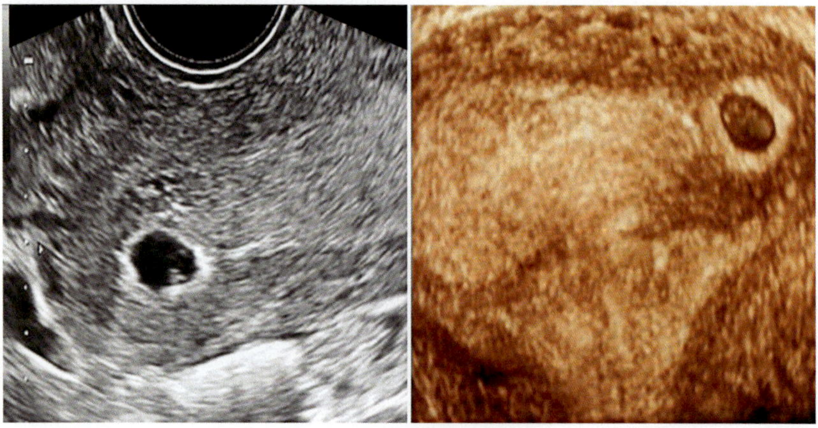

Fig. 34: Angular pregnancy.

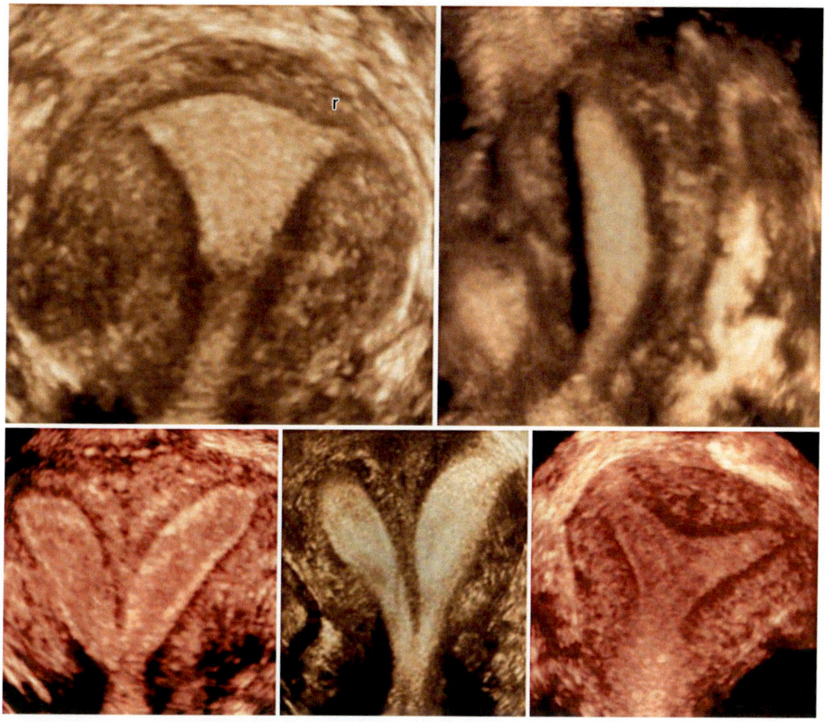

Fig. 35: Three-dimensional ultrasound of normal uterus and congenital uterine anomalies (unicornuate, bicornuate, subseptate, and arcuate).

Acquired Uterine Abnormalities

Fibroids

Fibroids are easily and reliably diagnosed by 2D and color Doppler. 3D US is done to precisely assess the relationship between submucous fibroid and endometrial cavity **(Fig. 36)**. As 3D US precisely shows the location of the fibroid, it will also be a guide to decide the route of surgery. 3D US is done in fibroids for follow-up in pregnancy, menopause, and when under gonadotropin-releasing hormone agonist (GnRH-a) treatment for volume measurement by VOCAL. These are the conditions which may show remarkable increase or decrease in size of the fibroid. In difficult cases, using 3D power Doppler angiomode can be used to differentiate between fibroids and adenomyosis. Circumferential vascular pattern suggests fibroid whereas radiating/penetrating vascular pattern suggests adenomyoma **(Fig. 37)**.

Polyp

Endometrial polyps are best seen on 2D US in periovulatory phase as solid isoechoic lesions in the endometrial cavity. They are at times difficult to

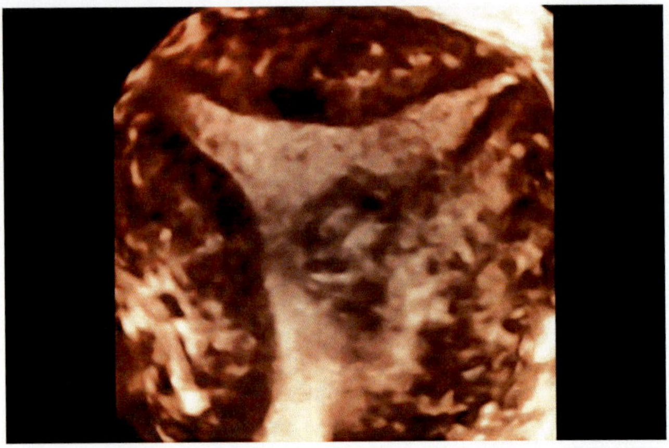

Fig. 36: Three-dimensional ultrasound of fibroid.

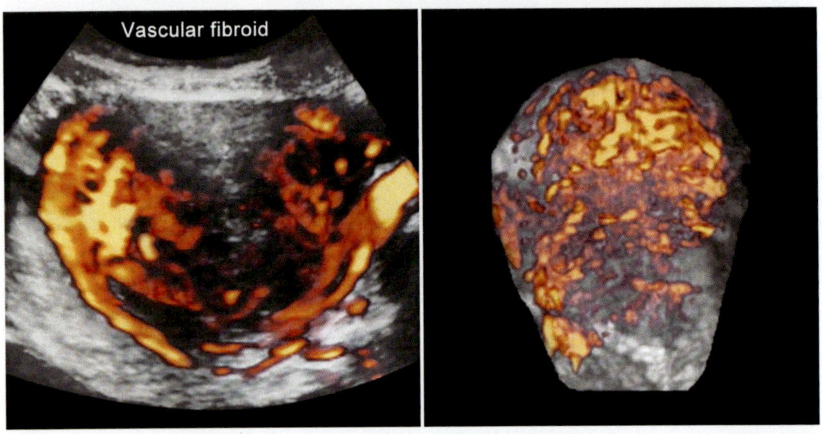

Fig. 37: *3D power Doppler:* Fibroid and adenomyosis.

differentiate from other endometrial lesions like hyperplasia, malignancy or synechiae. 3D US is the diagnostic tool for diagnosis of polyp **(Fig. 38)**. TUI in coronal plane shows the pedicle also and exact site of origin. It differentiates thus, polyp from hyperplasia and malignancy.

Synechiae

These are the most commonly missed lesions on 2D US. 3D US delineates and localizes the adhesions and helps surgical planning. In cases of bridging adhesions 3D gives exact assessment of extent of obliteration of cavity. Sonohysterography is a better tool to assess the extent of restriction of the cavity.

In cervical or uterine malignancies, 3D US helps to detect the invasion of surrounding organs and tissues. 3D PD shows typical chaotic vascular

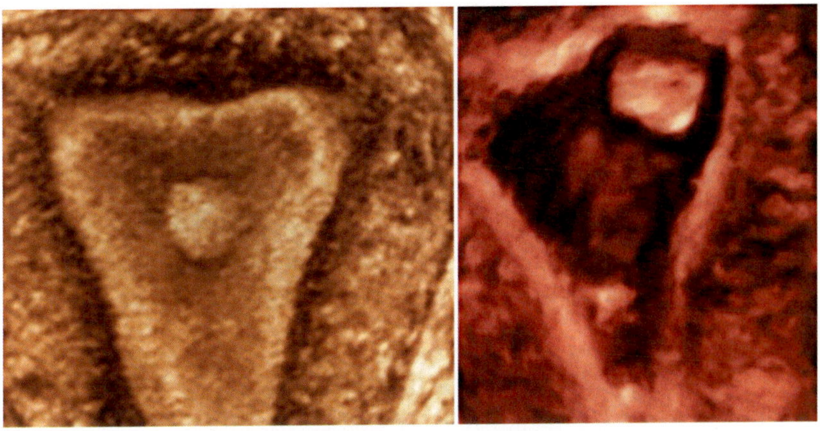

Fig. 38: Three-dimensional ultrasound—polyp.

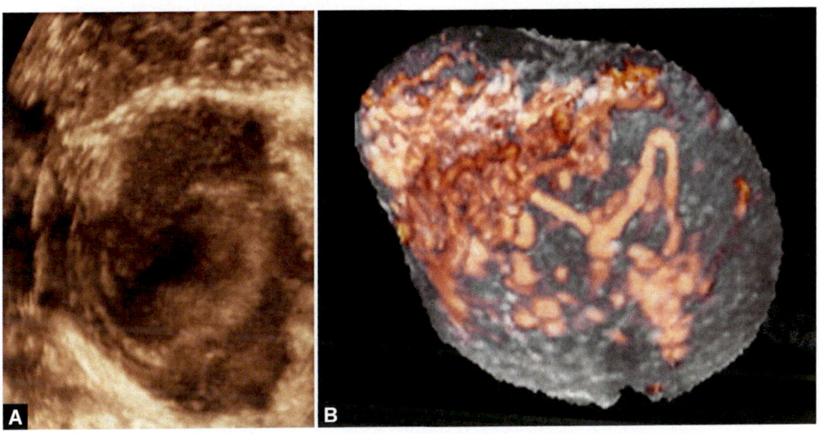

Figs. 39A and B: (A) Carcinoma cervix invading surrounding tissues; (B) *Three-dimensional power Doppler:* Endometrial carcinoma.

pattern of malignancy due to microaneurysms and arteriovenous fistulae **(Figs. 39A and B)**.

OVARIAN LESIONS

Ovarian Cysts

Three-dimensional is essential for any complex cyst of the ovary to define the wall thickness and wall characteristics. Solid projections and septae may sometimes only be defined by 3D US. As 3D may show all three orthogonal planes sometimes the cystic lesions considered to be ovarian cysts on 2D US may discover themselves as hydrosalpinx on 3D multiplanar or surface rendered mode by incomplete septae and sausage shape **(Fig. 40)**.

Three-dimensional PD is absolutely essential for any large or suspicious cyst or cyst in high-risk group females as even simple looking cysts may show tumor vascularity **(Fig. 41)**.

Dermoids

These are most likely of ovarian origin.

On US, they show thick wall with echogenic material in lumen. Regional diffuse bright echoes with or without acoustic shadowing may be seen due to hair clumps or fat in Rokitansky's protuberance. Fluid level due to sebaceous

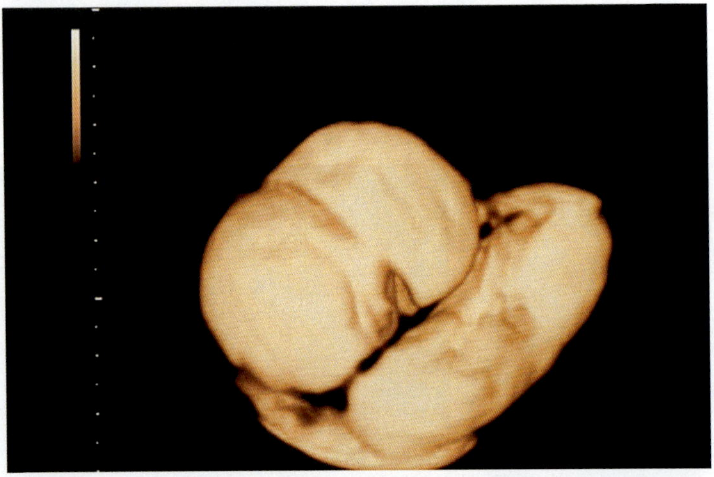

Fig. 40: Hydrosalpinx in inversion mode.

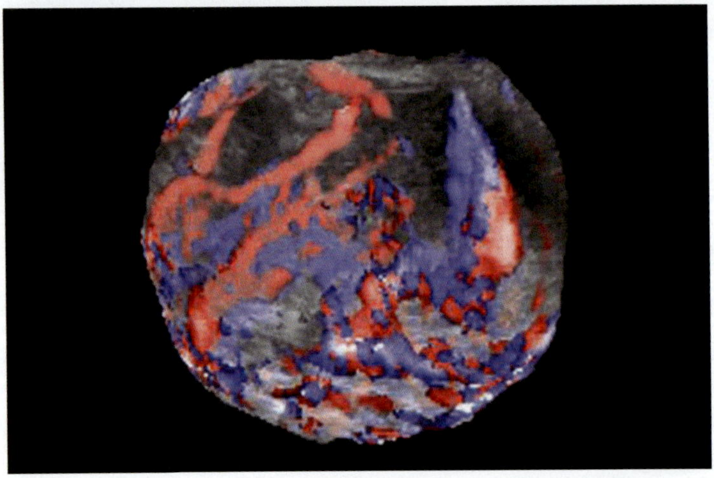

Fig. 41: Three-dimensional power Doppler angiomode rendering showing abundant vascularity of the ovarian mass.

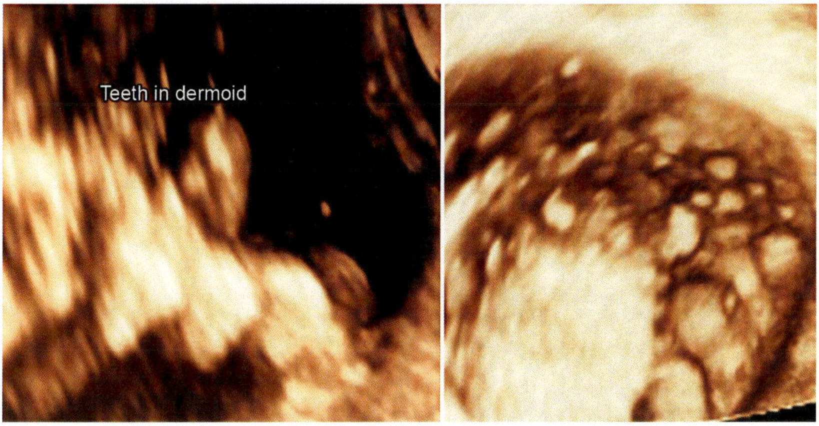

Fig. 42: *Three-dimensional ultrasound:* Dermoid.

material and hyperechoic lines and dots due to hair may be seen. 3D US shows these features better **(Fig. 42)**.

Infertility

Three-dimensional US is complementary to 2D US for the diagnosis of polycystic ovary syndrome (PCOS) for assessment of antral follicle count (AFC) by inversion mode, sonographic automatic volume calculation (SonoAVC) and stromal volume by threshold volume after VOCAL. Rendering by inversion mode is better which will show all antral follicles as solid balls **(Figs. 43A and B)**.

Kupesic has shown correlation in the ovarian stromal flow index (FI) and number of mature oocytes retrieved in an in vitro fertilization (IVF) cycles and pregnancy rates.[21]

Vascularity index (VI), FI, and vascularity flow index (VFI) are 3D PD histogram indices calculated by the computer from the volumes acquired with PD and defined by VOCAL.

- Vascularity index (abundance)—VI
- Flow index (intensity)—FI
- Vascularity flow index (perfusion)—VFI

PREOVULATORY SCAN

Follicular Assessment

Follicular volume is more reliable than follicular diameter. And volumes calculated by 3D VOCAL are more reliable than volumes calculated by 2D US, three diameter formula. The limits of agreement between the volume of the follicular aspirate and 3D volume of the follicle were +0.96 to -0.43 with

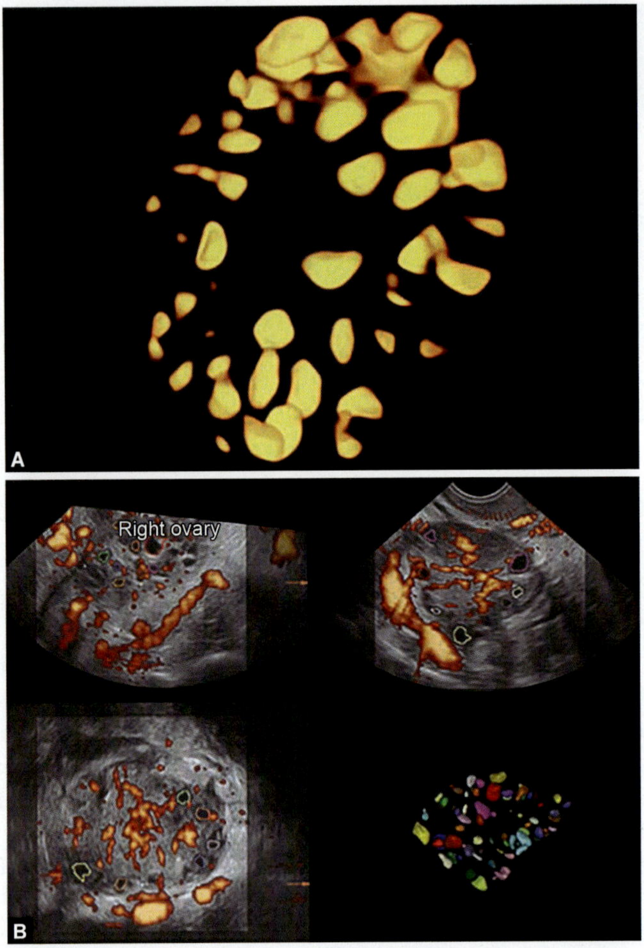

Figs. 43A and B: *Polycystic ovary:* Inversion mode and tomographic ultrasound imaging (TUI).

3D, and +3.47 to –2.42 by 2D volume estimation.[22] But for volumes of follicles of <10 mm diameter, the limits of agreement are too high. Follicular volumes of between 3 and 7 cc are optimum for oocyte retrieval.

Moreover, according to Kurjak et al. on the day of human chorionic gonadotropin (hCG) if cumulus-like echoes is not seen in all three planes in the follicle, it is less likely to be mature fertilizable oocyte.[23] It is possible to see the cumulus only in up to 40% of follicles by 2D US but using 3D rendering we have found that cumulus can be seen in more than 90% of the mature follicles **(Figs. 44A to D)**.

This study was done to find out if 3D and 3D PD indices for assessment of pre-hCG follicle and endometrium are better than 2D and color Doppler. One thousand plus superovulation with intrauterine insemination (IUI)

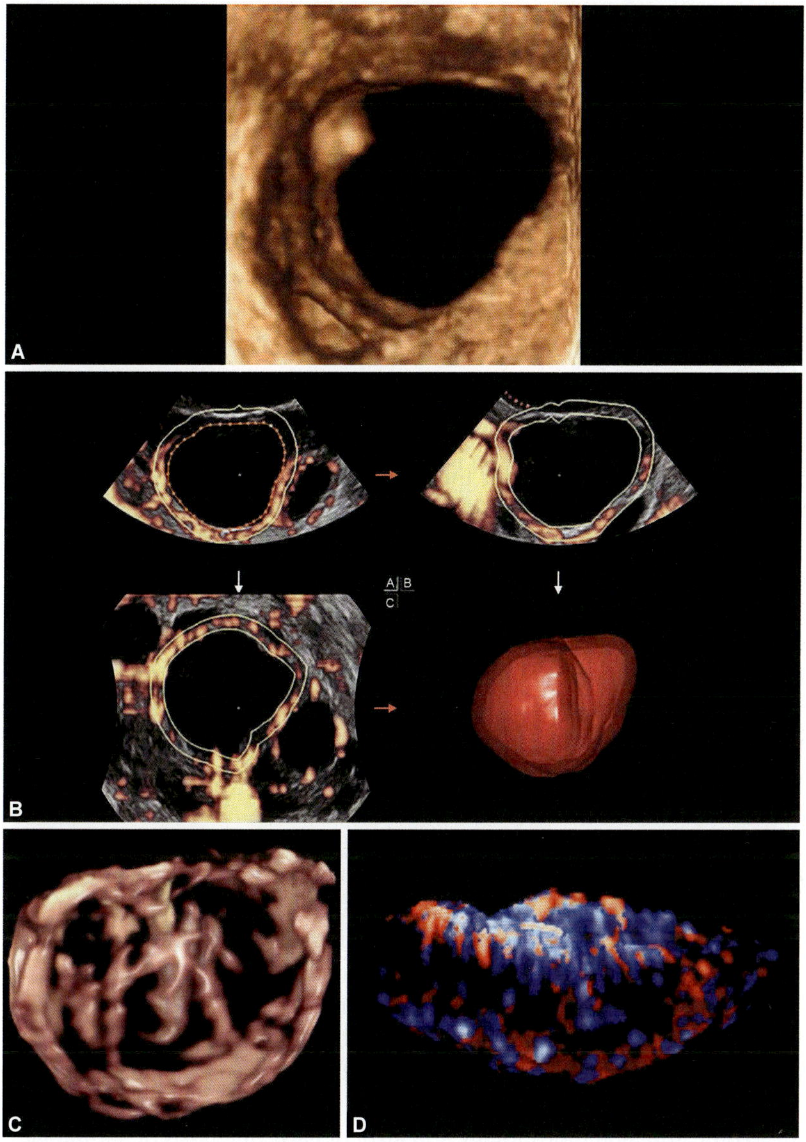

Figs. 44A to D: Virtual organ computer-aided analysis (VOCAL) of follicle with three-dimensional power Doppler (3D PD) angiomode. (A) Cumulus oophorus; (B) Endometrial vascular 3D PD; (C) 3D PD angiomode showing perifollicular vascularity; (D) 3D PD showing endometrial vascularity.

cycles were randomly studied, all of idiopathic infertility. Human chorionic gonadotropin was given for ovulation trigger when follicle and endometrium appeared mature by 2D and color Doppler parameters. 3D and 3D PD of follicle and endometrium was done for all patients.

We have found that even when 2D and color Doppler parameters were normal only a percentage of patients conceived who had following endometrial and follicular parameters.

Follicular volume 3-7-5 cc, follicular VI 6-20, follicular FI > 27, endometrial volume > 3, endometrial FI > 20, and endometrial VFI > 5.[24]

Similar values are suggested by different authors. More than 2.5 mL endometrial volume before hCG has a significantly higher pregnancy rates. Median values for a favorable endometrium is 4.28 ± 1.9 mL.

Volume US—VOCAL and color histogram—VI, FI, and VFI values in our experience have proved to be of added value in evaluation of ovarian response, endometrial receptivity, and pre-hCG follicular and endometrial evaluation. Though larger studies may be needed to standardize the techniques and values.

Ovarian volumes may also be useful in predicting the risk of ovarian hyperstimulation syndrome in the preovulatory phase. Even when the age of the patient and total number of follicles are similar, the ovarian volume was significantly higher in the patients who developed OHSS (271 ± 87 versus 157.30 ± 54.20 mL).[25]

Full potential of 3D is yet to be completely explored. Though storing volumes and studying predefined sections later on by different specialists is a boon. It is important to think and find out as to what information you want out of the stored volume and how to bring it out. Sectional plane studies such as CT or MRI can be done at a much lower cost, noninvasively and is much less troublesome to the patient. Initial scanning time may be longer but with increasing practice it decreases.

Volume US is an indispensable tool in any center for prenatal diagnosis. 3D sonography is a fundamental tool for complete neurosonographic examination of the fetus and can help to a better understanding of complex mechanisms leading to normal or abnormal brain development.

Rendering modes will allow better definition of anatomic spatial relationship between spine and ribs, visualization of clavicles and scapula, evaluation of abdominal masses diagnosed by 2D, and anomalies of genitalia. Multiplanar mode is useful for evaluation of thoracic vertebra and sternum.

Three-dimensional US is finding a new role in understanding of normal embryonic and fetal morphology and also for early diagnosis of pathologies.

3D-4D techniques are seen as powerful complement to conventional US, but not a substitution to it. 3D US is not a substitute for 2D US but is a useful complementary technique. All 3D tools must be used complementary with PD. It must be offered to all high-risk patients.

REFERENCES

1. Kurjak A, Kupesic S, Kosuta-Ivanevic M. Three dimensional transvaginal ultrasound improves measurement of nuchal translucency. J Perinat Med. 1999;27:97-102.

2. Eppel W, Christof W, Frigo P, Lee A. Three versus two dimensional ultrasound for nuchal translucency thickness measurements: comparison of feasibility and levels of agreement. Prenat Diagn. 2001;21:596-601.
3. Peralta CFA, Falcon O, Wegrzyn P, Faro C, Nicolaides KH. Assessment of the gap between the fetal nasal bones at 11 to 13 + 6 weeks of gestation by three dimensional ultrasound. Ultrasound Obstet Gynecol. 2005;25(5):464-7.
4. Merz E, Weber G, Bahlmann F, Miric-Tesanic D. Application of transvaginal and abdominal three dimensional ultrasound for detection or exclusion of fetal malformations of fetal face. Ultrasound Obstet Gynecol. 1997;9:237-43.
5. Rotten D, Levaillant JM. Two- and three-dimensional sonographic assessment of the fetal face. Analysis of cleft lip, alveolus and palate. Ultrasound Obstet Gynecol. 2004;24(4):402-11.
6. Pilu G, Segata M. A novel technique for visualization of the normal and cleft fetal secondary palate: angled insonation and three-dimensional ultrasound. Ultrasound Obstet Gynecol. 2007;29(2):166-9.
7. Kurjak A, Azumendi G, Andonotopo W, Salihagic-Kadic A. Three- and four-dimensional ultrasonography for the structural and functional evaluation of the fetal face. Am J Obstet Gynecol. 2007;196(1):16-28.
8. Campbell S, Lees C, Moscoso G, Hall P. Ultrasound antenatal diagnosis of cleft palate by a new technique: the 3D "reverse face" view. Ultrasound Obstet Gynecol. 2005;25:12-8.
9. Sleurs E, Goncalves LF, Jhonson A, J Espinoza, P Devers, T Chaiworapongsa, et al. First trimester ultrasonic findings in a fetus with frontonasal malformation. J Matern Fetal Neonatal Med. 2004;16:187-97.
10. Paladini D, Morra T, Teodoro A, A Lamberti, F Tremolaterra, P Martinelli. Objective diagnosis of micrognathia in the fetus: The Jaw Index. Obstet Gynecol. 1999;93:382-6.
11. Dikkeboom CM, Roelfsema NM, Van Adrichem LN, Wladimiroff JW. The role of three-dimensional ultrasound in visualizing the fetal cranial sutures and fontanels during the second half of pregnancy. Ultrasound Obstet Gynecol. 2004;24(4):412-6.
12. Gonzales-Gomez F, Salamanca A, Padilla MC, Camara M, Sabatel RM. Alobar holoprosencephalic embryo detected via transvaginal sonography. Eur J Obstet Gynecol Reprod Biol. 1992;47:266-70.
13. Paladini D, Volpe P. Posterior fossa and vermian morphometry in the characterization of fetal cerebellar abnormalities: a perspective three dimensional ultrasound study. Ultrasound Obstet Gynecol. 2006;27:482-9.
14. Roelfsema NM, Grijseels EW, Hop WC, Wladimiroff JW. Three-dimensional sonography of prenatal skull-base development. Ultrasound Obstet Gynecol. 2007;29:372-7.
15. Roelf NM, Hop WC, van Adrichem LN, Wladimiroff JW. Craniofacial variability index in utero: a three-dimensional ultrasound study. Ultrasound Obstet Gynecol. 2007;29:258-64.
16. Kurjak A, Pooh RK, Merce LT, Carrera JM, Salihagic-Kadic A, Andonotopo W, et al. Structural and functional early human development assessed by three dimensional and four dimensional sonography. Fertil Steril. 2005;84:1285-99.
17. Gerards FA, Twisk JW, Bakker M, Barkhof F, van Vugt JMG. Fetal lung volume: three-dimensional ultrasonography compared with magnetic resonance imaging. Ultrasound Obstet Gynecol. 2007;29(5):533-6.
18. Fang KH, Wu JL, Chen M, Yeh GP, Chou PH, Hsu J-C. Prenatal sonographic features of hypospadia: two- and three-dimensional findings. Taiwan J Obstet Gynecol. 2006;45(1):53-5.
19. Benacerraf BR, Bromley B, Shipp TS. Can 3D volume sets alone be used to detect fetal malformations? New Jersey, United States: John Wiley & Sons; 2006.

20. Bega G, Wapner R, Lev-Toaff A, Kuhlman K. Diagnosis of conjoined twins at 10 weeks using three-dimensional ultrasound: a case report. Ultrasound Obstet Gynecol. 2000;16(4):388-90.
21. Kupesic S, Kurjak A. Predictors of IVF outcome by three-dimensional ultrasound. Hum Reprod. 2002;17:950-5.
22. Kyei-Mensah A, Maconochie N, Zaidi J, Pittrof R, Campbell S, Tan SL. Transvaginal three-dimensional ultrasound: reproducibility of ovarian and endometrial volume measurements. Fertil Steril. 1996;66:718-22.
23. Poehl M, Hohlagschwandtner M, Doerner V, Dillinger B, Feichtinger W. Cumulus assessment by three-dimensional ultrasound for in vitro fertilization. Ultrasound Obstet Gynecol. 2000;16:251-3.
24. Sonal P, Nagori CB. Can 3D PD be a better tool for assessing the pre-hCG follicle and endometrium. New Jersey, United States: John Wiley & Sons; 2006.
25. Oyesanya OA, Parsons JH, Collins WP, Campbell S. Total ovarian volume before human chorionic gonadotrophin administration for ovulation induction may predict the hyperstimulation syndrome. Hum Reprod. 1995;10:3211-2.

Index

Page numbers followed by *b* refer to box, *f* refer to figure, *fc* refer to flowchart, and *t* refer to table.

A

Abdomen 298, 314, 499
  axial section of 312*f*
  coronal section of 316*f*
  transverse section of 313*f*
Abdominal abnormalities 330
Abdominal cavity 245
Abdominal circumference
  measurement 438*f*
  stomach section for 298
Abdominal diameter 441, 442
Abdominal ectopic pregnancy 286, 287*f*
Abdominal scan 203
Abnormal early pregnancy, evaluation of 279
Abortion 142
  early missed 280
Abruption, chronic 436
Absent central hyperechoic 206*f*
Absent corpus callosum 382*f*
Abstinence 6
Achondroplasia 333, 334*f*
Acidemia 459
Acidosis 459
Acquired thrombophilia 150
Acquired uterine abnormalities 208, 505
Acrania 293, 294*f*, 323, 325, 326*f*
Active married life 4
Acupuncture 131
Adenomyomas 209
Adenomyosis 209, 213, 234, 506*f*
  B-mode of 143*f*
  uterus 214*f*
Adenosine triphosphate 447
Adnexa 195, 246
  thickening of 195
Adnexal diseases 230
Adnexal lesions 230, 231
Adnexal malignancy, detection of 245*t*
Adnexal mass 285
Adrenal dysfunction 23
  manifestation of 23
Adrenal glands 16
Adrenal hyperplasia, congenital 123
Adrenocorticotropic hormone 16
Agonists 33
Alcohol 120
  bad effects of 120
Alloimmunity 154, 162
Alpha-fetoprotein 445
Alyce's forceps 69
American Fertility Society 138
American Thyroid Association 159
Amniotic band syndrome 334
Amniotic fluid index 317, 318, 439
  assessment of 319*f*, 440*f*, 443
Amniotic membrane 291
Anastrozole 42
Androgen 38, 125
  diffuses 56
Androstenedione 16
Anechoic myometrial cysts 213
Anemia 338
Anencephaly 323, 325
Aneuploidies 351
Angiomode 484
Angular pregnancy 504*f*
Antagonist 26
  protocol 54
Antagonist-agonist protocol 55
Anteverted anteflexed uterus 189*f*
Anteverted retroflexed uterus 189*f*
Antiandrogenic properties 26
Antibodies, presence of 73
Anticytokine effect 145
Antiestrogenic agent 26
Antiestrogenic effect 29, 30
Antigen-receptor interactions 155
Anti-inflammatory drugs 126
Anti-müllerian hormone 17*t*, 18, 54, 55, 69, 114, 259
  applications of 19
Antinuclear antibody 147, 148
Antioxidants 127, 128
  dosage of 132
Antiphospholipid antibodies,
  diagnosis of 146
  syndrome 435

Antiphospholipid syndrome 145, 162
Antiserotonin agents 126
Antithyroid antibody 147
Antral follicle 17
  arrangement of 254
  in vitro fertility cycles 260
  number of 254, 260
Antral follicle count 12, 48, 49, 69, 255, 260
  assessment of 509
Aortic arch 298
Aortic end-diastolic flow, absent 453*f*
Aortic isthmus 457*f*
  flow 455
Apert syndrome 366
Aplastic uterus 207
Arachnoid cyst 369, 370
Arginine 129
Aromatase 38
  inhibitors 127
Artifacts 183
Artificial insemination, failed 63
Ascites 334
Aseptic technique 73
Aspirin 34, 147, 152
  low dose 34
Assisted reproductive technology 5, 53, 90
  protocols for 53
Asthenospermia 128
Atrioventricular septal defect 329, 329*f*
Atypical endometrium 253
Autocrine-paracrine mechanism 127
Autoimmune diseases 441
Autosomal recessive trait 150

B

Basal body temperature chart 87
Baseline scoring system 49*t*
Basic probe movements 186
Basic transvaginal sonography 173
Beak sign 231, 249*f*
Benzyl alcohol 90
Beta-human chorionic gonadotropin 245, 279, 322
Bicarbonate 75
Bicorporeal septate uterus 203, 204*f*
Bicorporeal uterus 140*f*, 141, 188, 202, 203, 205, 205*f*
  complete 204*f*
Binocular diameter 307
Biophysical profile 443
  role of 461
Biopsy attachment 185*f*
Biparietal diameter 300, 369, 375, 437, 441
Bird's nest appearance 235*f*
Bladder 298
  exstrophy of 332
  with dimple 207*f*
Blake's pouch cyst 372
Blastocyst transfer 51
Blood
  flow 261
  vessels 182*f*
Body mass index 40, 49, 106
Bones, short long 351
Bowel atresia 351
Brain development 387
Breast and ovarian cancer 30
Breast cancer, risk of 30
Broad ligament 245
  fibroid 230, 247
Bromocriptine 11, 32
Butterfly sign 387

C

Caffeine 120
Calculating risk 353
Captopril 126
Cardiac abnormalities 294, 329, 338, 340
Cardiac activity 290, 291
Cardiac anomaly 352
Cardiac disease 435
Cardiovascular abnormalities 323
Carotenoids 131
Carpenter syndrome 366
Cavum septi pellucidi 372, 373*f*
Cavum septum pellucidum 300, 366, 369, 371
Cell-free fetal deoxyribonucleic acid 354
Central hyperechoic mucosa 242
Central nervous system 494
  abnormalities of 362
Centrifuge machine 78
Cephalometric analysis 309
Cerebellar hypoplasia 372
Cerebellar transverse diameter 375
Cerebellum 305, 366, 371, 377
  banana sign of 306, 377, 378*f*

Cerebral artery
- Doppler, middle 449
- middle 373, 374*f*, 447, 452*f*, 459
- resistance, low middle 453*f*

Cerebral circulation 373, 373*f*
Cerebral hypoxia 453
Cerebral index 441
Cerebral vasculature 496*f*
- study of 373

Cerebroplacental ratio 451
Cervical
- anomalies 199
- aplasia, unilateral 207
- factor, counseling for 5
- fibroid 227*f*
- glands 191
- incompetence 144
- index 144
- lesions 208, 225
- malignancies 225, 506
- mucosa 191
- polyps 227*f*
- pregnancy 285*f*
- secretions 6

Cervix 29, 189, 191, 195
- carcinoma 507*f*
- normal 207
- normal double 208*f*
- single normal 208*f*
- with septum 208*f*

Chaotic vascular architecture 239
Chest 498, 499*f*
Chocolate cyst 234
Chorioangioma 295, 295*f*
Chorionic tissue, abnormal 221
Chorionic villus sampling 357
Choroid plexus 368
- cyst 301*f*, 348, 348*f*, 349*t*

Chromosomal abnormalities 152, 436
Chromosomal anomalies 337
- fetal screening for 321

Chromosomal markers 334
Cilia, movements of 7
Cingulate gyrus 382
Circle of Willis 374, 374*f*, 380
Cirrhosis 472
Cisterna magna 305, 366, 371, 372, 377, 377*f*
- depth of 375

Cleft lip 327, 328*f*, 491*f*
Cleft palate 323, 327, 328*f*, 491*f*
Clinical pregnancy rate 55
Clomiphene 26, 34, 166
- failure patients 47
- resistant patients 46
- treatment, extended 31

Clomiphene citrate 26, 32-35, 42, 45, 63, 107, 110, 122, 124
- contraindications 27
- cycles 13
- dose of 28*t*, 166
- indications of 26
- mechanism of action 26
- monitoring 28
- resistant 39
- risks of 30
- side effects 29
- treatment
  - alternatives 31
  - regimes 27

Club feet 334*f*, 501*f*
Coenzyme Q10 130
- natural source of 130

Cogwheel sign 245
Collagen vascular disease 435
Color Doppler 177, 197, 212, 266, 277
- aliasing in 183

Common testicular abnormalities 469
Conception rates 115*f*, 115*t*
Congenital anomalies 30
Congenital infections 351
Congenital uterine abnormalities 504
Conjoined twins 503
Contingent sequential screening 358
Corifollitropin alpha 56
Coronal plane 298, 314, 379, 385
Coronal spine 386*f*
Corpus callosum 368, 382
- agenesis of 368*f*

Corpus luteal 278*f*
- function 15
- normal 88*f*

Corpus luteum 84, 232, 233, 233*f*, 246, 247*f*, 270, 271*f*, 277, 278*f*
- rescue of 86

Cranial abnormalities 493
Cranial sutures 494*f*
Craniofacial variability index 496

Crown-rump length 335, 435,
  measurement of 335*f*
Cryptorchidism 469
Cumulus oophorus 265*f*, 511*f*
Cyclopia 328
Cyproheptadine hydrochloric acid 126
Cystic atrophy 225*f*
Cystic hygroma 335, 340, 340*f*
  milder cases of 340
Cystic lesion 249*f*
  in prostate, large 478*f*
Cysts with internal echogenicities 231, 232
Cytochrome 38
Cytomegalovirus 351, 436

D

Dandy-Walker
  malformation 372, 372*f*, 377
  variation 372
Degenerated heterogeneous fibroid 211*f*
Dehydroandrosterone 16
Dehydroepiandrosterone 16
  sulfate 15, 31
Density gradient methods 79
Deoxyribonucleic acid 127, 154
Dermoids 237, 238*f*, 508
Dexamethasone 31
Dextrocardia 294
Diabetes mellitus 159
  severe 435
Diastematomyelia 387, 387*f*
Dichorionic diamniotic twins 287*f*, 503*f*
Diencephalon, development of 494
Diethylstilbestrol 139, 199*f*
Doppler angle 181
Doppler assessment, technique of 448
Doppler findings, obstetric management on 459
Doppler settings 177
  making correct 179
Double bubble sign 331, 331*f*
Double intrauterine insemination 68
Down's fetuses 340
Down's syndrome 321, 342, 343, 349, 357, 358*t*
  diagnosis of 342
Drugs 120
  dosage of 131
Dual trigger 99
Ductus arch 298
Ductus venosus 341, 358, 459
  flow 335, 341, 341*f*, 343
    abnormal 341*f*
    normal 454*f*, 456*f*
Duodenal atresia 323, 331, 352
Duodenum, dilated 500*f*
Dysmorphic uterus 139, 140, 199, 201*f*
Dysovulatory infertility 9, 26, 62

E

Ear
  low placed 329*f*
  short low placed 323, 328
Earle's balance
  media 74
  salt 75
Ebstein's anomaly 295*f*, 329, 329*f*
Echogenic cardiac focus 349
Echogenic mass 238*f*
Echogenic walls 247*f*
Ectopic pregnancies 7, 245, 247*f*, 280, 504
Effervescent progesterone vaginal tablets 92*f*
Eight weeks pregnancy 292*f*
Ejaculation, disorders of 123
Ejaculatory ducts 477
  fibrosis of 479
Ellis-Van creveld syndrome 372
Embryo 7, 29, 278
  transfer 252
Empiric therapy 124
Encephalocele 325*f*
Enclomiphene 26
  proportion of 26
End-diastolic flow in umbilical artery, absent 452*f*
Endocrine
  causes 158
  workup 23
Endocrinological reports, normal 8
Endometrial biopsy 29, 87
Endometrial calcification 221, 223*f*
  flecks of 217*f*
Endometrial carcinoma 221
Endometrial cavitiy 203, 213, 220
  blood in 221*f*

fresh blood in 221*f*
one-third 203*f*
Endometrial fibroid 218, 219*f*
Endometrial grading 265
Endometrial hyperplasia 215, 218*f*
Endometrial lesions 208, 220
differential diagnosis of 217
Endometrial malignancy 221
Endometrial mass 224*f*
Endometrial metaplasia 223
Endometrial morphology 189
Endometrial pathologies 215, 220
Endometrial polyp 216, 218*f*
Endometrial stroma 225
Endometrial synechiea 143*f*
Endometrial thickness 278
Endometrial tuberculosis 7
Endometrioid tumors 237
Endometrioma 232, 234, 235*f*
diagnosis of 235
Endometriomyometrial junction 217*f*
thickness of 191
Endometriosis 157, 234
cases of 157
mild to moderate 62
Endometritis 215
acute 215, 216*f*
chronic 215
Endometrium 29, 189, 197, 215, 223, 265, 266*f*, 268, 270, 272
effects of 223
mature 264
normal multilayered 190*f*
persistently thin 215
poor 32
thick 216*f*
thin 217*f*
Endoscopy, normal 8
Epidermal growth factor 84
Epididymal ductal ectasia 477*f*
Epididymal lesions 473
Epididymis 467*f*
Epithelial tumors 237, 238
Equipment settings 173
Estimated fetal weight 438
Estradiol benzoate 88
Estrogen 26, 31, 38
therapy 472
European Society for Gynecological Endoscopy 139, 198
European Society of Human Reproduction and Embryology 139

F

Facial abnormalities 490
Facial angle, inferior 309
Facial anomalies 327
Fallopian tube 245, 282
inflammation of 242
Fallot's tetralogy 329
Feet, normal 501*f*
Female genital tract anomalies, classification of 139*t*
Femur length 316, 441, 442
Fertility 251
treatment, withholding 19
Fetal blood pressure, continuous rise in 446
Fetal cardiac output, continuous rise in 446
Fetal central nervous system 495
Fetal faces 490*f*
Fetal growth restriction 435
management of 435
Fetal head-brain, primary assessment of 363
Fetal heart rate 455
Fetal kidneys 333
Fetal medicine foundation 297, 322*f*, 335, 337
Fetal organ biometry 441
Fetal pole 290
Fetal spine, qualitative evaluation of 374
Fetal thrombophilia 151
Fetal well-being, assessment of 458
Fetus scratching ear 497*f*
Fibrinogen deficiency 150
Fibrinolytic factors 149
Fibroid 209, 213*f*, 476, 505, 506*f*
classification of 211
cystic degeneration of 211*f*
location of 212, 212*f*
three-dimensional ultrasound of 143*f*, 506*f*
typical of 218
Folate 127
Folic acid 128
Follicle
fertilization of 264
mature 262, 262*f*, 264

Follicle-stimulating hormone 11, 12*f*, 38, 45, 48*f*, 50, 51, 55, 64*f*, 107, 122, 125, 166, 252*f*, 256
Follicular atresia 257
Follicular cyst 232, 232*f*
Follicular growth, monitoring of 273
Follicular maturation 56
Follicular maturing drugs 159
Follicular maturity 13
Follicular ring sign 236, 237*f*
Follicular volume 512
Folliculogenesis 38
Follitropin alpha 53
Forearm, absent 502*f*
Frontomaxillary facial angle 308, 344, 344*f*
Frozen embryo transfer 94
Functional rudimentary horn 206*f*

G

G sperm 77
Galactorrhea 15, 32
Galen aneurysm, vein of 369, 370, 370*f*
Gastroschisis 332, 332*f*
Generalized cystic pattern 257
Genetic causes 152, 162
Genetic scan 323
Genital tract
  infections 123
  tuberculosis 479
Genital tuberculosis 479
Genitourinary anomalies 332
Genomic hybridization, comparative 152
Germ cell failure 22
Gestational age 297, 316, 435
  small for 435
Gestational sac 281, 285, 285*f*, 288, 352
  location of 282
  measuring 288*f*
  normally implanted 282*f*
  volume 289*f*
Giant mitochondria 84
Glucocorticoids 31, 110, 148
Glutamine, substitution of 150
Glutathione 129
Gonadotropin 33, 42, 45, 47, 53, 58, 63-65, 109, 110, 122
  addition of metformin to 109
  agonist 113
  antagonist protocol 112
  deficiency, severe 56
  low doses of 106
  specific bioactivity of 110, 110*t*
  stimulated cycles 97
  theory, two-cell-two 56
  types of 52*t*
Gonadotropin therapy 46
  indications of 46
  principles of 46
Gonadotropin-releasing hormone 12*f*, 26, 54, 55, 65
  agonist 13, 33, 98, 99, 505
    and antagonist, role of 65
Granulosa cell 18
  tumors 20
Great arteries, transposition of 330
Growth restriction intervention trial 458
Gynecological couch 184

H

Haematococcus pluvialis 128
Hairballs in cyst 238*f*
Hampered villous microcirculation 446
Hand, movements of 497*f*
Hands and fingers, normal 501*f*
Head
  circumference 441, 443
  qualitative
    evaluation of 364
    examination of 366, 375
  shape and calvarium 366
Heart, four chamber of 298, 310, 310*f*
Helicobacter pylori 145
Hemiuterus 142, 188, 205
Hemivertebrae 386
Hemorrhagic cyst 232, 233, 246
Heparin 147
  dose of 148
  inhibits 152
  mechanism of action of 148
Hepatitis C 145
Hernia, diaphragmatic 323, 330, 331*f*, 498
Heterogeneous myometrium 214*f*
Heterogeneous testis, small 471*f*
Hippocampal gyrus 373, 373*f*
Holoprosencephaly 294*f*, 324*f*
Hormone-dependent cancers 40

Human chorionic gonadotropin 32, 41, 47*f*, 48*f*, 55, 64*f*-66*f*, 85, 86, 99, 112*f*, 124, 125, 152, 166, 264, 510
 disadvantages of 95
 supplementation 94, 160
 trigger 98
Human immunodeficiency virus 82, 145
Human menopausal gonadotropin 22, 45, 52, 63, 110, 111, 123
Human serum albumin 74
Hydrocephalus 301*f*, 326
Hydrocephaly, severe 369
Hydrosalpinx 243
Hydrothorax 334
Hyperandrogenism 253
Hyperechoic bowel 350, 351*f*
Hyperhomocysteinemia 150
Hyperplasia 215
Hyperprolactinemia 22, 123, 160
Hyperstimulation, suspected risk of 14
Hypertension 441
 chronic 435
 pregnancy-induced 148, 435, 447*f*
Hypervolemia 339
Hypoechoic cervical glands 192*f*
Hypoechoic heterogeneous testis 472*f*
Hypogonadotropic hypogonadism 46, 56, 122
Hypopituitary disorders 472
Hypoplastic uterus 201*f*
Hypoproteinemia 338
Hypothalamo-pituitary
 dysfunction 96
 ovarian axis 11
 testicular axis 12*f*
Hypothalamus 15, 26
Hypoxemia, stage of 450

I

Idiopathic infertility, treatment for 8
Idiopathic normogonadotropic oligozoospermia 125
Idiopathic oligozoospermia 125
Immature follicles 257
Immunization, active 155
Immunological causes 123, 436
In situ hybridization, multiplex fluorescence 152
In vitro fertilization 11, 18, 33, 41, 49, 62, 120, 509
 counseling for 9
In vitro maturation 116
Inadequate corpus luteal function 272*f*
Inadequate trophoblastic invasion 446
Indomethacin 126
Infection 157, 436
Infertile couple
 counseling of 3
 hormonal assessment of 11
Infertile women, investigations for 11
Infertility 509
Infertility management 62, 166
 backbone of 3
 drugs 166
 investigations 167
 meaningless for 11
 prescription 169
 procedures 168
 ultrasonography 169
Infertility treatment
 assessment for 251
 regular 5
Infrequent anomalies 207
Iniencephaly 323, 326, 326*f*
Innate immune system 154
Insemination, timing of 68
Insulin
 lowering drugs 108
 resistance 20
  severe 20
Insulin-like growth factor 18, 38, 84, 114, 259
Intact hypoechoic endometriomyometrial junction 190*f*
Intensive luteal support 99
Intercourse, continuous unprotected 4
Internal carbohydrate complexity 53
International ovarian tumor analysis 230
Intracranial translucency 306*f*, 327, 346, 346*f*
Intracytoplasmic sperm injection 14, 75, 109, 120, 169
Intramuscular progesterone 90
Intraovarian cystic lesion 241*f*
Intraovarian lesion 231*f*
Intrauterine adhesions 144

Intrauterine contraceptive device 221
Intrauterine gestational sac 285
Intrauterine growth restriction 303, 332, 372, 460*t*
- baby, history of 435
- risk factors for 441
- ultrasound diagnosis of 441

Intrauterine insemination 8, 27, 42, 47, 49, 62, 69, 73, 78, 112*f*, 121, 252, 510
- counseling for 8
- indications of 62
- steps of 63

Intravenous immunoglobulin 148
Intravenous pyelography 138
Ishidori's regimen 167
Isoechoic walls 247*f*
Isomerism 330

J

Jejunal atresia 334

K

Ketotifen 126
Kidneys 298
Klinefelter's syndrome 472

L

L-acetylcarnitine 129
Laparoscopic ovarian drilling 114
Laparoscopic tubal ligation 8
Laparoscopic-assisted myomectomy 144
Last menstrual period 435
L-carnitine 129
Left ventricle, echogenic focus in 349*f*
Left ventricular outflow tract 298, 310
Leiomyosarcoma 209, 212
Lemon sign 378
Lemon skull 301*f*, 367*f*
- sign 378*f*

Lenses 298
Lesions
- benign 242*t*
- malignant 242*t*

Letrozole 38, 42, 45, 65, 107, 108, 166
- advantages of 39, 41
- characteristics of 39
- doses 40
- indications 39
- side effects 41
- step-up protocol 41
- stimulated cycle 97
- therapy, extended 41

Leukemia inhibitory factor 84, 98, 155
Leuprolide acetate 54
Limb 298, 315
- abnormalities 293, 499
- body wall complex 334
- reduction abnormalities 324, 333

Lip 298, 307
- lower 308*f*

Lissencephaly, absence indicates 373
Localized fluid collection 195
Low birth weight 435
Low pulse repetition frequency 183*f*
Low resistance ovarian stromal flow 259*f*
Low-dose protocol, chronic 48, 65, 111
Lower limbs, fusion of 334
Low-molecular-weight heparin 147
Luteal gap 98
Luteal phase defect 27, 84, 159, 272, 272*f*, 273*f*
- cause of 96
- diagnosis of 87
- pathophysiology of 85

Luteal phase estradiol 85
Luteal support, duration of 101
Luteinized unruptured follicle 232, 233, 234*f*, 271, 272*f*
Luteinizing hormone 11, 12*f*, 26, 38, 45, 56, 65, 106, 252*f*, 256
- ceiling effect 57
- releasing hormone 39
- supplementation 56, 57
- threshold 56

Lycopene 131
Lymphatic drainage, development of 338

M

Macroadenoma 15
Magicut 485*f*
Male infertility 467
- laboratory investigations for 21
- management of 22
- medical management in 120, 121
- ultrasonography in 465

Male subfertility 62
Marfan syndrome 366
Mass lesion 190, 195
Maxilla, plane of 307
Maxillary plane 297
Mayer-Rokitansky-Küster-Hauser syndrome 207
Meckel-Gruber syndrome 372
Meconium ileus 351
Mega cystitis 324
Megacystis 333*f*, 350
Meigs' syndrome 236
Meiotic division 45
Meningocele 386*f*
Menstrual cycle 252*f*
  phases of 191
Mesencephalon, development of 494
Metformin 33, 34, 109
  after conception 109
  alternatives 109
  effectiveness of 109
  therapy 20
Microadenoma 15
Micrognathia 323, 328, 328*f*
Microlithiasis 472
Midline vessels on Doppler 383*f*
Midluteal serum progesterone 14
Miscarriage 30
Misconception 6
Modern infertility practice 7
Modulating secretory transformation 84*b*
Motile sperms 73
Motility, decrease 79
Müllerian abnormalities 198
  classification for 198, 200*f*
Müllerian duct 198, 205
  abnormalities 138, 198, 199, 202
    class U0 199
    class U1 199
    incidence of 198
  incidence of 198
  normal fusion of 202
Müllerian malformations 205
Multifollicular development 41
  causes 26
Multiple anomaly syndromes 436
Multiple antral follicles 253, 254
Multiple follicles 14
Multiple gestation 287*f*, 436
  early detection of 279, 286
Multiple pregnancy 30, 65
  early 280
Myocardial performance index 461
Myomas 142
Myometrial calcification 217*f*
Myometrial cysts 215
Myometrial lesions 208
Myometrium 190, 209, 213, 215
  anterior 193
  homogenicity of 190
  innermost layer of 189
  posterior 193

N

Nabothian cysts 225, 227*f*
Nasal bone 298, 327, 336, 342, 343, 343*f*, 346*f*
  length 308, 335
Natural cycle, luteal support in 96
Negative predictive value 235
Neural tube anomalies 324
Neuromuscular defects 338
Nonapoptotic sperm selection 82
Non-assisted reproductive technology 167
Non-hyperactivated sperms 79*f*
Non-in vitro fertilization 95
Nonseptated clear cysts 231
Noonan's syndrome 340
Nostrils 308*f*
Nuchal fold thickness 339
Nuchal scan 488
Nuchal translucency 327, 335, 338, 339, 343, 346*f*, 354, 489*f*
  causes of increased 337
  measuring 335
Nuclear channel system 84

O

Occupational and environmental hazards 120
Ocular abnormalities 323, 328
Oligoasthenospermia, antioxidants for 128*t*
Oligoasthenoteratozoospermia 21
Oligoasthenozoospermia, role in 129
Oligomenorrhea 160
Oligospermia 128

Oligozoospermia 124*b*
  medical management of 120
Omega-3 fatty acids 131
Omphalocele 313*f*, 324, 331, 331*f*
Oocyte numbers, reduced 12
Open spinal canal 386
  defect 386*f*, 387*f*
Optimal fertility 17
Oral contraceptive 100
  treatment with 34
Oral sustained-release tablets 89
Orchitis 472, 472*f*
Outpatient department 3
Ovarian area 258
Ovarian artery perfusion 273
Ovarian cancer 242*t*
Ovarian causes, counseling for 8
Ovarian cysts 507
Ovarian drilling 113, 168
  advantage of 113
  indications of 113
  newer methods for 115
Ovarian ectopic pregnancy 246, 285, 286*f*
Ovarian fibroma 236*f*
Ovarian follicular development 26
Ovarian hyperstimulation syndrome 14, 30, 47, 55
  controlled 19, 40, 47
  high risk of 106
  incidence of 65
  risk of 41, 168
Ovarian lesions 230, 231, 507
  classification of 231
Ovarian response 56*t*
  predictors of 55
Ovarian stimulation, controlled 18, 45, 55
Ovarian stroma 197
  resistance index 48
Ovarian stromal flow, measurement of 261
Ovarian suppression, assess 13
Ovarian torsion 237*f*
Ovarian volume 48, 258, 512
Ovaries 29, 203, 245
  baseline scan of 252
  enlarged 253
  simple cyst of 232
  three-dimensional ultrasound of 258*f*
Ovulation
  mechanism of induction of 38
  physiology of 46
Ovum 29
  donation 69

P

Panhypopituitarism 22
Paramesonephric ducts 198
Paraovarian cyst 230, 247, 248, 249*f*
Parental lymphocyte immunization 156
Partial mole 221
Partial septum-subseptate uterus 202
Peak systolic velocity 49, 66*f*, 277, 450
Pedunculated fibromas 236
Pelvic inflammatory disease 242, 244*f*
Pelvic mass 188
Pelvic organs
  anatomical relationship of 175
  orientation of 184
  sonography of 184
Pelvis 205*f*
Penicillin 74, 75
Pentalogy of cantrell 329, 330
Pentoxifylline 129
Peripheral cystic pattern 257, 257*f*
Peritoneal ectopic pregnancy 286
Peritoneal inclusion cyst 230, 247, 248, 248*f*
Periurethral cysts 478
Placenta 499
  anterior 318*f*
Placental apoptosis, induction of 145
Placental bleeding 436
Placental growth factor, low 445
Placental infarct 435
Placental infections 436
Placental mosaicism, confined 436
Placental perfusion, reduced 446
Placental vasculature on angiomode, normal 484*f*
Placental vessels, widening of 446
Placental villi, continuous maturation of 446
Platyspondyly 387
Pneumonia 145
Polycystic ovarian syndrome 26, 39, 47, 65, 106, 112*f*, 160, 163, 253, 256, 509
  diagnosis of 11, 258

evolution of 256
principles of treatment 106
treatment modalities in 106
Polycystic ovary 9, 18, 48, 169, 251, 253, 255*f*, 257*f*, 510*f*
diagnosis of 12
three-dimensional volume of 255*f*
Polymerase chain reaction 7
Polyp 144, 216, 505
Porencephalic cyst 369, 370, 370*f*
Positive predictive value 235
Postcoital test 5
normal 6
Postcurettage endometrial collection 220
Postmenopausal bleeding 221
Pouch of Douglas 271
Power Doppler 178
Predominant hyperechoic stroma 257
Pregnancy
abnormal first-trimester 277
abnormal location of 284
confirmation of 279
first trimester of 277
growth of 287
location of 279
monitoring 154
normal 154
normal first-trimester 277
progress of 279, 287
six weeks 291*f*
twelve weeks 293*f*
Pregnancy loss 160
anatomical causes 138
in thrombophilia, pathophysiology of 150
recurrent 137, 153, 157, 161
Pregnancy-associated plasma protein-A 322
Pre-human chorionic gonadotropin endometrial parameters 67*f*
Preimplantation genetic
diagnosis, role of 153
screening 161
Prenatal tests, noninvasive 354
Preovulation luteinizing hormone 84
Preovulatory scan 251, 261, 509
Progesterone 89, 93, 113, 159
gel 93
in luteal phase, role of 84*b*
induced blocking factor 159
injectable 90
micronized 34
natural micronized 91*b*
preparations 89
production of 85*fc*
resistance 100
vaginal effervescent tablets 92
Prostatic cysts 478*f*
Prostatic inflammation 479
Protein
C deficiency 149
S deficiency 149
Prothrombotic states 435
Pseudo sac 279*t*, 280*f*
Pulmonary atresia 330
Pulmonary hypoplasia 330
Pulsatility index 259, 374
Pulse repetition frequency 179, 448, 468
higher 180*f*
Pulsed wave Doppler 179
Punctures, number of 115
Puresperm 81

R

Radial aplasia 333
Recombinant deoxyribonucleic acid 49
Recombinant follicle-stimulating hormone 49, 50, 52, 53, 56, 111, 123
types of 52
Recombinant human luteinizing hormone 57, 58
Recombinant luteinizing hormone 57
Rectal placement 184
Rectovaginal septum 234
Recurrent pregnancy loss, causes of 137
Region of interest 179
Renal disease 435
Renal pelvic diameter, assessment of 313*f*
Renal pelvis 313*f*
plane 312
Renal pyelectasis 350, 350*f*
Residual endometrial cavity 280*f*
Resistance index 212
Retroflexed fundus 188
Retrograde ejaculation 22, 82
Retroverted anteflexed uterus 189*f*
Retroverted retroflexed uterus 189*f*

Rhombencephalon 388*f*
  development of 494
Ribonucleoprotein 154
Right ventricular outflow tract 298, 310, 311*f*
Rim sign 231
Robert syndrome 366
Rokitansky's tubercle, large 238*f*
Rubin's test 4
Rupture of follicle, physiology of 68

S

Sacrum
  transverse 298
    section of 314*f*
Sagittal leg and foot 298
Saline infusion sonohysterography 198
Salpingitis 245
Satisfactory fertility 17
Scandinavian method 81
Scar tissues 190
Scrotal ultrasound 465
Secretory endometrial flow, normal 88*f*
Secretory endometrium 271*f*, 278*f*
Secretory scan 251, 270
Selenium 129
Semen
  analysis 121
    counseling for 4
    normal 8
  collection jar 74
  normal 121*t*
  parameters, normal 121*t*
  preparation 63, 69
    complications 70
  sample, collection of 73
Seminal plasma 75
Seminal vesicle 476
  cysts 476
Seminal vesiculitis 476
Septal defect 295*f*
Septate uterus 140*f*, 141, 202
Septo-optic dysplasia 369
Serosa 190
  anterior 193
  posterior 193
Serum
  albumin 75
  anti-müllerian hormone 17
  cortisol 23
  dehydroepiandrosterone sulfate 16
  estradiol 13
  follicle-stimulating hormone 11
  luteinizing hormone 13
  progesterone 14, 87, 159
  prolactin 15, 20, 23
  testosterone 16, 23
  thyroid-stimulation hormone 20
Sex hormone-binding globulin 23, 130
Shirodkar's operation 145
Simple cyst 232
Single-strand annealing 154
Single-stranded binding 154
Singleton pregnancies 33
Sirenomelia 334
Situs inversus 294
Skeletal abnormalities 333
Skeletal dysplasias 436
Sliding organ sign 195
Smoking 120
  and poor nutrition 435
  bad effects of 120
Smoothness of contour 190
Sodium
  bicarbonate 74
  pyruvate 74
Solid lesions 231, 236
Sonohysterography 138, 220
Speckle reduction imaging 177, 178*f*
Sperm 8
  abnormal 5
  capacitation 76
  count 5
  damage 73
  morphology, abnormal 160
  motility 130
    lower 73
  preparation 73, 74
    laboratory 74
    media 74, 77, 77*t*
    methods 75
Spermatid arrest 22
Spermatogonia arrest 22
Spermatozoa 6, 69
  motility of 128
Spina bifida 323, 326
  occulta 386
  with hydrocephalus 327*f*
Spinal abnormalities 497
Spinal canal defects 387*f*

Spinal defects 295
Spine 298
  abnormalities, multiple 387*f*
  coronal planes of 384*f*
  coronal section of 315*f*
  longitudinal 375*f*
    section of 375, 385*f*
  normal 498*f*
  qualitative evaluation of 364
  three-dimensional ultrasound of 384*f*
  vertebra 498*f*
Spiral arteries 197, 266
Spiral vessels, normal 213
Split ejaculation 74
Spontaneous abortion 157
Steelman-Pohley bioassay 53
Stepwise sequential screening 358
Stimulate follicular estradiol 26
Stimulates hypothalamus 45
Stomach, dilated 500*f*
Strassman's operation 142
Strawberry-shaped skull 348, 348*f*, 367*f*
Streptomycin 75
Streptopenicillin 75
Stress, role of 158
Stricture urethra 479
Stromal abundance 253
Stromal area 258
Stromal predominance 254
Stromal volume 258
Subclavian artery, aberrant right 346, 355
Subcutaneous aqueous progesterone 90
Subendometrial vascularity 216*f*
Submucous fibroid 213
Submucous myomas 142
Subnuclear glycogen deposit 84
Superovulation 63
Suprasperm 80
  method for 80
Swim-up from ejaculate 76, 77
Sylvian fissure 374
Sylvius, aqueduct of 336
Synechiae 219, 506
Synthetic progesterones 93
Synthetic serum replacement 74

T

Tamoxifen 125, 223
  effects of 223
Tender loving care, role of 158
Teratogens 436
Testicular atrophy 470
Testicular infarction 472
Testicular neoplasms 472
Testicular sperm extraction 124
Testicular torsion 472
Testicular trauma 473
Testis, normal 467*f*
Testosterone 16, 125
  deficiency, isolated 123
  high 21
  low 22
  normal 21
  sources of 16*t*
  undecanoate 125
Thermal balloon ablation 216
Thorax 298
Thromboelastography 149
Thrombophilia 148, 150, 162, 163
  screening for 151
Thrombosis 150
Thumb, infolding of 502*f*
Thyroid 158
  dysfunction 22
  function 158
    tests 20
Timor-Tritsch sign 195
Tissue
  hormones 126
  interface, maintenance of 190
Total motile sperm 62
Total ovarian stromal area 260
Total ovarian volume 260
Total oxyradical scavenging capacity 130
Traditional Chinese herbal medicine 131
Transabdominal route 184
Transabdominal scan 195
Transcaudate coronal plane 380*f*
Transcerebellar plane 371*f*, 381*f*
Transdermal progesterone 90
Transforming growth factor 17, 84
Transfrontal coronal plane 379*f*
Transfrontal plane 297, 306, 379
Transrectal route 184
Transrectal ultrasound 473
Transthalamic coronal plane 380*f*
Transthalamic plane 297, 300, 364, 372, 380

Transvaginal route 184
Transvaginal scan 184, 188*f*
  interpretation of 187
  method of 363
Transvaginal sonography 198, 251, 277
Tricuspid flow, normal 345*f*
Tricuspid regurgitation 344, 346
Trimester scan, second 297
Triploidy 338
Trisomy 18 303, 321, 333, 338
Trisomy 21 321, 354*t*
True gestational sac 279*f*
True sac 279*t*
Tubal ectopic pregnancy 247*f*, 285, 286*f*
Tubal factor, counseling for 7
Tubal inflammation 245*t*
Tubal lesions 230, 242
Tubal ligation 8
Tuberculosis 215
Tuberculous endometritis 215
Tuberculous orchitis 479
Tubo-ovarian
  abscess 245
  complex 245
  lesions 230
Tumors 239, 334
  malignant 239
Turner's syndrome 332, 338
Twin-to-twin transfusion 436
Typical bird's nest appearance 235
Typical golf-club appearance 316

U

Umbilical artery 449*f*, 454*f*, 458
  Doppler 448
  flow 320
  normal 445
  single 352*f*
Umbilical cord 312, 317
  abnormalities 351
  cyst 296*f*
  insertion 298, 312
  placental attachment of 317
Umbilical hypoxemia 446
Undescended testis 469
Unexplained infertility 8, 27
  trial 64
Unicornuate uterus 140*f*, 142
Uniparental disomies 332
Unprotected intercourse 4
Upper lip 308*f*
Urinary follicle-stimulating hormone 50, 52, 56
Urinary tract infection 145
Uterine abnormalities 198, 199*f*
Uterine aplasia 207*f*
Uterine artery 195, 212, 270, 445
  anatomy of 448*f*
  Doppler 448
  flow 268*f*, 444*f*
    high resistance 259*f*
  spectral Doppler of 320*f*
Uterine blood flow 273
Uterine cornu 245
Uterine diseases, ultrasound in 198
Uterine factor, counseling for 7
Uterine malignancies 506
Uterine natural killer cells 155
Uterine pass effect, first 91*f*
Uterine pathologies 198
Uterine scar 225
Uterine vasodilatation, absence of 446
Uterine vessels, entry of 191
Uterocervical length 261*f*
  physiological 192
Uteroplacental dysfunction 435
Uterus 184, 188, 195, 206, 213, 245, 261
  abnormality of 188
  aplasia 207
  infantalis 140, 200
  layer of 190
  normal 191*f*, 199, 201*f*
  partial bicorporeal 203, 204*f*
  section of 193*f*
  systematic assessment of 189
  thickness of 193
  T-shaped 139, 140, 199, 201*f*

V

Vaginal absorption 92*f*
Vaginal anomalies 199
Vaginal aplasia 207
Vaginal progesterone 90, 101
  rings 93
Vaginal suppositories 90
Varicocele 22, 466
  correction 132
  ultrasound grading of 470*t*
Vas deferens 474
  congenital absence of 473

Vascular endothelial growth factor 18, 84, 114, 259
Vascularity flow index 509
Vena cava, inferior 294, 453, 466
Venous congestion 338
Venous Doppler, abnormal 459
Ventricular atrium 303, 375, 376
Vermis, absent inferior 372*f*
Vesicular mole 221, 295
Vessel compliance, continuous changes in 446
Virtual organ computer-aided analysis 485
Vitamin
  B_{12} 128
  C 127, 128
  D 130
  E 127, 128
Volume transvaginal probe 185*f*

W

Weak cesarean scar 226*f*
White blood cell 73

Y

Y-chromosome deletion 472
Yolk sac 288, 288*f*
  large 290*f*
  solid 290*f*
  thick-walled 290*f*
  tiny 290*f*

Z

Zinc 125
Zuclomiphene 26
  proportion of 26
Zygoma 336